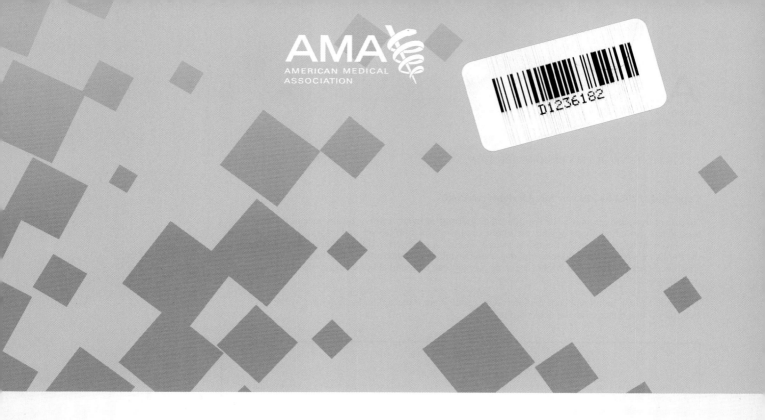

AMA
AMERICAN MEDICAL ASSOCIATION

HCPCS Level II

Professional 2021

AMA publications fund initiatives that drive improvements in patient health, practice innovation and medical education.

AMAstore.com

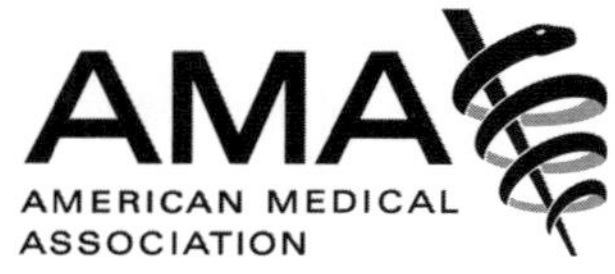

2021 HCPCS LEVEL II, PROFESSIONAL EDITION ISBN: 978-1-64016-090-3

Notice

Practitioners and researchers must always rely on their own experience and knowledge in evaluating and using any information, methods, compounds or experiments described herein. Because of rapid advances in the medical sciences, in particular, independent verification of diagnoses and drug dosages should be made. To the fullest extent of the law, no responsibility is assumed by Elsevier, authors, editors or contributors for any injury and/or damage to persons or property as a matter of products liability, negligence or otherwise, or from any use or operation of any methods, products, instructions, or ideas contained in the material herein.

Previous editions copyrighted 2020, 2019, 2018, 2017, 2016, 2015, 2014, 2013, 2012, 2011, 2010, 2009, 2008, 2007, 2006, 2005, 2004, 2003, 2002, 2001, 2000

International Standard Book Number: 978-1-64016-090-3

Our Commitment to Accuracy
The American Medical Association (AMA) is committed to producing accurate and reliable materials. To report corrections, please call the AMA Unified Service Center at (800) 621-8335. AMA publication and product updates, errata, and addenda can be found at amaproductupdates.org.

To purchase additional copies, contact the AMA at 800-621-8335 or visit the AMA store at amastore.com. Refer to item number **OP231521**.

Senior Content Strategist: Brandi Graham
Senior Content Development Manager: Luke E. Held
Senior Content Development Specialist: Joshua S. Rapplean
Publishing Services Manager: Julie Eddy
Senior Project Manager: Tracey Schriefer
Senior Book Designer: Maggie Reid

Printed in Canada

Last digit is the print number: 9 8 7 6 5 4 3 2 1

DEVELOPMENT OF THIS EDITION

Lead Technical Collaborator

Jackie L. Koesterman, CPC

Coder III/Reimbursement Specialist

Grand Forks, North Dakota

CONTENTS

INTRODUCTION v

GUIDE TO USING THE 2021 HCPCS LEVEL II CODES vi

SYMBOLS AND CONVENTIONS vii

2021 HCPCS UPDATES xiii

ANATOMY ILLUSTRATIONS xv

2021 HCPCS INDEX 1

2021 TABLE OF DRUGS 45

2021 HCPCS LEVEL II MODIFIERS 102

2021 HCPCS LEVEL II NATIONAL CODES 113

Appendix A—Jurisdiction List for DMEPOS HCPCS Codes 433

Appendix B—General Correct Coding Policies for National Correct Coding Initiative Policy Manual for Medicare Services 439

Figure Credits 454

Updates will be posted on codingupdates.com when available.

Check codingupdates.com for Practitioner and Facility Medically Unlikely Edits (MUEs) and Column 1 and Column 2 Edits.

Check the Centers for Medicare & Medicaid Services (www.cms.gov/Manuals/IOM/list.asp) website and codingupdates.com for full and select IOMs.

Notice: 2021 DMEPOS updates were unavailable at the time of printing. Check codingupdates.com for updates and DMEPOS Modifiers in January.

INTRODUCTION

2021 HCPCS quarterly updates available on the companion website at: www.codingupdates.com

The Centers for Medicare & Medicaid Services (CMS) (formerly Health Care Financing Administration [HCFA]) Healthcare Common Procedure Coding System (HCPCS) is a collection of codes and descriptors that represent procedures, supplies, products, and services that may be provided to Medicare beneficiaries and to individuals enrolled in private health insurance programs. The codes are divided as follows:

Level I: Codes and descriptors copyrighted by the American Medical Association's (AMA's) Current Procedural Terminology, ed. 4 (CPT-4). These are five-digit numeric codes representing physician and nonphysician services.

Level II: Includes codes and descriptors copyrighted by the American Dental Association's current dental terminology, seventh edition (CDT-7/8). These are five-digit alphanumeric codes comprising the D series. All other Level II codes and descriptors are alphanumeric and approved and maintained jointly by the editorial panel (consisting of CMS, the Health Insurance Association of America, and the Blue Cross Blue Shield Association). These are five-digit alphanumeric codes representing primarily items and nonphysician services that are not represented in the Level I codes.

Level III: The CMS eliminated Level III local codes. See Program Memorandum AB-02-113.

Headings are provided as a means of grouping similar or closely related items. The placement of a code under a heading does not indicate additional means of classification, nor does it relate to any health insurance coverage categories.

HCPCS also contains modifiers, which are two-digit codes and descriptors used to indicate that a service or procedure that has been performed has been altered by some specific circumstance but unchanged in its definition or code. Modifiers are grouped by levels. Level I modifiers and descriptors are copyrighted by the AMA. Level II modifiers are HCPCS modifiers. Modifiers in the D series are copyrighted by the ADA.

HCPCS is designed to promote uniform reporting and statistical data collection of medical procedures, supplies, products, and services.

HCPCS Disclaimer

Inclusion or exclusion of a procedure, supply, product, or service does not imply any health insurance coverage or reimbursement policy.

HCPCS makes as much use as possible of generic descriptions, but the inclusion of brand names to describe devices or drugs is intended only for indexing purposes; it is not meant to convey endorsement of any particular product or drug.

Updating HCPCS

The primary updates are made annually. Quarterly updates are also issued by CMS.

GUIDE TO USING THE 2021 HCPCS LEVEL II CODES

Medical coding has long been a part of the health care profession. Through the years medical coding systems have become more complex and extensive. Today, medical coding is an intricate and immense process that is present in every health care setting. The increased use of electronic submissions for health care services only increases the need for coders who understand the coding process.

2021 HCPCS Level II was developed to help meet the needs of today's coder.

All material adheres to the latest government versions available at the time of printing.

Annotated

Throughout this text, revisions and additions are indicated by the following symbols:

- ▶ **New:** Additions to the previous edition are indicated by the color triangle.
- ⮐ **Revised:** Revisions within the line or code from the previous edition are indicated by the color arrow.
- ✔ **Reinstated** indicates a code that was previously deleted and has now been reactivated.
- ✖ ~~Deleted~~ words have been removed from this year's edition.

HCPCS Symbols

- ◌ **Special coverage instructions** apply to these codes. Usually these special coverage instructions are included in the Internet Only Manuals (IOM). References to the IOM locations are given in the form of Medicare Pub. 100 reference numbers listed below the code. IOM select references are located at codingupdates.com.
- ⃠ **Not covered or valid by Medicare** is indicated by the "No" symbol. Usually the reason for the exclusion is included in the Internet Only Manuals (IOM) select references at codingupdates.com.
- * **Carrier discretion** is an indication that you must contact the individual third-party payers to find out the coverage available for codes identified by this symbol.
- *Other* Drugs approved for Medicare Part B and other FDA-approved drugs are listed as Other.
- A2-Z3 **ASC Payment Indicators** identify the 2019 final payment for the code. A list of Payment Indicators is listed in the front matter of this text.
- A-Y **OPPS Status Indicators** identify the 2019 final status assigned to the code. A list of Status Indicators is listed in the front matter of this text.
- Ⓑ Bill Part B MAC.
- Ⓑ Bill DME MAC.
- Coding Clinic Indicates the American Hospital Association *Coding Clinic®* for HCPCS references by year, quarter, and page number.
- ♿ DMEPOS identifies durable medical equipment, prosthetics, orthotics, and supplies that may be eligible for payment from CMS.
- ♀ Indicates a code for female only.
- ♂ Indicates a code for male only.
- A Indicates a code with an indication of age.
- MIPS Indicates a code included in the MIPS Quality Measure Specifications.
- Qp Indicates there is a maximum allowable number of units of service, per day, per patient for physician/provider services (*see* codingupdates.com for Practitioner Medically Unlikely Edits).
- Qh Indicates there is a maximum allowable number of units of service, per day, per patient in the outpatient hospital setting (*see* codingupdates.com for Hospital Medically Unlikely Edits).

Red, green, and blue typeface terms within the Table of Drugs and tabular section are terms added by the publisher and do not appear in the official code set. Information supplementing the official HCPCS Index produced by CMS is *italicized*.

SYMBOLS AND CONVENTIONS

HCPCS Symbols

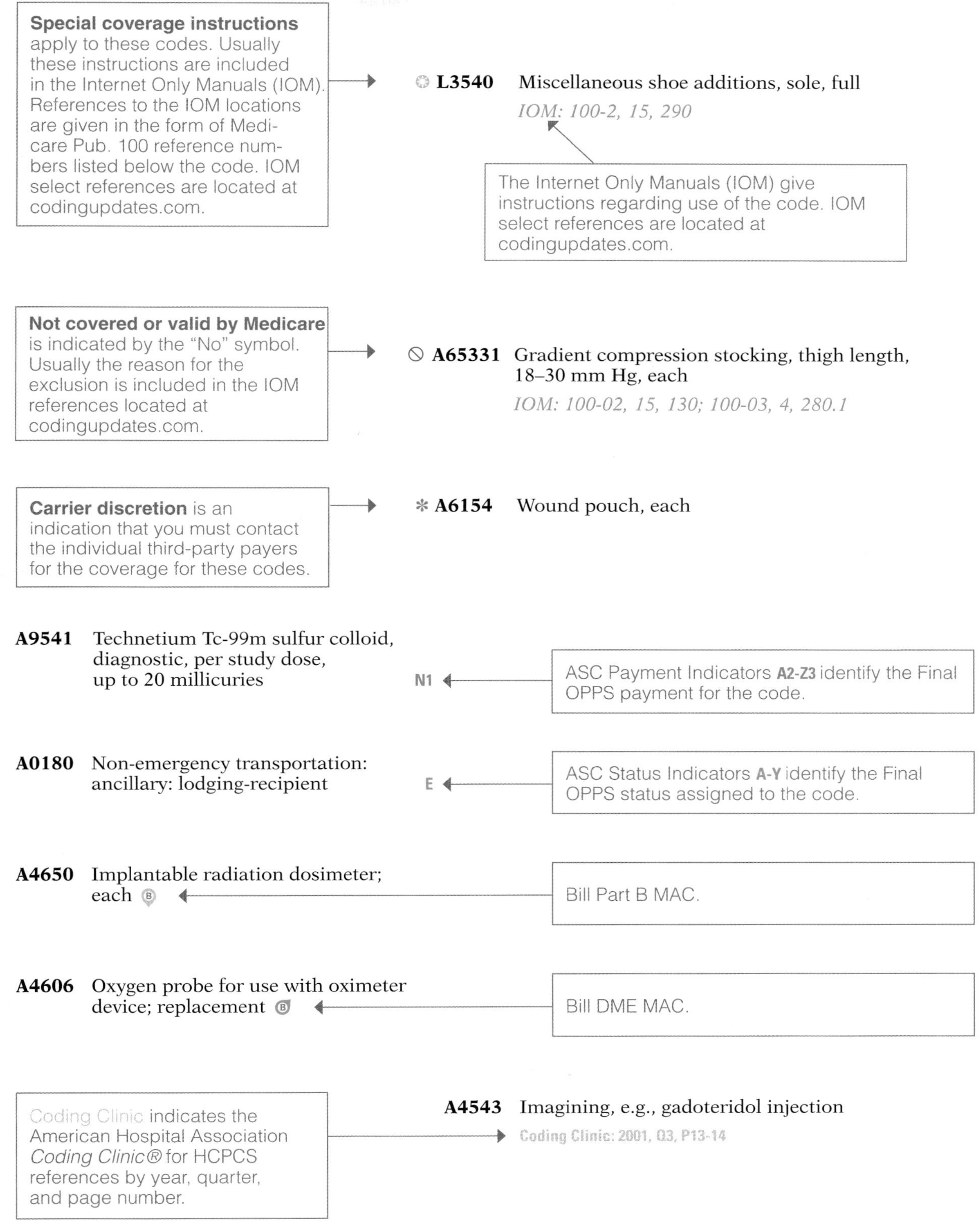

Special coverage instructions apply to these codes. Usually these instructions are included in the Internet Only Manuals (IOM). References to the IOM locations are given in the form of Medicare Pub. 100 reference numbers listed below the code. IOM select references are located at codingupdates.com.
L3540 Miscellaneous shoe additions, sole, full
IOM: 100-2, 15, 290
The Internet Only Manuals (IOM) give instructions regarding use of the code. IOM select references are located at codingupdates.com.
Not covered or valid by Medicare is indicated by the "No" symbol. Usually the reason for the exclusion is included in the IOM references located at codingupdates.com.
A65331 Gradient compression stocking, thigh length, 18–30 mm Hg, each
IOM: 100-02, 15, 130; 100-03, 4, 280.1
Carrier discretion is an indication that you must contact the individual third-party payers for the coverage for these codes.
* A6154 Wound pouch, each
A9541 Technetium Tc-99m sulfur colloid, diagnostic, per study dose, up to 20 millicuries
N1
ASC Payment Indicators A2-Z3 identify the Final OPPS payment for the code.
A0180 Non-emergency transportation: ancillary: lodging-recipient
E
ASC Status Indicators A-Y identify the Final OPPS status assigned to the code.
A4650 Implantable radiation dosimeter; each
Bill Part B MAC.
A4606 Oxygen probe for use with oximeter device; replacement
Bill DME MAC.
Coding Clinic indicates the American Hospital Association Coding Clinic® for HCPCS references by year, quarter, and page number.
A4543 Imagining, e.g., gadoteridol injection
Coding Clinic: 2001, Q3, P13-14

Codes shown are for illustration purposes only and may not be current codes.

DMEPOS symbol identifies durable medical equipment, prosthetics, orthotics, and supplies that may be eligible for payment from CMS.

E2210 Wheelchair accessory, bearings, any type, replacement only, each ♿

✻ **A4233** Replacement battery, alkaline (other than J cell), for use with medically necessary home blood glucose monitor owned by patient, each ♿

If "incident to" physician service, do not bill; otherwise bill DME MAC

On DMEPOS Fee Schedule.

B9000 Enteral nutrition infusion pump - without alarm Qp Y

Pump will be denied as not medically necessary if medical necessity of pump is not documented

IOM: 100-02, 15, 120; 100-03, 3, 180.2; 100-04, 20, 100.2.2

PEN: On Fee Schedule

On the Parenteral and Enteral Nutrition Items or Services (PEN) with modifier(s) from current PEN Fee Schedule.

A4261 Cervical cap for contraceptive use ♀

Indicates for female only.

A4267 Contraceptive supply, condom, male, each ♂

Indicates for male only.

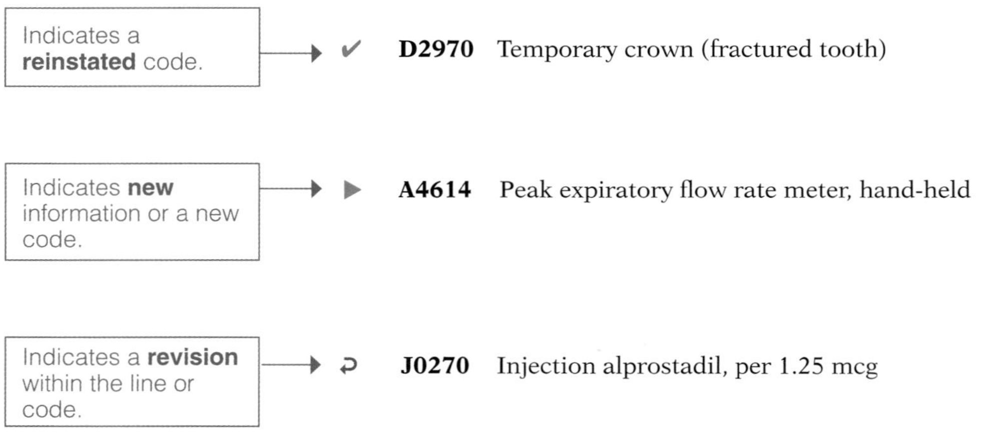
Indicates a **reinstated** code.
✔ **D2970** Temporary crown (fractured tooth)
Indicates **new** information or a new code.
▶ **A4614** Peak expiratory flow rate meter, hand-held
Indicates a **revision** within the line or code.
↩ **J0270** Injection alprostadil, per 1.25 mcg

Codes shown are for illustration purposes only and may not be current codes.

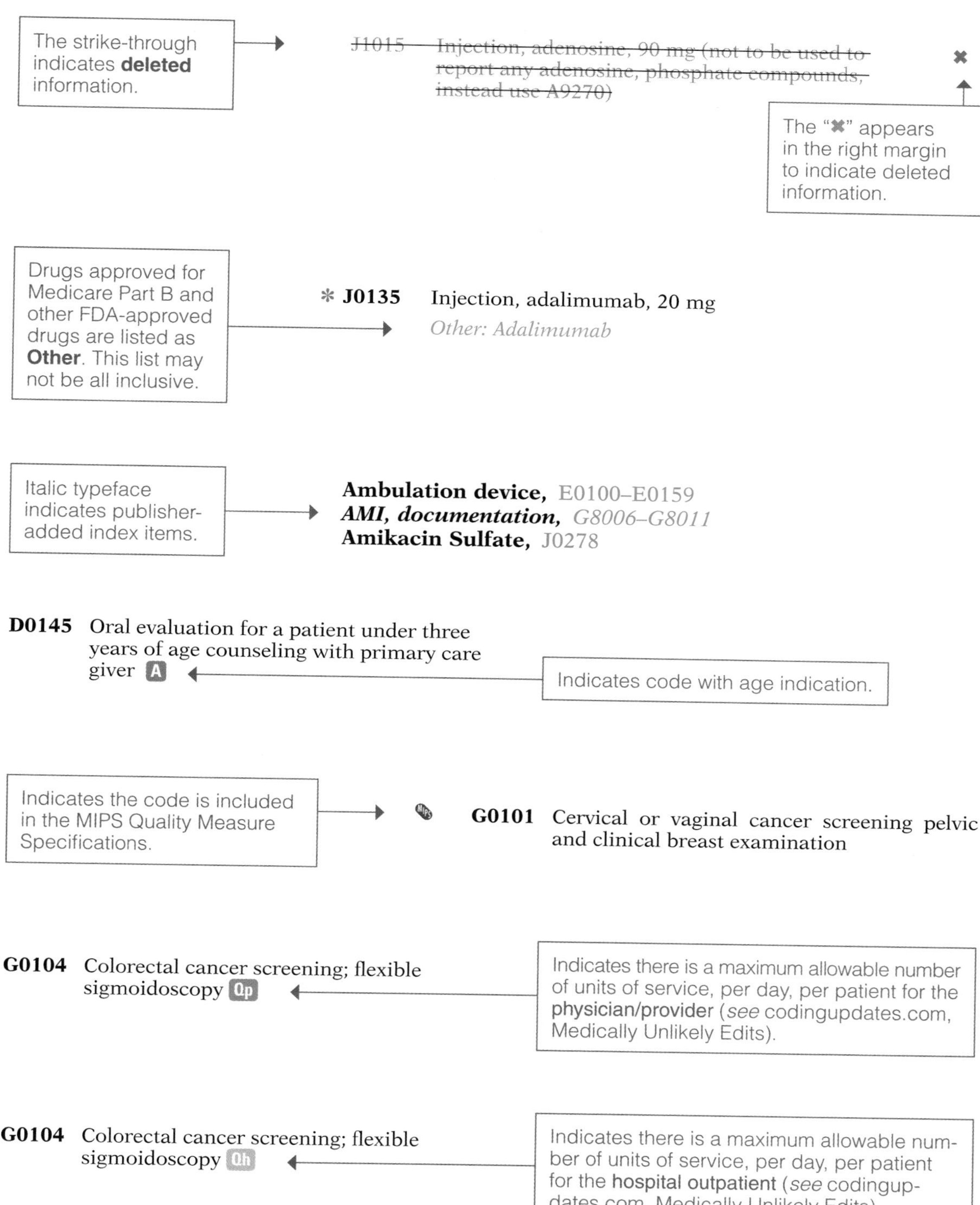
The strike-through indicates **deleted** information.
~~J1015 Injection, adenosine, 90 mg (not to be used to report any adenosine, phosphate compounds, instead use A9270)~~
✖
The "✖" appears in the right margin to indicate deleted information.
Drugs approved for Medicare Part B and other FDA-approved drugs are listed as **Other**. This list may not be all inclusive.
✻ **J0135** Injection, adalimumab, 20 mg
Other: Adalimumab
Italic typeface indicates publisher-added index items.
Ambulation device, E0100–E0159
AMI, documentation, *G8006–G8011*
Amikacin Sulfate, J0278
D0145 Oral evaluation for a patient under three years of age counseling with primary care giver A
Indicates code with age indication.
Indicates the code is included in the MIPS Quality Measure Specifications.
MIPS
G0101 Cervical or vaginal cancer screening pelvic and clinical breast examination
G0104 Colorectal cancer screening; flexible sigmoidoscopy Qp
Indicates there is a maximum allowable number of units of service, per day, per patient for the **physician/provider** (*see* codingupdates.com, Medically Unlikely Edits).
G0104 Colorectal cancer screening; flexible sigmoidoscopy Qh
Indicates there is a maximum allowable number of units of service, per day, per patient for the **hospital outpatient** (*see* codingupdates.com, Medically Unlikely Edits).

Codes shown are for illustration purposes only and may not be current codes.

A2-Z3 ASC Payment Indicators

Final ASC Payment Indicators for CY 2021	
Payment Indicator	**Payment Indicator Definition**
A2	Surgical procedure on ASC list in CY 2007; payment based on OPPS relative payment weight.
B5	Alternative code may be available; no payment made.
D5	Deleted/discontinued code; no payment made.
F4	Corneal tissue acquisition, hepatitis B vaccine; paid at reasonable cost.
G2	Non-office-based surgical procedure added in CY 2008 or later; payment based on OPPS relative payment weight.
H2	Brachytherapy source paid separately when provided integral to a surgical procedure on ASC list; payment OPPS rate.
J7	OPPS pass-through device paid separately when provided integral to a surgical procedure on ASC list; payment contractor-priced.
J8	Device-intensive procedure; paid at adjusted rate.
K2	Drugs and biologicals paid separately when provided integral to a surgical procedure on ASC list; payment based on OPPS rate.
K5	Drugs and biologicals for which pricing information is not yet available.
K7	Unclassified drugs and biologicals; payment contractor-priced.
L1	Influenza vaccine; pneumococcal vaccine. Packaged item/service; no separate payment made.
L6	New Technology Intraocular Lens (NTIOL); special payment.
N1	Packaged service/item; no separate payment made.
P2	Office-based surgical procedure added to ASC list in CY 2008 or later with MPFS nonfacility PE RVUs; payment based on OPPS relative payment weight.
P3	Office-based surgical procedure added to ASC list in CY 2008 or later with MPFS nonfacility PE RVUs; payment based on MPFS nonfacility PE RVUs.
R2	Office-based surgical procedure added to ASC list in CY 2008 or later without MPFS nonfacility PE RVUs; payment based on OPPS relative payment weight.
Z2	Radiology or diagnostic service paid separately when provided integral to a surgical procedure on ASC list; payment based on OPPS relative payment weight.
Z3	Radiology or diagnostic service paid separately when provided integral to a surgical procedure on ASC list; payment based on MPFS nonfacility PE RVUs.
CMS-1717-FC, Final Changes to the ASC Payment System and CY 2021 Payment Rates, http://www.cms.gov/Medicare/Medicare-Fee-for-Service-Payment/ASCPayment/ASC-Regulations-and-Notices.html.	

A-Y OPPS Status Indicators

Final OPPS Payment Status Indicators for CY 2021		
Indicator	**Item/Code/Service**	**OPPS Payment Status**
A	Services furnished to a hospital outpatient that are paid under a fee schedule or payment system other than OPPS,* for example:	Not paid under OPPS. Paid by MACs under a fee schedule or payment system other than OPPS. Services are subject to deductible or coinsurance unless indicated otherwise.
	• Ambulance Services	
	• Separately Payable Clinical Diagnostic Laboratory Services	Not subject to deductible or coinsurance.
	• Separately Payable Non-Implantable Prosthetics and Orthotics	
	• Physical, Occupational, and Speech Therapy	
	• Diagnostic Mammography	
	• Screening Mammography	Not subject to deductible or coinsurance.
B	Codes that are not recognized by OPPS when submitted on an outpatient hospital Part B bill type (12x and 13x)	Not paid under OPPS. • May be paid by MACs when submitted on a different bill type, for example, 75x (CORF), but not paid under OPPS. • An alternate code that is recognized by OPPS when submitted on an outpatient hospital Part B bill type (12x and 13x) may be available.
C	Inpatient Procedures	Not paid under OPPS. Admit patient. Bill as inpatient.
D	Discontinued Codes	Not paid under OPPS or any other Medicare payment system.
E1	Items, Codes and Services: • Not covered by any Medicare outpatient benefit category • Statutorily excluded by Medicare • Not reasonable and necessary	Not paid by Medicare when submitted on outpatient claims (any outpatient bill type).
E2	Items, Codes and Services: for which pricing information and claims data are not available	Not paid by Medicare when submitted on outpatient claims (any outpatient bill type).
F	Corneal Tissue Acquisition; Certain CRNA Services and Hepatitis B Vaccines	Not paid under OPPS. Paid at reasonable cost.
G	Pass-Through Drugs and Biologicals	Paid under OPPS; separate APC payment.
H	Pass-Through Device Categories	Separate cost-based pass-through payment; not subject to copayment.
J1	Hospital Part B services paid through a comprehensive APC	Paid under OPPS; all covered Part B services on the claim are packaged with the primary "J1" service for the claim, except services with OPPS status indicator of "F," "G," "H," "L," and "U"; ambulance services; diagnostic and screening mammography; all preventive services; and certain Part B inpatient services.
J2	Hospital Part B Services That May Be Paid Through a Comprehensive APC	Paid under OPPS; Addendum B displays APC assignments when services are separately payable. (1) Comprehensive APC payment based on OPPS comprehensive-specific payment criteria. Payment for all covered Part B services on the claim is packaged into a single payment for specific combinations of services, except services with OPPS status indicator of "F," "G," "H," "L," and "U"; ambulance services; diagnostic and screening mammography; all preventive services; and certain Part B inpatient services. (2) Packaged APC payment if billed on the same claim as a HCPCS code assigned status indicator "J1." (3) In other circumstances, payment is made through a separate APC payment or packaged into payment for other services.

A-Y OPPS Status Indicators—cont'd

Final OPPS Payment Status Indicators for CY 2021		
Indicator	**Item/Code/Service**	**OPPS Payment Status**
K	Non-Pass-Through Drugs and Non-Implantable Biologicals, including Therapeutic Radiopharmaceuticals	Paid under OPPS: separate APC payment.
L	Influenza Vaccine; Pneumococcal Pneumonia Vaccine	Not paid under OPPS. Paid at reasonable cost; not subject to deductible or coinsurance.
M	Items and Services Not Billable to the MAC	Not paid under OPPS.
N	Items and Services Packaged into APC Rates	Paid under OPPS; payment is packaged into payment for other services. Therefore, there is no separate APC payment.
P	Partial Hospitalization	Paid under OPPS; per diem APC payment.
Q1	STV-Packaged Codes	Paid under OPPS; Addendum B displays APC assignments when services are separately payable. (1) Packaged APC payment if billed on the same claim as a HCPCS code assigned status indicator "S," "T," or "V." (2) Composite APC payment if billed with specific combinations of services based on OPPS composite-specific payment criteria. Payment is packaged into a single payment for specific combinations of services. (3) In other circumstances, payment is made through a separate APC payment.
Q2	T-Packaged Codes	Paid under OPPS; Addendum B displays APC assignments when services are separately payable. (1) Packaged APC payment if billed on the same claim as a HCPCS code assigned status indicator "T." (2) In other circumstances, payment is made through a separate APC payment.
Q3	Codes That May Be Paid Through a Composite APC	Paid under OPPS; Addendum B displays APC assignments when services are separately payable. Addendum M displays composite APC assignments when codes are paid through a composite APC. (1) Composite APC payment based on OPPS composite-specific payment criteria. Payment is packaged into a single payment for specific combinations of service. (2) In other circumstances, payment is made through a separate APC payment or packaged into payment for other services.
Q4	Conditionally packaged laboratory tests	Paid under OPPS or CLFS. (1) Packaged APC payment if billed on the same claim as a HCPCS code assigned published status indicator "J1," "J2," "S," "T," "V," "Q1," "Q2," or "Q3." (2) In other circumstances, laboratory tests should have an SI=A and payment is made under the CLFS.
R	Blood and Blood Products	Paid under OPPS; separate APC payment.
S	Procedure or Service, Not Discounted when Multiple	Paid under OPPS; separate APC payment.
T	Procedure or Service, Multiple Procedure Reduction Applies	Paid under OPPS; separate APC payment.
U	Brachytherapy Sources	Paid under OPPS; separate APC payment.
V	Clinic or Emergency Department Visit	Paid under OPPS; separate APC payment.
Y	Non-Implantable Durable Medical Equipment	Not paid under OPPS. All institutional providers other than home health agencies bill to a DME MAC.

*** Note — Payments "under a fee schedule or payment system other than OPPS" may be contractor priced.**

CMS-1717-FC, Final Changes to the ASC Payment System and CY 2021 Payment Rates, http://www.cms.gov/Medicare/Medicare-Fee-for-Service-Payment/HospitalOutpatientPPS/Hospital-Outpatient-Regulations-and-Notices.html.

2021 HCPCS UPDATES

2021 HCPCS New/Revised/Deleted Codes and Modifiers

HCPCS quarterly updates are posted on the companion website (www.codingupdates.com) when available.

NEW CODES/MODIFIERS

J5
V4
A9591
C1052
C1062
C1748
C1825
C1849
C9053
C9056
C9057
C9058
C9059
C9061
C9063
C9065
C9067
C9068
C9069
C9070
C9071
C9072
C9073
C9122
C9759
C9760
C9761
C9762
C9763
C9764
C9765
C9766
C9767
C9768
C9769
C9770
C9771
C9772
C9773
C9774
C9775
C9803
G0088
G0089
G0090
G1012
G1013
G1214
G1015
G1016
G1017
G1018
G1019
G1020
G1021
G1022
G1023
G2023
G2024
G2025
G2168
G2170
G2171
G2173
G2174
G2175
G2176
G2177
G2178
G2179
G2180
G2181
G2182
G2183
G2184
G2185
G2186
G2187
G2188
G2189
G2190
G2191
G2192
G2193
G2194
G2195
G2196
G2197
G2198
G2199
G2200
G2201
G2202
G2203
G2204
G2205
G2206
G2207
G2208
G2209
G2210
G2211
G2212
G2213
G2214
G2215
G2216
G2250
G2251
G2252
J0223
J0591
J0691
J0693
J0742
J0791
J0896
J1201
J1429
J1437
J1558
J1632
J1738
J1823
J3032
J3241
J3399
J7169
J7204
J7212
J7333
J7351
J7352
J9144
J9177
J9198
J9223
J9227
J9246
J9281
J9304
J9316
J9317
J9358
K1006
K1007
K1009
K1010
K1011
K1012
M0239
M0243
M1145
M1146
M1147
M1148
M1149
Q0239
Q0243
Q4227
Q4228
Q4229
Q4230
Q4231
Q4232
Q4233
Q4234
Q4235
Q4236
Q4237
Q4238
Q4239
Q4240
Q4241
Q4242
Q4244
Q4245
Q4246
Q4247
Q4248
Q4249
Q4250
Q4254
Q4255
Q5119
Q5120
Q5121
Q5122
Q9001
Q9002
Q9003
S0013
T2047
U0001
U0002
U0003
U0004
U0005
V2524

REVISED CODES/MODIFIERS

CS
C9760
G0068
G0069
G0070
G2097
G2115
G2116
G2118
G2125
G2126
G2127
G2140
G2151
G2152
G2167
G8430
G8601
G8650
G8654
G8658
G8694
G8709
G8924
G8938
G8969
G9299
G9355
G9356
G9401
G9402
G9415
G9448
G9537
G9550
G9642
G9659
G9660
G9661
G9663
G9666
G9703
G9716
G9717
G9722
G9727
G9729
G9731
G9938
G9945
J7189
J7321
J9245
M1003
M1041
M1045
M1046
M1051
M1108
M1109
M1110
M1113
M1114
M1115
M1118
M1119
M1120
M1123
M1124
M1125
M1128
M1129
M1130
M1132
M1133
M1134
M1141
Q4176

DELETED CODES/MODIFIERS

C9041
C9053
C9054
C9056
C9057
C9058
C9060
C9062
C9064
C9066
C9745
C9747
C9449
C9754
C9755
C9754
G0297
G1005
G1006
G2058
G2089
G2102
G2103
G2104
G2114
G2117
G2119
G2120
G2123
G2124
G2130
G2131
G2132
G2133
G2134
G2135
G2153
G2154
G2155
G2156
G2157
G2158
G2159
G2160
G2161
G2162
G2163
G2164
G2165
G2166
G8398
G8442
G8509
G8571
G8572
G8573
G8574
G8627
G8628
G8671
G8672
G8674
G8730
G8731
G8732
G8809
G8810
G8811
G8872
G8873
G8874
G8939
G8959
G8960
G8973
G8974
G8975
G8976
G9232
G9239
G9240
G9241
G9256
G9257
G9258
G9259
G9260
G9261
G9262
G9263
G9264
G9265
G9266
G9300
G9301
G9302
G9303
G9304
G9326
G9327
G9329
G9340
G9365
G9366
G9389
G9390
G9469
G9503
G9523
G9524
G9525
G9526
G9532
G9558
G9559
G9560
G9573
G9574
G9600
G9601
G9602
G9615
G9616
G9617
G9701
G9738
G9739
G9747
G9748
G9749
G9750
G9759
G9798
G9799
G9800
G9801
G9802
G9803
G9804
G9814
G9815
G9816
G9817
G9825
G9826
G9827
G9828
G9829
G9833
G9834
G9835
G9836
G9837
G9849
G9850
G9851
G9855
G9856
G9857
G9924
G9933
G9934
G9935
G9936
G9937
G9966
G9967
J9199
M1015
M1023
M1024
M1033
M1061
M1062
M1063
M1064
M1065
M1066
M1136
M1137
M1138
M1139
M1140
M1144

NEW, REVISED, AND DELETED DENTAL CODES

New
D0604
D0605
D0701
D0702
D0703
D0704
D0705
D0706
D0707
D0708
D0709
D1321
D1255
D2928
D3471
D3472
D3473
D3501
D3502
D3503
D5995
D5996
D6191
D6192
D7961
D7993
D7994

Revised
D0120
D0150
D1110
D1120
D2960
D2961
D2962
D5225
D5226
D5820
D5821
D6011
D6091
D6098
D9971

Deleted
D3427
D5994
D6052
D7960

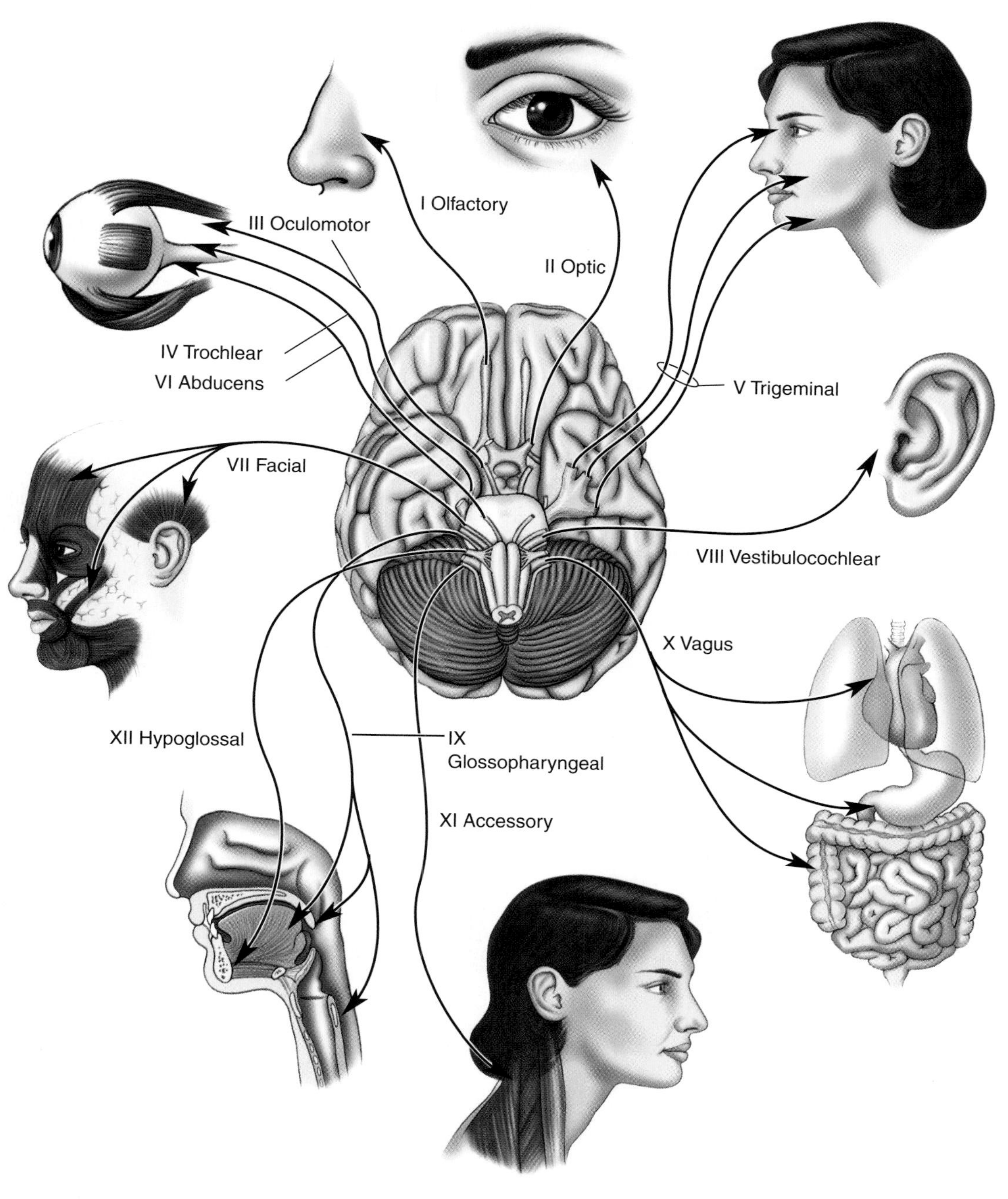
I Olfactory
III Oculomotor
II Optic
IV Trochlear
VI Abducens
V Trigeminal
VII Facial
VIII Vestibulocochlear
X Vagus
XII Hypoglossal
IX
Glossopharyngeal
XI Accessory

Plate 1 Cranial Nerves (12 pairs) are known by their numbers (Roman numerals) and names. (Herlihy BL: The Human Body in Health and Illness, ed 6, St. Louis, 2018, Elsevier.)

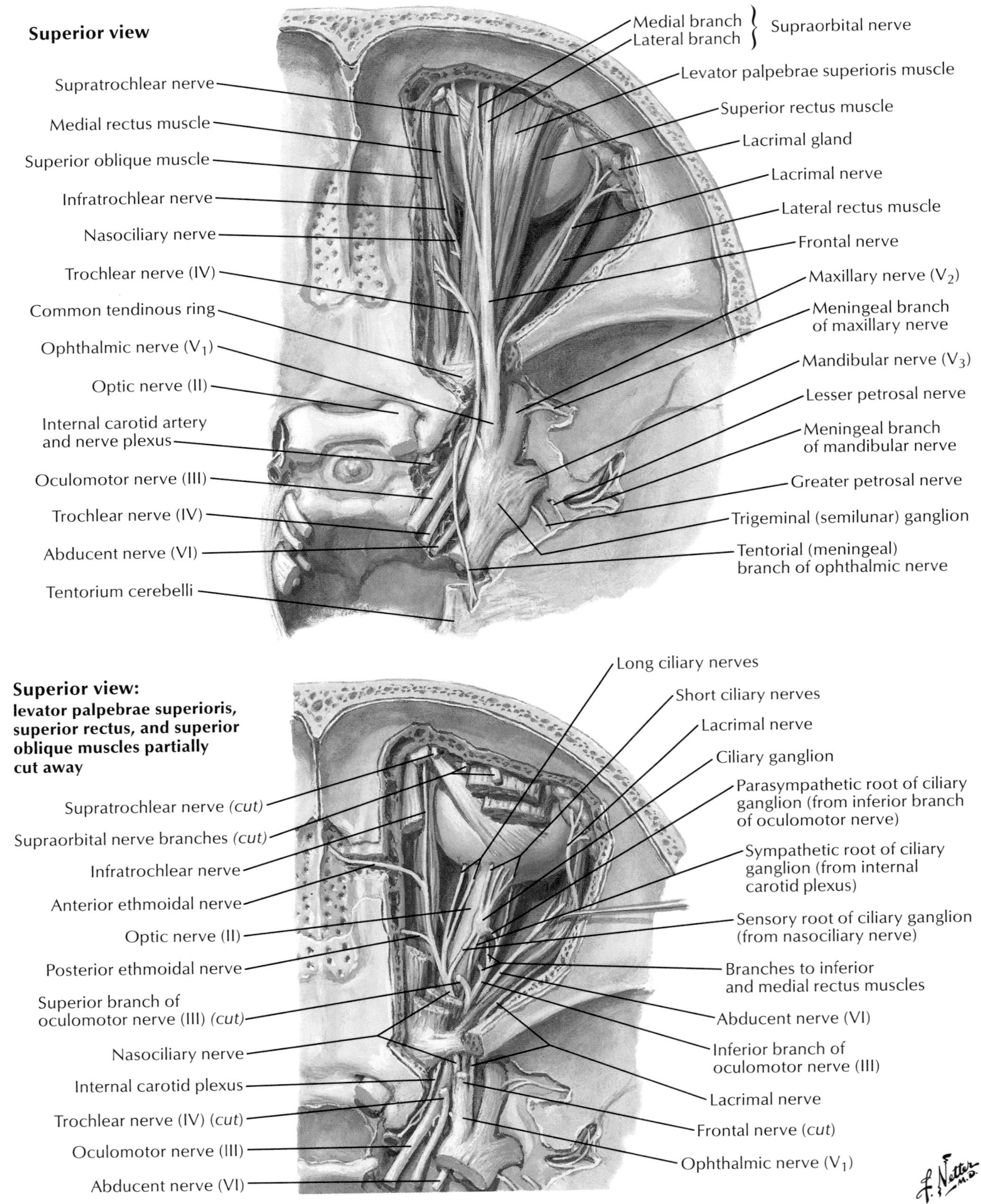

Superior view
Medial branch
Lateral branch
Supraorbital nerve
Supratrochlear nerve
Levator palpebrae superioris muscle
Medial rectus muscle
Superior rectus muscle
Superior oblique muscle
Lacrimal gland
Infratrochlear nerve
Lacrimal nerve
Lateral rectus muscle
Nasociliary nerve
Frontal nerve
Trochlear nerve (IV)
Maxillary nerve (V_2)
Common tendinous ring
Meningeal branch of maxillary nerve
Ophthalmic nerve (V_1)
Mandibular nerve (V_3)
Optic nerve (II)
Lesser petrosal nerve
Internal carotid artery and nerve plexus
Meningeal branch of mandibular nerve
Oculomotor nerve (III)
Greater petrosal nerve
Trochlear nerve (IV)
Trigeminal (semilunar) ganglion
Abducent nerve (VI)
Tentorial (meningeal) branch of ophthalmic nerve
Tentorium cerebelli
Superior view: levator palpebrae superioris, superior rectus, and superior oblique muscles partially cut away
Long ciliary nerves
Short ciliary nerves
Lacrimal nerve
Ciliary ganglion
Supratrochlear nerve (cut)
Parasympathetic root of ciliary ganglion (from inferior branch of oculomotor nerve)
Supraorbital nerve branches (cut)
Infratrochlear nerve
Sympathetic root of ciliary ganglion (from internal carotid plexus)
Anterior ethmoidal nerve
Sensory root of ciliary ganglion (from nasociliary nerve)
Optic nerve (II)
Posterior ethmoidal nerve
Branches to inferior and medial rectus muscles
Superior branch of oculomotor nerve (III) (cut)
Abducent nerve (VI)
Inferior branch of oculomotor nerve (III)
Nasociliary nerve
Internal carotid plexus
Lacrimal nerve
Trochlear nerve (IV) (cut)
Frontal nerve (cut)
Oculomotor nerve (III)
Ophthalmic nerve (V_1)
Abducent nerve (VI)
F. Netter M.D.

Plate 2 Nerves of Orbit.

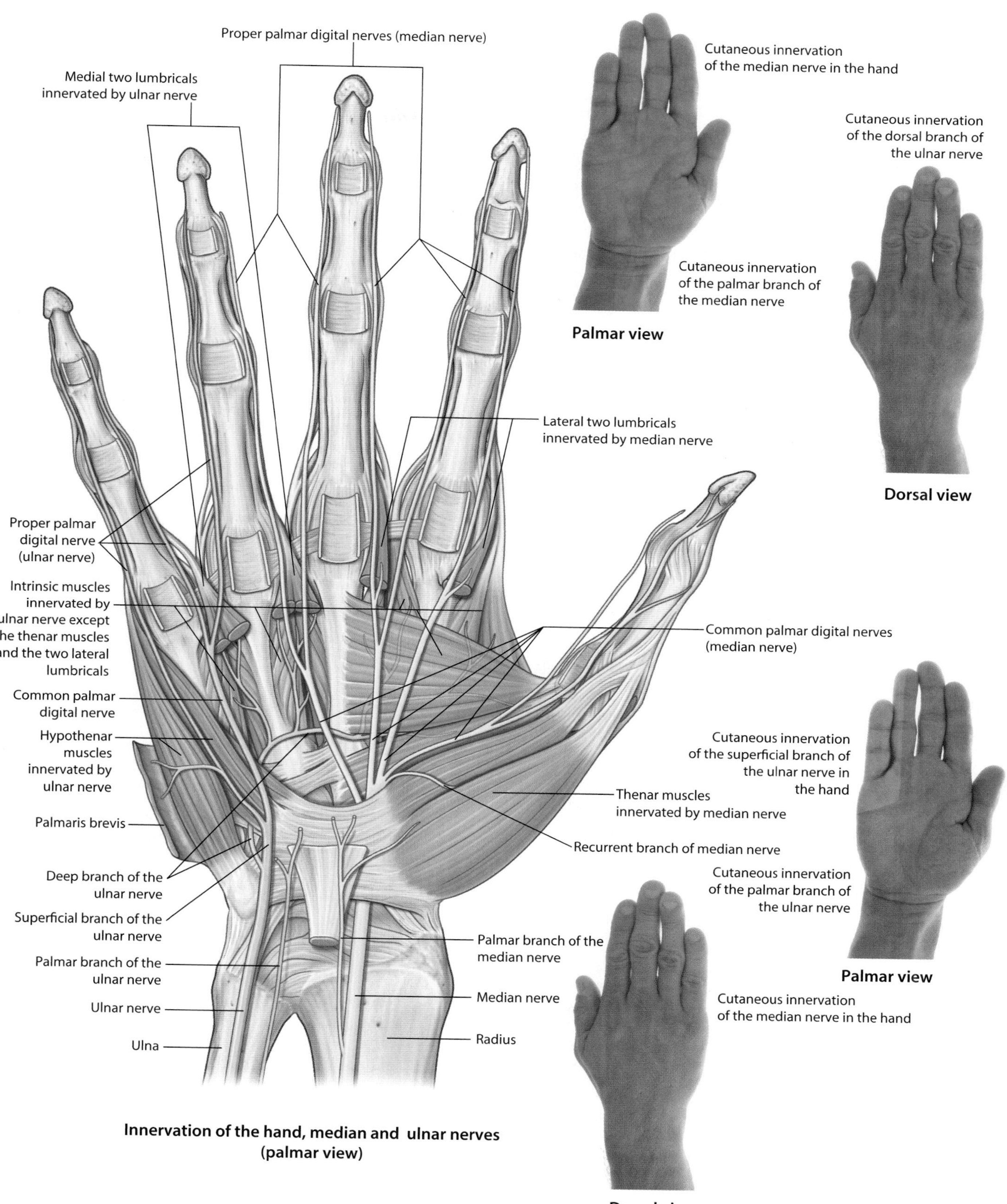

Proper palmar digital nerves (median nerve)
Medial two lumbricals innervated by ulnar nerve
Lateral two lumbricals innervated by median nerve
Proper palmar digital nerve (ulnar nerve)
Intrinsic muscles innervated by ulnar nerve except the thenar muscles and the two lateral lumbricals
Common palmar digital nerves (median nerve)
Common palmar digital nerve
Hypothenar muscles innervated by ulnar nerve
Thenar muscles innervated by median nerve
Palmaris brevis
Recurrent branch of median nerve
Deep branch of the ulnar nerve
Superficial branch of the ulnar nerve
Palmar branch of the median nerve
Palmar branch of the ulnar nerve
Median nerve
Ulnar nerve
Radius
Ulna
Innervation of the hand, median and ulnar nerves (palmar view)
Cutaneous innervation of the median nerve in the hand
Cutaneous innervation of the palmar branch of the median nerve
Palmar view
Cutaneous innervation of the dorsal branch of the ulnar nerve
Dorsal view
Cutaneous innervation of the superficial branch of the ulnar nerve in the hand
Cutaneous innervation of the palmar branch of the ulnar nerve
Palmar view
Cutaneous innervation of the median nerve in the hand
Dorsal view

Plate 3 Innervation of the Hand: Median and Ulnar Nerves (From Drake RL, Vogl AW, Mitchell AWM, Tibbitts RM, Richardson PE: Gray's Atlas of Anatomy, ed 2, Philadelphia, 2015, Churchill Livingstone.)

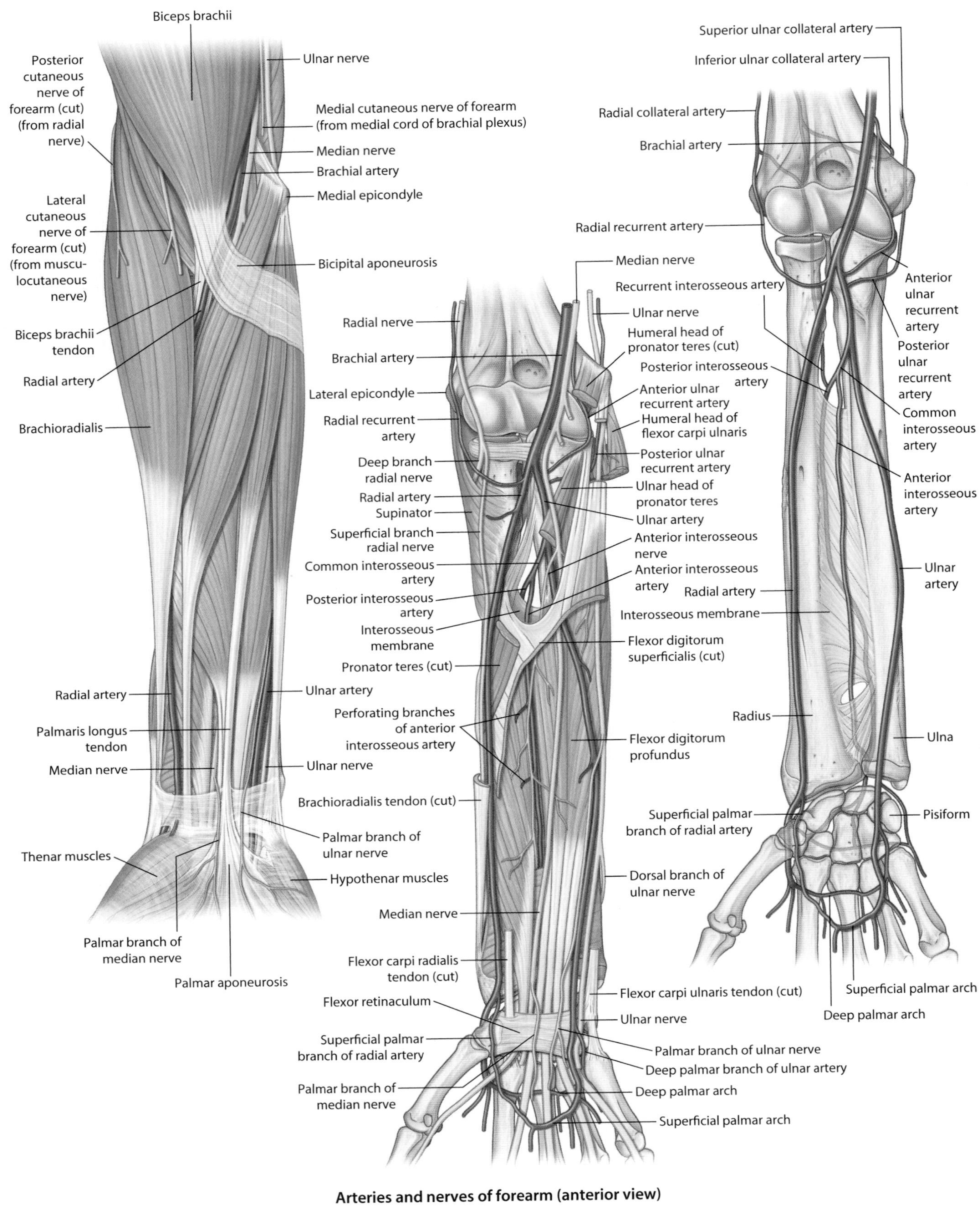

Biceps brachii
Posterior cutaneous nerve of forearm (cut) (from radial nerve)
Ulnar nerve
Medial cutaneous nerve of forearm (from medial cord of brachial plexus)
Median nerve
Brachial artery
Medial epicondyle
Lateral cutaneous nerve of forearm (cut) (from musculocutaneous nerve)
Bicipital aponeurosis
Biceps brachii tendon
Radial artery
Brachioradialis
Radial artery
Ulnar artery
Palmaris longus tendon
Median nerve
Ulnar nerve
Thenar muscles
Palmar branch of ulnar nerve
Hypothenar muscles
Palmar branch of median nerve
Palmar aponeurosis
Median nerve
Recurrent interosseous artery
Radial nerve
Ulnar nerve
Humeral head of pronator teres (cut)
Brachial artery
Posterior interosseous artery
Lateral epicondyle
Anterior ulnar recurrent artery
Radial recurrent artery
Humeral head of flexor carpi ulnaris
Deep branch radial nerve
Posterior ulnar recurrent artery
Radial artery
Ulnar head of pronator teres
Supinator
Ulnar artery
Superficial branch radial nerve
Anterior interosseous nerve
Common interosseous artery
Anterior interosseous artery
Posterior interosseous artery
Interosseous membrane
Flexor digitorum superficialis (cut)
Pronator teres (cut)
Perforating branches of anterior interosseous artery
Flexor digitorum profundus
Brachioradialis tendon (cut)
Dorsal branch of ulnar nerve
Median nerve
Flexor carpi radialis tendon (cut)
Flexor carpi ulnaris tendon (cut)
Flexor retinaculum
Ulnar nerve
Superficial palmar branch of radial artery
Palmar branch of ulnar nerve
Deep palmar branch of ulnar artery
Palmar branch of median nerve
Deep palmar arch
Superficial palmar arch
Superior ulnar collateral artery
Inferior ulnar collateral artery
Radial collateral artery
Brachial artery
Radial recurrent artery
Anterior ulnar recurrent artery
Posterior ulnar recurrent artery
Common interosseous artery
Anterior interosseous artery
Ulnar artery
Radial artery
Interosseous membrane
Radius
Ulna
Superficial palmar branch of radial artery
Pisiform
Superficial palmar arch
Deep palmar arch

Arteries and nerves of forearm (anterior view)

Plate 4 Arteries and Nerves of the Forearm (Anterior View) (From Drake RL, Vogl AW, Mitchell AWM, Tibbitts RM, Richardson PE: Gray's Atlas of Anatomy, ed 2, Philadelphia, 2015, Churchill Livingstone.)

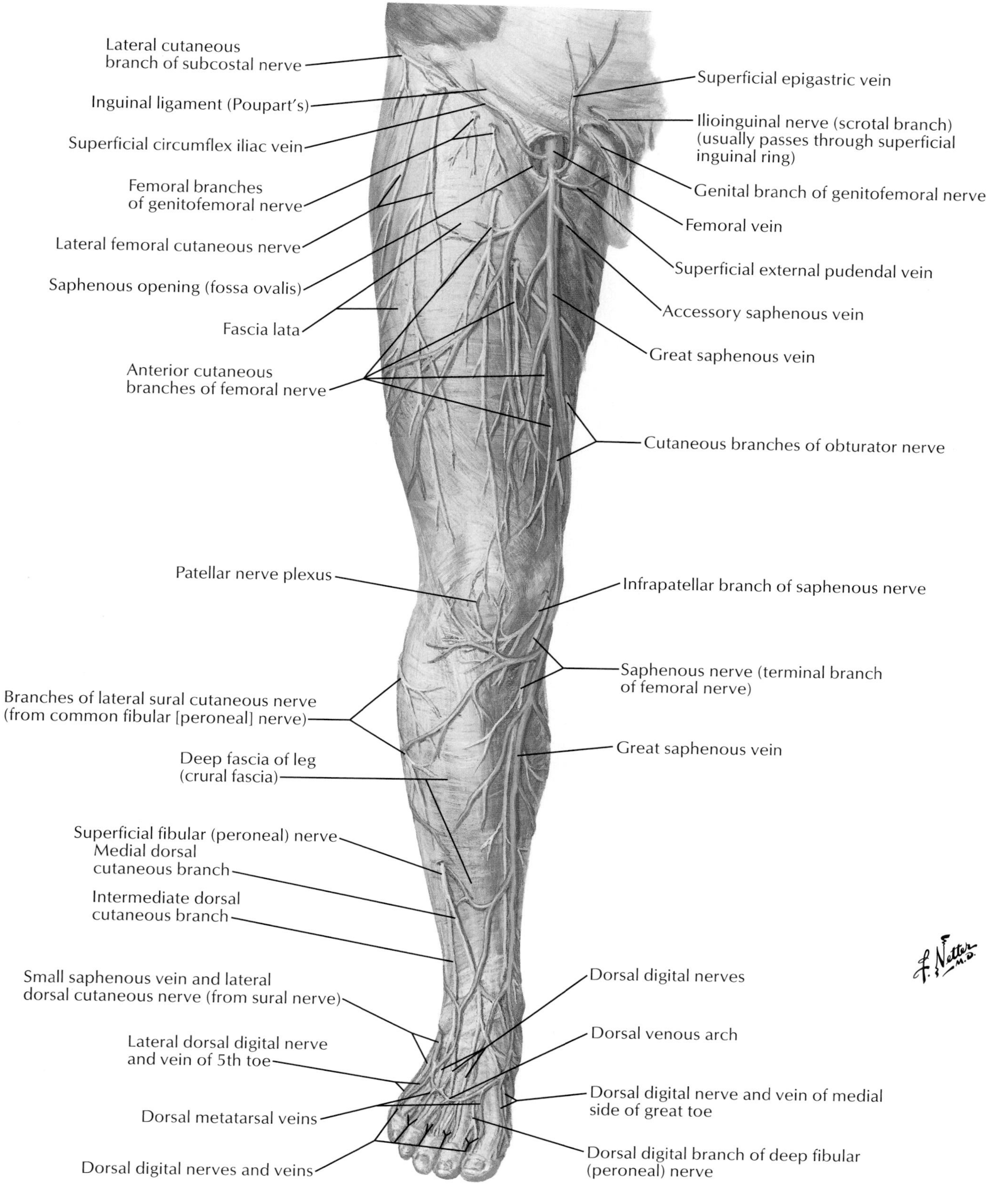
Lateral cutaneous branch of subcostal nerve
Inguinal ligament (Poupart's)
Superficial circumflex iliac vein
Femoral branches of genitofemoral nerve
Lateral femoral cutaneous nerve
Saphenous opening (fossa ovalis)
Fascia lata
Anterior cutaneous branches of femoral nerve
Superficial epigastric vein
Ilioinguinal nerve (scrotal branch) (usually passes through superficial inguinal ring)
Genital branch of genitofemoral nerve
Femoral vein
Superficial external pudendal vein
Accessory saphenous vein
Great saphenous vein
Cutaneous branches of obturator nerve
Patellar nerve plexus
Infrapatellar branch of saphenous nerve
Saphenous nerve (terminal branch of femoral nerve)
Branches of lateral sural cutaneous nerve (from common fibular [peroneal] nerve)
Great saphenous vein
Deep fascia of leg (crural fascia)
Superficial fibular (peroneal) nerve
Medial dorsal cutaneous branch
Intermediate dorsal cutaneous branch
Small saphenous vein and lateral dorsal cutaneous nerve (from sural nerve)
Lateral dorsal digital nerve and vein of 5th toe
Dorsal metatarsal veins
Dorsal digital nerves and veins
Dorsal digital nerves
Dorsal venous arch
Dorsal digital nerve and vein of medial side of great toe
Dorsal digital branch of deep fibular (peroneal) nerve
F. Netter M.D.

ANATOMY ILLUSTRATIONS

Plate 5 Superficial Nerves and Veins of Lower Limb: Anterior View. (Copyright 2020 Elsevier Inc. All rights reserved. www.netterimages.com. Image ID: 4846.)

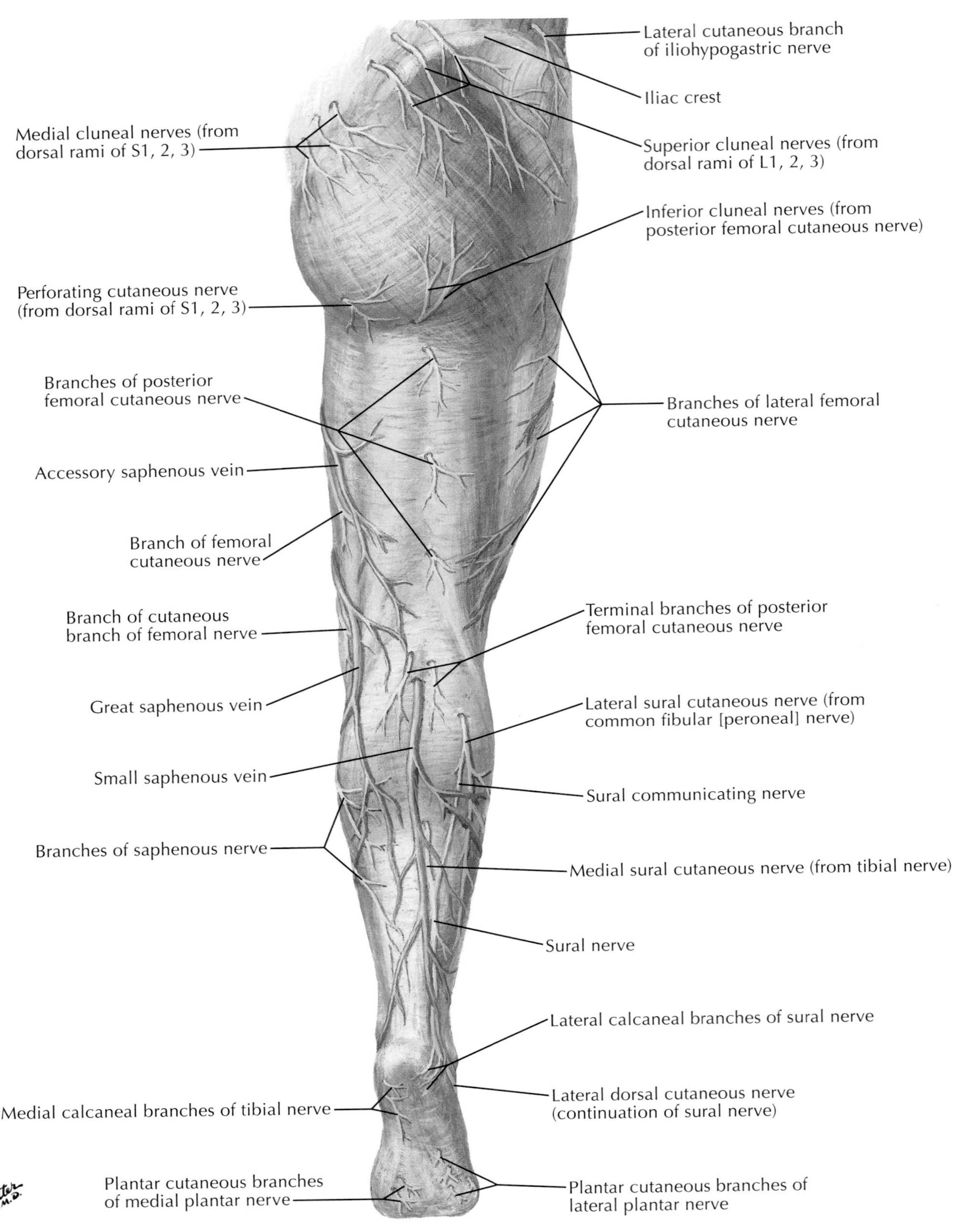
Lateral cutaneous branch of iliohypogastric nerve
Iliac crest
Medial cluneal nerves (from dorsal rami of S1, 2, 3)
Superior cluneal nerves (from dorsal rami of L1, 2, 3)
Inferior cluneal nerves (from posterior femoral cutaneous nerve)
Perforating cutaneous nerve (from dorsal rami of S1, 2, 3)
Branches of posterior femoral cutaneous nerve
Branches of lateral femoral cutaneous nerve
Accessory saphenous vein
Branch of femoral cutaneous nerve
Branch of cutaneous branch of femoral nerve
Terminal branches of posterior femoral cutaneous nerve
Great saphenous vein
Lateral sural cutaneous nerve (from common fibular [peroneal] nerve)
Small saphenous vein
Sural communicating nerve
Branches of saphenous nerve
Medial sural cutaneous nerve (from tibial nerve)
Sural nerve
Lateral calcaneal branches of sural nerve
Medial calcaneal branches of tibial nerve
Lateral dorsal cutaneous nerve (continuation of sural nerve)
Plantar cutaneous branches of medial plantar nerve
Plantar cutaneous branches of lateral plantar nerve
Netter M.D.

Plate 6 Superficial Nerves and Veins of Lower Limb: Posterior View.

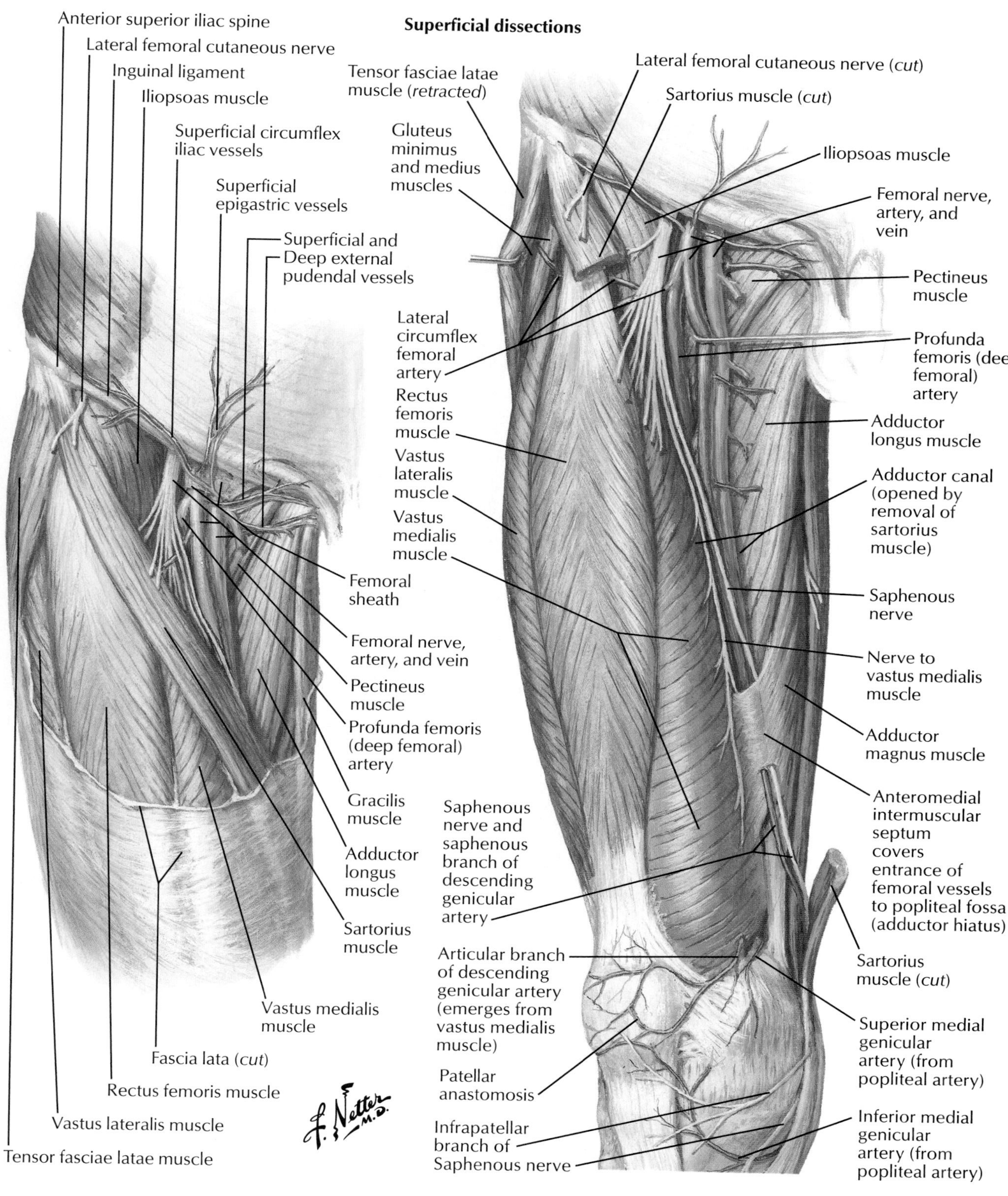
Superficial dissections
Anterior superior iliac spine
Lateral femoral cutaneous nerve
Inguinal ligament
Iliopsoas muscle
Superficial circumflex iliac vessels
Superficial epigastric vessels
Superficial and Deep external pudendal vessels
Femoral sheath
Femoral nerve, artery, and vein
Pectineus muscle
Profunda femoris (deep femoral) artery
Gracilis muscle
Adductor longus muscle
Sartorius muscle
Vastus medialis muscle
Fascia lata (cut)
Rectus femoris muscle
Vastus lateralis muscle
Tensor fasciae latae muscle
Tensor fasciae latae muscle (retracted)
Gluteus minimus and medius muscles
Lateral circumflex femoral artery
Rectus femoris muscle
Vastus lateralis muscle
Vastus medialis muscle
Saphenous nerve and saphenous branch of descending genicular artery
Articular branch of descending genicular artery (emerges from vastus medialis muscle)
Patellar anastomosis
Infrapatellar branch of Saphenous nerve
Lateral femoral cutaneous nerve (cut)
Sartorius muscle (cut)
Iliopsoas muscle
Femoral nerve, artery, and vein
Pectineus muscle
Profunda femoris (deep femoral) artery
Adductor longus muscle
Adductor canal (opened by removal of sartorius muscle)
Saphenous nerve
Nerve to vastus medialis muscle
Adductor magnus muscle
Anteromedial intermuscular septum covers entrance of femoral vessels to popliteal fossa (adductor hiatus)
Sartorius muscle (cut)
Superior medial genicular artery (from popliteal artery)
Inferior medial genicular artery (from popliteal artery)
F. Netter M.D.

Plate 7 Arteries and Nerves of Thigh: Anterior Views. (Copyright 2020 Elsevier Inc. All rights reserved. www.netterimages.com. Image ID: 4475.)

ANATOMY ILLUSTRATIONS

Deep dissection

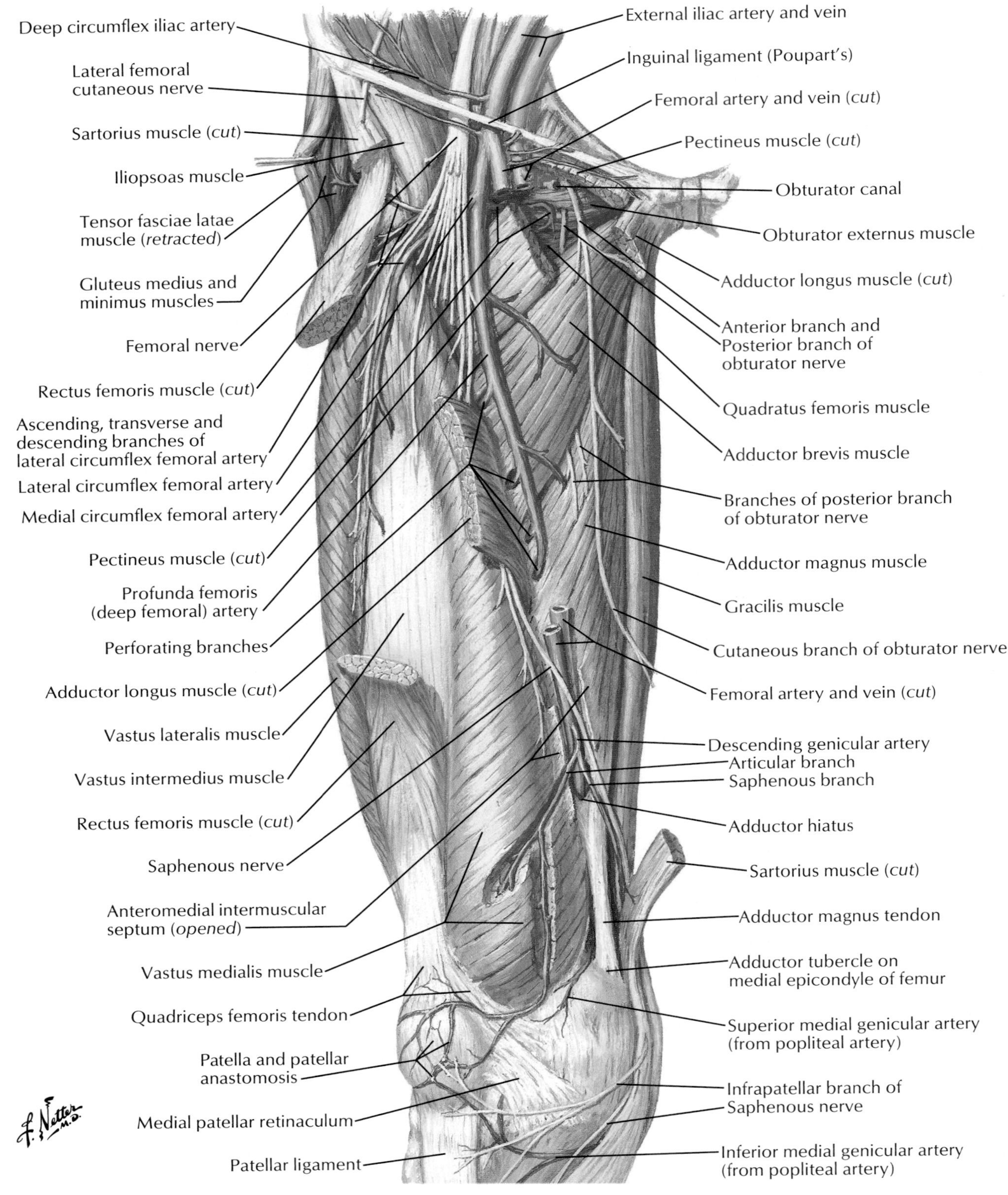
Deep circumflex iliac artery
Lateral femoral cutaneous nerve
Sartorius muscle (*cut*)
Iliopsoas muscle
Tensor fasciae latae muscle (*retracted*)
Gluteus medius and minimus muscles
Femoral nerve
Rectus femoris muscle (*cut*)
Ascending, transverse and descending branches of lateral circumflex femoral artery
Lateral circumflex femoral artery
Medial circumflex femoral artery
Pectineus muscle (*cut*)
Profunda femoris (deep femoral) artery
Perforating branches
Adductor longus muscle (*cut*)
Vastus lateralis muscle
Vastus intermedius muscle
Rectus femoris muscle (*cut*)
Saphenous nerve
Anteromedial intermuscular septum (*opened*)
Vastus medialis muscle
Quadriceps femoris tendon
Patella and patellar anastomosis
Medial patellar retinaculum
Patellar ligament
External iliac artery and vein
Inguinal ligament (Poupart's)
Femoral artery and vein (*cut*)
Pectineus muscle (*cut*)
Obturator canal
Obturator externus muscle
Adductor longus muscle (*cut*)
Anterior branch and Posterior branch of obturator nerve
Quadratus femoris muscle
Adductor brevis muscle
Branches of posterior branch of obturator nerve
Adductor magnus muscle
Gracilis muscle
Cutaneous branch of obturator nerve
Femoral artery and vein (*cut*)
Descending genicular artery
Articular branch
Saphenous branch
Adductor hiatus
Sartorius muscle (*cut*)
Adductor magnus tendon
Adductor tubercle on medial epicondyle of femur
Superior medial genicular artery (from popliteal artery)
Infrapatellar branch of Saphenous nerve
Inferior medial genicular artery (from popliteal artery)
F. Netter M.D.

ANATOMY ILLUSTRATIONS

Plate 8 Arteries and Nerves of Thigh: Posterior View. (Copyright 2020 Elsevier Inc. All rights reserved. www.netterimages.com. Image ID: 49316.)

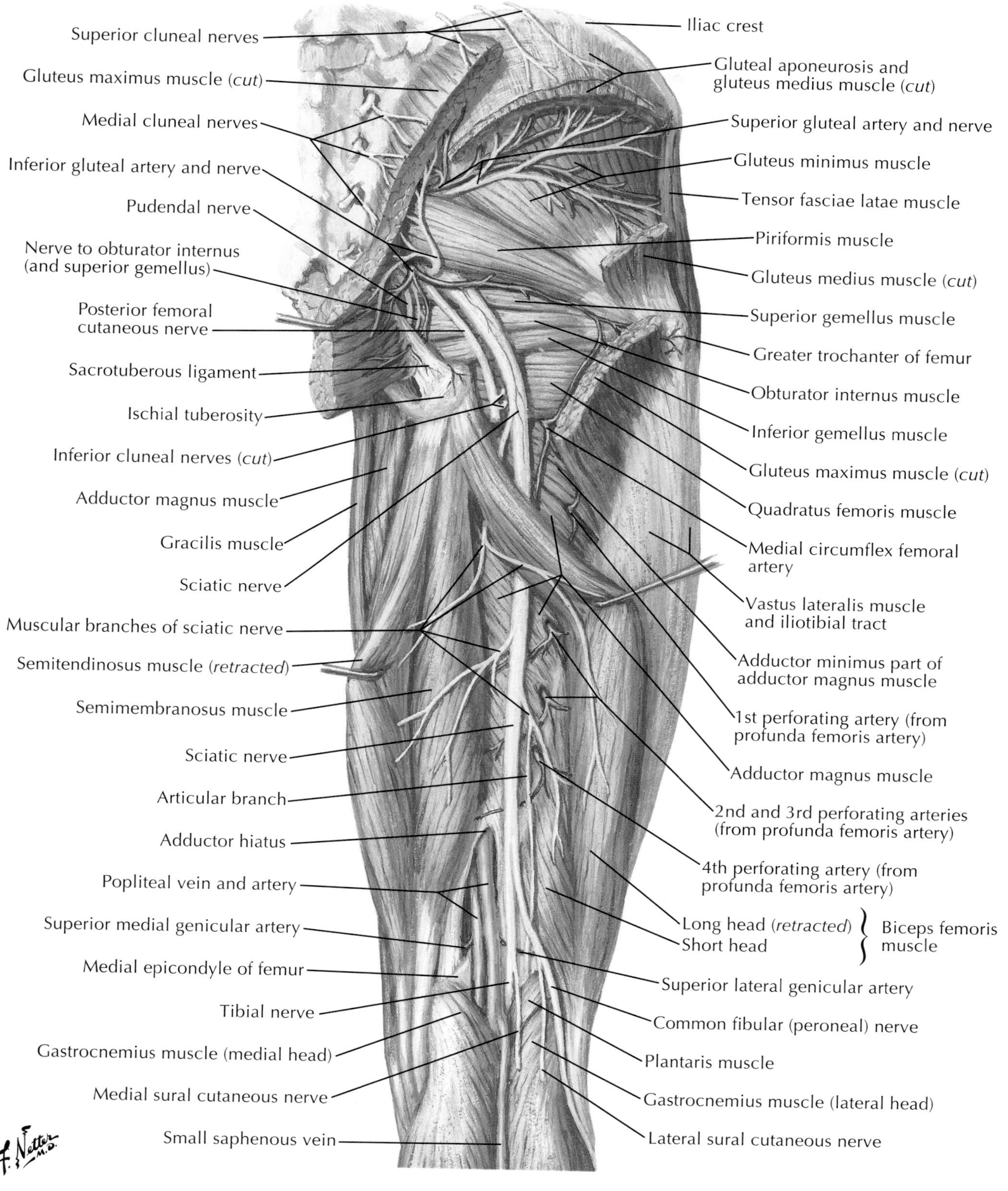
Deep dissection
Superior cluneal nerves
Gluteus maximus muscle (cut)
Medial cluneal nerves
Inferior gluteal artery and nerve
Pudendal nerve
Nerve to obturator internus
(and superior gemellus)
Posterior femoral
cutaneous nerve
Sacrotuberous ligament
Ischial tuberosity
Inferior cluneal nerves (cut)
Adductor magnus muscle
Gracilis muscle
Sciatic nerve
Muscular branches of sciatic nerve
Semitendinosus muscle (retracted)
Semimembranosus muscle
Sciatic nerve
Articular branch
Adductor hiatus
Popliteal vein and artery
Superior medial genicular artery
Medial epicondyle of femur
Tibial nerve
Gastrocnemius muscle (medial head)
Medial sural cutaneous nerve
Small saphenous vein
Iliac crest
Gluteal aponeurosis and
gluteus medius muscle (cut)
Superior gluteal artery and nerve
Gluteus minimus muscle
Tensor fasciae latae muscle
Piriformis muscle
Gluteus medius muscle (cut)
Superior gemellus muscle
Greater trochanter of femur
Obturator internus muscle
Inferior gemellus muscle
Gluteus maximus muscle (cut)
Quadratus femoris muscle
Medial circumflex femoral
artery
Vastus lateralis muscle
and iliotibial tract
Adductor minimus part of
adductor magnus muscle
1st perforating artery (from
profunda femoris artery)
Adductor magnus muscle
2nd and 3rd perforating arteries
(from profunda femoris artery)
4th perforating artery (from
profunda femoris artery)
Long head (retracted)
Short head
Biceps femoris
muscle
Superior lateral genicular artery
Common fibular (peroneal) nerve
Plantaris muscle
Gastrocnemius muscle (lateral head)
Lateral sural cutaneous nerve
F. Netter M.D.

Plate 9 Arteries and Nerves of Thigh: Posterior View. Image ID: 49317.)

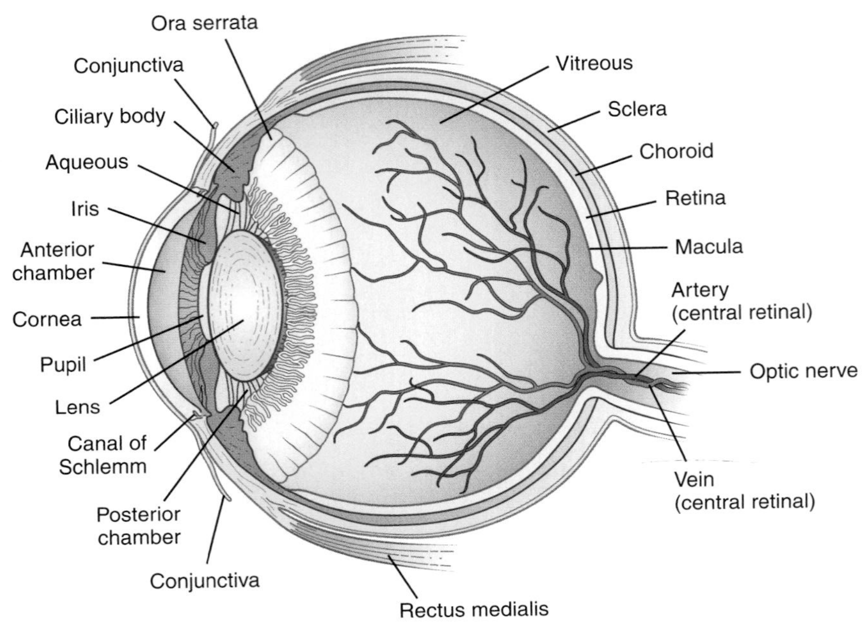
Ora serrata
Conjunctiva
Ciliary body
Aqueous
Iris
Anterior chamber
Cornea
Pupil
Lens
Canal of Schlemm
Posterior chamber
Conjunctiva
Rectus medialis
Vitreous
Sclera
Choroid
Retina
Macula
Artery (central retinal)
Optic nerve
Vein (central retinal)

Plate 10 Anatomy of the Eye. (Dehn RW, Asprey DP: Essential Clinical Procedures, ed 3, Philadelphia, 2013, Saunders.)

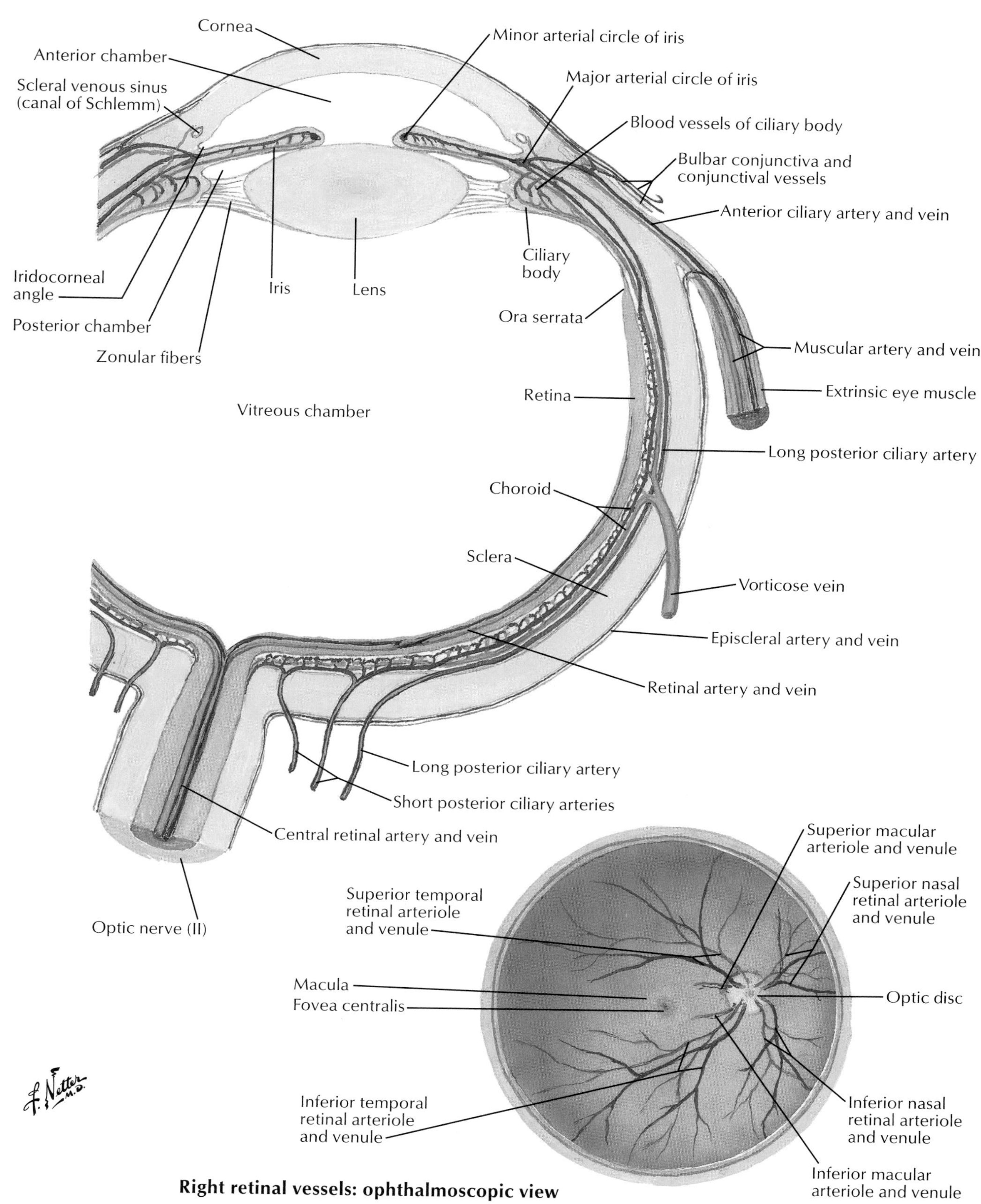
Cornea
Anterior chamber
Scleral venous sinus
(canal of Schlemm)
Minor arterial circle of iris
Major arterial circle of iris
Blood vessels of ciliary body
Bulbar conjunctiva and
conjunctival vessels
Anterior ciliary artery and vein
Iridocorneal
angle
Posterior chamber
Zonular fibers
Iris
Lens
Ciliary
body
Ora serrata
Muscular artery and vein
Extrinsic eye muscle
Retina
Vitreous chamber
Long posterior ciliary artery
Choroid
Sclera
Vorticose vein
Episcleral artery and vein
Retinal artery and vein
Long posterior ciliary artery
Short posterior ciliary arteries
Central retinal artery and vein
Optic nerve (II)
Superior macular
arteriole and venule
Superior nasal
retinal arteriole
and venule
Superior temporal
retinal arteriole
and venule
Macula
Fovea centralis
Optic disc
Inferior temporal
retinal arteriole
and venule
Inferior nasal
retinal arteriole
and venule
Inferior macular
arteriole and venule
Right retinal vessels: ophthalmoscopic view
F. Netter M.D.

Plate 11 Intrinsic Arteries and Veins of Eye. (Copyright 2020 Elsevier Inc. All rights reserved. www.netterimages.com. Image ID: 49107.)

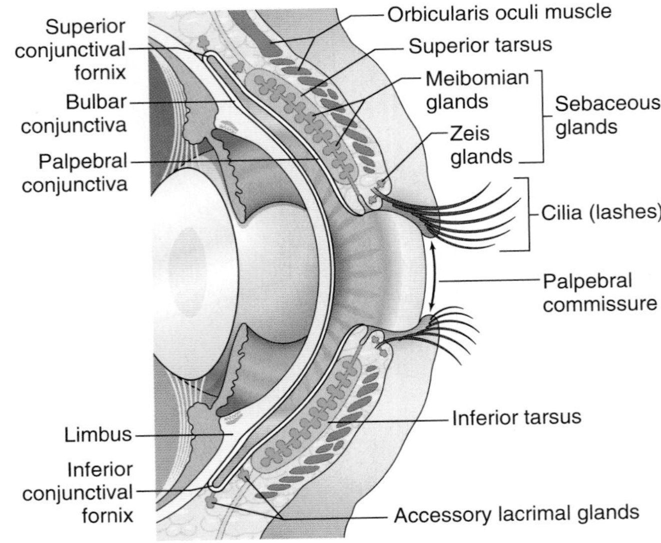
Superior
conjunctival
fornix
Bulbar
conjunctiva
Palpebral
conjunctiva
Limbus
Inferior
conjunctival
fornix
Orbicularis oculi muscle
Superior tarsus
Meibomian
glands
Zeis
glands
Sebaceous
glands
Cilia (lashes)
Palpebral
commissure
Inferior tarsus
Accessory lacrimal glands

Plate 12 Anatomy of the Conjunctiva and Eyelids. (Kumar V, Abbas AK, Aster JC: Robbins and Cotran Pathologic Basis of Disease, ed 9, Philadelphia, 2015, Saunders.)

ANATOMY ILLUSTRATIONS

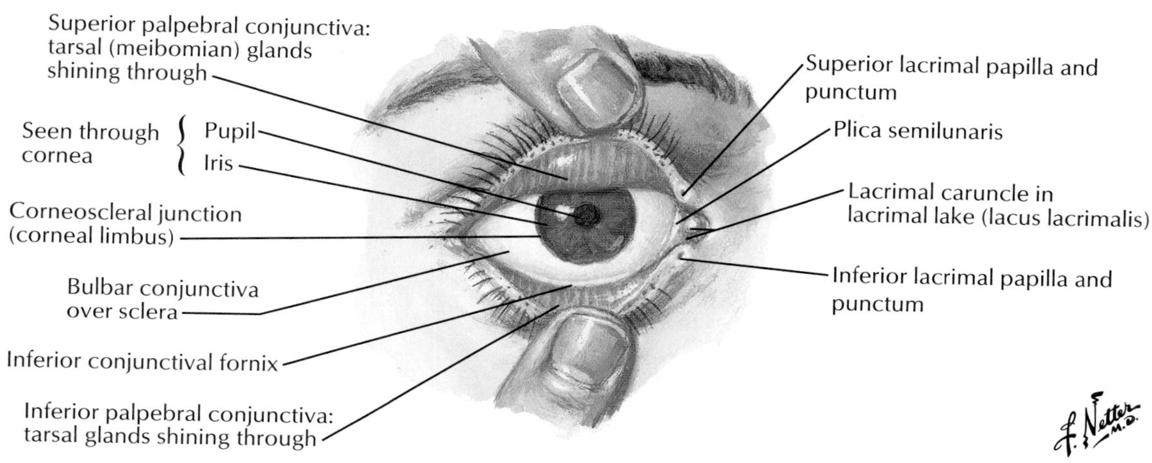
Superior palpebral conjunctiva: tarsal (meibomian) glands shining through
Seen through cornea
Pupil
Iris
Corneoscleral junction (corneal limbus)
Bulbar conjunctiva over sclera
Inferior conjunctival fornix
Inferior palpebral conjunctiva: tarsal glands shining through
Superior lacrimal papilla and punctum
Plica semilunaris
Lacrimal caruncle in lacrimal lake (lacus lacrimalis)
Inferior lacrimal papilla and punctum

Plate 13 Eyelid. (Copyright 2020 Elsevier Inc. All rights reserved. www.netterimages.com. Image ID: 4557.)

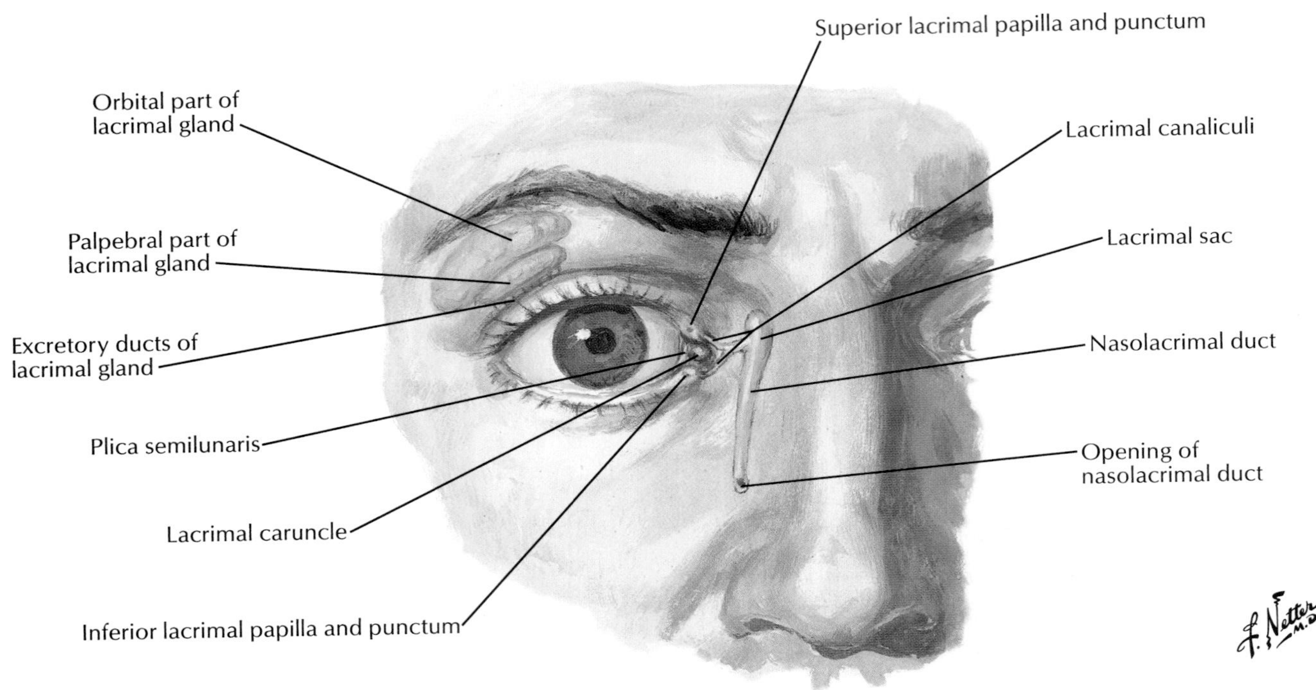
Superior lacrimal papilla and punctum
Orbital part of lacrimal gland
Lacrimal canaliculi
Lacrimal sac
Palpebral part of lacrimal gland
Excretory ducts of lacrimal gland
Nasolacrimal duct
Plica semilunaris
Opening of nasolacrimal duct
Lacrimal caruncle
Inferior lacrimal papilla and punctum
F. Netter M.D.

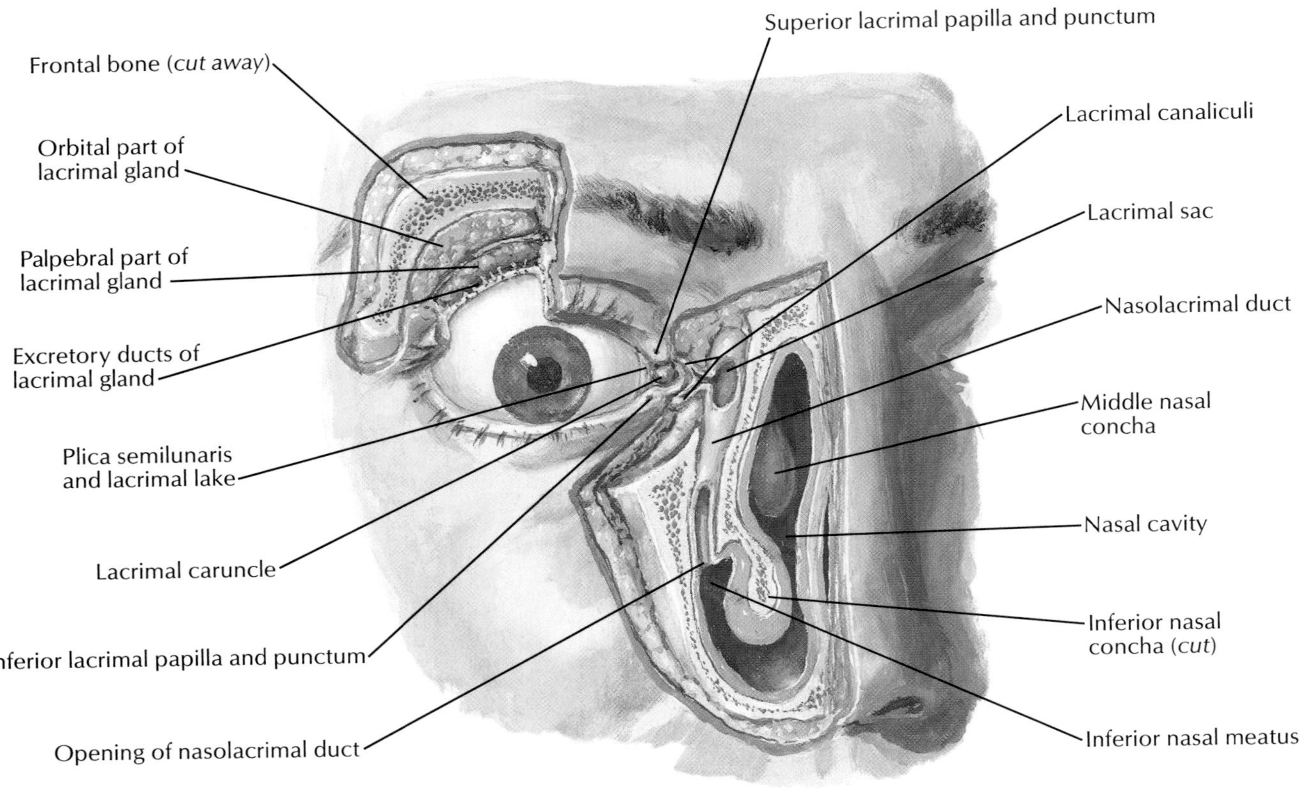
Superior lacrimal papilla and punctum
Frontal bone (*cut away*)
Lacrimal canaliculi
Orbital part of lacrimal gland
Lacrimal sac
Palpebral part of lacrimal gland
Nasolacrimal duct
Excretory ducts of lacrimal gland
Middle nasal concha
Plica semilunaris and lacrimal lake
Nasal cavity
Lacrimal caruncle
Inferior nasal concha (*cut*)
Inferior lacrimal papilla and punctum
Inferior nasal meatus
Opening of nasolacrimal duct

Plate 14 Lacrimal Apparatus.

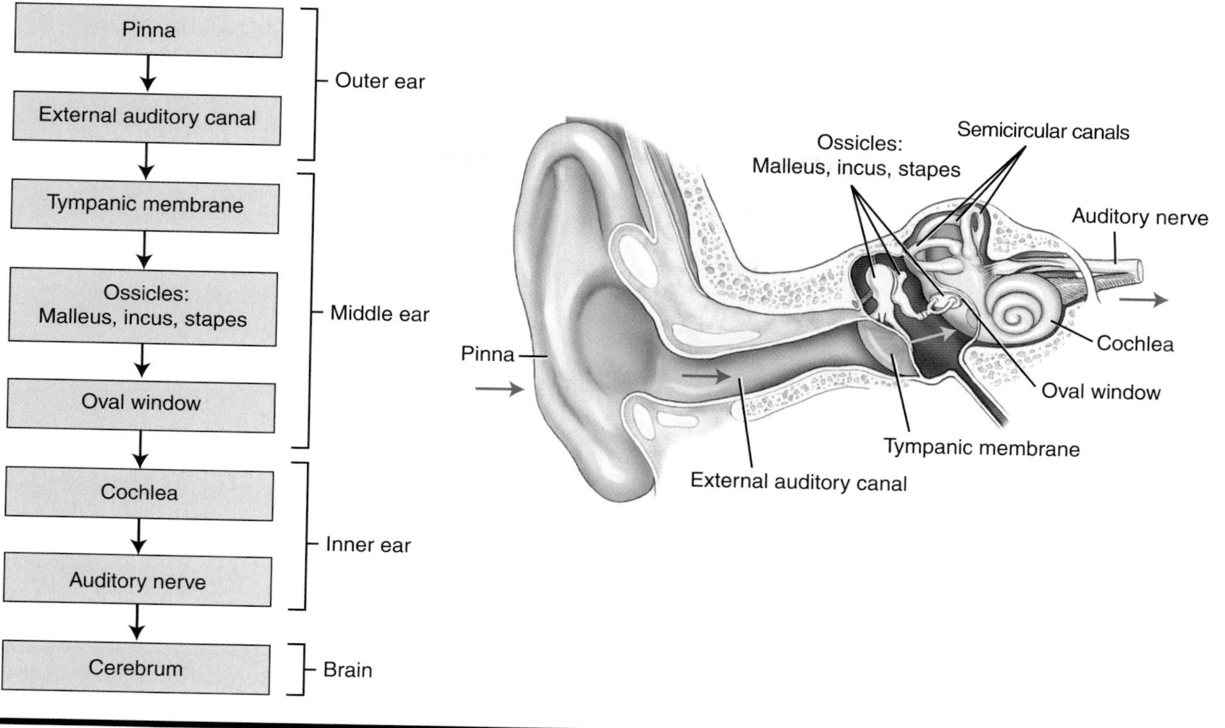
Pinna
External auditory canal
Tympanic membrane
Ossicles:
Malleus, incus, stapes
Oval window
Cochlea
Auditory nerve
Cerebrum
Outer ear
Middle ear
Inner ear
Brain
Ossicles:
Malleus, incus, stapes
Semicircular canals
Auditory nerve
Cochlea
Oval window
Tympanic membrane
External auditory canal
Pinna

Plate 15 Pathway of Sound. (LaFleur Brooks D, LaFleur Brooks M: Basic Medical Language, ed 4, St. Louis, 2013, Mosby.)

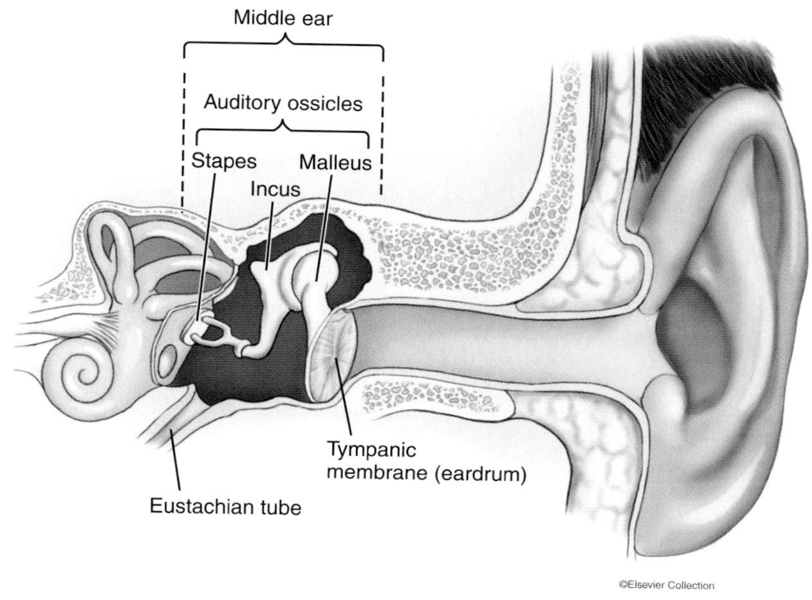
Middle ear
Auditory ossicles
Stapes
Malleus
Incus
Tympanic
membrane (eardrum)
Eustachian tube
©Elsevier Collection

Plate 16 Middle Ear Structures. (©Elsevier Collection.)

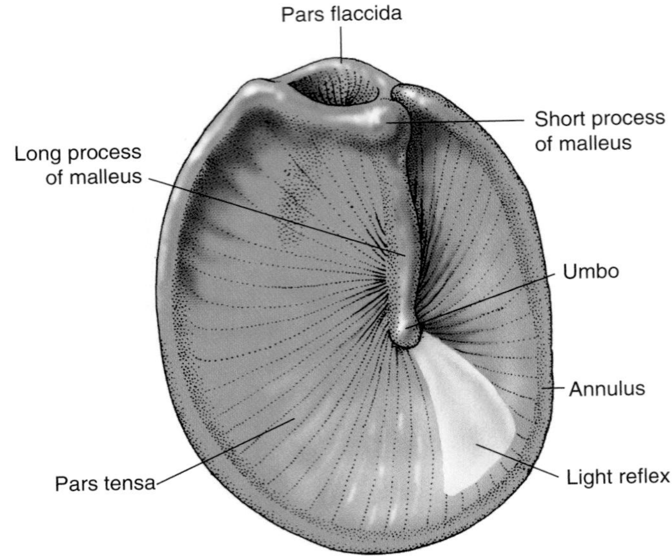
RIGHT TYMPANIC MEMBRANE
Pars flaccida
Short process
of malleus
Long process
of malleus
Umbo
Annulus
Pars tensa
Light reflex

Plate 17 Structural Landmarks of Tympanic Membrane. (Ignatavicius DD, Workman ML: Medical-Surgical Nursing: Patient-Centered Collaborative Care, ed 7, St. Louis, 2013, Saunders.)

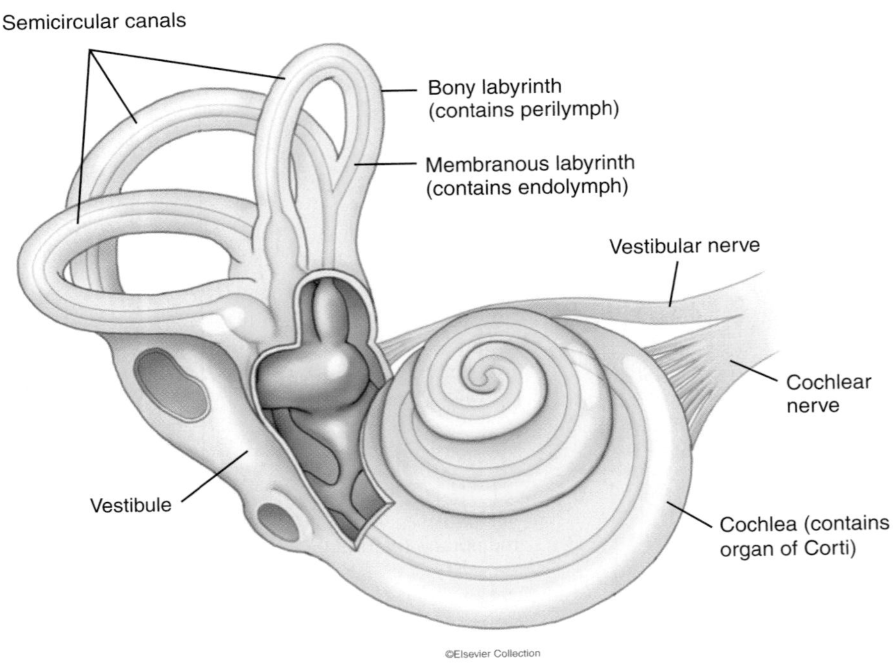
Semicircular canals
Bony labyrinth
(contains perilymph)
Membranous labyrinth
(contains endolymph)
Vestibular nerve
Cochlear
nerve
Vestibule
Cochlea (contains
organ of Corti)
©Elsevier Collection

Plate 18 Inner Ear Structures. (©Elsevier Collection.)

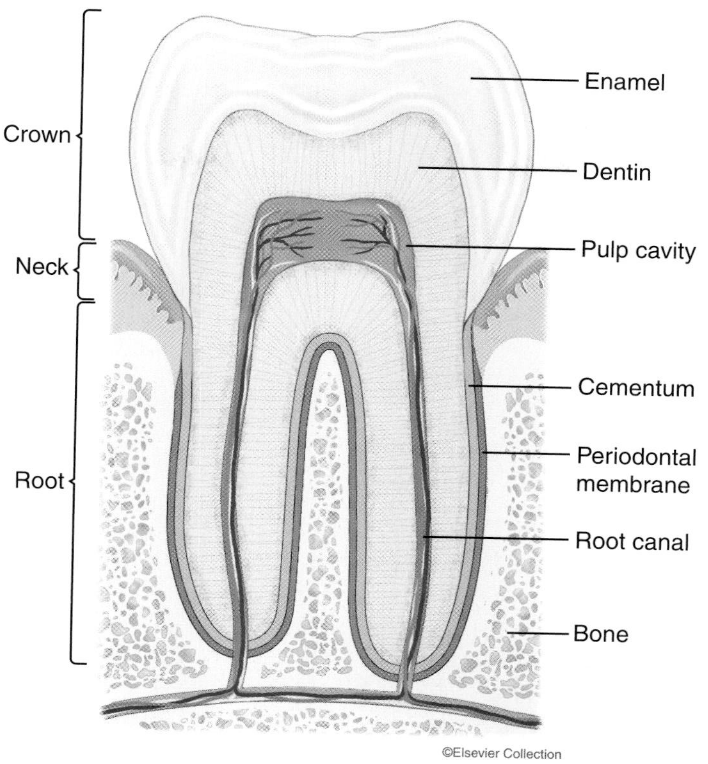
Crown
Neck
Root
Enamel
Dentin
Pulp cavity
Cementum
Periodontal membrane
Root canal
Bone
©Elsevier Collection

Plate 19 The Tooth. (©Elsevier Collection).

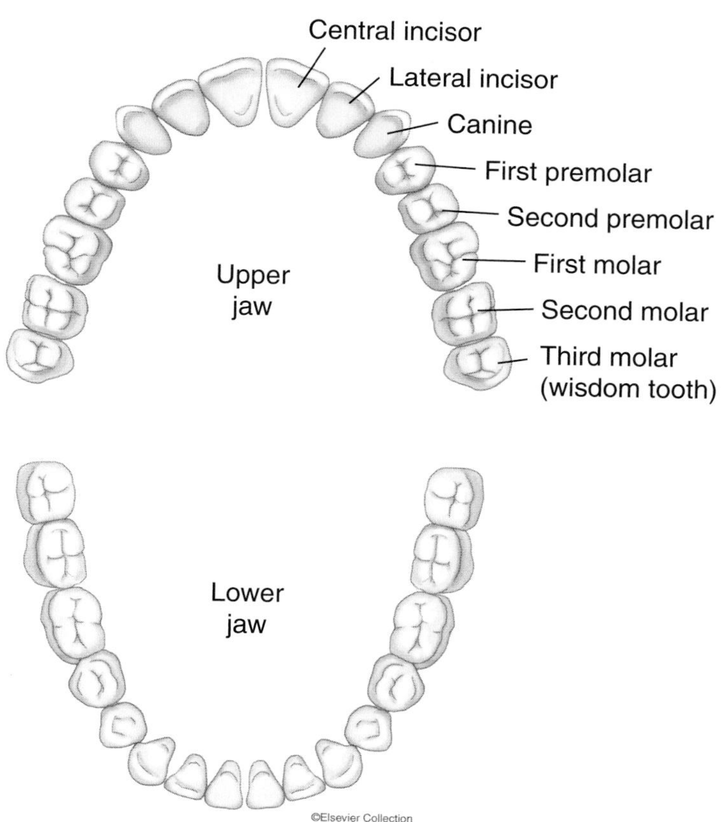
Central incisor
Lateral incisor
Canine
First premolar
Second premolar
First molar
Second molar
Third molar (wisdom tooth)
Upper jaw
Lower jaw
©Elsevier Collection

Plate 20 Adult Teeth. (©Elsevier Collection).

ANATOMY ILLUSTRATIONS

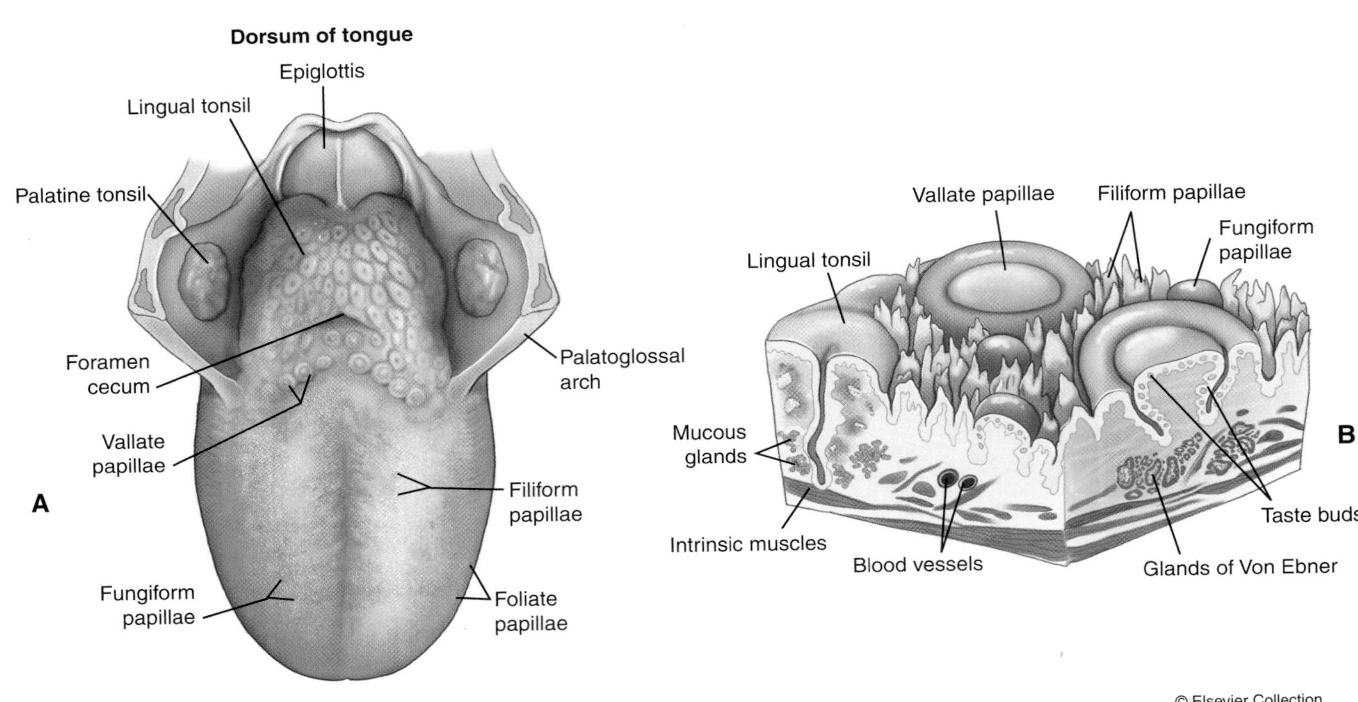

Dorsum of tongue
Epiglottis
Lingual tonsil
Palatine tonsil
Foramen
cecum
Vallate
papillae
A
Fungiform
papillae
Palatoglossal
arch
Filiform
papillae
Foliate
papillae
Vallate papillae
Filiform papillae
Fungiform
papillae
Lingual tonsil
Mucous
glands
Intrinsic muscles
Blood vessels
Glands of Von Ebner
Taste buds
B

Plate 21 A, Dorsal view of tongue showing the roughened large lingual tonsils on the posterior of the tongue and the foliate papillae on the side. B, Section of dorsal of the tongue showing a cutaway through lingual papillae and showing von Ebner's glands at the base of the vallate papilla. (Brand RW, Isselhard DE: Anatomy of Orofacial Structures: A Comprehensive Approach, ed 8, St. Louis, 2019, Elsevier.)

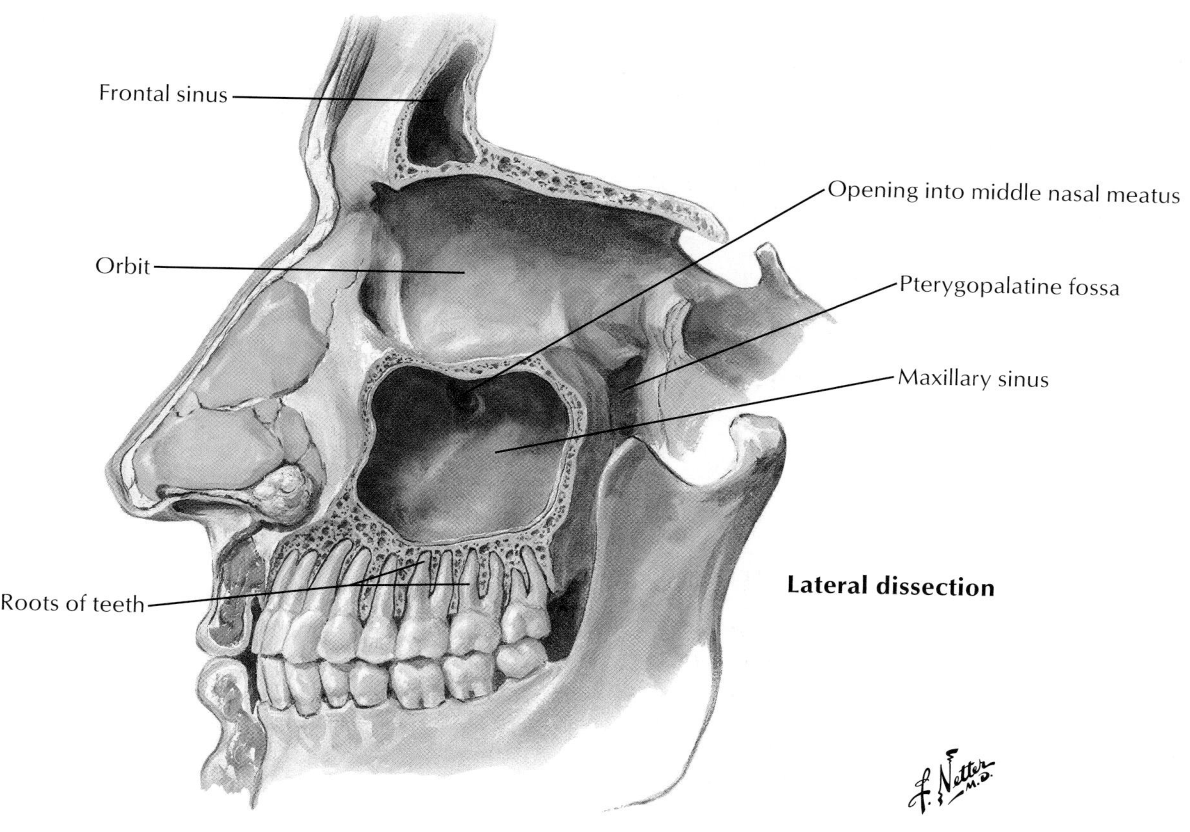
Frontal sinus
Opening into middle nasal meatus
Orbit
Pterygopalatine fossa
Maxillary sinus
Roots of teeth
Lateral dissection

Plate 22 Paranasal Sinuses.

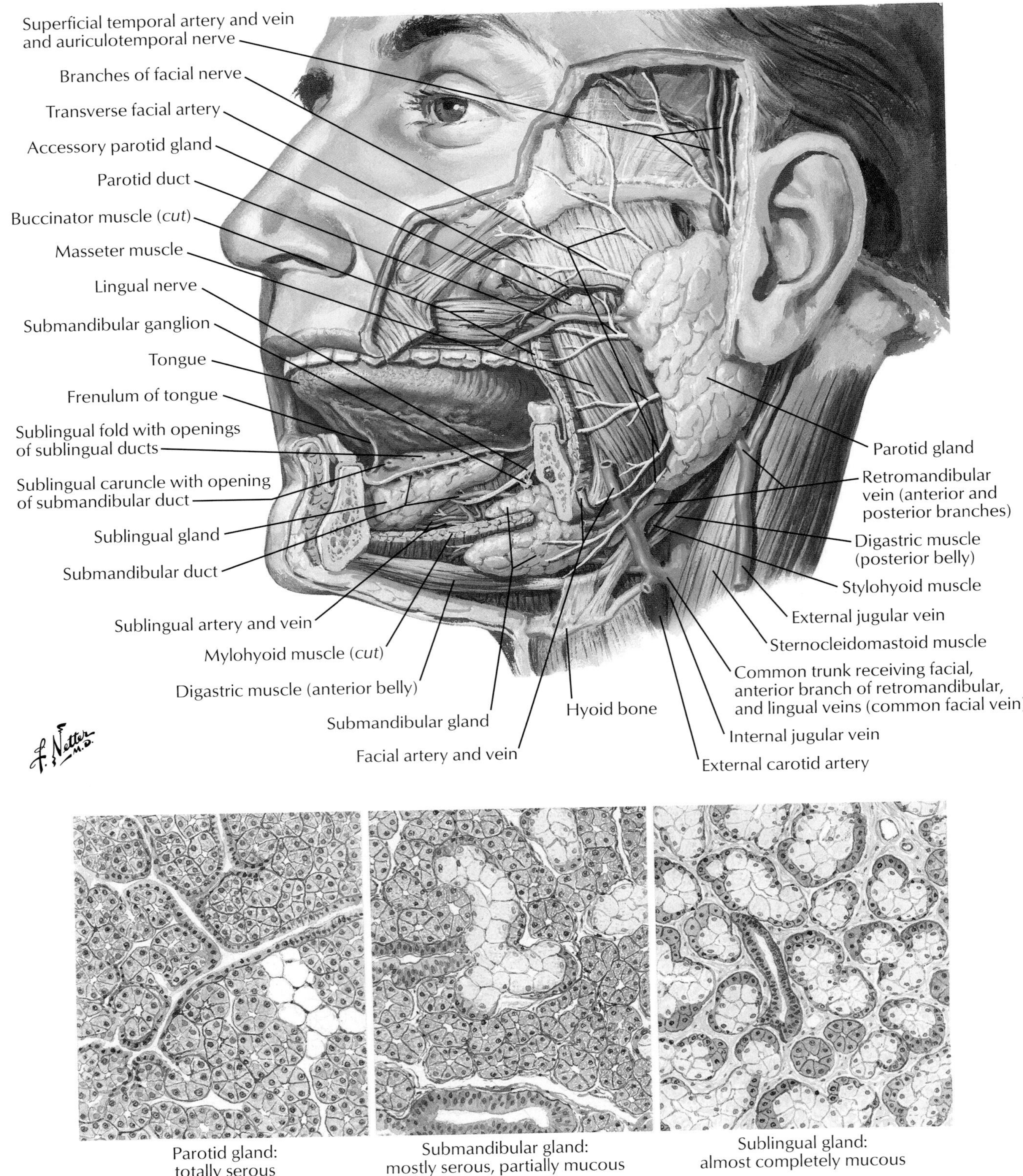
Superficial temporal artery and vein and auriculotemporal nerve
Branches of facial nerve
Transverse facial artery
Accessory parotid gland
Parotid duct
Buccinator muscle (*cut*)
Masseter muscle
Lingual nerve
Submandibular ganglion
Tongue
Frenulum of tongue
Sublingual fold with openings of sublingual ducts
Sublingual caruncle with opening of submandibular duct
Sublingual gland
Submandibular duct
Sublingual artery and vein
Mylohyoid muscle (*cut*)
Digastric muscle (anterior belly)
Submandibular gland
Facial artery and vein
Hyoid bone
External carotid artery
Internal jugular vein
Common trunk receiving facial, anterior branch of retromandibular, and lingual veins (common facial vein)
Sternocleidomastoid muscle
External jugular vein
Stylohyoid muscle
Digastric muscle (posterior belly)
Retromandibular vein (anterior and posterior branches)
Parotid gland
F. Netter M.D.

Parotid gland: totally serous

Submandibular gland: mostly serous, partially mucous

Sublingual gland: almost completely mucous

Plate 23 Salivary Glands. (Copyright 2020 Elsevier Inc. All rights reserved. www.netterimages.com. Image ID: 4396.)

Coronary Arteries: Arteriographic Views

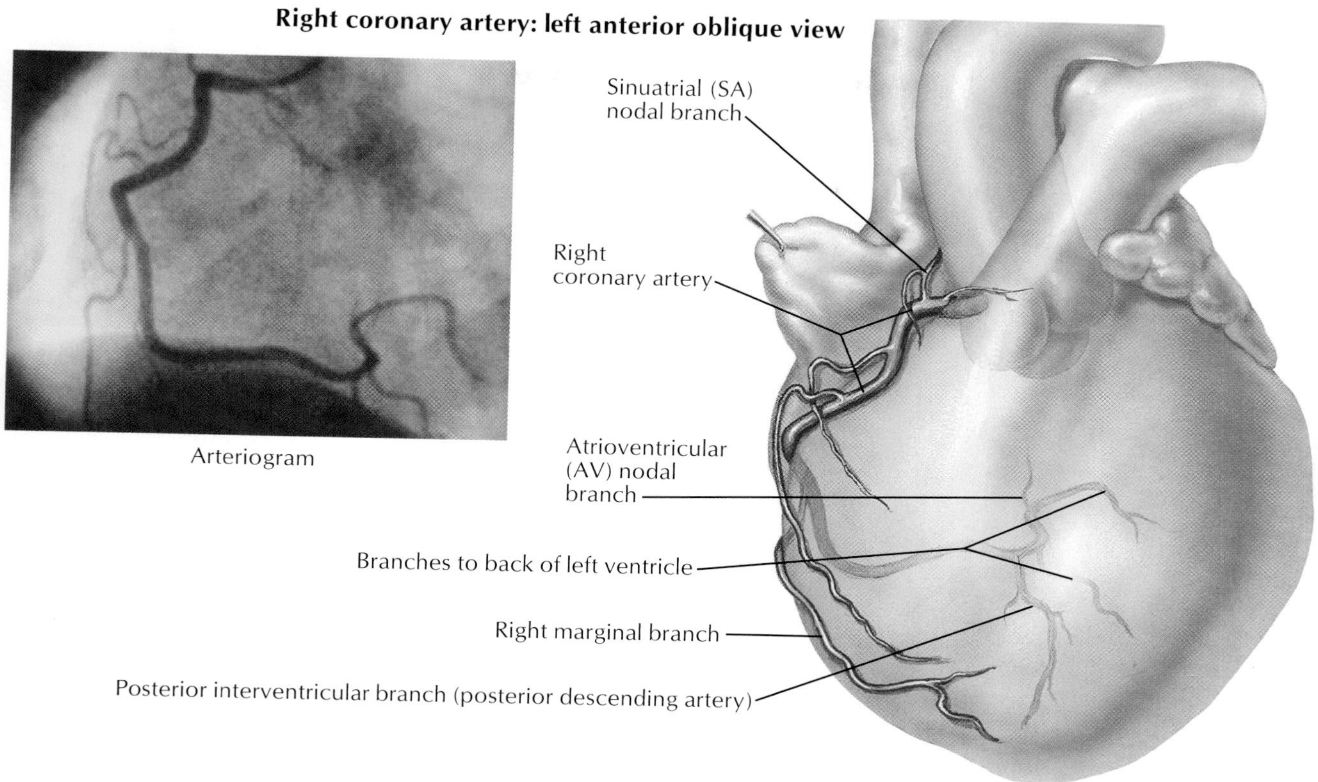
Right coronary artery: left anterior oblique view
Arteriogram
Sinuatrial (SA) nodal branch
Right coronary artery
Atrioventricular (AV) nodal branch
Branches to back of left ventricle
Right marginal branch
Posterior interventricular branch (posterior descending artery)

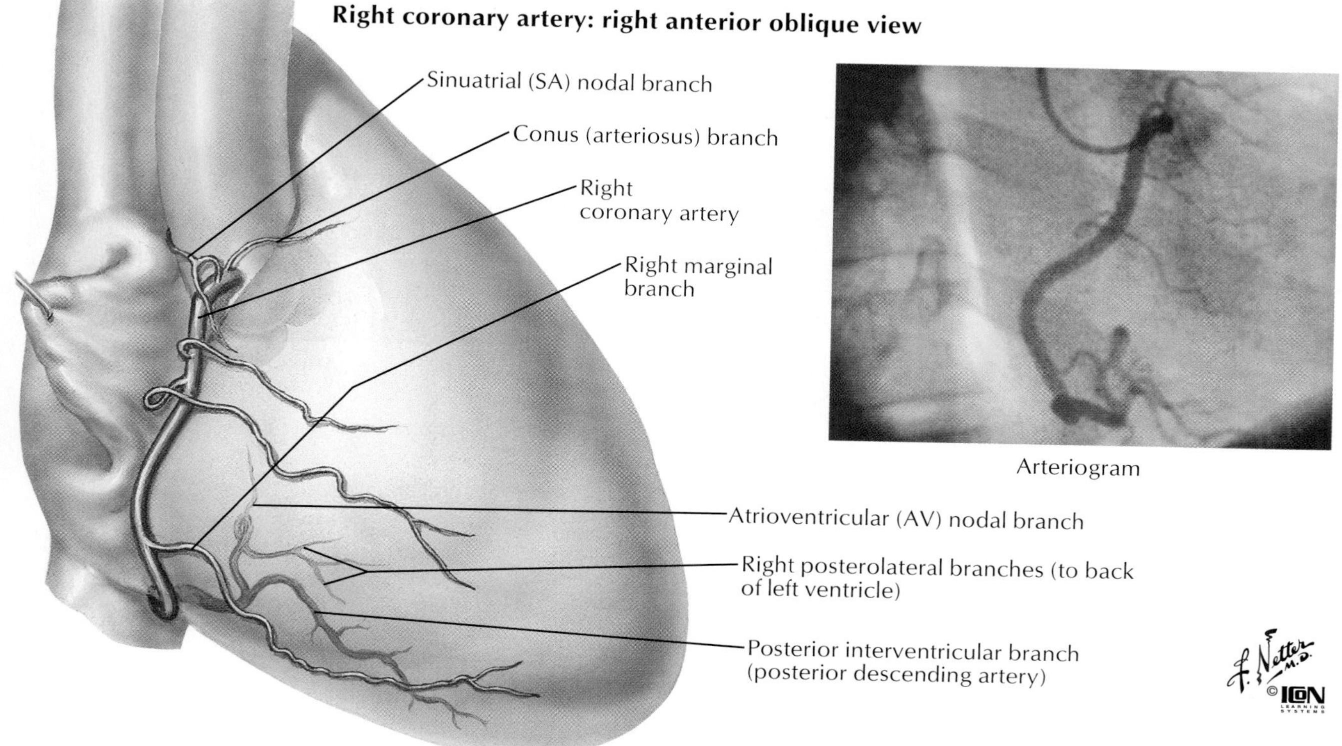
Right coronary artery: right anterior oblique view
Sinuatrial (SA) nodal branch
Conus (arteriosus) branch
Right coronary artery
Right marginal branch
Arteriogram
Atrioventricular (AV) nodal branch
Right posterolateral branches (to back of left ventricle)
Posterior interventricular branch (posterior descending artery)
F. Netter M.D.
© ICON LEARNING SYSTEMS

ANATOMY ILLUSTRATIONS

Plate 24 Coronary Arteries: Arteriographic Views. Image ID: 4725.)

Left coronary artery: left anterior oblique view

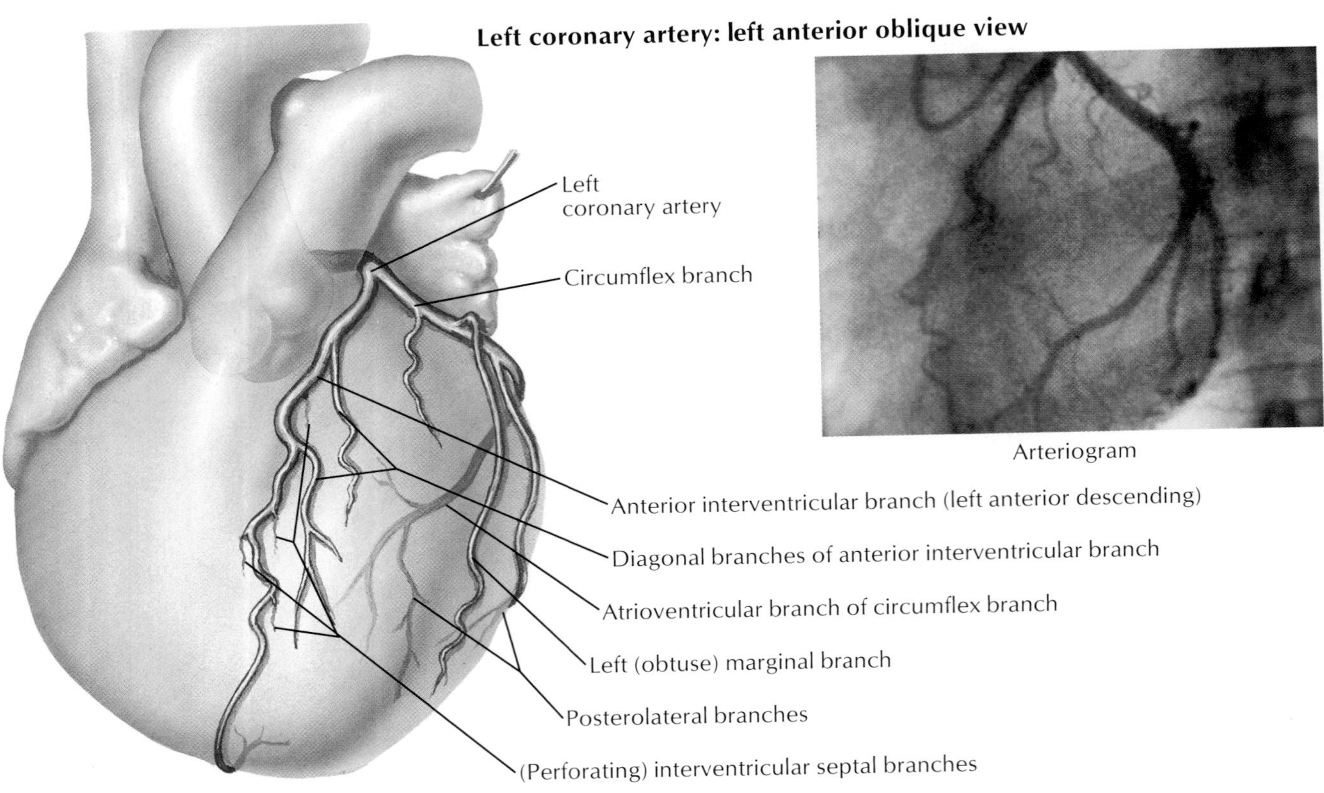
Left
coronary artery
Circumflex branch
Arteriogram
Anterior interventricular branch (left anterior descending)
Diagonal branches of anterior interventricular branch
Atrioventricular branch of circumflex branch
Left (obtuse) marginal branch
Posterolateral branches
(Perforating) interventricular septal branches

Left coronary artery: right anterior oblique view

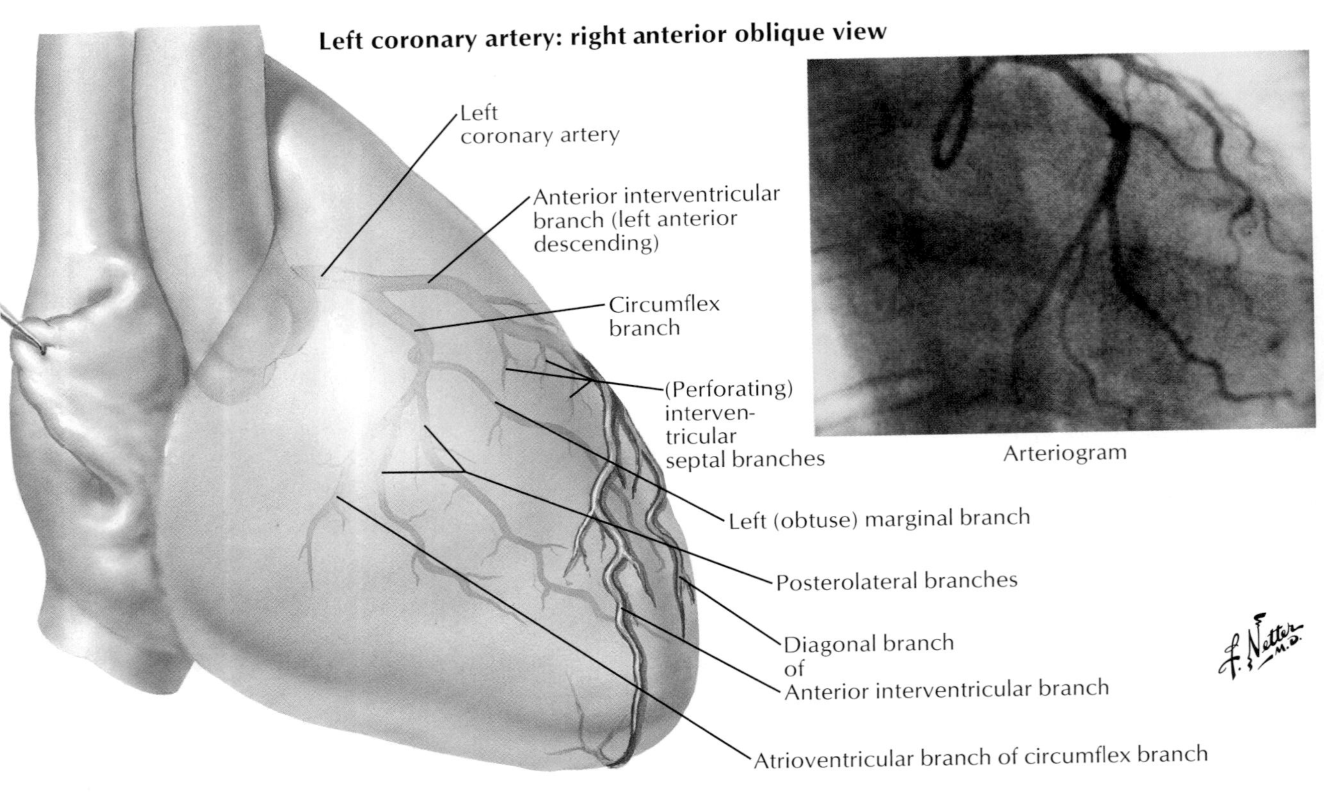
Left
coronary artery
Anterior interventricular
branch (left anterior
descending)
Circumflex
branch
(Perforating)
interven-
tricular
septal branches
Arteriogram
Left (obtuse) marginal branch
Posterolateral branches
Diagonal branch
of
Anterior interventricular branch
Atrioventricular branch of circumflex branch

Plate 25 Coronary Arteries: Arteriographic Views. Image ID: 4542.)

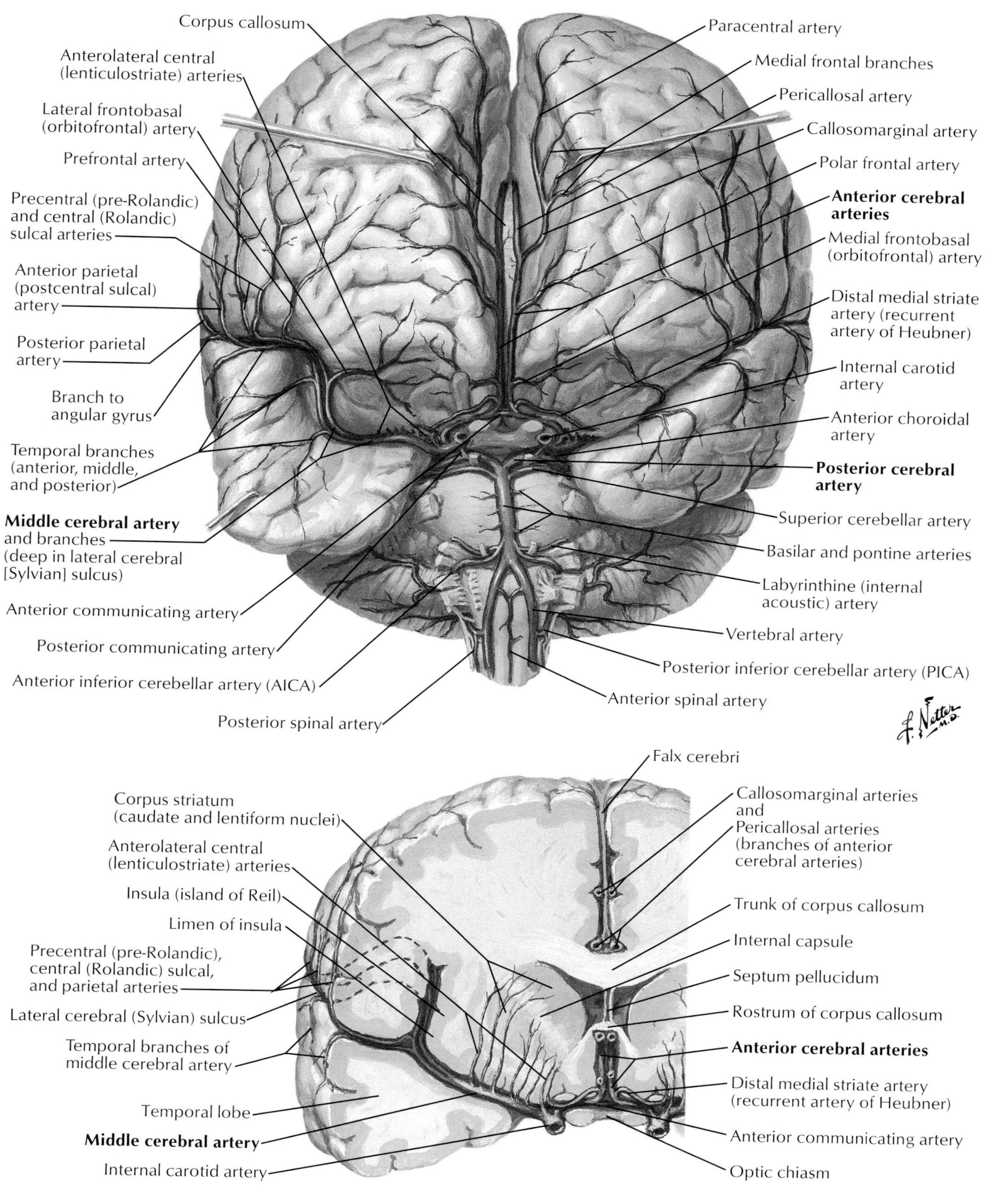
Corpus callosum
Anterolateral central (lenticulostriate) arteries
Lateral frontobasal (orbitofrontal) artery
Prefrontal artery
Precentral (pre-Rolandic) and central (Rolandic) sulcal arteries
Anterior parietal (postcentral sulcal) artery
Posterior parietal artery
Branch to angular gyrus
Temporal branches (anterior, middle, and posterior)
Middle cerebral artery and branches (deep in lateral cerebral [Sylvian] sulcus)
Anterior communicating artery
Posterior communicating artery
Anterior inferior cerebellar artery (AICA)
Posterior spinal artery
Paracentral artery
Medial frontal branches
Pericallosal artery
Callosomarginal artery
Polar frontal artery
Anterior cerebral arteries
Medial frontobasal (orbitofrontal) artery
Distal medial striate artery (recurrent artery of Heubner)
Internal carotid artery
Anterior choroidal artery
Posterior cerebral artery
Superior cerebellar artery
Basilar and pontine arteries
Labyrinthine (internal acoustic) artery
Vertebral artery
Posterior inferior cerebellar artery (PICA)
Anterior spinal artery
F. Netter M.D.
Falx cerebri
Corpus striatum (caudate and lentiform nuclei)
Anterolateral central (lenticulostriate) arteries
Insula (island of Reil)
Limen of insula
Precentral (pre-Rolandic), central (Rolandic) sulcal, and parietal arteries
Lateral cerebral (Sylvian) sulcus
Temporal branches of middle cerebral artery
Temporal lobe
Middle cerebral artery
Internal carotid artery
Callosomarginal arteries and Pericallosal arteries (branches of anterior cerebral arteries)
Trunk of corpus callosum
Internal capsule
Septum pellucidum
Rostrum of corpus callosum
Anterior cerebral arteries
Distal medial striate artery (recurrent artery of Heubner)
Anterior communicating artery
Optic chiasm

Plate 26 Arteries of Brain: Frontal View and Section. (Copyright 2020 Elsevier Inc. All rights reserved. www.netterimages.com. Image ID: 4588.)

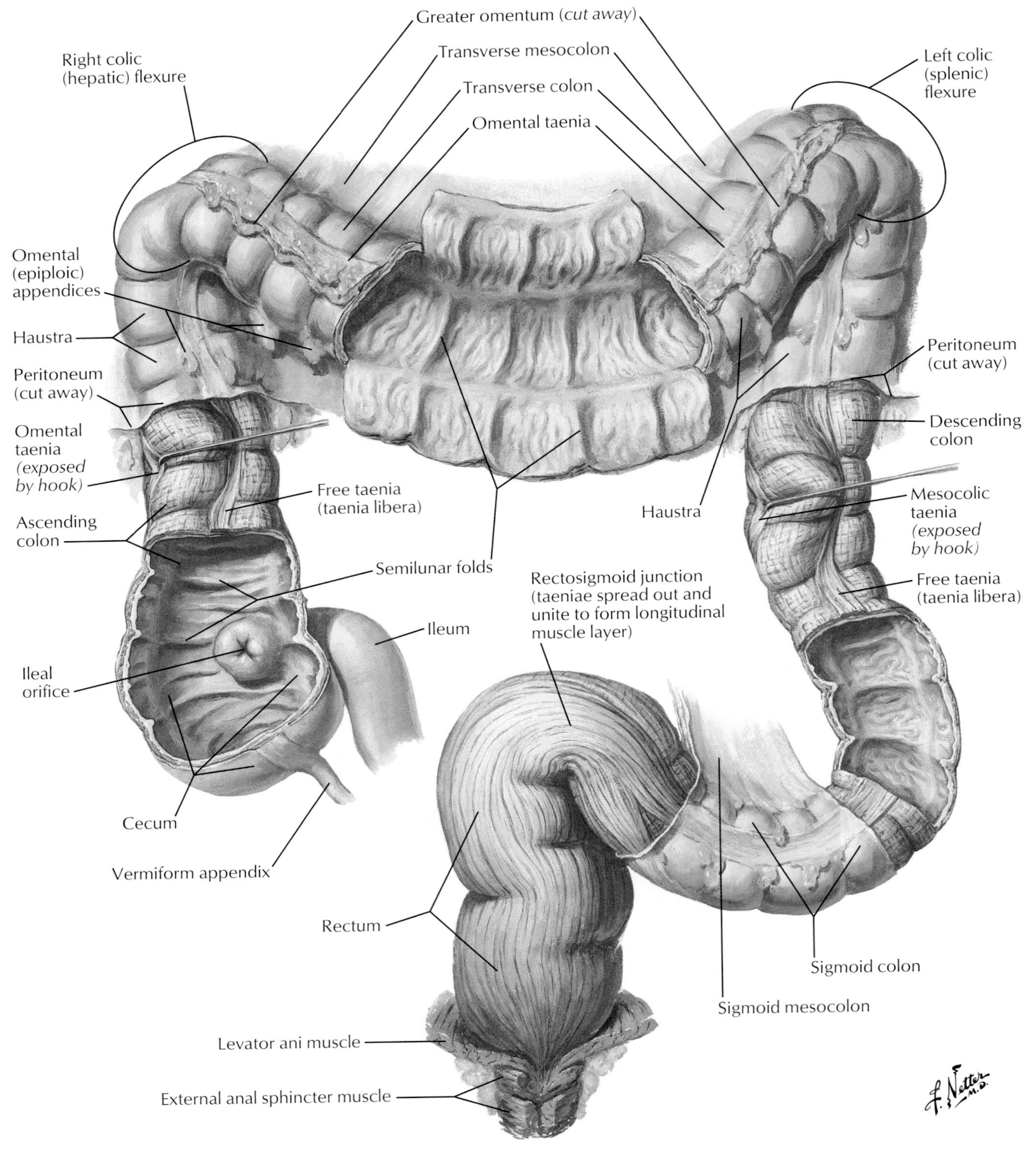
Greater omentum (cut away)
Transverse mesocolon
Transverse colon
Omental taenia
Right colic (hepatic) flexure
Left colic (splenic) flexure
Omental (epiploic) appendices
Haustra
Peritoneum (cut away)
Omental taenia (exposed by hook)
Free taenia (taenia libera)
Ascending colon
Semilunar folds
Ileum
Ileal orifice
Cecum
Vermiform appendix
Haustra
Peritoneum (cut away)
Descending colon
Mesocolic taenia (exposed by hook)
Free taenia (taenia libera)
Rectosigmoid junction (taeniae spread out and unite to form longitudinal muscle layer)
Rectum
Sigmoid colon
Sigmoid mesocolon
Levator ani muscle
External anal sphincter muscle

Plate 27 Mucosa and Musculature of Large Intestine. Image ID: 4778.)

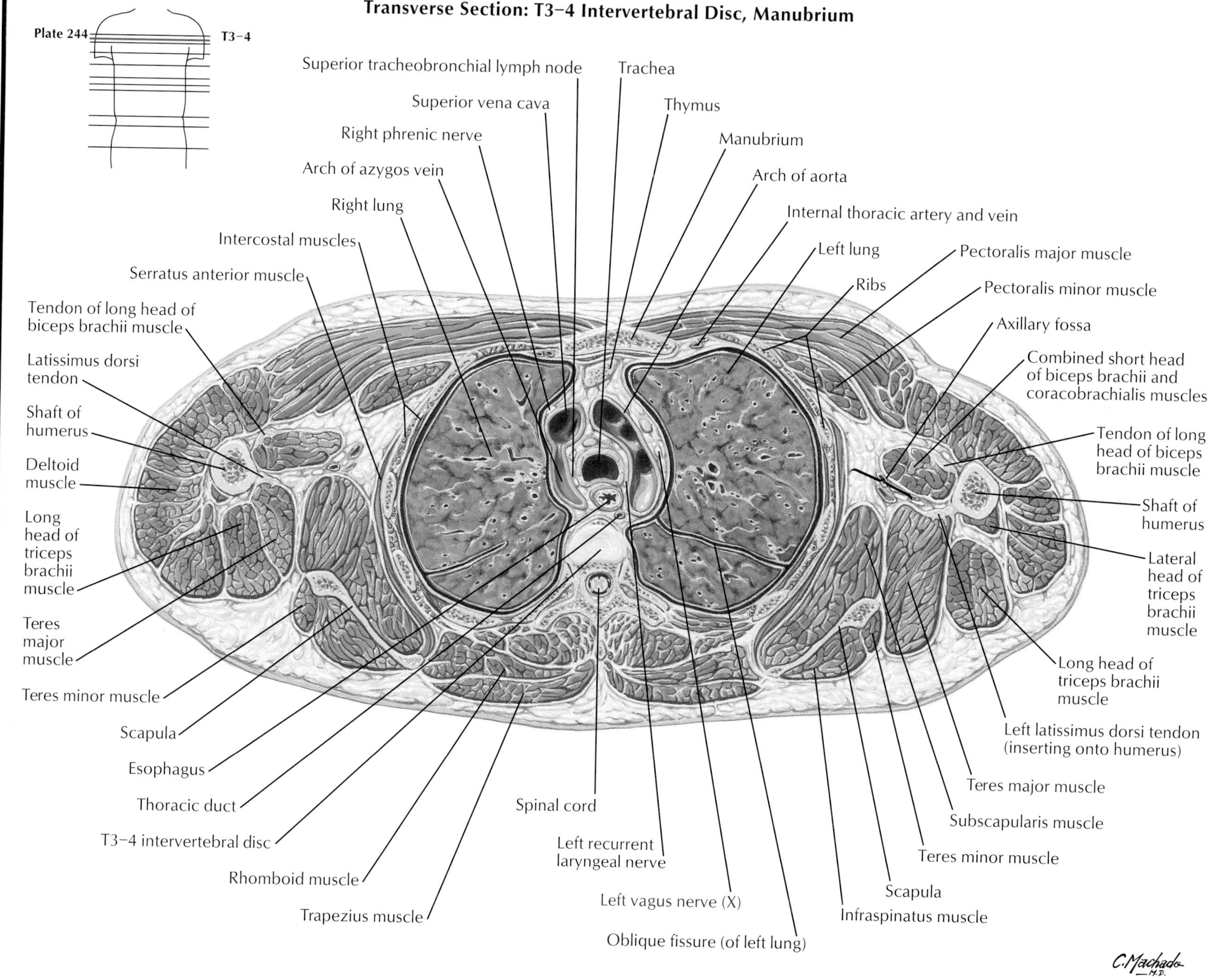
Transverse Section: T3–4 Intervertebral Disc, Manubrium
Plate 244
T3–4
Superior tracheobronchial lymph node
Trachea
Superior vena cava
Thymus
Right phrenic nerve
Manubrium
Arch of azygos vein
Arch of aorta
Right lung
Internal thoracic artery and vein
Intercostal muscles
Left lung
Pectoralis major muscle
Serratus anterior muscle
Ribs
Pectoralis minor muscle
Tendon of long head of biceps brachii muscle
Axillary fossa
Latissimus dorsi tendon
Combined short head of biceps brachii and coracobrachialis muscles
Shaft of humerus
Tendon of long head of biceps brachii muscle
Deltoid muscle
Shaft of humerus
Long head of triceps brachii muscle
Lateral head of triceps brachii muscle
Teres major muscle
Long head of triceps brachii muscle
Teres minor muscle
Scapula
Left latissimus dorsi tendon (inserting onto humerus)
Esophagus
Teres major muscle
Thoracic duct
Spinal cord
Subscapularis muscle
T3–4 intervertebral disc
Left recurrent laryngeal nerve
Teres minor muscle
Rhomboid muscle
Scapula
Left vagus nerve (X)
Trapezius muscle
Infraspinatus muscle
Oblique fissure (of left lung)
C.Machado M.D.

Plate 28 Cross Section of Thorax at T3-4 Disc Level. (Copyright 2020 Elsevier Inc. All rights reserved. www.netterimages.com. Image ID: 4880.)

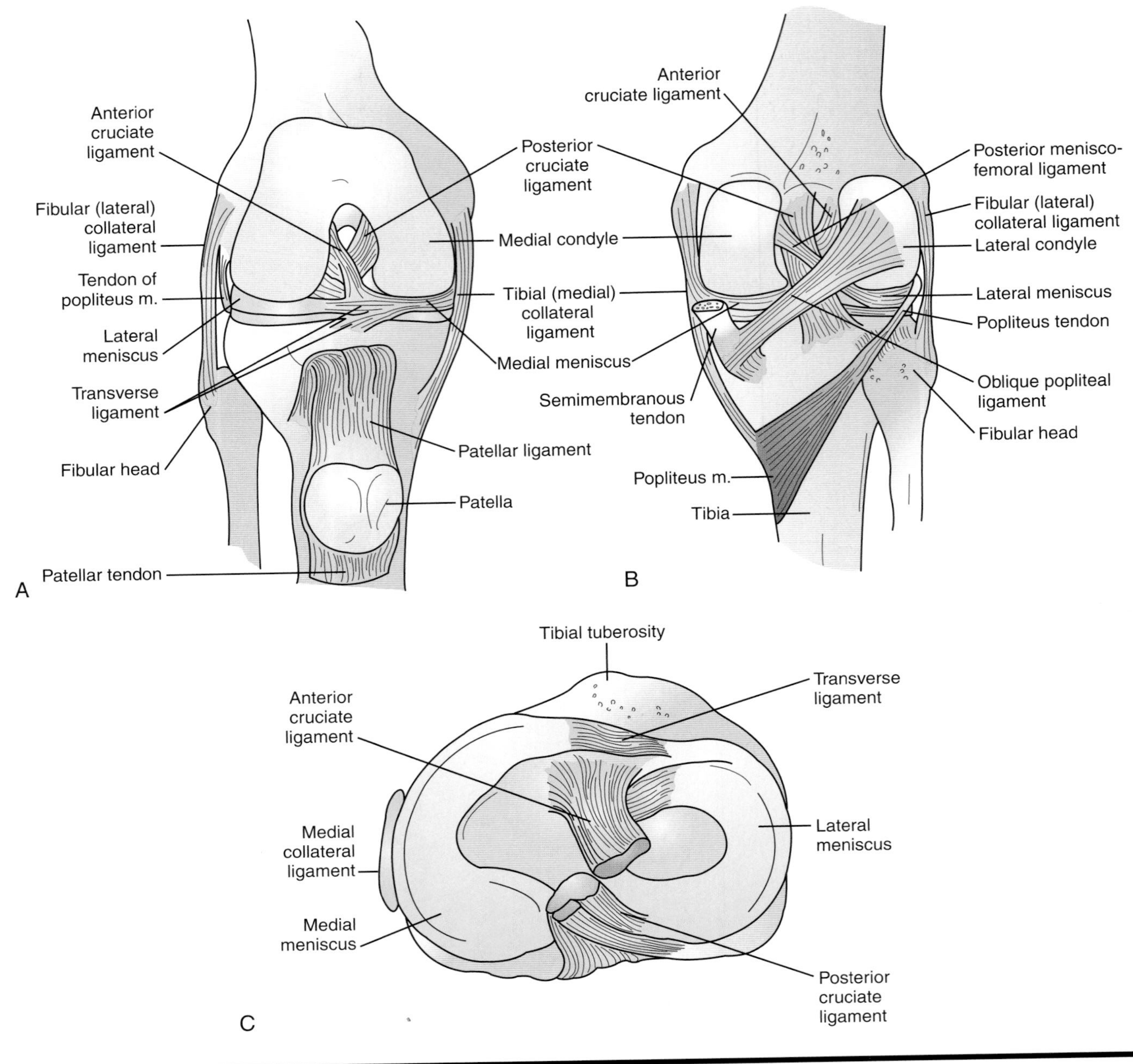

Anterior cruciate ligament
Fibular (lateral) collateral ligament
Tendon of popliteus m.
Lateral meniscus
Transverse ligament
Fibular head
Patellar tendon
A
Posterior cruciate ligament
Medial condyle
Tibial (medial) collateral ligament
Medial meniscus
Patellar ligament
Patella
Anterior cruciate ligament
Semimembranous tendon
Popliteus m.
Tibia
B
Posterior menisco-femoral ligament
Fibular (lateral) collateral ligament
Lateral condyle
Lateral meniscus
Popliteus tendon
Oblique popliteal ligament
Fibular head
Tibial tuberosity
Anterior cruciate ligament
Medial collateral ligament
Medial meniscus
Transverse ligament
Lateral meniscus
Posterior cruciate ligament
C

Plate 29 Knee joint opened; anterior, posterior, and proximal views. A, Anterior view of the knee joint, opened by folding the patella and patellar ligament inferiorly. On the lateral side is the fibular collateral ligament, separated by the popliteal tendon from the lateral meniscus. On the medial side, the tibial collateral ligament is attached to the medial meniscus. The anterior and posterior cruciate ligaments are seen between the femoral condyles. B, Posterior view of the opened knee joint with a more complete view of the posterior cruciate ligament. C, The femur is removed, showing the proximal (articular) end of the right tibia. On the medial side is the gently curved medial meniscus; on the lateral side is the more tightly curved lateral meniscus. The anterior end of the medial meniscus is anchored to the surface of the tibia by the transverse ligament. The cut ends of the anterior and posterior cruciate ligaments are shown, as well as the meniscofemoral ligament. (Fritz S: Mosby's Essential Sciences for Therapeutic Massage: Anatomy, Physiology, Biomechanics, and Pathology, ed 5, St. Louis, 2017, Elsevier.)

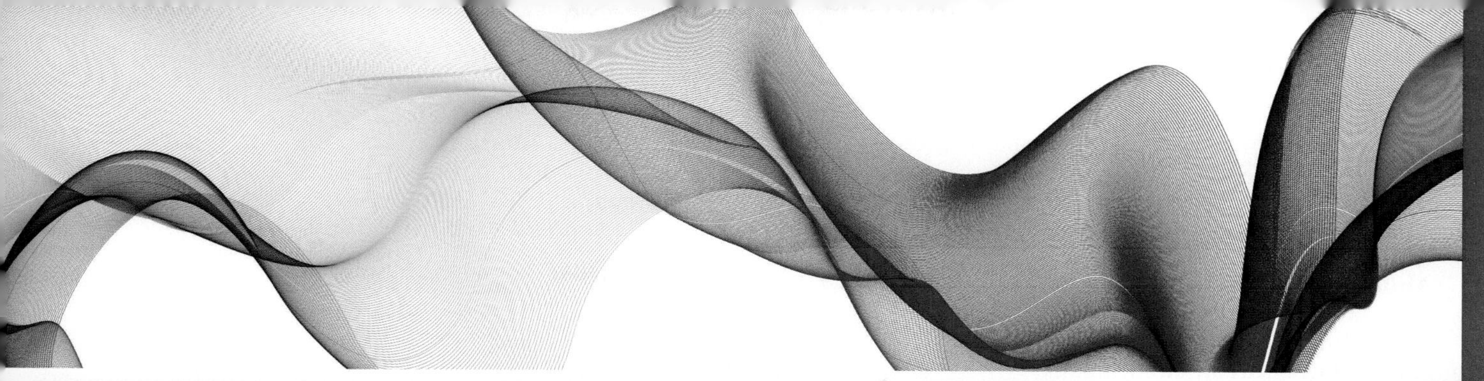

HCPCS 2021

INDEX

A

Abatacept, J0129
Abciximab, J0130
Abdomen
dressing holder/binder, A4462
pad, low profile, L1270
Abduction control, each, L2624
Abduction restrainer, *A4566*
Abduction rotation bar, foot, L3140–L3170
adjustable shoe style positioning device, L3160
including shoes, L3140
plastic, heel-stabilizer, off-shelf, L3170
without shoes, L3150
AbobotulinumtoxintypeA, J0586
Absorption dressing, A6251–A6256
Access, site, occlusive, device, *G0269*
Access system, A4301
Accessories
ambulation devices, E0153–E0159
crutch attachment, walker, E0157
forearm crutch, platform attachment, E0153
leg extension, walker, E0158
replacement, brake attachment, walker, E0159
seat attachment, walker, E0156
walker, platform attachment, E0154
wheel attachment, walker, per pair, E0155
artificial kidney and machine; (see also ESRD), E1510–E1699
adjustable chair, ESRD patients, E1570
automatic peritoneal dialysis system, intermittent, E1592
bath conductivity meter, hemodialysis, E1550
blood leak detector, hemodialysis, replacement, E1560
blood pump, hemodialysis, replacement, E1620
cycler dialysis machine, peritoneal, E1594
deionizer water system, hemodialysis, E1615
delivery/installation charges, hemodialysis equipment, E1600
hemodialysis machine, E1590
hemostats, E1637
heparin infusion pump, hemodialysis, E1520
kidney machine, dialysate delivery system, E1510
peritoneal dialysis clamps, E1634
portable travel hemodialyzer, E1635
reciprocating peritoneal dialysis system, E1630
replacement, air bubble detector, hemodialysis, E1530
replacement, pressure alarm, hemodialysis, E1540
reverse osmosis water system, hemodialysis, E1610
scale, E1639
sorbent cartridges, hemodialysis, E1636
transducer protectors, E1575
unipuncture control system, E1580
water softening system, hemodialysis, E1625
wearable artificial kidney, E1632
Accessories *(Continued)*
beds, E0271–E0280, E0300–E0326
bed board, E0273
bed, board/table, E0315
bed cradle, E0280
bed pan, standard, E0275
bed side rails, E0305–E0310
bed-pan fracture, E0276
hospital bed, extra heavy duty, E0302, E0304
hospital bed, heavy duty, E0301–E0303
hospital bed, pediatric, electric, E0329
hospital bed, safety enclosure frame, E0316
mattress, foam rubber, E0272
mattress, innerspring, E0271
over-bed table, E0274
pediatric crib, E0300
powered pressure-reducing air mattress, E0277
wheelchairs, E0950–E1030, E1050–E1298, E2300–E2399, K0001–K0109
accessory tray, E0950
arm rest, E0994
back upholstery replacement, E0982
calf rest/pad, E0995
commode seat, E0968
detachable armrest, E0973
elevating leg rest, E0990
headrest cushion, E0955
lateral trunk/hip support, E0956
loop-holder, E0951–E0952
manual swingaway, E1028
manual wheelchair, adapter, amputee, E0959
manual wheelchair, anti-rollback device, E0974
manual wheelchair, anti-tipping device, E0971
manual wheelchair, hand rim with projections, E0967
manual wheelchair, headrest extension, E0966
manual wheelchair, lever-activated, wheel drive, E0988
manual wheelchair, one-arm drive attachment, E0958
manual wheelchair, power add-on, E0983–E0984
manual wheelchair, push activated power assist, E0986
manual wheelchair, solid seat insert, E0992
medial thigh support, E0957
modification, pediatric size, E1011
narrowing device, E0969
No. 2 footplates, E0970
oxygen related accessories, E1352–E1406
positioning belt/safety belt/pelvic strap, E0978
power-seating system, E1002–E1010
reclining back addition, pediatric size wheelchair, E1014
residual limb support system, E1020
safety vest, E0980
seat lift mechanism, E0985
seat upholstery replacement, E0981

Accessories *(Continued)*
wheelchairs *(Continued)*
shock absorber, E1015–E1018
shoulder harness strap, E0960
ventilator tray, E1029–E1030
wheel lock brake extension, manual, E0961
wheelchair, amputee, accessories, E1170–E1200
wheelchair, fully inclining, accessories, E1050–E1093
wheelchair, heavy duty, accessories, E1280–E1298
wheelchair, lightweight, accessories, E1240–E1270
wheelchair, semi-reclining, accessories, E1100–E1110
wheelchair, special size, E1220–E1239
wheelchair, standard, accessories, E1130–E1161
whirlpool equipment, E1300–E1310
***Ace type, elastic bandage,** A6448–A6450*
Acetaminophen, J0131
Acetazolamide sodium, J1120
Acetylcysteine
inhalation solution, J7604, J7608
injection, J0132
***Activity, therapy,** G0176*
Acyclovir, J0133
Adalimumab, J0135
Additions to
fracture orthosis, L2180–L2192
abduction bar, L2300–L2310
adjustable motion knee joint, L2186
anterior swing band, L2335
BK socket, PTB and AFO, L2350
disk or dial lock, knee flexion, L2425
dorsiflexion and plantar flexion, L2220
dorsiflexion assist, L2210
drop lock, L2405
drop lock knee joint, L2182
extended steel shank, L2360
foot plate, stirrup attachment, L2250
hip joint, pelvic band, thigh flange, pelvic belt, L2192
integrated release mechanism, L2515
lacer custom-fabricated, L2320–L2330
lift loop, drop lock ring, L2492
limited ankle motion, L2200
limited motion knee joint, L2184
long tongue stirrup, L2265
lower extremity orthrosis, L2200–L2397
molded inner boot, L2280
offset knee joint, L2390
offset knee joint, heavy duty, L2395
Patten bottom, L2370
pelvic and thoracic control, L2570–L2680
plastic shoe insert with ankle joints, L2180
polycentric knee joint, L2387
pre-tibial shell, L2340
quadrilateral, L2188
ratchet lock knee extension, L2430
reinforced solid stirrup, L2260

***Additions to** (Continued)*
fracture orthosis (Continued)
rocker bottom, custom fabricated, L2232
round caliper/plate attachment, L2240
split flat caliper stirrups, L2230
straight knee joint, heavy duty, L2385
straight knee, or offset knee joints, L2405–L2492
suspension sleeve, L2397
thigh/weight bearing, L2500–L2550
torsion control, ankle joint, L2375
torsion control, straight knee joint, L2380
varus/valgus correction, L2270–L2275
waist belt, L2190
general additions, orthosis, L2750–L2999
lower extremity, above knee section, soft interface, L2830
lower extremity, concentric adjustable torsion style mechanism, L2861
lower extremity, drop lock retainer, L2785
lower extremity, extension, per extension, per bar, L2760
lower extremity, femoral length sock, L2850
lower extremity, full kneecap, L2795
lower extremity, high strength, lightweight material, hybrid lamination, L2755
lower extremity, knee control, condylar pad, L2810
lower extremity, knee control, knee cap, medial or lateral, L2800
lower extremity orthrosis, non-corrosive finish, per bar, L2780
lower extremity orthrosis, NOS, L2999
lower extremity, plating chrome or nickel, per bar, L2750
lower extremity, soft interface, below knee, L2820
lower extremity, tibial length sock, L2840
orthotic side bar, disconnect device, L2768
Adenosine, J0151, J0153
Adhesive, A4364
bandage, A6413
disc or foam pad, A5126
remover, A4455, A4456
support, breast prosthesis, A4280
wound, closure, G0168
***Adjunctive, dental,** D9110–D9999*
***Administration, chemotherapy,** Q0083–Q0085*
both infusion and other technique, Q0085
infusion technique only, Q0084
other than infusion technique, Q0083
Administration, Part D
vaccine, hepatitis B, G0010
vaccine, influenza, G0008
vaccine, pneumococcal, G0009
Administrative, Miscellaneous and Investigational, A9000–A9999
alert or alarm device, A9280
artificial saliva, A9155
DME delivery set-up, A9901
exercise equipment, A9300

Administrative, Miscellaneous and Investigational *(Continued)*
external ambulatory insulin delivery system, A9274
foot pressure off loading/supportive device, A9283
helmets, A8000–A8004
home glucose disposable monitor, A9275
hot-water bottle, ice cap, heat wrap, A9273
miscellaneous DME, NOS, A9999
miscellaneous DME supply, A9900
monitoring feature/device, stand-alone or integrated, A9279
multiple vitamins, oral, per dose, A9153
non-covered item, A9270
non-prescription drugs, A9150
pediculosis treatment, topical, A9180
radiopharmaceuticals, A9500–A9700
reaching grabbing device, A9281
receiver, external, interstitial glucose monitoring system, A9278
sensor, invasive, interstitial continuous glucose monitoring, A9276
single vitamin/mineral trace element, A9152
spirometer, non-electronic, A9284
transmitter, interstitial continuous glucose monitoring system, A9277
wig, any type, A9282
wound suction, disposable, A9272
Admission, observation, *G0379*
Ado-trastuzumab, J9354
Adrenalin, J0171
Advanced life support, *A0390, A0426, A0427, A0433*
ALS2, A0433
ALS emergency transport, A0427
ALS mileage, A0390
ALS, non-emergency transport, A0426
Aerosol
compressor, E0571–E0572
compressor filter, *A7013–A7014*, K0178–K0179
mask, *A7015*, K0180
Afamelanotide implant, J7352 ◀
Aflibercept, J0178
AFO, E1815, E1830, L1900–L1990, L4392, L4396
Afstyla, J7210
Agalsidase beta, J0180
Aggrastat, J3245
A-hydroCort, J1710
Aid, hearing, *V5030–V5263*
Aide, home, health, *G0156, S9122, T1021*
home health aide/certified nurse assistant, in home, S9122
home health aide/certified nurse assistant, per visit, T1021
home health or hospital setting, G0156
Air bubble detector, dialysis, E1530
Air fluidized bed, E0194
Air pressure pad/mattress, E0186, E0197
Air travel and nonemergency transportation, A0140
Alarm
not otherwise classified, A9280
pressure, dialysis, E1540
Alatrofloxacin mesylate, J0200
Albumin, human, P9041, P9042
Albuterol
all formulations, inhalation solution, J7620
all formulations, inhalation solution, concentrated, J7610, J7611
all formulations, inhalation solution, unit dose, J7609, J7613
Alcohol, A4244
Alcohol wipes, A4245
Alcohol/substance, assessment, *G0396, G0397, H0001, H0003, H0049*
alcohol abuse structured assessment, greater than 30 min., G0397
alcohol abuse structured assessment, 15–30 min., G0396
alcohol and/or drug assessment, Medicaid, H0001
alcohol and/or drug screening; laboratory analysis, Medicaid, H0003
alcohol and/or drug screening, Medicaid, H0049
Aldesleukin (IL2), J9015
Alefacept, J0215
Alemtuzumab, J0202
Alert device, A9280
Alginate dressing, A6196–A6199
alginate, pad more than 48 sq. cm, A6198
alginate, pad size 16 sq. cm, A6196
alginate, pad size more than 16 sq. cm, A6197
alginate, wound filler, sterile, A6199
Alglucerase, J0205
Alglucosidase, J0220
Alglucosidase alfa, J0221
Allogen, Q4212
Alphanate, J7186
Alpha-1-proteinase inhibitor, human, J0256, J0257
Alprostadil
injection, J0270
urethral suppository, J0275
ALS mileage, *A0390*
Alteplase recombinant, J2997
Alternating pressure mattress/pad, A4640, E0180, E0181, E0277
overlay/pad, alternating, pump, heavy duty, E0181
powered pressure-reducing air mattress, E0277
replacement pad, owned by patient, A4640
Alveoloplasty, *D7310–D7321*
in conjunction with extractions, four or more teeth, D7310
in conjunction with extractions, one to three teeth, D7311
not in conjunction with extractions, four or more teeth, D7320
not in conjunction with extractions, one to three teeth, D7321
Amalgam dental restoration, *D2140–D2161*
four or more surfaces, primary or permanent, D2161
one surface, primary or permanent, D2140
three surfaces, primary or permanent, D2160
two surfaces, primary or permanent, D2150

◀ New ⮌ Revised ✔ Reinstated ~~deleted~~ Deleted

Ambulance, A0021–A0999
air, A0430, A0431, A0435, A0436
conventional, transport, one way, fixed wing, A0430
conventional, transport, one way, rotary wing, A0431
fixed wing air mileage, A0435
rotary wing air mileage, A0436
disposable supplies, A0382–A0398
ALS routine disposable supplies, A0398
ALS specialized service disposable supplies, A0394
ALS specialized service, esophageal intubation, A0396
BLS routine disposable, A0832
BLS specialized service disposable supplies, defibrillation, A0384, A0392
non-emergency transport, fixed wing, S9960
non-emergency transport, rotary wing, S9961
oxygen, A0422
Ambulation device, E0100–E0159
brake attachment, wheeled walker replacement, E0159
cane, adjustable or fixed, with tip, E0100
cane, quad or three prong, adjustable or fixed, with tip, E0105
crutch attachment, walker, E0157
crutch forearm, each, with tips and handgrips, E0111
crutch substitute, lower leg platform, with or without wheels, each, E0118
crutch, underarm, articulating, spring assisted, each, E0117
crutches forearm, pair, tips and handgrips, E0110
crutches, underarm, other than wood, pair, with pads, tips and handgrips, E0114
crutches, underarm, other than wood, with pad, tip, handgrip, with or without shock absorber, each, E0116
crutches, underarm, wood, each, with pad, tip and handgrip, E0113
leg extensions, walker, set (4), E0158
platform attachment, forearm crutch, each, E0153
platform attachment, walker, E0154
seat attachment, walker, E0156
walker, enclosed, four-sided frame, wheeled, posterior seat, E0144
walker, folding, adjustable or fixed height, E0135
walker, folding, wheeled, adjustable or fixed height, E0143
walker, heavy duty, multiple braking system, variable wheel resistance, E0147
walker, heavy duty, wheeled, rigid or folding, E0149
walker, heavy duty, without wheels, rigid or folding, E0148
walker, rigid, adjustable or fixed height, E0130
walker, rigid, wheeled, adjustable or fixed height, E0141
walker, with trunk support, adjystable or fixed height, any, E0140
wheel attachment, rigid, pick up walker, per pair, E0155
Amikacin Sulfate, J0278
Aminolevulinate, J7309
Aminolevulinic acid HCl, J7308
Aminophylline, J0280
Aminolevulinic
Ameluz, J7345
Amiodarone HCl, J0282
Amitriptyline HCl, J1320
Ammonia N-13, A9526
Ammonia test paper, A4774
Amnioiwrap2, Q4221
Amnion Bio, Q4211
Amniotic membrane, V2790
Amobarbital, J0300
Amphotericin B, J0285
Lipid Complex, J0287–J0289
Ampicillin
sodium, J0290
sodium/sulbactam sodium, J0295
Amputee
adapter, wheelchair, E0959
prosthesis, L5000–L7510, L7520, L7900, L8400–L8465
above knee, L5200–L5230
additions to exoskeletal knee-shin systems, L5710–L5782
additions to lower extremity, L5610–L5617
additions to socket insert and suspension, L5654–L5699
additions to socket variations, L5630–L5653
additions to test sockets, L5618–L5629
additions/replacements feet-ankle units, L5700–L5707
ankle, L5050–L5060
below knee, L5100–L5105
component modification, L5785–L5795
endoskeletal, L5810–L5999
endoskeleton, below knee, L5301–L5312
endoskeleton, hip disarticulation, L5331–L5341
fitting endoskeleton, above knee, L5321
fitting procedures, L5400–L5460
hemipelvectomy, L5280
hip disarticulation, L5250–L5270
initial prosthesis, L5500–L5505
knee disarticulation, L5150–L5160
male vacuum erection system, L7900
partial foot, L5000–L5020
preparatory prosthesis, L5510–L5600
prosthetic socks, L8400–L8485
repair, prosthetic device, L7520
tension ring, vacuum erection device, L7902
upper extremity, battery components, L7360–L7368
upper extremity, other/repair, L7400–L7510
upper extremity, preparatory, elbow, L6584–L6586
upper limb, above elbow, L6250
upper limb, additions, L6600–L6698
upper limb, below elbow, L6100–L6130
upper limb, elbow disarticulation, L6200–L6205
upper limb, endoskeletal, above elbow, L6500
upper limb, endoskeletal, below elbow, L6400
upper limb, endoskeletal, elbow disarticulation, L6450
upper limb, endoskeletal, interscapular thoracic, L6570

Amputee *(Continued)*
prosthesis *(Continued)*
upper limb, endoskeletal, shoulder disarticulation, L6550
upper limb, external power, device, L6920–L6975
upper limb, interscapular thoracic, L6350–L6370
upper limb, partial hand, L6000–L6025
upper limb, postsurgical procedures, L6380–L6388
upper limb, preparatory, shoulder, interscapular, L6588–L6590
upper limb, preparatory, wrist, L6580–L6582
upper limb, shoulder disarticulation, L6300–L6320
upper limb, terminal devices, L6703–L6915, L7007–L7261
upper limb, wrist disarticulation, L6050–L6055
stump sock, L8470–L8485
single ply, fitting above knee, L8480
single ply, fitting, below knee, L8470
single ply, fitting, upper limb, L8485
wheelchair, E1170–E1190, E1200, K0100
detachable arms, swing away detachable elevating footrests, E1190
detachable arms, swing away detachable footrests, E1180
detachable arms, without footrests or legrest, E1172
detachable elevating legrest, fixed full length arms, E1170
fixed full length arms, swing away detachable footrest, E1200
heavy duty wheelchair, swing away detachable elevating legrests, E1195
without footrests or legrest, fixed full length arms, E1171
Amygdalin, J3570
Anadulafungin, J0348
Analgesia, dental, *D9230*
Analysis
saliva, D0418
semen, G0027
Angiography, iliac, artery, *G0278*
Angiography, renal, non-selective, *G0275*
non-ophthalmic fluorescent vascular, C9733
reconstruction, G0288
Anistreplase, J0350
Ankle splint, recumbent, K0126–K0130
Ankle-foot orthosis (AFO), L1900–L1990, L2106–L2116, L4361, L4392, L4396
ankle gauntlet, custom fabricated, L1904
ankle gauntlet, prefabricated, off-shelf, L1902
double upright free plantar dorsiflexion, olid stirrup, calf-band/cuff, custom, L1990
fracture orthrosis, tibial fracture, thermoplastic cast material, custom, L2106
multiligamentus ankle support, prefabricated, off-shelf, L1906
plastic or other material, custom fabricated, L1940
plastic or other material, prefabricated, fitting and adjustment, L1932, L1951

Ankle-foot orthosis *(Continued)*
plastic or other material, with ankle joint, prefabricated, fitting and adjustment, L1971
plastic, rigid anterior tibial section, custom fabricated, L1945
plastic, with ankle joint, custom, L1970
posterior, single bar, clasp attachment to shoe, L1910
posterior, solid ankle, plastic, custom, L1960
replacement, soft interface material, static AFO, L4392
single upright free plantar dorsiflection, solid stirrup, calf-band/cuff, custom, L1980
single upright with static or adjustable stop, custom, L1920
spiral, plastic, custom fabricated, L1950
spring wire, dorsiflexion assist calf band, L1900
static or dynamic AFO, adjustable for fit, minimal ambulation, L4396
supramalleolar with straps, custom fabricated, L1907
tibial fracture cast orthrosis, custom, L2108
tibial fracture orthrosis, rigid, prefabricated, fitting and adjustment, L2116
tibial fracture orthrosis, semi-rigid, prefabricated, fitting and adjustment, L2114
tibial fracture orthrosis, soft prefabricated, fitting and adjustment, L2112
walking boot, prefabricated, off-the-shelf, L4361
Anterior-posterior-lateral orthosis, L0700, L0710
Antibiotic, *G8708–G8712*
antibiotic not prescribed or dispensed, G8712
patient not prescribed or dispensed antibiotic, G8708
patient prescribed antibiotic, documented condition, G8709
patient prescribed or dispensed antibiotic, G8710
prescribed or dispensed antibiotic, G8711
Antidepressant, documentation, *G8126–G8128*
Anti-emetic, oral, J8498, J8597, Q0163–Q0181
antiemetic drug, oral NOS, J8597
antiemetic drug, rectal suppository, NOS, J8498
diphenhydramine hydrochloride, 50 mg, oral, Q0163
dolasetron mesylate, 100 mg, oral, Q0180
dronabinol, 2.5 mg, Q0167
granisetron hydrochloride, 1 mg, oral, Q0166
hydroxyzine pomoate, 25 mg, oral, Q0177
perphenazine, 4 mg, oral, Q0175
prochlorperazine maleate, 5 mg, oral, Q0164
promethazine hydrochloride, 12.5 mg, oral, Q0169
thiethylperazine maleate, 10 mg, oral, Q0174
trimethobenzamide hydrochloride, 250 mg, oral, Q0173
unspecified oral dose, Q0181
Anti-hemophilic factor (Factor VIII), J7190–J7192
Anti-inhibitors, per I.U., J7198
Antimicrobial, prophylaxis, documentation, *D4281, G8201*
Anti-neoplastic drug, NOC, J9999
Antithrombin III, J7197
Antithrombin recombinant, J7196

◀ New ⮌ Revised ✔ Reinstated ~~deleted~~ Deleted

Antral fistula closure, oral, *D7260*
Apexification, dental, *D3351–D3353*
Apicoectomy, *D3410–D3426*
anterior, periradicular surgery, D3410
biscuspid (first root), D3421
(each additional root), D3426
molar (first root), D3425
Apomorphine, J0364
Appliance
cleaner, A5131
pneumatic, E0655–E0673
non-segmental pneumatic appliance, E0655, E0660, E0665, E0666
segmental gradient pressure, pneumatic appliance, E0671–E0673
segmental pneumatic appliance, E0656–E0657, E0667–E0670
Application, heat, cold, *E0200–E0239*
electric heat pad, moist, E0215
electric heat pad, standard, E0210
heat lamp with stand, E0205
heat lamp without stand, E0200
hydrocollator unit, pads, E0225
hydrocollator unit, portable, E0239
infrared heating pad system, E0221
non-contact wound warming device, E0231
paraffin bath unit, E0235
phototherapy (bilirubin), E0202
pump for water circulating pad, E0236
therapeutic lightbox, E0203
warming card, E0232
water circulating cold pad with pump, E0218
water circulating heat pad with pump, E0217
Aprotinin, J0365
Aqueous
shunt, L8612
sterile, J7051
ARB/ACE therapy, *G8473–G8475*
Arbutamine HCl, J0395
Arch support, L3040–L3100
hallus-valgus night dynamic splint, off-shelf, L3100
intralesional, J3302
non-removable, attached to shoe, longitudinal, L3070
non-removable, attached to shoe, longitudinal/ metatarsal, each, L3090
non-removable, attached to shoe, metatarsal, L3080
removable, premolded, longitudinal, L3040
removable, premolded, longitudinal/metatarsal, each, L3060
removable, premolded, metatarsal, L3050
Arformoterol, J7605
Argatroban, J0883–J0884
Aripiprazole, J0400, J0401
Aripiprazol lauroxil, (aristada), J1944
aristada initio, H1943
Arm, wheelchair, E0973
Arsenic trioxide, J9017
Artacent cord, Q4216
Arthrography, injection, sacroiliac, joint, *G0259, G0260*
Arthroscopy, knee, surgical, *G0289, S2112*
chondroplasty, different compartment, knee, G0289
harvesting of cartilage, knee, S2112
Artificial
cornea, L8609
heart system, miscellaneous component, supply or accessory, L8698
kidney machines and accessories (see also Dialysis), E1510–E1699
larynx, L8500
saliva, A9155
Ascent, Q4213
Asparaginase, J9019–J9020
Aspirator, VABRA, *A4480*
Assessment
alcohol/substance (see also Alcohol/substance, assessment), G0396, G0397, H0001, H0003, H0049
assessment for hearing aid, V5010
audiologic, V5008–V5020
cardiac output, M0302
conformity evaluation, V5020
fitting/orientation, hearing aid, V5014
hearing screening, V5008
repair/modification hearing aid, V5014
speech, V5362–V5364
Assistive listening devices and accessories, V5281–V5290
FMlDM system, monaural, V5281
Astramorph, J2275
Atezolizumab, J9022
Atherectomy, PTCA, *C9602, C9603*
Atropine
inhalation solution, concentrated, J7635
inhalation solution, unit dose, J7636
Atropine sulfate, J0461
Attachment, walker, *E0154–E0159*
brake attachment, wheeled walker, replacement, E0159
crutch attachment, walker, E0157
leg extension, walker, E0158
platform attachment, walker, E0154
seat attachment, walker, E0156
wheel attachment, rigid pick up walker, E0155
Audiologic assessment, V5008–V5020
Auditory osseointegrated device, L8690–L8694
Auricular prosthesis, *D5914, D5927*
Aurothioglucose, J2910
Avelumab, J9023
Axobiomembrane, Q4211
Axolotl ambient or axolotl cryo, Q4215
Axolotl graft or axolotl dualgraft, Q4210
Azacitidine, J9025
Azathioprine, J7500, J7501
Azithromycin injection, J0456

B

Back supports, L0621–L0861, L0960
lumbar orthrosis, L0625–L0627
lumbar orthrosis, sagittal control, L0641–L0648
lumbar-sacral orthrosis, L0628–L0640
lumbar-sacral orthrosis, sagittal-coronal control, L0640, L0649–L0651
sacroiliac orthrosis, L0621–L0624
Baclofen, J0475, J0476
Bacterial sensitivity study, P7001
Bag
drainage, A4357
enema, A4458
irrigation supply, A4398
urinary, A4358, A5112
Bandage, conforming
elastic, >5", A6450
elastic, >3", <5", A6449
elastic, load resistance 1.25 to 1.34 foot pounds, >3", <5", A6451
elastic, load resistance <1.35 foot pounds, >3", <5", A6452
elastic, <3", A6448
non-elastic, non-sterile, >5", A6444
non-elastic, non-sterile, width greater than or equal to 3", <5", A6443
non-elastic, non-sterile, width <3", A6442
non-elastic, sterile, >5", A6447
non-elastic, sterile, >3" and <5", A6446
Basiliximab, J0480
Bath, aid, *E0160–E0162, E0235, E0240–E0249*
bath tub rail, floor base, E0242
bath tub wall rail, E0241
bath/shower chair, with/without wheels, E0240
pad for water circulating heat unit, replacement, E0249
paraffin bath unit, portable, E0235
raised toilet seat, E0244
sitz bath chair, E0162
sitz type bath, portable, with faucet attachment, E0161
sitz type bath, portable, with/without commode, E0160
toilet rail, E0243
transfer bench, tub or toilet, E0248
transfer tub rail attachment, E0246
tub stool or bench, E0245
Bathtub
chair, E0240
stool or bench, E0245, E0247–E0248
transfer rail, E0246
wall rail, E0241–E0242
Battery, L7360, L7364–L7368
charger, E1066, L7362, L7366
replacement for blood glucose monitor, A4233–A4236
Battery *(Continued)*
replacement for cochlear implant device, L8618, L8623–L8625
replacement for TENS, A4630
ventilator, A4611–A4613
~~**BCG live, intravesical, J9031**~~
Beclomethasone inhalation solution, J7622
Bed
accessories, E0271–E0280, E0300–E0326
bed board, E0273
bed cradle, E0280
bed pan, fracture, metal, E0276
bed pan, standard, metal, E0275
mattress, foam rubber, E0272
mattress innerspring, E0271
over-bed table, E0274
power pressure-reducing air mattress, E0277
air fluidized, E0194
cradle, any type, E0280
drainage bag, bottle, A4357, A5102
hospital, E0250–E0270, E0300–E0329
pan, E0275, E0276
rail, E0305, E0310
safety enclosure frame/canopy, E0316
Behavioral, health, treatment services (Medicaid), *H0002–H2037*
activity therapy, H2032
alcohol/drug services, H0001, H0003, H0005–H0016, H0020–H0022, H0026–H0029, H0049–H0050, H2034–H2036
assertive community treatment, H0040
community based wrap-around services, H2021–H2022
comprehensive community support, H2015–H2016
comprehensive medication services, H2010
comprehensive multidisciplinary evaluation, H2000
crisis intervention, H2011
day treatment, per diem, H2013
day treatment, per hour, H2012
developmental delay prevention activities, dependent child of client, H2037
family assessment, H1011
foster care, child, H0041–H0042
health screening, H0002
hotline service, H0030
medication training, H0034
mental health clubhouse services, H2030–H2031
multisystemic therapy, juveniles, H2033
non-medical family planning, H1010
outreach service, H0023
partial hospitalization, H0035
plan development, non-physician, H0033
prenatal care, at risk, H1000–H1005
prevention, H0024–H0025
psychiatric supportive treatment, community, H0036–H0037
psychoeducational service, H2027
psychoscial rehabilitation, H2017–H2018

◀ **New** ⮐ **Revised** ✔ **Reinstated** ~~deleted~~ **Deleted**

Behavioral, health, treatment services (Medicaid) *(Continued)*
rehabilitation program, H2010
residential treatment program, H0017–H0019
respite care, not home, H0045
self-help/peer services, H0039
sexual offender treatment, H2028–H2029
skill training, H2014
supported employment, H2024–H2026
supported housing, H0043–H0044
therapeutic behavioral services, H2019–H2020
Behavioral therapy, cardiovascular disease, *G0446*
Belatacept, J0485
Belimumab, J0490
Bellacell, Q4220
Belt
belt, strap, sleeve, garment, or covering, any type, A4467
extremity, E0945
ostomy, A4367
pelvic, E0944
safety, K0031
wheelchair, E0978, E0979
Bench, bathtub; (see also Bathtub), E0245
Bendamustine HCl
Bendeka, 1 mg, J9034
Treanda, 1 mg, J9033
Bendamustine HCI (Belrapzo/bendamustine), J9036
Benesch boot, L3212–L3214
Benztropine, J0515
Beta-blocker therapy, *G9188–G9192*
Betadine, A4246, A4247
Betameth, J0704
Betamethasone
acetate and betamethasone sodium phosphate, J0702
inhalation solution, J7624
Bethanechol chloride, J0520
Bevacizumab, J9035, Q2024
bvzr (Zirabez), Q5118
Bezlotoxuman, J0565
Bicuspid (excluding final restoration), *D3320*
retreatment, by report, D3347
surgery, first root, D3421
Bifocal, glass or plastic, V2200–V2299
aniseikonic, bifocal, V2218
bifocal add-over 3.25 d, V2220
bifocal seg width over 28 mm, V2219
lenticular, bifocal, myodisc, V2215
lenticular lens, V2221
specialty bifocal, by report, V2200
sphere, bifocal, V2200–V2202
spherocylinder, bifocal, V2203–V2214
Bilirubin (phototherapy) light, E0202
Binder, A4465
Biofeedback device, E0746
Bioimpedance, electrical, cardiac output, M0302
Biosimilar (infliximab), Q5102–Q5121 ⤼
BioWound, Q4217
Biperiden lactate, J0190
Bitewing, *D0270–D0277*
four radiographic images, D0274
single radiographic image, D0270
three radiographic images, D0273
two radiographic images, D0272
vertical bitewings, 7–8 radiographic images, D0277
Bitolterol mesylate, inhalation solution
concentrated, J7628
unit dose, J7629
Bivalirudin, J0583
Bivigam, 500 mg, *J1556*
Bladder calculi irrigation solution, Q2004
Bleomycin sulfate, J9040
Blood
count, G0306, G0307, S3630
complete CBC, automated, without platelet count, G0307
complete CBC, automated without platelet count, automated WBC differential, G0306
eosinophil count, blood, direct, S3630
component/product not otherwise classified, P9099
fresh frozen plasma, P9017
glucose monitor, E0607, E2100, E2101, *S1030*, *S1031*, *S1034*
blood glucose monitor, integrated voice synthesizer, E2100
blood glucose monitor with integrated lancing/blood sample, E2101
continuous noninvasive device, purchase, S1030
continuous noninvasive device, rental, S1031
home blood glucose monitor, E0607
glucose test, A4253
glucose, test strips, dialysis, A4772
granulocytes, pheresis, P9050
ketone test, A4252
leak detector, dialysis, E1560
leukocyte poor, P9016
mucoprotein, P2038
platelets, P9019
platelets, irradiated, P9032
platelets, leukocytes reduced, P9031
platelets, leukocytes reduced, irradiated, P9033
platelets, pheresis, P9034, P9072, P9073, P9100
platelets, pheresis, irradiated, P9036
platelets, pheresis, leukocytes reduced, P9035
platelets, pheresis, leukocytes reduced, irradiated, P9037
pressure monitor, A4660, A4663, A4670
pump, dialysis, E1620
red blood cells, deglycerolized, P9039
red blood cells, irradiated, P9038
red blood cells, leukocytes reduced, P9016
red blood cells, leukocytes reduced, irradiated, P9040

◀ New ⤼ Revised ✔ Reinstated ~~deleted~~ Deleted

Blood *(Continued)*
red blood cells, washed, P9022
strips, A4253
supply, P9010–P9022
testing supplies, A4770
tubing, A4750, A4755
Blood collection devices accessory, A4257, E0620
BMI, *G8417–G8422*
Body jacket
scoliosis, L1300, L1310
Body mass index, *G8417–G8422*
Body sock, L0984
Bond or cement, ostomy skin, A4364
Bone
density, study, G0130
Boot
pelvic, E0944
surgical, ambulatory, L3260
Bortezomib, J9041
Brachytherapy radioelements, Q3001
brachytherapy, LDR, prostate, G0458
brachytherapy planar source, C2645
brachytherapy, source, hospital outpatient, C1716–C1717, C1719
Breast prosthesis, L8000–L8035, L8600
adhesive skin support, A4280
custom breast prosthesis, post mastectomy, L8035
garment with mastectomy form, post mastectomy, L8015
implantable, silicone or equal, L8600
mastectomy bra, with integrated breast prosthesis form, unilateral, L8001
mastectomy bra, with prosthesis form, bilateral, L8002
mastectomy bra, without integrated breast prosthesis form, L8000
mastectomy form, L8020
mastectomy sleeve, L8010
nipple prosthesis, L8032
silicone or equal, with integral adhesive, L8031
silicone or equal, without integral adhesive, L8030
Breast pump
accessories, A4281–A4286
adapter, replacement, A4282
cap, breast pump bottle, replacement, A4283
locking ring, replacement, A4286
polycarbonate bottle, replacement, A4285
shield and splash protector, replacement, A4284
tubing, replacement, A4281
electric, any type, E0603
heavy duty, hospital grade, E0604
manual, any type, E0602
Breathing circuit, A4618
Brentuximab Vedotin, J9042
Brexanolone, J1632 ◀
Bridge
repair, by report, D6980
replacement, D6930
Brolucizumab-dbll, J0179
Brompheniramine maleate, J0945
Budesonide inhalation solution, J7626, J7627, J7633, J7634
Bulking agent, L8604, L8607
Buprenorphine hydrochlorides, J0592
Buprenorphine/Naloxone, J0571–J0575
Burn, compression garment, *A6501–A6513*
bodysuit, head-foot, A6501
burn mask, face and/or neck, A6513
chin strap, A6502
facial hood, A6503
foot to knee length, A6507
foot to thigh length, A6508
glove to axilla, A6506
glove to elbow, A6505
glove to wrist, A6504
lower trunk, including leg openings, A6511
trunk, including arms, down to leg openings, A6510
upper trunk to waist, including arm openings, A6509
Bus, nonemergency transportation, A0110
Busulfan, J0594, J8510
Butorphanol tartrate, J0595
Bypass, graft, coronary, artery
surgery, S2205–S2209

C

C-1 Esterase Inhibitor, J0596–J0598
Cabazitaxel, J9043
Cabergoline, oral, J8515
Cabinet/System, ultraviolet, *E0691–E0694*
multidirectional light system, 6 ft. cabinet, E0694
timer and eye protection, 4 foot, E0692
timer and eye protection, 6 foot, E0693
ultraviolet light therapy system, treatment area 2 sq ft., E0691
Caffeine citrate, J0706
Calaspargase pegol injection-mknl, J9118
Calcitonin-salmon, J0630
Calcitriol, J0636, *S0169*
Calcium
disodium edetate, J0600
gluconate, J0610
glycerophosphate and calcium lactate, J0620
lactate and calcium glycerophosphate, J0620
leucovorin, J0640
Calibrator solution, A4256
Canakinumab, J0638
Cancer, screening
cervical or vaginal, G0101
colorectal, G0104–G0106, G0120–G0122, G0328
alternative to screening colonoscopy, barium enema, G0120
alternative to screening sigmoidoscopy, barium enema, G0106
barium enema, G0122
colonoscopy, high risk, G0105

◀ New ⮌ Revised ✔ Reinstated ~~deleted~~ Deleted

Cancer, screening *(Continued)*
colorectal (Continued)
colonoscopy, not at high-risk, G0121
fecal occult blood test,1-3 simultaneous, G0328
flexible sigmoidoscopy, G0104
prostate, G0102, G0103
Cane, E0100, E0105
accessory, A4636, A4637
Canister
disposable, used with suction pump, A7000
non-disposable, used with suction pump, A7001
Cannula, nasal, A4615
Capecitabine, oral, J8520, J8521
Capsaicin patch, J7336
Carbidopa 5 mg/levodopa 20 mg enteral suspension, J7340
Carbon filter, A4680
Carboplatin, J9045
Cardia Event, recorder, implantable, E0616
Cardiokymography, Q0035
Cardiovascular services, M0300–M0301
Fabric wrapping abdominal aneurysm, M0301
IV chelation therapy, M0300
Cardioverter-defibrillator, *G0448*
Care, coordinated, *G9001–G9011*, *H1002*
coordinated care fee, home monitoring, G9006
coordinated care fee, initial rate, G9001
coordinated care fee, maintenance rate, G9002
coordinated care fee, physician coordinated care oversight, G9008
coordinated care fee, risk adjusted high, initial, G9003
coordinated care fee, risk adjusted low, initial, G9004
coordinated care fee, risk adjusted maintenance, G9005
coordinated care fee, risk adjusted maintenance, level 3, G9009
coordinated care fee, risk adjusted maintenance, level 4, G9010
coordinated care fee, risk adjusted maintenance, level 5, G9011
coordinated care fee, scheduled team conference, G9007
prenatal care, at-risk, enhanced service, care coordination, H1002
Care plan, *G0162*
Carfilzomib, J9047
Caries susceptibility test, *D0425*
Carmustine, J9050
Case management, T1016, T1017
dental, D9991–D9994
Caspofungin acetate, J0637
Cast
diagnostic, dental, D0470
hand restoration, L6900–L6915
materials, special, A4590
supplies, A4580, A4590, Q4001–Q4051
body cast, adult, Q4001–Q4002
cast supplies (e.g., plaster), A4580
cast supplies, unlisted types, Q4050
Cast *(Continued)*
supplies *(Continued)*
finger splint, static, Q4049
gauntlet cast, adult, Q4013–Q4014
gauntlet cast, pediatric, Q4015–Q4016
hip spica, adult, Q4025–Q4026
hip spica, pediatric, Q4027–Q4028
long arm cast, adult, Q4005–Q4006
long arm cast, pediatric, Q4007–Q4008
long arm splint, adult, Q4017–Q4018
long arm splint, pediatric, Q4019–Q4020
long leg cast, adult, Q4029–Q4030
long leg cast, pediatric, Q4031–Q4032
long leg cylinder cast, adult, Q4033–Q4034
long leg cylinder cast, pediatric, Q4035–Q4036
long leg splint, adult, Q4041–Q4042
long leg splint, pediatric, Q4043–Q4044
short arm cast, adult, Q4009–Q4010
short arm cast, pediatric, Q4011–Q4012
short arm splint, adult, Q4021–Q4022
short arm splint, pediatric, Q4023–Q4024
short leg cast, adult, Q4037–Q4038
short leg cast, pediatric, Q4039–Q4040
short leg splint, adult, Q4045–Q4046
short leg splint, pediatric, Q4047–Q4048
shoulder cast, adult, Q4003–Q4004
special casting material (fiberglass), A4590
splint supplies, miscellaneous, Q4051
thermoplastic, L2106, L2126
Caster
front, for power wheelchair, K0099
wheelchair, E0997, E0998
Catheter, A4300–A4355
anchoring device, A4333, A4334, A5200
cap, disposable (dialysis), A4860
external collection device, A4327–A4330, A4347–A7048
female external, A4327–A4328
indwelling, A4338–A4346
insertion tray, A4354
insulin infusion catheter, A4224
intermittent with insertion supplies, A4353
irrigation supplies, A4355
male external, A4324, A4325, *A4326*, A4348
oropharyngeal suction, A4628
starter set, A4329
trachea (suction), A4609, A4610, A4624
transluminal angioplasty, C2623
transtracheal oxygen, A4608
vascular, A4300–A4301
Catheterization, specimen collection, P9612, P9615
CBC, *G0306, G0307*
Cefazolin sodium, J0690
Cefepime HCl, J0692
Cefiderocol, J0693 ◀
Cefotaxime sodium, J0698
Ceftaroline fosamil, J0712
Ceftazidime, J0713, J0714

◀ New ⮐ Revised ✔ Reinstated ~~deleted~~ Deleted

Ceftizoxime sodium, J0715
Ceftolozane 50 mg and tazobactam 25 mg, J0695
Ceftriaxone sodium, J0696
Cefuroxime sodium, J0697
CellCept, K0412
Cellesta cord, Q4214
Cellesta or cellesta duo, Q4184
Cellular therapy, M0075
Cement, ostomy, A4364
Cemiplimab injection-rwlc, J9119
Centrifuge, A4650
Centruroides Immune F(ab), J0716
Cephalin Floculation, blood, P2028
Cephalothin sodium, J1890
Cephapirin sodium, J0710
Certification, physician, home, health (per calendar month), *G0179–G0182*
Physician certification, home health, G0180
Physician recertification, home health, G0179
Physician supervision, home health, complex care, 30 min or more, G0181
Physician supervision, hospice 30 min or more, G0182
Certolizumab pegol, J0717
Cerumen, removal, *G0268*
Cervical
cancer, screening, G0101
cytopathology, G0123, G0124, G0141–G0148
screening, automated thin layer, manual rescreening, physician supervision, G0145
screening, automated thin layer preparation, cytotechnologist, physician interpretation, G0143
screening, automated thin layer preparation, physician supervision, G0144
screening, by cytotechnologist, physician supervision, G0123
screening, cytopathology smears, automated system, physician interpretation, G0141
screening, interpretation by physician, G0124
screening smears, automated system, manual rescreening, G0148
screening smears, automated system, physician supervision, G0147
halo, L0810–L0830
head harness/halter, E0942
orthosis, L0100–L0200
cervical collar molded to patient, L0170
cervical, flexible collar, L0120–L0130
cervical, multiple post collar, supports, L0180–L0200
cervical, semi-rigid collar, L0150–L0160, L0172, L0174
cranial cervical, L0112–L0113
traction, E0855, E0856
Cervical cap contraceptive, A4261
Cervical-thoracic-lumbar-sacral orthosis (CTLSO), L0700, L0710
Cetuximab, J9055
Chair
adjustable, dialysis, E1570
lift, E0627
rollabout, E1031
sitz bath, E0160–E0162
transport, E1035–E1039
chair, adult size, heavy duty, greater than 300 pounds, E1039
chair, adult size, up to 300 pounds, E1038
chair, pediatric, E1037
multi-positional patient transfer system, extra-wide, greater than 300 pounds, E1036
multi-positional patient transfer system, up to 300 pounds, E1035
Chelation therapy, M0300
Chemical endarterectomy, M0300
Chemistry and toxicology tests, P2028–P3001
Chemotherapy
administration (hospital reporting only), Q0083–Q0085
drug, oral, not otherwise classified, J8999
drugs; (see also drug by name), J9000–J9999
Chest shell (cuirass), E0457
Chest Wall Oscillation System, E0483
hose, replacement, A7026
vest, replacement, A7025
Chest wrap, E0459
Chin cup, cervical, L0150
Chloramphenicol sodium succinate, J0720
Chlordiazepoxide HCl, J1990
Chloromycetin sodium succinate, J0720
Chloroprocaine HCl, J2400
Chloroquine HCl, J0390
Chlorothiazide sodium, J1205
Chlorpromazine HCl, J3230
Chlorpromazine HCL, 5 mg, oral, Q0161
Chorionic gonadotropin, J0725
Choroid, lesion, destruction, *G0186*
Chromic phosphate P32 suspension, A9564
Chromium CR-51 sodium chromate, A9553
Cidofovir, J0740
Cilastatin sodium, imipenem, J0743
Cinacalcet, J0604
Ciprofloxacin
for intravenous infusion, J0744
octic suspension, J7342
Cisplatin, J9060
Cladribine, J9065
Clamp
dialysis, A4918
external urethral, A4356
Cleanser, wound, A6260
Cleansing agent, dialysis equipment, A4790
Clofarabine, J9027
Clonidine, J0735
Closure, wound, adhesive, tissue, *G0168*
Clotting time tube, A4771
Clubfoot wedge, L3380

Cochlear prosthetic implant, L8614
accessories, L8615–L8617, *L8618*
batteries, L8621–L8624
replacement, L8619, L8627–L8629
external controller component, L8628
external speech processor and controller, integrated system, L8619
external speech processor, component, L8627
transmitting coil and cable, integrated, L8629
Codeine phosphate, J0745
Cold/Heat, application, *E0200–E0239*
bilirubin light, E0202
electric heat pad, moist, E0215
electric heat pad, standard, E0210
heat lamp with stand, E0205
heat lamp, without stand, E0200
hydrocollator unit, E0225
hydrocollator unit, portable, E0239
infrared heating pad system, E0221
non-contact wound warming device, E0231
paraffin bath unit, E0235
pump for water circulating pad, E0236
therapeutic lightbox, E0203
warming card, non-contact wound warming device, E0232
water circulating cold pad, with pump, E0218
water circulating heat pad, with pump, E0217
Colistimethate sodium, J0770
Collagen
meniscus implant procedure, G0428
skin test, G0025
urinary tract implant, L8603
wound dressing, A6020–A6024
Collagenase, Clostridium histolyticum, J0775
Collar, cervical
multiple post, L0180–L0200
nonadjust (foam), L0120
Collection and preparation, saliva, *D0417*
Colorectal, screening, cancer, *G0104–G0106, G0120–G0122, G0328*
Coly-Mycin M, J0770
Comfort items, A9190
Commode, E0160–E0175
chair, E0170–E0171
lift, E0172, E0625
pail, E0167
seat, wheelchair, E0968
Complete, blood, count, *G0306, G0307*
Composite dressing, A6200–A6205
Compressed gas system, E0424–E0446
oximeter device, E0445
portable gaseous oxygen system, purchase, E0430
portable gaseous oxygen system, rental, E0431
portable liquid oxygen, rental, container/supplies, E0434
portable liquid oxygen, rental, home liquefier, E0433
portable liquid oxygen system, purchase, container/refill adapter, E0435
Compressed gas system *(Continued)*
portable oxygen contents, gaseous, 1 month, E0443
portable oxygen contents, liquid, 1 month, E0444
stationary liquid oxygen system, purchase, use of reservoir, E0440
stationary liquid oxygen system, rental, container/supplies, E0439
stationary oxygen contents, gaseous, 1 month, E0441
stationary oxygen contents, liquid, 1 month, E0442
stationary purchase, compressed gas system, E0425
stationary rental, compressed gaseous oxygen system, E0424
topical oxygen delivery system, NOS, E0446
Compression
bandage, A4460
burn garment, A6501–A6512
stockings, A6530–A6549
Compressor, E0565, E0650–E0652, E0670–E0672
aerosol, E0572, E0575
air, E0565
nebulizer, E0570–E0585
pneumatic, E0650–E0676
Conductive gel/paste, *A4558*
Conductivity meter, bath, dialysis, E1550
Conference, team, *G0175, G9007, S0220, S0221*
coordinate care fee, scheduled team conference, G9007
medical conference/physician/interdisciplinary team, patient present, 30 min, S0220
medical conference physician/interdisciplinary team, patient present, 60 min, S0221
scheduled interdisciplinary team conference, patient present, G0175
Congo red, blood, P2029
Consultation, S0285, S0311, T1040, T1041
dental, D9311
Telehealth, G0425–G0427
Contact layer, A6206–A6208
Contact lens, V2500–V2599
Continent device, A5081, A5082, A5083
Continuous glucose monitoring system
receiver, A9278, *S1037*
sensor, A9276, *S1035*
transmitter, A9277, *S1036*
Continuous passive motion exercise device, E0936
Continuous positive airway pressure device(CPAP), E0601
compressor, K0269
Contraceptive
cervical cap, A4261
condoms, A4267, A4268
diaphragm, A4266
intratubal occlusion device, A4264
intrauterine, copper, J7300
intrauterine, levonorgestrel releasing, J7296–J7298, J7301
patch, J7304
spermicide, A4269
supply, A4267–A4269
vaginal ring, J7303

◀ New ⤾ Revised ✔ Reinstated ~~deleted~~ Deleted

C

Contracts, maintenance, ESRD, A4890
Contrast, *Q9951–Q9969*
HOCM, Q9958–Q9964
injection, iron based magnetic resonance, per ml, Q9953
injection, non-radioactive, non-contrast, visualization adjunct, Q9968
injection, octafluoropropane microspheres, per ml, Q9956
injection, perflexane lipid microspheres, per ml, Q9955
injection, perflutren lipid microspheres, per ml, Q9957
LOCM, Q9965–Q9967
LOCM, 400 or greater mg/ml iodine, per ml, Q9951
oral magnetic resonance contrast, Q9954
Tc-99m per study dose, Q9969
Contrast material
injection during MRI, A4643
low osmolar, A4644–A4646
Coordinated, care, *G9001–G9011*
CORF, registered nurse- face-face, G0128
Corneal tissue processing, V2785
Corset, spinal orthosis, L0970–L0976
LSO, corset front, L0972
LSO, full corset, L0976
TLSO, corset front, L0970
TLSO, full corset, L0974
Corticorelin ovine triflutate, J0795
Corticotropin, J0800
Corvert (see Ibutilide fumarate)
Cosyntropin, J0833, J0834
Cough stimulating device, A7020, E0482
Counseling
alcohol misuse, G0443
cardiovascular disease, G0448
control of dental disease, D1310, D1320
obesity, G0447
sexually transmitted infection, G0445
Count, blood, *G0306, G0307*
Counterpulsation, external, *G0166*
Cover, wound
alginate dressing, A6196–A6198
foam dressing, A6209–A6214
hydrogel dressing, A6242–A6248
non-contact wound warming cover, and accessory, A6000, E0231, E0232
specialty absorptive dressing, A6251–A6256
CPAP (continuous positive airway pressure) device, E0601
headgear, K0185
humidifier, A7046
intermittent assist, E0452
Cradle, bed, E0280
Cranial electrotherapy stimulation (CES), K1002
Crib, E0300
Cromolyn sodium, inhalation solution, unit dose, J7631, J7632
Crotalidae polyvalent immune fab, J0840
Crowns, *D2710–D2983, D4249, D6720–D6794*
clinical crown lengthening-hard tissue, D4249
fixed partial denture retainers, crowns, D6710–D6794
single restoration, D2710–D2983
Crutches, E0110–E0118
accessories, A4635–A4637, K0102
crutch substitute, lower leg, E0118
forearm, E0110–E0111
underarm, E0112–E0117
Cryoprecipitate, each unit, P9012
CTLSO, L0700, L0710, L1000–L1120
addition, axilla sling, L1010
addition, cover for upright, each, L1120
addition, kyphosis pad, L1020
addition, kyphosis pad, floating, L1025
addition, lumbar bolster pad, L1030
addition, lumbar rib pad, L1040
addition, lumbar sling, L1090
addition, outrigger, L1080
addition, outrigger bilateral, vertical extensions, L1085
addition, ring flange, L1100
addition, ring flange, molded to patient model, L1110
addition, sternal pad, L1050
addition, thoracic pad, L1060
addition, trapezius sling, L1070
anterior-posterior-lateral control, molded to patient model (CTLSO), L0710
cervical, thoracic, lumbar, sacral orthrosis (CTLSO), L0700
furnishing initial orthrosis, L1000
immobilizer, infant size, L1001
tension based scoliosis orthosis, fitting, L1005
Cuirass, E0457
Culture sensitivity study, P7001
Cushion, wheelchair, E0977
Cyanocobalamin Cobalt C057, A9559
Cycler dialysis machine, E1594
Cyclophosphamide, J9070
oral, J8530
Cyclosporine, J7502, J7515, J7516
Cytarabine, J9100
liposome, J9098
Cytomegalovirus immune globulin (human), J0850
Cytopathology, cervical or vaginal, *G0123, G0124,* G0141–G0148

D

Dacarbazine, J9130
Daclizumab, J7513
Dactinomycin, J9120
Dalalone, J1100
Dalbavancin, 5mg, J0875
Dalteparin sodium, J1645
Daptomycin, J0878
Daratumumab, J9144, J9145 ⮐

◀ New ⮐ Revised ✔ Reinstated ~~deleted~~ Deleted

Darbepoetin Alfa, J0881–J0882
Daunorubicin
Citrate, J9151
HCl, J9150
DaunoXome (see Daunorubicin citrate)
Decitabine, J0894
Decubitus care equipment, E0180–E0199
air fluidized bed, E0194
air pressure mattress, E0186
air pressure pad, standard mattress, E0197
dry pressure mattress, E0184
dry pressure pad, standard mattress, E0199
gel or gel-like pressure pad mattress, standard, E0185
gel pressure mattress, E0196
heel or elbow protector, E0191
positioning cushion, E0190
power pressure reducing mattress overlay, with pump, E0181
powered air flotation bed, E0193
pump, alternating pressure pad, replacement, E0182
synthetic sheepskin pad, E0189
water pressure mattress, E0187
water pressure pad, standard mattress, E0198
Deferoxamine mesylate, J0895
Defibrillator, external, E0617, K0606
battery, K0607
electrode, K0609
garment, K0608
Degarelix, J9155
Deionizer, water purification system, E1615
Delivery/set-up/dispensing, A9901
Denileukin diftitox, J9160
Denosumab, J0897
Density, bone, study, *G0130*
Dental procedures
adjunctive general services, D9110–D9999
alveoloplasty, D7310–D7321
analgesia, D9230
diagnostic, D0120–D0999
endodontics, D3000–D3999
evaluations, D0120–D0180
implant services, D6000–D6199
implants, D3460, D5925, D6010–D6067, D6075–D6199
laboratory, D0415–D0999
maxillofacial, D5900–D5999
orthodontics, D8000–D8999
periodontics, D4000–D4999
preventive, D1000–D1999
prosthetics, D5911–D5960, D5999
prosthodontics, fixed, D6200–D6999
prosthodontics, removable, D5000–D5999
restorative, D2000–D2999
scaling, D4341–D4346, D6081
Dentures, *D5110–D5899*
Depo-estradiol cypionate, J1000
Dermacell, dermacell awn or dermacell awn porous, Q4122
Dermal filler injection, *G0429*
Desmopressin acetate, J2597
Destruction, lesion, choroid, *G0186*
Detector, blood leak, dialysis, E1560
Developmental testing, *G0451*
Devices, other orthopedic, *E1800–E1841*
assistive listening device, V5267–V5290
Dexamethasone
acetate, J1094
inhalation solution, concentrated, J7637
inhalation solution, unit dose, J7638
intravitreal implant, J7312
lacrimal ophthalmic insert, J1096
oral, J8540
sodium phosphate, J1100
Dextran, J7100
Dextrose
saline (normal), J7042
water, J7060, J7070
Dextrose, 5% in lactated ringers infusion, J7121
Dextrostick, A4772
Diabetes
evaluation, G0245, G0246
shoes (fitting/modifications), A5500–A5508
deluxe feature, depth-inlay shoe, A5508
depth inlay shoe, A5500
molded from cast patient's foot, A5501
shoe with metatarsal bar, A5505
shoe with off-set heel(s), A5506
shoe with rocker or rigid-bottom rocker, A5503
shoe with wedge(s), A5504
specified modification NOS, depth-inlay shoe, A5507
training, outpatient, G0108, G0109
Diagnostic
dental services, D0100–D0999
florbetaben, Q9983
flutemetamol F18, Q9982
mammography, digital image, G9899, G9900
radiology services, R0070–R0076
Dialysate
concentrate additives, A4765
solution, *A4720*–A4728
testing solution, A4760
Dialysis
air bubble detector, E1530
bath conductivity, meter, E1550
chemicals/antiseptics solution, A4674
disposable cycler set, A4671
emergency, G0257
equipment, E1510–E1702
extension line, A4672–A4673
filter, A4680
fluid barrier, E1575
home, S9335, S9339
kit, A4820
pressure alarm, E1540

◀ New ↩ Revised ✔ Reinstated ~~deleted~~ Deleted

D

Dialysis *(Continued)*
shunt, A4740
supplies, A4650–A4927
tourniquet, A4929
unipuncture control system, E1580
unscheduled, G0257
venous pressure clamp, A4918
Dialyzer, A4690
Diaper, T1500, T4521–T4540, T4543, T4544
adult incontinence garment, A4520, A4553
incontinence supply, rectal insert, any type, each, A4337
disposable penile wrap, T4545
Diathermy low frequency ultrasonic treatment device for home use, K1004
Diazepam, J3360
Diazoxide, J1730
Diclofenac, J1130
Dicyclomine HCl, J0500
Diethylstilbestrol diphosphate, J9165
Digoxin, J1160
Digoxin immune fab (ovine), J1162
Dihydroergotamine mesylate, J1110
Dimenhydrinate, J1240
Dimercaprol, J0470
Dimethyl sulfoxide (DMSO), J1212
Diphenhydramine HCl, J1200
Dipyridamole, J1245
Disarticulation
lower extremities, prosthesis, L5000–L5999
above knee, L5200–L5230
additions exoskeletal-knee-shin system, L5710–L5782
additions to lower extremities, L5610–L5617
additions to socket insert, L5654–L5699
additions to socket variations, L5630–L5653
additions to test sockets, L5618–L5629
additions/replacements, feet-ankle units, L5700–L5707
ankle, L5050–L5060
below knee, L5100–L5105
component modification, L5785–L5795
endoskeletal, L5810–L5999
endoskeletal, above knee, L5321
endoskeletal, hip disarticulation, L5331–L5341
endoskeleton, below knee, L5301–L5312
hemipelvectomy, L5280
hip disarticulation, L5250–L5270
immediate postsurgical fitting, L5400–L5460
initial prosthesis, L5500–L5505
knee disarticulation, L5150–L5160
partial foot, L5000–L5020
preparatory prosthesis, L5510–L5600
upper extremities, prosthesis, L6000–L6692
above elbow, L6250
additions to upper limb, L6600–L6698
below elbow, L6100–L6130
elbow disarticulation, L6200–L6205

Disarticulation *(Continued)*
upper extremities, prosthesis *(Continued)*
endoskeletal, below elbow, L6400
endoskeletal, interscapular thoracic, L6570–L6590
endoskeletal, shoulder disarticulation, L6550
immediate postsurgical procedures, L6380–L6388
interscapular/thoracic, L6350–L6370
partial hand, L6000–L6026
shoulder disarticulation, L6300–L6320
wrist disarticulation, L6050–L6055
Disease
status, oncology, G9063–G9139
Dispensing, fee, pharmacy, *G0333, Q0510–Q0514, S9430*
dispensing fee inhalation drug(s), 30 days, Q0513
dispensing fee inhalation drug(s), 90 days, Q0514
inhalation drugs, 30 days, as a beneficiary, G0333
initial immunosuppressive drug(s), post transplanr, G0510
oral anti-cancer, oral anti-emetic, immunosuppressive, first prescription, Q0511
oral anti-cancer, oral anti-emetic, immunosuppressive, subsequent preparation, Q0512
Disposable collection and storage bag for breast milk, K1005
Disposable supplies, ambulance, A0382, A0384, A0392–A0398
DME
miscellaneous, A9900–A9999
DME delivery, set up, A9901
DME supple, NOS, A9999
DME supplies, A9900
DMSO, J1212
Dobutamine HCl, J1250
Docetaxel, J9171
Documentation
antidepressant, G8126–G8128
blood pressure, G8476–G8478
bypass, graft, coronary, artery, documentation, G8160–G8163
CABG, G8160–G8163
dysphagia, G8232
dysphagia, screening, G8232, V5364
ECG, 12-lead, G8705, G8706
eye, functions, G8315–G8333
influenza, immunization, G8482–G8484
pharmacologic therapy for osteoporosis, G8635
physician for DME, G0454
prophylactic antibiotic, G8702, G8703
prophylactic parenteral antibiotic, G8629–G8632
prophylaxis, DVT, G8218
prophylaxis, thrombosis, deep, vein, G8218
urinary, incontinence, G8063, G8267
Dolasetron mesylate, J1260
Dome and mouthpiece (for nebulizer), A7016
Dopamine HCl, J1265
Doripenem, J1267

Dornase alpha, inhalation solution, unit dose form, J7639
Doxercalciferol, J1270
Doxil, J9001
Doxorubicin HCl, J9000, J9002
Drainage
bag, A4357, A4358
board, postural, E0606
bottle, A5102
Dressing; (see also Bandage), A6020–A6406
alginate, A6196–A6199
collagen, A6020–A6024
composite, A6200–A6205
contact layer, A6206–A6208
foam, A6209–A6215
gauze, A6216–A6230, A6402–A6406
holder/binder, A4462
hydrocolloid, A6234–A6241
hydrogel, A6242–A6248
specialty absorptive, A6251–A6256
transparent film, A6257–A6259
tubular, A6457
wound, K0744–K0746
Droperidol, J1790
and fentanyl citrate, J1810
Dropper, A4649
Drugs; (see also Table of Drugs)
administered through a metered dose inhaler, J3535
antiemetic, J8498, J8597, Q0163–Q0181
chemotherapy, J8500–J9999
disposable delivery system, 50 ml or greater per hour, A4305
disposable delivery system, 5 ml or less per hour, A4306
immunosuppressive, J7500–J7599
infusion supplies, A4221, A4222, A4230–A4232
inhalation solutions, J7608–J7699
non-prescription, A9150
not otherwise classified, J3490, J7599, J7699, J7799, J7999, J8499, J8999, J9999
oral, NOS, J8499
prescription, oral, J8499, J8999
Dry pressure pad/mattress, E0179, E0184, E0199
Durable medical equipment (DME), E0100–E1830, K Codes
additional oxygen related equipment, E1352–E1406
arm support, wheelchair, E2626–E2633
artificial kidney machines/accessories, E1500–E1699
attachments, E0156–E0159
bath and toilet aides, E0240–E0249
canes, E0100–E0105
commodes, E0160–E0175
crutches, E0110–E0118
decubitus care equipment, E0181–E0199
DME, respiratory, inexpensive, purchased, A7000–A7509
gait trainer, E8000–E8002
heat/cold application, E0200–E0239
Durable medical equipment *(Continued)*
hospital beds and accessories, E0250–E0373
humidifiers/nebulizers/compressors, oxygen IPPB, E0550–E0585
infusion supplies, E0776–E0791
IPPB machines, E0500
jaw motion rehabilitation system, E1700–E1702
miscellaneous, E1902–E2120
monitoring equipment, home glucose, E0607
negative pressure, E2402
other orthopedic devices, E1800–E1841
oxygen/respiratory equipment, E0424–E0487
pacemaker monitor, E0610–E0620
patient lifts, E0621–E0642
pneumatic compressor, E0650–E0676
rollout chair/transfer system, E1031–E1039
safety equipment, E0700–E0705
speech device, E2500–E2599
suction pump/room vaporizers, E0600–E0606
temporary DME codes, regional carriers, K0000–K9999
TENS/stimulation device(s), E0720–E0770
traction equipment, E0830–E0900
trapeze equipment, fracture frame, E0910–E0948
walkers, E0130–E0155
wheelchair accessories, E2201–E2397
wheelchair, accessories, E0950–E1030
wheelchair, amputee, E1170–E1200
wheelchair cusion/protection, E2601–E2621
wheelchair, fully reclining, E1050–E1093
wheelchair, heavy duty, E1280–E1298
wheelchair, lightweight, E1240–E1270
wheelchair, semi-reclining, E1100–E1110
wheelchair, skin protection, E2622–E2625
wheelchair, special size, E1220–E1239
wheelchair, standard, E1130–E1161
whirlpool equipment, E1300–E1310
Duraclon, (see Clonidine)
Dyphylline, J1180
Dysphagia, screening, documentation, *G8232, V5364*
Dystrophic, nails, trimming, *G0127*

E

Ear mold, V5264, *V5265*
Ecallantide, J1290
Echocardiography injectable contrast material, A9700
ECG, 12–lead, G8704
Eculizumab, J1300
ED, visit, *G0380–G0384*
Edetate
calcium disodium, J0600
disodium, J3520
Educational Services
chronic kidney disease, G0420, G0421
Eggcrate dry pressure pad/mattress, E0184, E0199

◀ New ⮌ Revised ✔ Reinstated ~~deleted~~ Deleted

EKG, *G0403–G0405*
Elbow
disarticulation, endoskeletal, L6450
orthosis (EO), E1800, L3700–L3740, L3760, L3671
dynamic adjustable elbow flexion device, E1800
elbow arthrosis, L3702–L3766
protector, E0191
Electric hand, *L7007–L7008*
Electric, nerve, stimulator, transcutaneous, *A4595, E0720–E0749*
conductive garment, E0731
electric joint stimulation device, E0762
electrical stimulator supplies, A4595
electromagnetic wound treatment device, E0769
electronic salivary reflex stimulator, E0755
EMG, biofeedback device, E0746
functional electrical stimulator, nerve and/or muscle groups, E0770
functional stimulator sequential muscle groups, E0764
incontinence treatment system, E0740
nerve stimulator (FDA), treatment nausea and vomiting, E0765
osteogenesis stimulator, electrical, surgically implanted, E0749
osteogenesis stimulator, low-intensity ultrasound, E0760
osteogenesis stimulator, non-invasive, not spinal, E0747
osteogenesis stimulator, non-invasive, spinal, E0748
radiowaves, non-thermal, high frequency, E0761
stimulator, electrical shock unit, E0745
stimulator for scoliosis, E0744
TENS, four or more leads, E0730
TENS, two lead, E0720
Electrical stimulation device used for cancer treatment, E0766
Electrical work, dialysis equipment, A4870
Electrodes, per pair, A4555, A4556
Electromagnetic, therapy, *G0295, G0329*
Electronic medication compliance, *T1505*
Electronic positional obstructive sleep apnea treatment, K1001
Elevating leg rest, K0195
Elliotts B solution, J9175
Elotuzumab, J9176
Emapalumab injection-lzsg, J9210
Emergency department, visit, *G0380–G0384*
EMG, E0746
Eminase, J0350
Endarterectomy, chemical, M0300
Endodontic procedures, *D3000–D3999*
periapical services, D3410–D3470
pulp capping, D3110, D3120
root canal therapy, D3310–D3353
therapy, D3310–D3330
Endodontics, dental, *D3000–D3999*
Endoscope sheath, A4270
Endoskeletal system, addition, L5848, L5856–L5857, L5925, *L5961*, L5969
Enema, bag, *A4458*
Enfuvirtide, J1324
Enoxaparin sodium, J1650
Enteral
feeding supply kit (syringe) (pump) (gravity), B4034–B4036
formulae, B4149–B4156, *B4157–B4162*
nutrition infusion pump (with alarm) (without), B9000, B9002
therapy, supplies, B4000–B9999
enteral and parenteral pumps, B9002–B9999
enteral formula/medical supplies, B0434–B4162
parenteral solutions/supplies, B4164–B5200
Epinephrine, J0171
Epirubicin HCl, J9178
Epoetin alpha, J0885, Q4081
Epoetin alpha-epbx, (Retacrit) (for ESRD on dialysis), Q5105
Epoetin alpha-epbx, (Retacrit) (non-ESRD use), Q5106
Epoetin beta, J0887–J0888
Epoprostenol, J1325
Eptinezumab-jjmr, J3032 ◀
Equipment
decubitus, E0181–E0199
exercise, A9300, E0935, E0936
orthopedic, E0910–E0948, E1800–E8002
oxygen, E0424–E0486, E1353–E1406
pump, E0781, E0784, E0791
respiratory, E0424–E0601
safety, E0700, E0705
traction, E0830–E0900
transfer, E0705
trapeze, E0910–E0912, E0940
whirlpool, E1300, E1310
Eravacycline injection, J0122
Erection device, tension ring, *L7902*
Ergonovine maleate, J1330
Eribulin mesylate, J9179
Ertapenem sodium, J1335
Erythromycin lactobionate, J1364
Esketamine, nasal spray, S0013 ◀
ESRD (End-Stage Renal Disease); (see also Dialysis)
machines and accessories, E1500–E1699
adjustable chair, ESRD, E1570
centrifuge, dialysis, E1500
dialysis equipment, NOS, E1699
hemodialysis, air bubble detector, replacement, E1530
hemodialysis, bath conductivity meter, E1550
hemodialysis, blood leak detector, replacement, E1560
hemodialysis, blood pump, replacement, E1620
hemodialysis equipment, delivery/installation charges, E1600
hemodialysis, heparin infusion pump, E1520

ESRD *(Continued)*
machines and accessories *(Continued)*
hemodialysis machine, E1590
hemodialysis, portable travel hemodialyzer system, E1635
hemodialysis, pressure alarm, E1540
hemodialysis, reverse osmosis water system, E1615
hemodialysis, sorbent cartridges, E1636
hemodialysis, transducer protectors, E1575
hemodialysis, unipuncture control system, E1580
hemodialysis, water softening system, E1625
hemostats, E1637
peritoneal dialysis, automatic intermittent system, E1592
peritoneal dialysis clamps, E1634
peritoneal dialysis, cycler dialysis machine, E1594
peritoneal dialysis, reciprocating system, E1630
scale, E1639
wearable artificial kidney, E1632
plumbing, A4870
supplies, A4651–A4929
acetate concentrate solution, hemodialysis, A4708
acid concentrate solution, hemodialysis, A4709
activated carbon filters, hemodialysis, A4680
ammonia test strip, dialysis, A4774
automatic blood pressure monitor, A4670
bicarbonate concentrate, powder, hemodialysis, A4707
bicarbonate concentrate, solution, A4706
blood collection tube, vaccum, dialysis, A4770
blood glucose test strip, dialysis, A4772
blood pressure cuff only, A4663
blood tubing, arterial and venous, hemodialysis, A4755
blood tubing, arterial or venous, hemodialysis, A4750
chemicals/antiseptics solution, clean dialysis equipment, A4674
dialysate solution, non-dextrose, A4728
dialysate solution, peritoneal dialysis, A4720–A4726, A4760–A4766
dialyzers, hemodialysis, A4690
disposable catheter tips, peritoneal dialysis, A4860
disposable cycler set, dialysis machine, A4671
drainage extension line, dialysis, sterile, A4672
extension line easy lock connectors, dialysis, A4673
fistula cannulation set, hemodialysis, A4730
injectable anesthetic, dialysis, A4737
occult blood test strips, dialysis, A4773
peritoneal dialysis, catheter anchoring device, A4653
protamine sulfate, hemodialysis, A4802
serum clotting timetube, dialysis, A4771
shunt accessory, hemodialysis, A4740
sphygmomanometer, cuff and stethoscope, A4660
syringes, A4657
topical anesthetic, dialysis, A4736
treated water, peritoneal dialysis, A4714
"Y set" tubing, peritoneal dialysis, A4719
Estrogen conjugated, J1410
Estrone (5, Aqueous), J1435
Etelcalcetide, J0606
Eteplirsen, J1428
Ethanolamine oleate, J1430
Etidronate disodium, J1436
Etonogestrel implant system, J7307
Etoposide, J9181
oral, J8560
Euflexxa, J7323
Evaluation
conformity, V5020
contact lens, S0592
dental, D0120–D0180
diabetic, G0245, G0246
footwear, G8410–G8416
hearing, S0618, V5008, V5010
hospice, G0337
multidisciplinary, H2000
nursing, T1001
ocularist, S9150
performance measurement, S3005
resident, T2011
speech, S9152
team, T1024
Everolimus, J7527
Examination
gynecological, S0610–S0613
ophthalmological, S0620, S0621
oral, D0120–D0160
pinworm, Q0113
Exercise
class, S9451
equipment, A9300
External
ambulatory infusion pump, E0781, E0784
ambulatory infusion pump continuous glucose sensing, E0787
ambulatory insulin delivery system, A9274
power, battery components, L7360–L7368
power, elbow, L7160–L7191
urinary supplies, A4356–A4359
Extractions; (see also Dental procedures), *D7111–D7140, D7251*
Extremity
belt/harness, E0945
traction, E0870–E0880
Eye
case, V2756
functions, documentation, G8315–G8333
lens (contact) (spectacle), V2100–V2615
pad, patch, A6410–A6412
prosthetic, V2623, V2629
service (miscellaneous), V2700–V2799

F

Face tent, oxygen, A4619
Faceplate, ostomy, A4361

Factor IX, J7193, J7194, J7195, J7200–J7202
Factor VIIA coagulation factor, recombinant, J7189, J7205, J7212 ⊋
Factor VIII, anti-hemophilic factor, J7182, J7185, J7190–J7192, J7207–J7209
Factor X, J7175
Factor XIII, anti-hemophilic factor, J7180, J7188
Factor XIII, A-subunit, J7181
Family Planning Education, H1010
Fee
coordinated care, G9001–G9011
dispensing, pharmacy, G0333, Q0510–Q0514, S9430
Fentanyl citrate, J3010
and droperidol, J1810
Fern test, Q0114
Ferric derisomaltose, J1437 ◀
Ferric pyrophosphate citrate powder, J1444
Ferumoxytol, Q0138, Q0139
Filgrastim (G-CSF & TBO), J1442, J1447, Q5101
Filler, wound
alginate dressing, A6199
foam dressing, A6215
hydrocolloid dressing, A6240, A6241
hydrogel dressing, A6248
not elsewhere classified, A6261, A6262
Film, transparent (for dressing), A6257–A6259
Filter
aerosol compressor, A7014
dialysis carbon, A4680
ostomy, A4368
tracheostoma, A4481
ultrasonic generator, A7014
Fistula cannulation set, A4730
Flebogamma, J1572
Florbetapir F18, A9586
Flowmeter, E0440, E0555, E0580
Floxuridine, J9200
Fluconazole, injection, J1450
Fludarabine phosphate, J8562, J9185
Fluid barrier, dialysis, E1575
Fluid flow, Q4206
Flunisolide inhalation solution, J7641
Fluocinolone, J7311, J7313
(Yutiq), J7314
Fluoride treatment, *D1201–D1205*
Fluorodeoxyglucose F-18 FDG, A9552
Fluoroestradiol F 18, A9591 ◀
Fluorouracil, J9190
Fluphenazine decanoate, *J2680*
Foam
dressing, A6209–A6215
pad adhesive, A5126
Folding walker, E0135, E0143
Foley catheter, A4312–A4316, A4338–A4346
indwelling catheter, specialty type, A4340
indwelling catheter, three-way, continuous irrigation, A4346
indwelling catheter, two-way, all silicone, A4344
indwelling catheter, two-way latex, A4338

Foley catheter *(Continued)*
insertion tray with drainage bag, A4312
insertion tray with drainage bag, three-way, continuous irrigation, A4316
insertion tray with drainage bag, two-way latex, A4314
insertion tray with drainage bag, two-way, silicone, A4315
insertion tray without drainage bag, A4313
Fomepizole, J1451
Fomivirsen sodium intraocular, J1452
Fondaparinux sodium, J1652
Foot care, *G0247*
Footdrop splint, L4398
Footplate, E0175, E0970, L3031
Footwear, orthopedic, L3201–L3265
additional charge for split size, L3257
Benesch boot, pair, child, L3213
Benesch boot, pair, infant, L3212
Benesch boot, pair, junior, L3214
custom molded shoe, prosthetic shoe, L3250
custom shoe, depth inlay, L3230
ladies' shoe, depth inlay, L3216
ladies' shoe, hightop, L3217
ladies' shoe, oxford, L3215
ladies' shoe, oxford/brace, L3224
men's shoe, depth inlay, L3221
men's shoe, hightop, L3222
men's shoe, oxford, L3219
men's shoe, oxford/brace, L3225
molded shoe, custom fitted, Plastazote, L3253
non-standard size or length, L3255
non-standard size or width, L3254
Plastazote sandal, L3265
shoe, hightop, child, L3206
shoe, hightop, infant, L3204
shoe, hightop, junior, L3207
shoe molded/patient model, Plastazote, L3252
shoe, molded/patient model, silicone, L3251
shoe, oxford, child, L3202
shoe, oxford, infant, L3201
shoe, oxford, junior, L3203
surgical boot, child, L3209
surgical boot, infant, L3208
surgical boot, junior, L3211
surgical boot/shoe, L3260
Forearm crutches, E0110, E0111
Formoterol, J7640
fumarate, J7606
Fosaprepitant, J1453
Foscarnet sodium, J1455
Fosphenytoin, Q2009
Fracture
bedpan, E0276
frame, E0920, E0930, E0946–E0948
attached to bed/weights, E0920
attachments for complex cervical traction, E0948
attachments for complex pelvic traction, E0947
dual, cross bars, attached to bed, E0946
free standing/weights, E0930

◀ New ⊋ Revised ✔ Reinstated ~~deleted~~ Deleted

Fracture *(Continued)*
orthosis, L2106–L2136, L3980–L3984
ankle/foot orthosis, fracture, L2106–L2128
KAFO, fracture orthosis, L2132–L2136
upper extremity, fracture orthosis, L3980–L3984
orthotic additions, L2180–L2192, L3995
addition to upper extremity orthosis, sock, fracture, L3995
additions lower extremity fracture, L2180–L2192
Fragmin, (see Dalteparin sodium), *J1645*
Frames (spectacles), V2020, V2025
deluxe frame, V2025
purchases, V2020
Fremanezumab-vfrm, J3031
Fulvestrant, J9395
Furosemide, J1940

G

Gadobutrol, A9585
Gadofosveset trisodium, A9583
Gadoxetate disodium, A9581
Gait trainer, E8000–E8002
Gallium Ga67, A9556
Gallium nitrate, J1457
Galsulfase, J1458
Gamma globulin, J1460, J1560
injection, gamma globulin (IM), 1cc, J1460
injection, gamma globulin (IM), over 10cc, J1560
Gammagard liquid, J1569
Gammaplex, J1557
Gamunex, J1561
Ganciclovir
implant, J7310
sodium, J1570
Garamycin, J1580
Gas system
compressed, E0424, E0425
gaseous, E0430, E0431, E0441, E0443
liquid, E0434–E0440, E0442, E0444
Gastric freezing, hypothermia, *M0100*
Gatifloxacin, J1590
Gauze; (see also Bandage)
impregnated, A6222–A6233, A6266
non-impregnated, A6402–A6404
Gefitinib, J8565
Gel
conductive, A4558
pressure pad, E0185, E0196
Gemcitabine HCl, not otherwise specified, J9201
Infugem, J9198 ⮌
Gemtuzumab ozogamicin, J9203
Generator
neurostimulator (implantable), high frequency, C1822
ultrasonic with nebulizer, E0574–E0575
Gentamicin (Sulfate), J1580
Gingival procedures, *D4210–D4240*
gingival flap procedure, D4240–D4241
gingivectomy or gingivoplasty, D4210–D4212
Glasses
air conduction, V5070
binaural, V5120–V5150
behind the ear, V5140
body, V5120
glasses, V5150
in the ear, V5130
bone conduction, V5080
frames, V2020, V2025
hearing aid, V5230
Glaucoma
screening, G0117, G0118
Gloves, A4927
Glucagon HCl, J1610
Glucose
monitor includes all supplies, K0553
monitor with integrated lancing/blood sample collection, E2101
monitor with integrated voice synthesizer, E2100
receiver (monitor) dedicated, K0554
test strips, A4253, A4772
Gluteal pad, L2650
Glycopyrrolate, inhalation solution, concentrated, J7642
Glycopyrrolate, inhalation solution, unit dose, J7643
Gold
foil dental restoration, D2410–D2430
gold foil, one surface, D2410
gold foil, two surfaces, D2420
gold foil, three surfaces, D2430
sodium thiomalate, J1600
Golimumab, J1602
Gomco drain bottle, A4912
Gonadorelin HCl, J1620
Goserelin acetate implant; (see also Implant), J9202
Grab bar, trapeze, E0910, E0940
Grade-aid, wheelchair, E0974
Gradient, compression stockings, *A6530–A6549*
below knee, 18–30 mmHg, A6530
below knee, 30–40 mmHg, A6531
below knee, thigh length, 18–30 mmHg, A6533
full length/chap style, 18–30 mmHg, A6536
full length/chap style, 30–40 mmHg, A6537
full length/chap style, 40–50 mmHg, A6538
garter belt, A6544
non-elastic below knee, 30–50 mmhg, A6545
sleeve, NOS, A6549
thigh length, 30–40 mmHg, A6534
thigh length, 40–50 mmHg, A6535
waist length, 18–30 mmHg, A6539
waist length, 30–40 mmHg, A6540
waist length, 40–50 mmHg, A6541
Granisetron HCl, J1626
XR, J1627
Gravity traction device, E0941

◀ New ⮌ Revised ✔ Reinstated ~~deleted~~ Deleted

Gravlee jet washer, A4470
Guidelines, practice, oncology, *G9056–G9062*

H

Habilitation, prevocational, waiver, T2047 ◀
Hair analysis (excluding arsenic), P2031
Halaven, Injection, eribulin mesylate, 0.1 mg, J9179
Hallus-Valgus dynamic splint, L3100
Hallux prosthetic implant, L8642
Halo procedures, L0810–L0860
addition HALO procedure, MRI compatible systems, L0859
addition HALO procedure, replacement liner, L0861
cervical halo/jacket vest, L0810
cervical halo/Milwaukee type orthosis, L0830
cervical halo/plaster body jacket, L0820
Haloperidol, J1630
decanoate, J1631
Halter, cervical head, E0942
Hand finger orthosis, prefabricated, L3923
Hand restoration, L6900–L6915
orthosis (WHFO), E1805, E1825, L3800–L3805, L3900–L3954
partial prosthesis, L6000–L6020
partial hand, little and/or ring finger remaining, L6010
partial hand, no finger, L6020
partial hand, thumb remaining, L6000
transcarpal/metacarpal or partial hand disarticulation prosthesis, L6025
rims, wheelchair, E0967
Handgrip (cane, crutch, walker), A4636
Harness, E0942, E0944, E0945
Headgear (for positive airway pressure device), K0185
Hearing
aid, V5030–V5267, V5298
aid-body worn, V5100
assistive listening device, V5268–V5274, V5281–V5290
battery, use in hearing device, V5266
contralateral routing, V5171–V5172, V5181, V5211–V5115, V5221
dispensing fee, binaural, V5160
dispensing fee, monaural hearing aid, any type, V5241
dispensing fee, unspecified hearing aid, V5090
ear impression, each, V5275
ear mold/insert, disposable, any type, V5265
ear mold/insert, not disposable, V5264
glasses, air conduction, V5070
glasses, bone conduction, V5080
hearing aid, analog, binaural, CIC, V5248
hearing aid, analog, binaural, ITC, V5249
hearing aid, analog, monaural, CIC, V5242
hearing aid, analog, monaural, ITC, V5243
hearing aid, BICROS, V5210–V5240

Hearing *(Continued)*
aid (Continued)
hearing aid, binaural, V5120–V5150
hearing aid, CROS, V5170–V5200
hearing aid, digital, V5254–V5261
hearing aid, digitally programmable, V5244–V5247, V5250–V5253
hearing aid, disposable, any type, binaural, V5263
hearing aid, disposable, any type, monaural, V5262
hearing aid, monaural, V5030–V5060
hearing aid, NOC, V5298
hearing aid or assistive listening device/supplies/ accessories, NOS, V5267
hearing service, miscellaneous, V5299
semi-implantable, middle ear, V5095
assessment, S0618, V5008, V5010
devices, L8614, V5000–V5169, V5171–V5179, V5181–V5209, V5211–V5219, V5221–V5299
services, V5000–V5999
Heat
application, E0200–E0239
infrared heating pad system, A4639, E0221
lamp, E0200, E0205
pad, A9273, E0210, E0215, E0237, E0249
Heater (nebulizer), E1372
Heavy duty, wheelchair, *E1280–E1298, K0006, K0007, K0801–K0886*
detachable arms, elevating legrests, E1280
detachable arms, swing away detachable footrest, E1290
extra heavy duty wheelchair, K0007
fixed full length arms, elevating legrest, E1295
fixed full length arms, swing away detachable footrest, E1285
heavy duty wheelchair, K0006
power mobility device, not coded by DME PDAC or no criteria, K0900
power operated vehicle, group 2, K0806–K0808
power operated vehicle, NOC, K0812
power wheelchair, group 1, K0813–K0816
power wheelchair, group 2, K0820–K0843
power wheelchair, group 3, K0848–K0864
power wheelchair, group 4, K0868–K0886
power wheelchair, group 5, pediatric, K0890–K0891
power wheelchair, NOC, K0898
power-operated vehicle, group 1, K0800–K0802
special wheelchair seat depth and/or width, by construction, E1298
special wheelchair seat depth, by upholstery, E1297
special wheelchair seat height from floor, E1296
Heel
elevator, air, E0370
protector, E0191
shoe, L3430–L3485
stabilizer, L3170
Helicopter, ambulance; (see also Ambulance)
Helmet
cervical, L0100, L0110
head, A8000–A8004

Hemin, J1640
Hemipelvectomy prosthesis, L5280
Hemi-wheelchair, E1083–E1086
Hemodialysis machine, E1590
Hemodialyzer, portable, E1635
Hemofil M, J7190
Hemophilia clotting factor, J7190–J7198
anti-inhibitor, per IU, J7198
anti-thrombin III, human, per IU, J7197
Factor IX, complex, per IU, J7194
Factor IX, purified, non-recombinant, per IU, J7193
Factor IX, recombinant, J7195
Factor VIII, human, per IU, J7190
Factor VIII, porcine, per IU, J7191
Factor VIII, recombinant, per IU, NOS, J7192
injection, antithrombin recombinant, 50 i.u., J7196
NOC, J7199
Hemostats, A4850, *E1637*
Hemostix, A4773
Hepagam B
IM, J1571
IV, J1573
Heparin
infusion pump, dialysis, E1520
lock flush, J1642
sodium, J1644
Hepatitis B, vaccine, administration, *G0010*
Hep-Lock (U/P), J1642
Hexalite, A4590
High osmolar contrast material, Q9958–Q9964
HOCM, 400 or greater mg/ml iodine, Q9964
HOCM, 150–199 mg/ml iodine, Q9959
HOCM, 200–249 mg/ml iodine, Q9960
HOCM, 250–299 mg/ml iodine, Q9961
HOCM, 300–349 mg/ml iodine, Q9962
HOCM, 350–399 mg/ml iodine, Q9963
HOCM, up to 149 mg/ml iodine, Q9958
Hip
disarticulation prosthesis, L5250, L5270
orthosis (HO), L1600–L1690
Hip-knee-ankle-foot orthosis (HKAFO), L2040–L2090
Histrelin
acetate, J1675
implant, J9225
HKAFO, L2040–L2090
Home
certification, home health, G0180
glucose, monitor, E0607, E2100, E2101, S1030, S1031
health, aide, G0156, S9122, T1021
health, aide, in home, per hour, S9122
health, aide, per visit, T1021
health, clinical, social worker, G0155
health, hospice, each 15 min, G0156
health, occupational, therapist, G0152
Home *(Continued)*
health, physical therapist, G0151
health, physician, certification, G0179–G0182
health, respiratory therapy, S5180, S5181
recertification, home health, G0179
supervision, home health, G0181
supervision, hospice, G0182
therapist, speech, S9128
Home Health Agency Services, T0221, *T1022*
care improvement home visit assessment, G9187
Home sleep study test, *G0398–G0400*
HOPPS, *C1000–C9999*
Hospice care
assisted living facility, Q5002
hospice facility, Q5010
inpatient hospice facility, Q5006
inpatient hospital, Q5005
inpatient psychiatric facility, Q5008
long-term care facility, Q5007
nursing long-term facility, Q5003
patient's home, Q5001
skilled nursing facility, Q5004
Hospice, evaluation, pre-election, *G0337*
Hospice physician supervision, *G0182*
Hospital
bed, E0250–E0304, E0328, E0329
observation, G0378, G0379
outpatient clinic visit, assessment, G0463
Hospital Outpatient Payment System, *C1000–C9999*
Hot water bottle, A9273
Human fibrinogen concentrate, J7178
Humidifier, A7046, E0550–E0563
durable, diring IPPB treatment, E0560
durable, extensive, IPPB, E0550
durable glass bottle type, for regulator, E0555
heated, used with positive airway pressure device, E0562
non-heated, used with positive airway pressure, E0561
water chamber, humidifier, replacement, positive airway device, A7046
Hyalgan, J7321
Hyalomatrix, *Q4117*
Hyaluronan, J7326, J7327
derivative, J7332
durolane, J7318
gel-Syn, J7328
genvisc, J7320
hymovis, J7322
trivisc, J7329
Hyaluronate, sodium, J7317
Hyaluronidase, J3470, J9316 ↩
ovine, J3471–J3473
Hydralazine HCl, J0360
Hydraulic patient lift, E0630
Hydrocollator, E0225, E0239
Hydrocolloid dressing, A6234–A6241

◀ New ↩ Revised ✔ Reinstated ~~deleted~~ Deleted

H

Hydrocortisone
acetate, J1700
sodium phosphate, J1710
sodium succinate, J1720
Hydrogel dressing, A6231–A6233, A6242–A6248
Hydromorphone, J1170
Hydroxyprogesterone caproate, J1725–J1726, J1729
Hydroxyzine HCl, J3410
Hygienic item or device, disposable or non-disposable, any type, each, A9286
Hylan G-F 20, J7322
Hyoscyamine Sulfate, J1980
Hyperbaric oxygen chamber, topical, A4575
Hypertonic saline solution, J7130, *J7131*

I

Ibandronate sodium, J1740
Ibuprofen, J1741
Ibutilide Fumarate, J1742
Icatibant, J1744
Ice
cap, E0230
collar, E0230
Idarubicin HCl, J9211
Idursulfase, J1743
Ifosfamide, J9208
Iliac, artery, angiography, *G0278*
Iloprost, Q4074
Imaging, PET, *G0219, G0235*
any site, NOS, G0235
whole body, melanoma, non-covered indications, G0219
Imiglucerase, J1786
Immune globulin, J1575
Bivigam, 500 mg, J1556
Cuvitru, J1555
Flebogamma, J1572
Gammagard liquid, J1569
Gammaplex, J1557
Gamunex, J1561
HepaGam B, J1571
Hizentra, J1559
Intravenous services, supplies and accessories, Q2052
NOS, J1566
Octagam, J1568
Privigen, J1459
Rho(D), J2788, J2790, *J2791*
Rhophylac, J2791
Subcutaneous, J1562
Xembify, J1558 ◀
Immunosuppressive drug, not otherwise classified, J7599
Implant
access system, A4301
aqueous shunt, L8612
bimatoprost, intracameral implant, J7351 ◀
breast, L8600
buprenorphine implant, J0570

Implant *(Continued)*
cochlear, L8614, L8619
collagen, urinary tract, L8603
dental, D3460, D5925, D6010–D6067, D6075–D6199
crown, provisional, D6085
endodontic endosseous implant, D3460
facial augmentation implant prosthesis, D5925
implant supported prosthetics, D6055–D6067, D6075–D6077
other implant services, D6080–D6199
surgical placement, D6010–D6051
dextranomer/hyaluronic acid copolymer, L8604
ganciclovir, J7310
hallux, L8642
infusion pump, programmable, E0783, E0786
implantable, programmable, E0783
implantable, programmable, replacement, E0786
joint, L8630, L8641, L8658
interphalangeal joint spacer, silicone or equal, L8658
metacarpophalangeal joint implant, L8630
metatarsal joint implant, L8641
lacrimal duct, A4262, A4263
maintenance procedures, D6080
maxillofacial, D5913–D5937
auricular prosthesis, D5914
auricular prosthesis, replacement, D5927
cranial prosthesis, D5924
facial augmentation implant prosthesis, D5925
facial prosthesis, D5919
facial prosthesis, replacement, D5929
mandibular resection prosthesis, with guide flange, D5934
mandibular resection prosthesis, without guide flange, D5935
nasal prosthesis, D5913
nasal prosthesis, replacement, D5926
nasal septal prosthesis, D5922
obturator prosthesis, definitive, D5932
obturator prosthesis, modification, D5933
obturator prosthesis, surgical, D5931
obturator/prosthesis, interim, D5936
ocular prosthesis, D5916
ocular prosthesis, interim, D5923
orbital prosthesis, D5915
orbital prosthesis, replacement, D5928
trismus appliance, not for TM treatment, D5937
metacarpophalangeal joint, L8630
metatarsal joint, L8641
neurostimulator pulse generator, L8679, L8681–L8688
not otherwise specified, L8699
ocular, L8610
ossicular, L8613
osteogenesis stimulator, E0749
percutaneous access system, A4301
removal, dental, D6100
repair, dental, D6090
replacement implantable intraspinal catheter, E0785
synthetic, urinary, L8606
urinary tract, L8603, L8606
vascular graft, L8670

Implantable radiation dosimeter, A4650
Impregnated gauze dressing, A6222–A6230, *A6231–A6233*
Incobotulinumtoxin a, J0588
Incontinence
appliances and supplies, A4310, A4331, A4332, A4360, A5071–A5075, *A5081–A5093*, A5102–A5114
garment, A4520, T4521–T4543
adult sized disposable incontinence product, T4522–T4528
any type, e.g. brief, diaper, A4520
pediatric sized disposable incontinence product, T4529–T4532
youth sized disposable incontinence product, T4533–T4534
supply, A4335, A4356–A4360
bedside drainage bag, A4357
disposable external urethral clamp/compression device, A4360
external urethral clamp or compression device, A4356
incontinence supply, miscellaneous, A4335
urinary drainage bag, leg or abdomen, A4358
treatment system, E0740
Indium IN-111
carpromab pendetide, A9507
ibritumomab tiuxetan, A9542
labeled autologous platelets, A9571
labeled autologous white blood cells, A9570
oxyquinoline, A9547
pentetate, A9548
pentetreotide, A9572
satumomab, A4642
Inebilizumab-cdon, J1823 ◀
Infliximab injection, J1745
Influenza
afluria, Q2035
agriflu, Q2034
flulaval, Q2036
fluvirin, Q2037
fluzone, Q2038
immunization, documentation, G8482–G8484
not otherwise specified, Q2039
vaccine, administration, G0008
virus vaccine, Q2034–Q2039
Infusion
pump, ambulatory, with administrative equipment, E0781
pump, continuous glucose sensing supplies for maintenance, A4226
pump, heparin, dialysis, E1520
pump, implantable, E0782, E0783
pump, implantable, refill kit, A4220
pump, insulin, E0784
pump, mechanical, reusable, E0779, E0780
pump, uninterrupted infusion of Epiprostenol, K0455
replacement battery, A4602
saline, J7030–J7060
supplies, A4219, A4221, A4222, A4225, A4230–A4232, E0776–E0791
therapy, other than chemotherapeutic drugs, Q0081
Inhalation solution; (see also drug name), J7608–J7699, Q4074
Injection device, needle-free, *A4210*
Injections; (see also drug name), J0120–J2504, J0223, J0591, J0691, J0693, J0742, J0791, J0896, J1201, J2794, J2798, J1303, J1429, J1823, J1943–J1944, J2506, J3031, J3399, J7169, J7204, J7311, J7313, J7314, J7320, J7321, J7332, J7333, J7208, J9032, J9036, J9039, J9044, J9057, J9153, J9118, J9173, J9177, J9201, J9210, J9223, J9229, J9269, J9271, J9299, J9308, J9309, J9313, J9316, J9317, J9355, J9356, Q5112–Q5118, Q5122, Q9950, Q9991, Q9992 ⮐
ado-trastuzumab emtansine, 1 mg, J9354
aripiprazole, extended release, J0401
arthrography, sacroiliac, joint, G0259, G0260
carfilzomib, 1 mg, J9047
certolizumab pegol, J0717
dental service, D9610, D9630
other drugs/medicaments, by report, D9630
therapeutic parenteral drug, single administration, D9610
therapeutic parenteral drugs, two or more administrations, different medications, D9612
dermal filler (LDS), G0429
filgrastim, J1442
interferon beta-1a, IM, Q3027
interferon beta-1a, SC, Q3028
omacetaxtine mepesuccinate, 0.01 mg, J9262
pertuzumb, 1 mg, J9306
sculptra, 0.5 mg, Q2028
supplies for self-administered, A4211
vincristine, 1 mg, J9371
ziv-aflibercept, 1 mg, J9400
Inlay/onlay dental restoration, *D2510–D2664*
INR, monitoring, *G0248–G0250*
demonstration prior to initiation, home INR, G0248
physician review and interpretation, home INR, G0250
provision of test materials, home INR, G0249
Insertion tray, A4310–A4316
Instillation, hexaminolevulinate hydrochloride, A9589
Insulin, J1815, J1817, *S5550–S5571*
ambulatory, external, system, A9274
treatment, outpatient, G9147
Integra flowable wound matrix, *Q4114*
Interferon
Alpha, J9212–J9215
Beta-1a, J1826, Q3027, Q3028
Beta-1b, J1830
Gamma, J9216
Intermittent
assist device with continuous positive airway pressure device, E0470–E0472
limb compression device, E0676
peritoneal dialysis system, E1592
positive pressure breathing machine (IPPB), E0500
Interphalangeal joint, prosthetic implant, L8658, L8659

◀ New ⮐ Revised ✔ Reinstated ~~deleted~~ Deleted

Interscapular thoracic prosthesis
endoskeletal, L6570
upper limb, L6350–L6370
Intervention, alcohol/substance (not tobacco), *G0396–G0397*
Intervention, tobacco, *G9016*
Intraconazole, J1835
Intraocular
lenses, V2630–V2632
Intraoral radiographs, dental, *D0210–D0240*
intraoral-complete series, D0210
intraoral-occlusal image, D0420
intraoral-periapical-each additional image, D0230
intraoral-periapical-first radiographic image, D0220
Intrapulmonary percussive ventilation system, E0481
Intrauterine copper contraceptive, J7300
Inversion/eversion correction device, A9285
Iodine I-123
iobenguane, A9582
ioflupane, A9584
sodium iodide, A9509, A9516
Iodine I-125
serum albumin, A9532
sodium iodide, A9527
sodium iothalamate, A9554
Iodine I-131
iodinated serum albumin, A9524
sodium iodide capsule, A9517, A9528
sodium iodide solution, A9529–A9531
Iodine Iobenguane sulfate I-131, A9508
Iodine swabs/wipes, A4247
IPD
system, E1592
Ipilimumab, J9228
IPPB machine, E0500
Ipratropium bromide, inhalation solution, unit dose, J7644, J7645
Irinotecan, J9205, J9206
Iron
Dextran, J1750
sucrose, J1756
Irrigation solution for bladder calculi, Q2004
Irrigation supplies, A4320–A4322, A4355, A4397–A4400
irrigation supply, sleeve, each, A4397
irrigation syringe, bulb, or piston, each, A4320
irrigation tubing set, bladder irrigation, A4355
ostomy irrigation set, A4400
ostomy irrigation supply, bag, A4398
ostomy irrigation supply, cone/catheter, A4399
Irrigation/evacuation system, bowel
control unit, E0350
disposable supplies for, E0352
manual pump enema, A4459
Isatuximab-irfc, J9227 ◀
Isavuconazonium, J1833
Islet, transplant, *G0341–G0343*, *S2102*
Isoetharine HCl, inhalation solution
concentrated, J7647, J7648
unit dose, J7649, J7650
Isolates, B4150, B4152
Isoproterenol HCl, inhalation solution
concentrated, J7657, J7658
unit dose, J7659, J7660
Isosulfan blue, Q9968
Item, non-covered, *A9270*
IUD, *J7300, S4989*
IV pole, each, E0776, K0105
Ixabepilone, J9207

J

Jacket
scoliosis, L1300, L1310
Jaw, motion, rehabilitation system, *E1700–E1702*
Jenamicin, J1580
Jetria, (ocriplasmin), *J7316*

K

Kadcyla, ado-trastuzumab emtansine, 1 mg, *J9354*
Kanamycin sulfate, J1840, J1850
Kartop patient lift, toilet or bathroom; (see also Lift), E0625
Keramatrix or kerasorb, J4165
Ketorolac thomethamine, J1885
Kidney
ESRD supply, A4650–A4927
machine, E1500–E1699
machine, accessories, E1500–E1699
system, E1510
wearable artificial, E1632
Kits
enteral feeding supply (syringe) (pump) (gravity), B4034–B4036
fistula cannulation (set), A4730
parenteral nutrition, B4220–B4224
administration kit, per day, B4224
supply kit, home mix, per day, B4222
supply kit, premix, per day, B4220
surgical dressing (tray), A4550
tracheostomy, A4625
Knee
arthroscopy, surgical, G0289, S2112, S2300
knee, surgical, harvesting cartilage, S2112
knee, surgical, removal loose body, chondroplasty, different compartment, G0289
shoulder, surgical, thermally-induced, capsulorraphy, S2300
disarticulation, prosthesis, L5150, L5160
joint, miniature, L5826

◀ New ⮐ Revised ✔ Reinstated ~~deleted~~ Deleted

Knee *(Continued)*
orthosis (KO), E1810, L1800–L1885
dynamic adjustable elbow entension/flexion device, E1800
dynamic adjustable knee extension/flexion device, E1810
static-progressive devices, E1801, E1806, E1811, E1816–E1818, E1831, E1841
Knee-ankle-foot device with microprocessor control, L2006
Knee-ankle-foot orthosis (KAFO), K1007, L2000–L2039, L2126–L2136 ↩
addition, high strength, lightweight material, L2755
base procedure, used with any knee joint, double upright, double bar, L2020
base procedure, used with any knee joint, full plastic double upright, L2036
base procedure, used with any knee joint, single upright, single bar, L2000
foot orthrosis, double upright, double bar, without knee joint, L2030
foot orthrosis, single upright, single bar, without knee joint, L2010
Kovaltry, J7211
Kyphosis pad, L1020, L1025

L

Laboratory
dental, D0415–D0999
adjunctive pre-diagnostic tests, mucosal abnormalities, D0431
analysis saliva sample, D0418
caries risk assessment, low, D0601
caries risk assessment, moderate, D0602
caries susceptibility tests, D0425
collection and preparation, saliva sample, D0417
collection of microorganisms for culture and sensitivity, D0415
diagnostic casts, D0470
oral pathology laboratory, D0472–D0502
processing, D0414
pulp vitality tests, D0460
services, P0000–P9999
viral culture, D0416
Laboratory tests
chemistry, P2028–P2038
cephalin flocculation, blood, P2028
congo red, blood, P2029
hair analysis, excluding arsenic, P2031
mucoprotein, blood, P2038
thymol turbidity, blood, P2033
microbiology, P7001
miscellaneous, P9010–P9615, Q0111–Q0115
blood, split unit, P9011
blood, whole, transfusion, unit, P9010

Laboratory tests *(Continued)*
miscellaneous *(Continued)*
catheterization, collection specimen, multiple patients, P9615
catheterization, collection specimen, single patient, P9612
cryoprecipitate, each unit, P9012
fern test, Q0114
fresh frozen plasma, donor retested, each unit, P9060
fresh frozen plasma (single donor), frozen within 8 hours, P9017
fresh frozen plasma, within 8–24 hours of collection, each unit, P9059
granulocytes, pheresis, each unit, P9050
infusion, albumin (human), 25%, 20 ml, P9046
infusion, albumin (human), 25%, 50 ml, P9047
infusion, albumin (human), 5%, 250 ml, P9045
infusion, albumin (human), 5%, 50 ml, P9041
infusion, plasma protein fraction, human, 5%, 250 ml, P9048
infusion, plasma protein fraction, human, 5%, 50 ml, P9043
KOH preparation, Q0112
pinworm examinations, Q0113
plasma, cryoprecipitate reduced, each unit, P9044
plasma, pooled, multiple donor, frozen, P9023
platelet rich plasma, each unit, P9020
platelets, each unit, P9019
platelets, HLA-matched leukocytes reduced, apheresis/pheresis, each unit, P9052
platelets, irradiated, each unit, P9032
platelets, leukocytes reduced, CMV-neg, aphresis/pheresis, each unit, P9055
platelets, leukocytes reduced, each unit, P9031
platelets, leukocytes reduced, irradiated, each unit, P9033
platelets, pheresis, each unit, P9034
platelets, pheresis, irradiated, each unit, P9036
platelets, pheresis, leukocytes reduced, CMV-neg, irradiated, each unit, P9053
platelets, pheresis, leukocytes reduced, each unit, P9035
platelets, pheresis, leukocytes reduced, irradiated, each unit, P9037
post-coital, direct qualitative, vaginal or cervical mucous, Q0115
red blood cells, deglycerolized, each unit, P9039
red blood cells, each unit, P9021
red blood cells, frozen/deglycerolized/washed, leukocytes reduced, irradiated, each unit, P9057
red blood cells, irradiated, each unit, P9038
red blood cells, leukocytes reduced, CMV-neg, irradiated, each unit, P9058
red blood cells, leukocytes reduced, each unit, P9016

Laboratory tests *(Continued)*
miscellaneous *(Continued)*
red blood cells, leukocytes reduced, irradiated, each unit, P9040
red blood cells, washed, each unit, P9022
travel allowance, one way, specimen collection, home/nursing home, P9603, P9604
wet mounts, vaginal, cervical, or skin, Q0111
whole blood, leukocytes reduced, irradiated, each unit, P9056
whole blood or red blood cells, leukocytes reduced, CMV-neg, each unit, P9051
whole blood or red blood cells, leukocytes reduced, frozen, deglycerol, washed, each unit, P9054
toxicology, P3000–P3001, Q0091
Lacrimal duct, implant
permanent, A4263
temporary, A4262
Lactated Ringer's infusion, J7120
Laetrile, J3570
Lanadelumab-flyo, J0593
Lancet, A4258, A4259
Language, screening, V5363
Lanreotide, J1930
Laronidase, J1931
Larynx, artificial, L8500
Laser blood collection device and accessory, A4257, E0620
LASIK, S0800
Lead investigation, T1029
Lead wires, per pair, A4557
Leg
bag, A4358, A5105, A5112
leg or abdomen, vinyl, with/without tubes, straps, each, A4358
urinary drainage bag, leg bag, leg/abdomen, latex, with/without tube, straps, A5112
urinary suspensory, leg bag, with/without tube, each, A5105
extensions for walker, E0158
rest, elevating, K0195
rest, wheelchair, E0990
strap, replacement, A5113–A5114
Legg Perthes orthosis, L1700–L1755
Newington type, L1710
Patten bottom type, L1755
Scottish Rite type, L1730
Tachdjian type, L1720
Toronto type, L1700
Lens
aniseikonic, V2118, V2318
contact, V2500–V2599
gas permeable, V2510–V2513
hydrophilic, V2520–V2523
other type, V2599
PMMA, V2500–V2503
scleral, gas, V2530–V2531
Lens *(Continued)*
eye, V2100–V2615, V2700–V2799
bifocal, glass or plastic, V2200–V2299
contact lenses, V2500–V2599
low vision aids, V2600–V2615
miscellaneous, V2700–V2799
single vision, glass or plastic, V2100–V2199
trifocal, glass or plastic, V2300–V2399
variable asphericity, V2410–V2499
intraocular, V2630–V2632
anterior chamber, V2630
iris supported, V2631
new technology, category 4, IOL, Q1004
new technology, category 5, IOL, Q1005
posterior chamber, V2632
telescopic lens, C1840
low vision, V2600–V2615
hand held vision aids, V2600
single lens spectacle mounted, V2610
telescopic and other compound lens system, V2615
progressive, V2781
Lepirudin, J1945
Lesion, destruction, choroid, G0186
Leucovorin calcium, J0640
Leukocyte poor blood, each unit, P9016
Leuprolide acetate, J1950, J9217, J9218, J9219
for depot suspension, 7.5 mg, J9217
implant, 65 mg, J9219
injection, for depot suspension, per 3.75 mg, J1950
per 1 mg, J9218
Levalbuterol, all formulations, inhalation solution
concentrated, J7607, J7612
unit dose, J7614, J7615
Levetiracetam, J1953
Levocarnitine, J1955
Levofloxacin, J1956
Levoleucovorin injection, J0641
Levoleucovorin injection (khapzory), J0642
Levonorgestrel, (contraceptive), implants and supplies, J7306
Levorphanol tartrate, J1960
Lexidronam, A9604
Lidocaine HCl, J2001
Lift
patient (includes seat lift), E0621–E0635
bathroom or toilet, E0625
mechanism incorporated into a combination lift-chair, E0627
patient lift, electric, E0635
patient lift, hydraulic or mechanical, E0630
separate seat lift mechanism, patient owned furniture, non-electric, E0629
sling or seat, canvas or nylon, E0621
shoe, L3300–L3334
lift, elevation, heel, L3334
lift, elevation, heel and sole, cork, L3320
lift, elevation, heel and sole, Neoprene, L3310

Lift *(Continued)*
shoe *(Continued)*
lift, elevation, heel, tapered to metatarsals, L3300
lift, elevation, inside shoe, L3332
lift, elevation, metal extension, L3330
Lightweight, wheelchair, *E1087–E1090, E1240–E1270*
detachable arms, swing away detachable, elevating leg rests, E1240
detachable arms, swing away detachable footrest, E1260
fixed full length arms, swing away detachable elevating legrests, E1270
fixed full length arms, swing away detachable footrest, E1250
high strength, detachable arms desk, E1088
high strength, detachable arms desk or full length, E1090
high strength, fixed full length arms, E1087
high strength, fixed length arms swing away footrest, E1089
Lincomycin HCl, J2010
Linezolid, J2020
Liquid barrier, ostomy, A4363
Listening devices, assistive, *V5281–V5290*
personal Bluetooth FM/DM, V5286
personal FM/DM adapter/boot coupling device for receiver, V5289
personal FM/DM binaural, 2 receivers, V5282
personal FM/DM, direct audio input, V5285
personal FM/DM, ear level receiver, V5284
personal FM/DM monaural, 1 receiver, V5281
personal FM/DM neck, loop induction receiver, V5283
personal FM/DM transmitter assistive listening device, V5288
transmitter microphone, V5290
Lodging, recipient, escort nonemergency transport, A0180, A0200
LOPS, *G0245–G0247*
follow-up evaluation and management, G0246
initial evaluation and management, G0245
routine foot care, G0247
Lorazepam, J2060
Loss of protective sensation, *G0245–G0247*
Low osmolar contrast material, Q9965–Q9967
Loxapine, for inhalation, J2062
LSO, L0621–L0640
Lubricant, A4332, A4402
Lumbar flexion, L0540
Lumbar-sacral orthosis (LSO), L0621–L0640
LVRS, services, *G0302–G0305*
Lymphocyte immune globulin, J7504, J7511

M

Machine
IPPB, E0500
kidney, E1500–E1699
Magnesium sulphate, J3475
Maintenance contract, ESRD, A4890
Mammography, screening, *G9899, G9900*
Mannitol, J2150, J7665
Marker, tissue, *A4648*
Mask
aerosol, K0180
oxygen, A4620
Mastectomy
bra, L8000
form, L8020
prosthesis, L8030, L8600
sleeve, L8010
Matristem, *Q4118*
micromatrix, 1 mg, Q4118
Mattress
air pressure, E0186
alternating pressure, E0277
dry pressure, E0184
gel pressure, E0196
hospital bed, E0271, E0272
non-powered, pressure reducing, E0373
overlay, E0371–E0372
powered, pressure reducing, E0277
water pressure, E0187
Measurement period
left ventricular function testing, G8682
Mecasermin, J2170
Mechlorethamine HCl, J9230
Medicaid, codes, *T1000–T9999*
Medical and surgical supplies, A4206–A8999
Medical nutritional therapy, *G0270, G0271*
Medical services, other, *M0000–M9999*
Medroxyprogesterone acetate, J1050
Meloxicam, J1738 ◀
Melphalan NOS, J9245, J9246 ⮐
~~HCl, J9245~~ ✖
Melphalan oral, J8600 ⮐
Membrane graft/wrap, Q4205
Mental, health, training services, *G0177*
Meperidine, J2175
and promethazine, J2180
Mepivacaine HCl, J0670
Mepolizumab, J2182
Meropenem, J2185
Mesna, J9209
Metacarpophalangeal joint, prosthetic implant, L8630, L8631
Metaproterenol sulfate, inhalation solution
concentrated, J7667, J7668
unit dose, J7669, J7670
Metaraminol bitartrate, J0380
Metatarsal joint, prosthetic implant, L8641
Meter, bath conductivity, dialysis, E1550
Methacholine chloride, J7674
Methadone HCl, J1230
Methergine, *J2210*
Methocarbamol, J2800

◀ New ⮐ Revised ✔ Reinstated ~~deleted~~ Deleted

Methotrexate
oral, J8610
sodium, J9250, J9260
Methyldopate HCl, J0210
Methylene blue, Q9968
Methylnaltrexone, J2212
Methylprednisolone
acetate, J1020–J1040
injection, 20 mg, J1020
injection, 40 mg, J1030
injection, 80 mg, J1040
oral, J7509
sodium succinate, J2920, J2930
Metoclopramide HCl, J2765
Micafungin sodium, J2248
Microbiology test, P7001
Midazolam HCl, J2250
Mileage
ALS, A0390
ambulance, A0380, A0390
Milrinone lactate, J2260
Mini-bus, nonemergency transportation, A0120
Minocycline hydrochloride, J2265
Miscellaneous and investigational, *A9000–A9999*
Mitomycin, J7315, J9280, J9281 ⤾
Mitoxantrone HCl, J9293
MNT, *G0270, G0271*
Mobility device, physician, service, *G0372*
Modalities, with office visit, M0005–M0008
Mogamulizumab injection-kpkc, J9201
Moisture exchanger for use with invasive mechanical ventilation, A4483
Moisturizer, skin, A6250
Molecular pathology procedure, *G0452*
Mometasone furoate sinus implant, J7401
Monitor
blood glucose, home, E0607
blood pressure, A4670
pacemaker, E0610, E0615
Monitoring feature/device, A9279
Monitoring, INR, *G0248–G0250*
demonstration prior to initiation, G0248
physician review and interpretation, G0250
provision of test materials, G0249
Monoclonal antibodies, J7505
Morphine sulfate, J2270
epidural or intrathecal use, J2274
Motion, jaw, rehabilitation system, *E1700–E1702*
motion rehabilitation system, E1700
replacement cushions, E1701
replacement measuring scales, E1702
Mouthpiece (for respiratory equipment), A4617
Moxetumomab pasudotox-tdfx, J9313
Moxifloxacin, J2280
Mucoprotein, blood, P2038
Multiaxial ankle, L5986
Multidisciplinary services, H2000–H2001, T1023–T1028
Multiple post collar, cervical, L0180–L0200
occipital/mandibular supports, adjustable, L0180
occipital/mandibular supports, adjustable cervical bars, L0200
SQMI, Guilford, Taylor types, L0190
Multi-Podus type AFO, L4396
Muromonab-CD3, J7505
Mycophenolate mofetil, J7517
Mycophenolic acid, J7518
MyOwn skin, Q4226

N

Nabilone, J8650
Nails, trimming, dystrophic, *G0127*
Nalbuphine HCl, J2300
Naloxone HCl, J2310
Naltrexone, J2315
Nandrolone
decanoate, J2320
Narrowing device, wheelchair, E0969
Nasal
application device, K0183
pillows/seals (for nasal application device), K0184
vaccine inhalation, J3530
Nasogastric tubing, B4081, B4082
Natalizumab, J2323
Nebulizer, E0570–E0585
aerosol compressor, E0571, *E0572*
aerosol mask, A7015
corrugated tubing, disposable, A7010
filter, disposable, A7013
filter, non-disposable, A7014
heater, E1372
large volume, disposable, prefilled, A7008
large volume, disposable, unfilled, A7007
not used with oxygen, durable, glass, A7017
pneumatic, administration set, A7003, A7005, A7006
pneumatic, nonfiltered, A7004
portable, E0570
small volume, A7003–A7005
ultrasonic, E0575
ultrasonic, dome and mouthpiece, A7016
ultrasonic, reservoir bottle, non-disposable, A7009
water collection device, large volume nebulizer, A7012
Necitumumab, J9295
Needle, A4215
bone marrow biopsy, C1830
non-coring, A4212
with syringe, A4206–A4209
Negative pressure wound therapy pump, E2402
accessories, A6550
Nelarabine, J9261
Neonatal transport, ambulance, base rate, A0225
Neostigmine methylsulfate, J2710

◀ New ⤾ Revised ✔ Reinstated ~~deleted~~ Deleted

Nerve, conduction, sensory, test, *G0255*
Nerve stimulator with batteries, E0765
Nesiritide injection, J2324, *J2325*
Neupogen, injection, filgrastim, 1 mcg, *J1442*
Neuromuscular stimulator, E0745
Neurophysiology, intraoperative, monitoring, *G0453*
Neurostimulator
battery recharging system, L8695
external antenna, L8696
implantable pulse generator, L8679
pulse generator, L8681–L8688
dual array, non-rechargeable, with extension, L8688
dual array, rechargeable, with extension, L8687
patient programmer (external), replacement only, L8681
radiofrequency receiver, L8682
radiofrequency transmitter (external), sacral root receiver, bowel and bladder management, L8684
radiofrequency transmitter (external), with implantable receiver, L8683
single array, rechargeable, with extension, L8686
Nipple prosthesis, custom fabricated, reusable, L8033
Nipple prosthesis, prefabricated, reusable, L8032
Nitrogen N-13 ammonia, A9526
NMES, *E0720–E0749*
Nonchemotherapy drug, oral, NOS, J8499
Noncovered services, A9270
Nonemergency transportation, A0080–A0210
Nonimpregnated gauze dressing, A6216–A6221, A6402–A6404
Nonprescription drug, A9150
Not otherwise classified drug, J3490, J7599, J7699, J7799, J8499, J8999, J9999, Q0181
Novafix, Q4208
NPH, J1820
NPWT, pump, *E2402*
NTIOL category 3, Q1003
NTIOL category 4, Q1004
NTIOL category 5, Q1005
Nursing care, T1030–T1031
Nursing service, direct, skilled, outpatient, *G0128*
Nusinersen, J2326
Nutrition
counseling, dental, D1310, D1320
enteral infusion pump, B9002
parenteral infusion pump, B9004, B9006
parenteral solution, B4164–B5200
therapy, medical, G0270, G0271

O

O & P supply/accessory/service, L9900
Observation
admission, G0379
hospital, G0378
Obturator prosthesis
definitive, D5932
interim, D5936
surgical, D5931
Occipital/mandibular support, cervical, L0160
Occlusive device, placement, *G0269*
Occupational, therapy, *G0129, S9129*
Ocrelizumab, J2350
Ocriplasmin, J7316
Octafluoropropane, Q9956
Octagam, J1568
Octreotide acetate, J2353, J2354
Ocular prosthetic implant, L8610
Ofatumumab, J9302
Olanzapine, J2358
Olaratumab, J9285
Omacetaxine Mepesuccinate, J9262
Omadacycline, J0121
Omalizumab, J2357
Omegaven, B4187
OnabotulinumtoxinA, J0585
Oncology
disease status, G9063–G9139
practice guidelines, G9056–G9062
visit, G9050–G9055
Ondansetron HCl, J2405
Ondansetron oral, Q0162
One arm, drive attachment, K0101
Ophthalmological examination, refraction, *S0621*
Oprelvekin, J2355
Oral and maxillofacial surgery, *D7111–D7999*
alveoloplasty, D7310–D7321
complicated suturing, D7911–D7912
excision of bone tissue, D7471–D7490
extractions, local, D7111–D7140
other repair procedures, D7920–D7999
other surgical procedures, D7260–D7295
reduction of dislocation/TMJ dysfunction, D7810–D7899
repair of traumatic wounds, D7910
surgical excision, intra-osseous lesions, D7440–D7465
surgical excision, soft tissue lesions, D7410–D7415
surgical extractions, D7210–D7251
surgical incision, D7510–D7560
treatment of fractures, compound, D7710–D7780
treatment of fractures, simple, D7610–D7680
vestibuloplasty, D7340–D7350
Oral device/appliance, E0485–E0486
Oral interface, A7047
Oral, NOS, drug, *J8499*
Oral/nasal mask, A7027
nasal pillows, A7029
oral cushion, A7028
Oritavancin, J2407
Oropharyngeal suction catheter, A4628
Orphenadrine, J2360
Orthodontics, *D8000–D8999*

Orthopedic shoes
arch support, L3040–L3100
footwear, *L3000–L3649*, L3201–L3265
insert, L3000–L3030
lift, L3300–L3334
miscellaneous additions, L3500–L3595
positioning device, L3140–L3170
transfer, L3600–L3649
wedge, L3340–L3420
Orthotic additions
carbon graphite lamination, L2755
fracture, L2180–L2192, L3995
halo, L0860
lower extremity, L2200–L2999, L4320
ratchet lock, L2430
scoliosis, L1010–L1120, L1210–L1290
shoe, L3300–L3595, L3649
spinal, L0970–L0984
upper limb, L3810–L3890, *L3900*, *L3901*, L3970–L3974, *L3975–L3978*, L3995
Orthotic devices
ankle-foot (AFO); (see also Orthopedic shoes), E1815, E1816, E1830, L1900–L1990, L2102–L2116, L3160, L4361, *L4397*
anterior-posterior-lateral, L0700, L0710
cervical, L0100–L0200
cervical-thoracic-lumbar-sacral (CTLSO), L0700, L0710
elbow (EO), E1800, E1801, L3700–L3740, L3760–L3761, *L3762*
fracture, L2102–L2136, L3980–L3986
halo, L0810–L0830
hand, (WHFO), E1805, E1825, L3807, L3900–L3954, *L3956*
hand, finger, prefabricated, L3923
hip (HO), L1600–L1690
hip-knee-ankle-foot (HKAFO), L2040–L2090
interface material, E1820
knee (KO), E1810, E1811, L1800–L1885
knee-ankle-foot (KAFO); (see also Orthopedic shoes), L2000–L2038, L2126–L2136
Legg Perthes, L1700–L1755
lumbar, L0625–L0651
multiple post collar, L0180–L0200
not otherwise specified, L0999, L1499, L2999, L3999, L5999, L7499, L8039, L8239
pneumatic splint, L4350–L4380
pronation/supination, E1818
repair or replacement, L4000–L4210
replace soft interface material, L4390–L4394
sacroiliac, L0600–L0620, *L0621–L0624*
scoliosis, L1000–L1499
shoe, (see Orthopedic shoes)
shoulder (SO), L1840, L3650, L3674, *L3678*
shoulder-elbow-wrist-hand (SEWHO), L3960–L3978
side bar disconnect, L2768
spinal, cervical, L0100–L0200
Orthotic devices *(Continued)*
spinal, DME, K0112–K0116
thoracic, L0210, *L0220*
thoracic-hip-knee-ankle (THKO), L1500–L1520
toe, E1830
wrist-hand-finger (WHFO), E1805, E1806, E1825, *L3806–L3809*, L3900–L3954, *L3956*
Orthovisc, J7324
Ossicula prosthetic implant, L8613
Osteogenesis stimulator, E0747–E0749, E0760
Osteotomy, segmented or subapical, *D7944*
Ostomy
accessories, A5093
belt, A4396
pouches, A4416–A4435, *A5056*, *A5057*
skin barrier, A4401–A4449, *A4462*
supplies, A4361–A4421, A5051–A5149, *A5200*
Otto Bock, prosthesis, *L7007*
Outpatient payment system, hospital, *C1000–C9999*
Overdoor, traction, *E0860*
Oxacillin sodium, J2700
Oxaliplatin, J9263
Oxygen
ambulance, A0422
battery charger, E1357
battery pack/cartridge, E1356
catheter, transtracheal, A7018
chamber, hyperbaric, topical, A4575
concentrator, E1390–E1391
DC power adapter, E1358
delivery system (topical), E0446
equipment, E0424–E0486, E1353–E1406
Liquid oxygen system, E0433
mask, A4620
medication supplies, A4611–A4627
rack/stand, E1355
regulator, E1352, E1353
respiratory equipment/supplies, E0424–E0480, A4611–A4627, *E0481*
supplies and equipment, E0425–E0444, E0455
tent, E0455
tubing, A4616
water vapor enriching system, E1405, E1406
wheeled cart, E1354
Oxymorphone HCl, J2410
Oxytetracycline HCl, J2460
Oxytocin, J2590

P

Pacemaker monitor, E0610, E0615
Paclitaxel, J9267
Paclitaxel protein-bound particles, J9264
Pad
correction, CTLSO, L1020–L1060
gel pressure, E0185, E0196

Pad *(Continued)*
heat, *A9273*, E0210, E0215, E0217, E0238, E0249
electric heat pad, moist, E0215
electric heat pad, standard, E0210
hot water bottle, ice cap or collar, heat and/or cold wrap, A9273
pad for water circulating heat unit, replacement only, E0249
water circulating heat pad with pump, E0217
orthotic device interface, E1820
sheepskin, E0188, E0189
water circulating cold with pump, E0218
water circulating heat unit, E0249
water circulating heat with pump, E0217
Pail, for use with commode chair, E0167
Pain assessment, *G8730–G8732*
Palate, prosthetic implant, L8618
Palifermin, J2425
Paliperidone palmitate, J2426
Palonosetron, J2469, J8655
Pamidronate disodium, J2430
Pan, for use with commode chair, E0167
Panitumumab, J9303
Papanicolaou screening smear (Pap), P3000, P3001, Q0091
cervical or vaginal, up to 3 smears, by technician, P3000
cervical or vaginal, up to 3 smears, physician interpretation, P3001
obtaining, preparing and conveyance, Q0091
Papaverine HCl, J2440
Paraffin, A4265
bath unit, E0235
Parenteral nutrition
administration kit, B4224
not otherwise specified, B4185
pump, B9004, B9006
solution, B4164, B4184, B4186
compounded amino acid and carbohydrates, with electrolytes, B4189–B4199, B5000–B5200
nutrition additives, homemix, B4216
nutrition administration kit, B4224
nutrition solution, amino acid, B4168–B4178
nutrition solution, carbohydrates, B4164, B4180
nutrition solution, per 10 grams, liquid, B4185
nutrition supply kit, homemix, B4222
supply kit, B4220, B4222
Paricalcitol, J2501
Parking fee, nonemergency transport, A0170
Partial Hospitalization, OT, *G0129*
Pasireotide long acting, J2502
Paste, conductive, A4558
Pathology and laboratory tests, miscellaneous, P9010–P9615
Pathology, surgical, *G0416*
Patient support system, E0636
Patient transfer system, E1035–E1036
Patisiran injection, J0222
Pediculosis (lice) treatment, *A9180*
PEFR, peak expiratory flow rate meter, A4614
Pegademase bovine, J2504
Pegaptanib, J2503
Pegaspargase, J9266
Pegfilgrastim, J2505, Q5122 ↩
Peginesatide, J0890
Pegloticase, J2507
Pelvic
belt/harness/boot, E0944
traction, E0890, E0900, E0947
Pemetrexed, J9304–J9305 ↩
Penicillin
G benzathine/G benzathine and penicillin G procaine, J0558, J0561
G potassium, J2540
G procaine, aqueous, J2510
Pentamidine isethionate, J2545, J7676
Pentastarch, 10% solution, J2513
Pentazocine HCl, J3070
Pentobarbital sodium, J2515
Pentostatin, J9268
Peramivir, J2547
Percussor, E0480
Percutaneous access system, A4301
Perflexane lipid microspheres, Q9955
Perflutren lipid microspheres, Q9957
Periapical service, *D3410–D3470*
apicoectomy, bicuspid, first root, D3421
apicoectomy, each additional root, D3426
apicoectomy, molar, first root, D3425
apicoectomy/periradicular surgery-anterior, D3410
biological materials, aid soft and osseous tissue regeneration/periradicular surgery, D3431
bone graft, per tooth, periradicular surgery, D3429
endodonic endosseous implant, D3460
guided tissue regeneration/periradicular surgery, D3432
intentional replantation, D3470
periradicular surgery without apicoectomy, D3427
retrograde filling, per root, D3430
root amputation, D3450
Periodontal procedures, *D4000–D4999*
Periodontics, dental, *D4000–D4999*
Peroneal strap, L0980
Peroxide, A4244
Perphenazine, J3310
Personal care services, T1019–T1021
home health aide or CAN, per visit, T1021
per diem, T1020
provided by home health aide or CAN, per 15 minutes, T1019
Pertuzumab, J9306, J9316 ↩
Pessary, A4561, A4562
PET, *G0219, G0235, G0252*
Pharmacologic therapy, *G8633*
Pharmacy, fee, *G0333*
Phenobarbital sodium, J2560
Phentolamine mesylate, J2760

◀ New ↩ Revised ✔ Reinstated ~~deleted~~ Deleted

P

Phenylephrine HCl, J2370
Phenylephrine/ketorolac ophthalmic solution, J1097
Phenytoin sodium, J1165
Phisohex solution, A4246
Photofrin, (see Porfimer sodium)
Photorefraction keratectomy, (PRK), *S0810*
Phototherapeutic keratectomy, (PTK), *S0812*
Phototherapy light, E0202
Phytonadione, J3430
Pillow, cervical, E0943
Pin retention (per tooth), *D2951*
Pinworm examination, Q0113
Plasma
multiple donor, pooled, frozen, P9023, P9070
single donor, fresh frozen, P9017, P9071
Plastazote, L3002, L3252, L3253, L3265, L5654–L5658
addition to lower extremity socket insert, L5654
addition to lower extremity socket insert, above knee, L5658
addition to lower extremity socket insert, below knee, L5655
addition to lower extremity socket insert, knee disarticulation, L5656
foot insert, removable, plastazote, L3002
foot, molded shoe, custom fitted, plastazote, L3253
foot, shoe molded to patient model, plastazote, L3252
plastazote sandal, L3265
Platelet, P9073, P9100
concentrate, each unit, P9019
rich plasma, each unit, P9020
Platelets, *P9031–P9037, P9052–P9053, P9055*
Platform attachment
forearm crutch, E0153
walker, E0154
Plazomicin injection, J0291
Plerixafor, J2562
Plicamycin, J9270
Plumbing, for home ESRD equipment, A4870
Pneumatic
appliance, E0655–E0673, L4350–L4380
compressor, E0650–E0652
splint, L4350–L4380
ventricular assist device, Q0477, Q0480–Q0505
Pneumatic nebulizer
administration set, small volume, filtered, A7006
administration set, small volume, nonfiltered, A7003
administration set, small volume, nonfiltered, nondisposable, A7005
small volume, disposable, A7004
Pneumococcal
vaccine, administration, G0009
Polatuzumab vedotin-piiq, J9309
Pontics, *D6210–D6252*
Porfimer, J9600
Portable
equipment transfer, R0070–R0076
gaseous oxygen, K0741, K0742
hemodialyzer system, E1635
liquid oxygen system, E0433
x-ray equipment, Q0092
Positioning seat, T5001
Positive airway pressure device, accessories, A7030–A7039, E0561–E0562
Positive expiratory pressure device, E0484
Post-coital examination, Q0115
Postural drainage board, E0606
Potassium
chloride, J3480
hydroxide preparation(KOH), Q0112
Pouch
fecal collection, A4330
ostomy, A4375–A4378, A5051–A5054, A5061–A5065
urinary, A4379–A4383, A5071–A5075
Practice, guidelines, oncology, *G9056–G9062*
Pralatrexate, J9307
Pralidoxime chloride, J2730
Prednisolone
acetate, J2650
oral, J7510
Prednisone, J7512
Prefabricated crown, *D2930–D2933*
Preparation kits, dialysis, A4914
Preparatory prosthesis, L5510–L5595
chemotherapy, J8999
nonchemotherapy, J8499
Pressure
alarm, dialysis, E1540
pad, A4640, E0180–E0199
Preventive dental procedures, *D1000–D1999*
Privigen, J1459
Procainamide HCl, J2690
Procedure
HALO, L0810–L0861
noncovered, G0293, G0294
scoliosis, L1000–L1499
Prochlorperazine, J0780
Progenamatrix, Q4222
Prolotherapy, M0076
Promazine HCl, J2950
Promethazine
and meperdine, J2180
HCl, J2550
Propranolol HCl, J1800
Prostate, cancer, screening, *G0102, G0103*
Prosthesis
artificial larynx battery/accessory, L8505
auricular, D5914
breast, L8000–L8035, L8600
dental, D5911–D5960, D5999
eye, L8610, L8611, V2623–V2629
fitting, L5400–L5460, L6380–L6388
foot/ankle one piece system, L5979

Prosthesis *(Continued)*
hand, L6000–L6020, L6026
implants, L8600–L8690
larynx, L8500
lower extremity, L5700–L5999, L8640–L8642
mandible, L8617
maxilla, L8616
maxillofacial, provided by a non-physician, L8040–L8048
miscellaneous service, L8499
obturator, D5931–D5933, D5936
ocular, V2623–V2629
repair of, L7520, L8049
socks (shrinker, sheath, stump sock), L8400–L8485
taxes, orthotic/prosthetic/other, L9999
tracheo-esophageal, L8507–L8509
upper extremity, L6000–L6999
vacuum erection system, L7900
Prosthetic additions
lower extremity, L5610–L5999
Powered Upper extremity range of motion assist device, L8701–L8702
upper extremity, L6600–L7405
Prosthetic, eye, *V2623*
Prosthodontic procedure
fixed, D6200–D6999
removable, D5000–D5899
Prosthodontics, removable, *D5110–D5899*
Protamine sulfate, J2720
Protectant, skin, A6250
Protector, heel or elbow, E0191
Protein C Concentrate, J2724
Protirelin, J2725
Psychotherapy, group, partial hospitalization, *G0410–G0411*
Pulp capping, *D3110, D3120*
Pulpotomy, *D3220*
partial, D3222
vitality test, D0460
Pulse generator, E2120
Pump
alternating pressure pad, E0182
ambulatory infusion, E0781, E0787 ⮌
ambulatory insulin, E0784
blood, dialysis, E1620
breast, E0602–E0604
enteral infusion, B9000, B9002
external infusion, E0779
heparin infusion, E1520
implantable infusion, E0782, E0783
implantable infusion, refill kit, A4220
infusion, supplies, A4226, A4230, A4232 ⮌
negative pressure wound therapy, E2402
parenteral infusion, B9004, B9006
suction, portable, E0600
water circulating pad, E0236
wound, negative, pressure, E2402
Purification system, E1610, E1615
Pyridoxine HCl, J3415

Q

Quad cane, E0105
Quinupristin/dalfopristin, J2770

R

Rack/stand, oxygen, E1355
Radiesse, Q2026
Radioelements for brachytherapy, Q3001
Radiograph, dental, *D0210–D0340*
Radiological, supplies, *A4641, A4642*
Radiology service, R0070–R0076
Radiopharmaceutical diagnostic and therapeutic imaging agent, A4641, A4642, A9500–A9699
Radiosurgery, robotic, *G0339–G0340*
Radiosurgery, stereotactic, *G0339, G0340*
Rail
bathtub, E0241, E0242, E0246
bed, E0305, E0310
toilet, E0243
Ranibizumab, J2778
Rasburicase, J2783
Ravulizumab injection-cwvz, J1303
Reaching/grabbing device, A9281
Reagent strip, A4252
Re-cement
crown, D2920
inlay, D2910
Reciprocating peritoneal dialysis system, E1630
Reclast, J3488, *J3489*
Reclining, wheelchair, *E1014, E1050–E1070, E1100–E1110*
Reconstruction, angiography, *G0288*
Rectal Control System for Vaginal insertion, A4563
Red blood cells, P9021, P9022
Regadenoson, J2785
Regular insulin, *J1815*, J1820
Regulator, oxygen, E1353
Rehabilitation
cardiac, S9472
program, H2001
psychosocial, H2017, H2018
pulmonary, S9473
system, jaw, motion, E1700–E1702
vestibular, S9476
Removal, cerumen, *G0268*
Repair
contract, ESRD, A4890
durable medical equipment, E1340
maxillofacial prosthesis, L8049
orthosis, L4000–L4130
prosthetic, L7500, L7510

◀ New ⮌ Revised ✔ Reinstated ~~deleted~~ Deleted

Replacement
battery, A4630
pad (alternating pressure), A4640
tanks, dialysis, A4880
tip for cane, crutches, walker, A4637
underarm pad for crutches, A4635
Resin dental restoration, *D2330–D2394*
Reslizumab, J2786
RespiGam, (see Respiratory syncytial virus immune globulin)
Respiratory
DME, A7000–A7527
equipment, E0424–E0601
function, therapeutic, procedure, G0237–G0239, S5180–S5181
supplies, A4604–A4629
Restorative dental procedure, *D2000–D2999*
Restraint, any type, E0710
Reteplase, J2993
Revascularization, *C9603–C9608*
Revefenacin inhalation solution, J7677
Rho(D) immune globulin, human, J2788, J2790, J2791, J2792
Rib belt, thoracic, A4572, L0220
Rilanocept, J2793
RimabotulinumtoxinB, J0587
Ring, ostomy, A4404
Ringers lactate infusion, J7120
Risk-adjusted functional status
elbow, wrist or hand, G8667–G8670
hip, G8651–G8654
lower leg, foot or ankle, G8655–G8658
lumbar spine, G8659–G8662
neck, cranium, mandible, thoracic spine, ribs, or other, G8671–G8674
shoulder, G8663–G8666
Risperidone (risperdal consta), J2794
(perseris), J2798
Rituximab, J9310
abbs (Truxina), Q5115
Robin-Aids, L6000, L6010, L6020, L6855, L6860
Rocking bed, E0462
Rolapitant, J8670
Rollabout chair, E1031
Romidepsin, J9315
Romiplostim, J2796
Romosozumab injection-aqqg, J3111
Root canal therapy, *D3310–D3353*
Ropivacaine HCl, J2795
Rubidium Rb-82, A9555

S

Sacituzumab govitecan-hziy, J9317 ◀
Sacral nerve stimulation test lead, A4290
Safety equipment, E0700
vest, wheelchair, E0980
Saline
hypertonic, J7130, *J7131*
infusion, J7030–J7060
solution, A4216–A4218, J7030–J7050
Saliva
artificial, A9155
collection and preparation, D0417
Samarium SM 153 Lexidronamm, A9605
Sargramostim (GM-CSF), J2820
Scale, E1639
Scoliosis, L1000–L1499
additions, L1010–L1120, L1210–L1290
Screening
alcohol misuse, G0442
cancer, cervical or vaginal, G0101
colorectal, cancer, G0104–G0106, G0120–G0122, G0328
cytopathology cervical or vaginal, G0123, G0124, G0141–G0148
depression, G0444
dysphagia, documentation, V5364
enzyme immunoassay, G0432
glaucoma, G0117, G0118
infectious agent antibody detection, G0433, G0435
language, V5363
mammography, digital image, G9899, G9900
prostate, cancer, G0102, G0103
speech, V5362
Sculptra, Q2028
Sealant
skin, A6250
tooth, D1351
Seat
attachment, walker, E0156
insert, wheelchair, E0992
lift (patient), E0621, E0627–E0629
upholstery, wheelchair, E0975, *E0981*
Sebelipase alfa , J2840
Secretin, J2850
Semen analysis, G0027
Semi-reclining, wheelchair, *E1100, E1110*
Sensitivity study, P7001
Sensory nerve conduction test, *G0255*
Sermorelin acetate, Q0515
Serum clotting time tube, A4771
Service
Allied Health, home health, hospice, G0151–G0161
behavioral health and/or substance abuse, H0001–H9999
hearing, V5000–V5999
laboratory, P0000–P9999
mental, health, training, G0177
non-covered, A9270
physician, for mobility device, G0372
pulmonary, for LVRS, G0302–G0305
skilled, RN/LPN, home health, hospice, G0162
social, psychological, G0409–G0411
speech-language, V5336–V5364
vision, V2020–V2799

◀ New ⮐ Revised ✔ Reinstated ~~deleted~~ Deleted

SEWHO, L3960–L3974, *L3975–L3978*
SEXA, *G0130*
Sheepskin pad, E0188, E0189
Shoes
arch support, L3040–L3100
for diabetics, A5500–A5514
insert, L3000–L3030, *L3031*
lift, L3300–L3334
miscellaneous additions, L3500–L3595
orthopedic, L3201–L3265
positioning device, L3140–L3170
transfer, L3600–L3649
wedge, L3340–L3485
Shoulder
disarticulation, prosthetic, L6300–L6320, L6550
orthosis (SO), L3650–L3674
spinal, cervical, L0100–L0200
Shoulder sling, A4566
Shoulder-elbow-wrist-hand orthosis (SEWHO), L3960–L3969, *L3971–L3978*
Shunt accessory for dialysis, A4740
aqueous, L8612
Sigmoidoscopy, cancer screening, G0104, G0106
Siltuximab, J2860
Sincalide, J2805
Sipuleucel-T, Q2043
Sirolimus, J7520
Sitz bath, E0160–E0162
Skin
barrier, ostomy, A4362, A4363, A4369–A4373, A4385, A5120
bond or cement, ostomy, A4364
sealant, protectant, moisturizer, A6250
substitute, Q4100–Q4248 ↩
~~*Skyla, 13.5 mg,* J7301~~ ✖
Sling, A4565
patient lift, E0621, E0630, E0635
Smear, Papanicolaou, screening, *P3000*, *P3001*, *Q0091*
SNCT, *G0255*
Social worker, clinical, home, health, *G0155*
Social worker, nonemergency transport, A0160
Social work/psychological services, CORF, *G0409*
Sock
body sock, L0984
prosthetic sock, *L8417*, L8420–L8435, L8470, L8480, L8485
stump sock, L8470–L8485
Sodium
chloride injection, J2912
ferric gluconate complex in sucrose, J2916
fluoride F-18, A9580
hyaluronate
Euflexxa, J7323
GELSYN-3, J7328
Hyalgan, J7321
Orthovisc, J7324
Supartz, J7321
Sodium *(Continued)*
hyaluronate *(Continued)*
Synvisc and Synvisc-One, J7325
Visco-3, J7321
phosphate P32, A9563
pyrophosphate, J1443
succinate, J1720
Solution
calibrator, A4256
dialysate, A4760
elliotts b, J9175
enteral formulae, B4149–B4156, *B4157–B4162*
parenteral nutrition, B4164–B5200
Solvent, adhesive remover, *A4455*
Somatrem, J2940
Somatropin, J2941
Sorbent cartridge, ESRD, E1636
Special size, wheelchair, *E1220–E1239*
Specialty absorptive dressing, A6251–A6256
Spectacle lenses, *V2100–V2199*
Spectinomycin HCl, J3320
Speech assessment, V5362–V5364
Speech generating device, E2500–E2599, K1009 ↩
Speech, pathologist, *G0153*
Speech-Language pathology, services, *V5336–V5364*
Spherocylinder, single vision, *V2100–V2114*
bifocal, V2203–V2214
trifocal, V2303–V2314
Spinal orthosis
cervical, L0100–L0200
cervical-thoracic-lumbar-sacral (CTLSO), L0700, L0710
DME, K0112–K0116
halo, L0810–L0830
multiple post collar, L0180–L0200
scoliosis, L1000–L1499
torso supports, L0960
Splint, A4570, L3100, L4350–L4380
ankle, L4390–L4398
dynamic, E1800, E1805, E1810, E1815, E1825, E1830, E1840
footdrop, L4398
supplies, miscellaneous, Q4051
Standard, wheelchair, *E1130*, *K0001*
Static progressive stretch, E1801, E1806, E1811, E1816, E1818, E1821
Status
disease, oncology, G9063–G9139
STELARA, ustekinumab, 1 mg, *J3357*
Stent, transcatheter, placement, *C9600*, *C9601*
Stereotactic, radiosurgery, *G0339*, *G0340*
Sterile cefuroxime sodium, J0697
Sterile water, A4216–A4217
Stimulation, electrical, non-attended, *G0281–G0283*
Stimulators
neuromuscular, E0744, E0745
osteogenesis, electrical, E0747–E0749
salivary reflex, E0755

◀ New ↩ Revised ✔ Reinstated ~~deleted~~ Deleted

Stimulators *(Continued)*
stoma absorptive cover, A5083
transcutaneous, electric, nerve, A4595, E0720–E0749
ultrasound, E0760
Stockings
gradient, compression, A6530–A6549
surgical, A4490–A4510
Stoma, plug or seal, *A5081*
Stomach tube, B4083
Streptokinase, J2995
Streptomycin, J3000
Streptozocin, J9320
Strip, blood glucose test, A4253–A4772
urine reagent, A4250
Strontium-89 chloride, supply of, A9600
Study, bone density, *G0130*
Stump sock, L8470–L8485
Stylet, A4212
Substance/Alcohol, assessment, *G0396, G0397, H0001, H0003, H0049*
Succinylcholine chloride, J0330
Suction pump
gastric, home model, E2000
portable, E0600
respiratory, home model, E0600
Sumatriptan succinate, J3030
Supartz, J7321
Supplies
battery, A4233–A4236, A4601, A4611–A4613, A4638
cast, A4580, A4590, Q4001–Q4051
catheters, A4300–A4306
contraceptive, A4267–A4269
diabetic shoes, A5500–A5513
dialysis, A4653–A4928
DME, other, A4630–A4640
dressings, A6000–A6513
enteral, therapy, B4000–B9999
incontinence, A4310–A4355, A5102–A5200
infusion, A4221, A4222, A4230–A4232, E0776–E0791
needle, A4212, A4215
needle-free device, A4210
ostomy, A4361–A4434, A5051–A5093, A5120–A5200
parenteral, therapy, B4000–B9999
radiological, A4641, A4642
refill kit, infusion pump, A4220
respiratory, A4604–A4629
self-administered injections, A4211
splint, Q4051
sterile water/saline and/or dextrose, A4216–A4218
surgical, miscellaneous, A4649
syringe, A4206–A4209, A4213, A4232
syringe with needle, A4206–A4209
urinary, external, A4356–A4360
Supply/accessory/service, A9900
Support
arch, L3040–L3090
cervical, L0100–L0200
Support *(Continued)*
spinal, L0960
stockings, L8100–L8239
Surederm, Q4220
Surgery, oral, *D7000–D7999*
Surgical
arthroscopy, knee, G0289, S2112
boot, L3208–L3211
dressing, A6196–A6406
procedure, noncovered, G0293, G0294
stocking, A4490–A4510
supplies, A4649
tray, A4550
Surgicord, Q4218–Q4219
Surgraft, Q4209
Swabs, betadine or iodine, A4247
Synojoynt, J7331
Synvisc and Synvisc-One, J7325
Syringe, A4213
with needle, A4206–A4209
System
external, ambulatory insulin, A9274
rehabilitation, jaw, motion, E1700–E1702
transport, E1035–E1039

T

Tables, bed, E0274, E0315
Tacrolimus
oral, J7503, J7507, J7508
parenteral, J7525
Tagraxofusp injections-erzs, J9269
Taliglucerase, J3060
Talimogene laheroareovec, J9325
Tape, *A4450–A4452*
Taxi, non-emergency transportation, A0100
Team, conference, *G0175, G9007, S0220, S0221*
Technetium TC 99M
Arcitumomab, A9568
Bicisate, A9557
Depreotide, A9536
Disofenin, A9510
Exametazine, A9521
Exametazine labeled autologous white blood cells, A9569
Fanolesomab, A9566
Glucepatate, A9550
Labeled red blood cells, A9560
Macroaggregated albumin, A9540
Mebrofenin, A9537
Mertiatide, A9562
Oxidronate, A9561
Pentetate, A9539, A9567
Pertechnetate, A9512
Pyrophosphate, A9538
Sestamibi, A9500
Succimer, A9551

Technetium TC 99M *(Continued)*
Sulfur colloid, A9541
Teboroxime, A9501
Tetrofosmin, A9502
Tilmanocept, A9520
Tedizolid phosphate, J3090
TEEV, J0900
Telavancin, J3095
Telehealth, Q3014
Telehealth transmission, T1014
Temozolomide
injection, J9328
oral, J8700
Temporary codes, *Q0000–Q9999,* S0009–S9999
Temporomandibular joint, *D0320, D0321*
Temsirolimus, J9330
Tenecteplase, J3101
Teniposide, Q2017
TENS, A4595, E0720–E0749
Tent, oxygen, E0455
Teprotumumab-trbw, J3241 ◀
Terbutaline sulfate, J3105
inhalation solution, concentrated, J7680
inhalation solution, unit dose, J7681
Teriparatide, J3110
Terminal devices, L6700–L6895
Test
sensory, nerve, conduction, G0255
Testosterone
cypionate and estradiol cypionate, J1071
enanthate, J3121
undecanoate, J3145
Tetanus immune globulin, human, J1670
Tetracycline, J0120
Thallous Chloride TL 201, A9505
Theophylline, J2810
Therapeutic lightbox, A4634, E0203
Therapy
activity, G0176
electromagnetic, G0295, G0329
endodontic, D3222–D3330
enteral, supplies, B4000–B9999
medical, nutritional, G0270, G0271
occupational, *G0129,* H5300, *S9129*
occupational, health, G0152
parenteral, supplies, B4000–B9999
respiratory, function, procedure, G0237–S0239, S5180, S5181
speech, home, G0153, S9128
wound, negative, pressure, pump, E2402
Theraskin, *Q4121*
Thermometer, A4931–A4932
dialysis, A4910
Thiamine HCl, J3411
Thiethylperazine maleate, J3280
Thiotepa, J9340
Thoracic orthosis, L0210
Thoracic-hip-knee-ankle (THKAO), L1500–L1520
Thoracic-lumbar-sacral orthosis (TLSO)
scoliosis, L1200–L1290
spinal, L0450–L0492
Thymol turbidity, blood, P2033
Thyrotropin Alfa, J3240
Tigecycline, J3243
Tinzarparin sodium, J1655
Tip (cane, crutch, walker) replacement, A4637
Tire, wheelchair, *E2211–E2225, E2381–E2395*
Tirofiban, J3246
Tisagenlecleucel, Q2040
Tissue marker, A4648
TLSO, L0450–L0492, L1200–L1290
Tobacco
intervention, G9016
Tobramycin
inhalation solution, unit dose, J7682, J7685
sulfate, J3260
Tocilizumab, J2362
Toe device, *E1831*
Toilet accessories, E0167–E0179, E0243, E0244, E0625
Tolazoline HCl, J2670
Toll, non emergency transport, A0170
Tomographic radiograph, dental, *D0322*
Topical hyperbaric oxygen chamber, A4575
Topotecan, J8705, J9351
Torsemide, J3265
Trabectedin, J9352
Tracheostoma heat moisture exchange system, A7501–A7509
Tracheostomy
care kit, A4629
filter, A4481
speaking valve, L8501
supplies, A4623, A4629, A7523–A7524
tube, A7520–A7522
Tracheotomy mask or collar, A7525–A7526
Traction
cervical, E0855, E0856
device, ambulatory, E0830
equipment, E0840–E0948
extremity, E0870–E0880
pelvic, E0890, E0900, E0947
Training
diabetes, outpatient, G0108, G0109
home health or hospice, G0162
services, mental, health, G0177
Transcutaneous electrical nerve stimulator (TENS), E0720–E0770
Transducer protector, dialysis, E1575
Transfer (shoe orthosis), L3600–L3640
Transfer system with seat, E1035
Transparent film (for dressing), A6257–A6259
Transplant
islet, G0341–G0343, S2102
Transport
chair, E1035–E1039
system, E1035–E1039
x-ray, R0070–R0076

◀ **New** ⮌ **Revised** ✔ **Reinstated** ~~deleted~~ **Deleted**

Transportation
ambulance, A0021–A0999, Q3019, Q3020
corneal tissue, V2785
EKG (portable), R0076
handicapped, A0130
non-emergency, A0080–A0210, T2001–T2005
service, including ambulance, A0021, A0999, T2006
taxi, non-emergency, A0100
toll, non-emergency, A0170
volunteer, non-emergency, A0080, A0090
x-ray (portable), R0070, R0075, *R0076*
Transportation services
air services, A0430, A0431, A0435, A0436
ALS disposable supplies, A0398
ALS mileage, A0390
ALS specialized service, A0392, A0394, A0396
ambulance, ALS, A0426, A0427, A0433
ambulance, outside state, Medicaid, A0021
ambulance oxygen, A0422
ambulance, waiting time, A0420
ancillary, lodging, escort, A0200
ancillary, lodging, recipient, A0180
ancillary, meals, escort, A0210
ancillary, meals, recipient, A0190
ancillary, parking fees, tolls, A0170
BLS disposable supplies, A0382
BLS mileage, A0380
BLS specialized service, A0384
emergency, neonatal, one-way, A0225
extra ambulance attendant, A0424
ground mileage, A0425
non-emergency, air travel, A0140
non-emergency, bus, A0110
non-emergency, case worker, A0160
non-emergency, mini-bus, A0120
non-emergency, no vested interest, A0080
non-emergency, taxi, A0100
non-emergency, wheelchair van, A0130
non-emergency, with vested interest, A0090
paramedic intercept, A0432
response and treat, no transport, A0998
specialty transport, A0434
Transtracheal oxygen catheter, A7018
Trapeze bar, E0910–E0912, E0940
Trauma, response, team, *G0390*
Tray
insertion, A4310–A4316
irrigation, A4320
surgical; (see also kits), A4550
wheelchair, E0950
Trastuzumab injection excludes biosimilar, J9316, J9355 ⮌
anns (kanjinti), Q5117
dkst (Ogivri), Q5114
dttb (Ontruzant), Q5112
fam-trastuzumab deruxtecan-nxki, J9358 ◀
pkrb (Herzuma), Q5113
qyyp (trazimera), Q5116
Trastuzumab and Hyaluronidase-oysk, J9356
Treatment
bone, G0412–G0415
pediculosis (lice), A9180
services, behavioral health, H0002–H2037
Treprostinil, J3285
Triamcinolone, J3301–J3303
acetonide, J3300, J3301
diacetate, J3302
hexacetonide, J3303
inhalation solution, concentrated, J7683
inhalation solution, unit dose, J7684
Triflupromazine HCl, J3400
Trifocal, glass or plastic, V2300–V2399
aniseikonic, V2318
lenticular, V2315, V2321
specialty trifocal, by report, V2399
sphere, plus or minus, V2300–V2302
spherocylinder, V2303–V2314
trifocal add-over 3.25d, V2320
trifocal, seg width over 28 mm, V2319
Trigeminal division block anesthesia, *D9212*
Triluron intraarticular injection, J7332
Trimethobenzamide HCl, J3250
Trimetrexate glucuoronate, J3305
Trimming, nails, dystrophic, *G0127*
Triptorelin pamoate, J3315
Trismus appliance, *D5937*
Truss, L8300–L8330
addition to standard pad, scrotal pad, L8330
addition to standard pad, water pad, L8320
double, standard pads, L8310
single, standard pad, L8300
Tube/Tubing
anchoring device, A5200
blood, A4750, A4755
corrugated tubing, non-disposable, used with large volume nebulizer,10 feet, A4337
drainage extension, A4331
gastrostomy, B4087, B4088
irrigation, A4355
larynectomy, A4622
nasogastric, B4081, B4082
oxygen, A4616
serum clotting time, A4771
stomach, B4083
suction pump, each, A7002
tire, K0091, K0093, K0095, K0097
tracheostomy, A4622
urinary drainage, K0280

U

Ultrasonic nebulizer, E0575
Ultrasound, *S8055, S9024*
paranasal sinus ultrasound, S9024
ultrasound guidance, multifetal pregnancy reduction, technical component, S8055

◀ New ⮌ Revised ✔ Reinstated ~~deleted~~ Deleted

Ultraviolet, cabinet/system, *E0691, E0694*
Ultraviolet light therapy system, A4633, E0691–E0694
light therapy system in 6 foot cabinet, E0694
replacement bulb/lamp, A4633
therapy system panel, 4 foot, E0692
therapy system panel, 6 foot, E0693
treatment area 2 sq feet or less, E0691
Unclassified drug, J3490
Underpads, disposable, *A4554*
Unipuncture control system, dialysis, E1580
Upper extremity addition, locking elbow, L6693
Upper extremity fracture orthosis, L3980–L3999
Upper limb prosthesis, L6000–L7499
Urea, J3350
Ureterostomy supplies, A4454–A4590
Urethral suppository, Alprostadil, J0275
Urinal, E0325, E0326
Urinary
catheter, A4338–A4346, A4351–A4353
indwelling catheter, A4338–A4346
intermittent urinary catheter, A4351–A4353
male external catheter, A4349
collection and retention (supplies), A4310–A4360
bedside drainage bag, A4357
disposable external urethral clamp, A4360
external urethral clamp, A4356
female external urinary collection device, A4328
insertion trays, A4310–A4316, A4354–A4355
irrigation syringe, A4322
irrigation tray, A4320
male external catheter/integral collection chamber, A4326
perianal fecal collection pouch, A4330
therapeutic agent urinary catheter irrigation, A4321
urinary drainage bag, leg/abdomen, A4358
supplies, external, A4335, A4356–A4358
bedside drainage bag, A4357
external urethral clamp/compression device, A4356
incontinence supply, A4335
urinary drainage bag, leg or abdomen, A4358
tract implant, collagen, L8603
tract implant, synthetic, L8606
Urine
sensitivity study, P7001
system, K1006 ◀
tests, A4250
Urofollitropin, J3355
Urokinase, J3364, J3365
Ustekinumab, J3357, J3758
U-V lens, V2755

V

Vabra aspirator, A4480
Vaccination, administration
flublok, Q2033
hepatitis B, G0010
Vaccination, administration *(Continued)*
influenza virus, G0008
pneumococcal, G0009
Vaccine
administration, influenza, G0008
administration, pneumococcal, G0009
hepatitis B, administration, G0010
Vaginal
cancer, screening, G0101
cytopathologist, G0123
cytopathology, G0123, G0124, G0141–G0148
screening, cervical/vaginal, thin-layer, cytopathologist, G0123
screening, cervical/vaginal, thin-layer, physician interpretation, G0124
screening cytopathology smears, automated, G0141–G0148
Vancomycin HCl, J3370
Vaporizer, E0605
Vascular
catheter (appliances and supplies), A4300–A4306
disposable drug delivery system, >50 ml/hr, A4305
disposable drug delivery system, <50 ml/hr, A4306
implantable access catheter, external, A4300
implantable access total, catheter, A4301
graft material, synthetic, L8670
Vasoxyl, J3390
Vedolizumab, J3380
Vehicle, power-operated, *K0800–K0899*
Velaglucerase alfa, J3385
Venous pressure clamp, dialysis, A4918
Ventilator
battery, A4611–A4613
home ventilator, any type, E0465, E0466
used with invasive interface (e.g., tracheostomy tube), E0465
used with non-invasive interface (e.g., mask, chest shell), E0466
moisture exchanger, disposable, A4483
Ventricular assist device, Q0478–Q0504, Q0506–Q0509
battery clips, electric or electric/pneumatic, replacement, Q0497
battery, lithium-ion, electric or electric/pneumatic, replacement, Q0506
battery, other than lithium-ion, electric or electric/pneumatic, replacement, Q0496
battery, pneumatic, replacement, Q0503
battery/power-pack charger, electric or electric/pneumatic, replacement, Q0495
belt/vest/bag, carry external components, replacement, Q0499
driver, replacement, Q0480
emergency hand pump, electric or electric/pneumatic, replacement, Q0494
emergency power source, electric, replacement, Q0490
emergency power source, electric/pneumatic, replacement, Q0491

Ventricular assist device *(Continued)*
emergency power supply cable, electric, replacement, Q0492
emergency power supply cable, electric/pneumatic, replacement, Q0493
filters, electric or electric/pneumatic, replacement, Q0500
holster, electric or electric/pneumatic, replacement, Q0498
leads (pneumatic/electrical), replacement, Q0487
microprocessor control unit, electric/pneumatic combination, replacement, Q0482
microprocessor control unit, pneumatic, replacement, Q0481
miscellaneous supply, external VAD, Q0507
miscellaneous supply, implanted device, Q0508
miscellaneous supply, implanted device, payment not made under Medicare Part A, Q0509
mobility cart, replacement, Q0502
monitor control cable, electric, replacement, Q0485
monitor control cable, electric/pneumatic, Q0486
monitor/display module, electric, replacement, Q0483
monitor/display module, electric/electric pneumatic, replacement, Q0484
power adapter, pneumatic, replacement, vehicle type, Q0504
power adapter, vehicle type, Q0478
power module, replacement, Q0479
power-pack base, electric, replacement, Q0488
power-pack base, electric/pneumatic, replacement, Q0489
shower cover, electric or electric/pneumatic, replacement, Q0501
Verteporfin, J3396
Vest, safety, wheelchair, E0980
Veteran Services Chaplain, Q9001–Q9003 ◀
Vinblastine sulfate, J9360
Vincristine sulfate, J9370, J9371
Vinorelbine tartrate, J9390
Vision service, V2020–V2799
bifocal, glass or plastic, V2200–V2299
contact lenses, V2500–V2599
frames, V2020–V2025
intraocular lenses, V2630–V2632
low-vision aids, V2600–V2615
miscellaneous, V2700–V2799
prosthetic eye, V2623–V2629
spectacle lenses, V2100–V2199
trifocal, glass or plastic, V2300–V2399
variable asphericity, V2410–V2499
Visit, emergency department, *G0380–G0384*
Visual, function, postoperative cataract surgery, *G0915–G0918*
Vitamin B-12 cyanocobalamin, J3420
Vitamin K, J3430
Voice
amplifier, L8510
prosthesis, L8511–L8514
Von Willebrand Factor Complex, human, J7179, J7183, J7187
Voriconazole, J3465

W

Waiver, T2012–T2050
assessment/plan of care development, T2024
case management, per month, T2022
day habilitation, per 15 minutes, T2021
day habilitation, per diem, T2020
habilitation, educational, per diem, T2012
habilitation, educational, per hour, T2013
habilitation, prevocational, per diem, T2014
habilitation, prevocational, per hour, T2015
habilitation, residential, 15 minutes, T2017
habilitation, residential, per diem, T2016
habilitation, supported employment, 15 minutes, T2019
habilitation, supported employment, per diem, T2018
targeted case management, per month, T2023
waiver services NOS, T2025
Walker, E0130–E0149
accessories, A4636, A4637
attachments, E0153–E0159
enclosed, four-sided frame, E0144
folding (pickup), E0135
folding, wheeled, E0143
heavy duty, multiple braking system, E0147
heavy duty, wheeled, rigid or folding, E0149
heavy duty, without wheels, E0148
rigid (pickup), E0130
rigid, wheeled, E0141
with trunk support, E0140
Walking splint, L4386
Washer, Gravlee jet, *A4470*
Water
dextrose, J7042, J7060, J7070
distilled (for nebulizer), A7018
pressure pad/mattress, E0187, E0198
purification system (ESRD), E1610, E1615
softening system (ESRD), E1625
sterile, A4714
WBC/CBC, *G0306*
Wedges, shoe, L3340–L3420
Wellness visit; annual, *G0438, G0439*
Wet mount, Q0111
Wheel attachment, rigid pickup walker, E0155
Wheelchair, E0950–E1298, K0001–K0108, *K0801–K0899*
accessories, E0192, E0950–E1030, E1065–E1069, E2211–E2230, E2300–E2399, *E2626–E2633*
amputee, E1170–E1200
back, fully reclining, manual, E1226
component or accessory, not otherwise specified, K0108
cushions, E2601–E2625

◀ New ⮌ Revised ✔ Reinstated ~~deleted~~ Deleted

Wheelchair *(Continued)*
custom manual wheelchair base, K0008
custom motorized/power base, K0013
dynamic positioning hardware for back, E2398
foot box, E0954
heavy duty, E1280–E1298, K0006, K0007, K0801–K0886
lateral thigh or knee support, E0953
lightweight, E1087–E1090, E1240–E1270
narrowing device, E0969
power add-on, E0983–E0984
reclining, fully, E1014, E1050–E1070, E1100–E1110
semi-reclining, E1100–E1110
shock absorber, E1015–E1018
specially sized, E1220, E1230
standard, E1130, K0001
stump support system, K0551
tire, E0999
transfer board or device, E0705
tray, K0107
van, non-emergency, A0130
youth, E1091
WHFO with inflatable air chamber, L3807
Whirlpool equipment, E1300–E1310
Whirlpool tub, walk-in, portable, K1003
WHO, wrist extension, L3914
Wig, A9282
Wipes, A4245, A4247
Wound
cleanser, A6260
closure, adhesive, G0168
cover
alginate dressing, A6196–A6198
collagen dressing, A6020–A6024
foam dressing, A6209–A6214
hydrocolloid dressing, A6234–A6239
hydrogel dressing, A6242–A6247
non-contact wound warming cover, and accessory, E0231–E0232
specialty absorptive dressing, A6251–A6256
Wound *(Continued)*
filler
alginate dressing, A6199
collagen based, A6010
foam dressing, A6215
hydrocolloid dressing, A6240–A6241
hydrogel dressing, A6248
not elsewhere classified, A6261–A6262
Woundfix, Woundfix Plus, Q4217
matrix, Q4114
pouch, A6154
therapy, negative, pressure, pump, E2402
wound suction, A9272, K0743
Wrapping, fabric, abdominal aneurysm, *M0301*
Wrist
disarticulation prosthesis, L6050, L6055
electronic wrist rotator, L7259
hand/finger orthosis (WHFO), E1805, E1825, L3800–L3954

X

Xenon Xe 133, A9558
X-ray
equipment, portable, Q0092, R0070, R0075
single, energy, absorptiometry (SEXA), G0130
transport, R0070–R0076
Xylocaine HCl, J2000

Y

Yttrium Y-90 ibritumomab, A9543

Z

Ziconotide, J2278
Zidovudine, J3485
Ziprasidone mesylate, J3486
Zoledronic acid, J3489

◀ New ↩ Revised ✔ Reinstated ~~deleted~~ Deleted

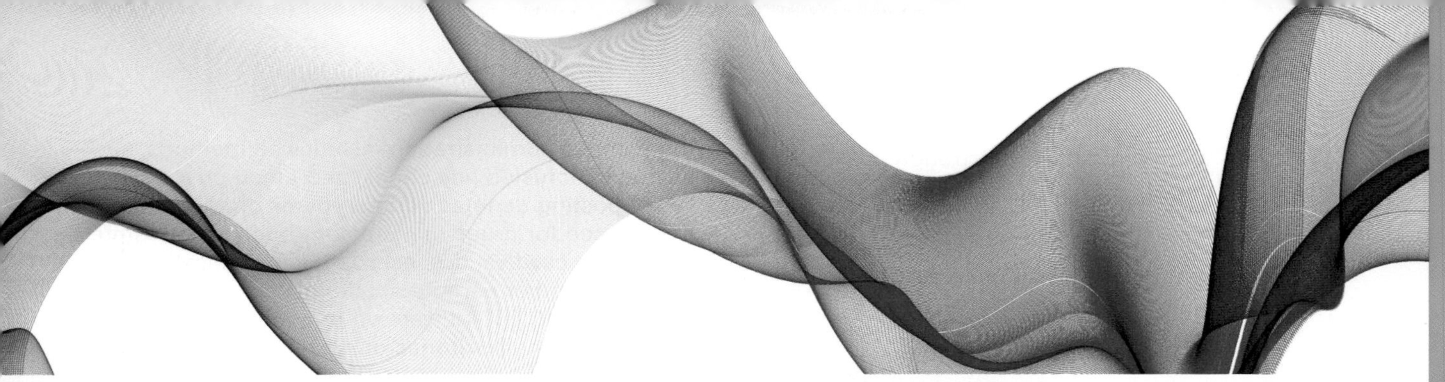

2021

TABLE OF DRUGS

IA	Intra-arterial administration
IU	International unit
IV	Intravenous administration
IM	Intramuscular administration
IT	Intrathecal
SC	Subcutaneous administration
INH	Administration by inhaled solution
VAR	Various routes of administration
OTH	Other routes of administration
ORAL	Administered orally

Intravenous administration includes all methods, such as gravity infusion, injections, and timed pushes. The "VAR" posting denotes various routes of administration and is used for drugs that are commonly administered into joints, cavities, tissues, or topical applications, in addition to other parenteral administrations. Listings posted with "OTH" indicate other administration methods, such as suppositories or catheter injections.

Blue typeface terms are added by publisher.

DRUG NAME	DOSAGE	METHOD OF ADMINISTRATION	HCPCS CODE
A			
Abatacept	10 mg	IV	**J0129**
Abbokinase	5,000 IU vial	IV	J3364
	250,000 IU vial	IV	J3365
Abbokinase, Open Cath	5,000 IU vial	IV	J3364
Abciximab	10 mg	IV	**J0130**
Abelcet	10 mg	IV	J0287-J0289
Abilify Maintena	1 mg		J0401
ABLC	50 mg	IV	J0285
AbobotulinumtoxintypeA	5 units	IM	**J0586**
Abraxane	1 mg		J9264
Accuneb	1 mg		J7613
Acetadote	100 mg		J0132
Acetaminophen	10 mg	IV	**J0131**
Acetazolamide sodium	up to 500 mg	IM, IV	**J1120**
Acetylcysteine			
injection	100 mg	IV	**J0132**
unit dose form	per gram	INH	**J7604, J7608**
Achromycin	up to 250 mg	IM, IV	J0120
Actemra	1 mg		J3262
ACTH	up to 40 units	IV, IM, SC	J0800
Acthar	up to 40 units	IV, IM, SC	J0800
Acthib			J3490
Acthrel	1 mcg		J0795
Actimmune	3 million units	SC	J9216
Activase	1 mg	IV	J2997

◀ New ⤺ Revised ✔ Reinstated ~~deleted~~ Deleted

DRUG NAME	DOSAGE	METHOD OF ADMINISTRATION	HCPCS CODE
Acyclovir	5 mg		**J0133**
			J8499
Adagen	25 IU		J2504
Adalimumab	20 mg	SC	**J0135**
Adcetris	1 mg	IV	J9042
Adenocard	1 mg	IV	J0153
Adenoscan	1 mg	IV	J0153
Adenosine	1 mg	IV	**J0153**
Ado-trastuzumab Emtansine	1 mg	IV	**J9354**
Adrenalin Chloride	up to 1 ml ampule	SC, IM	J0171
Adrenalin, epinephrine	0.1 mg	SC, IM	**J0171**
Adriamycin, PFS, RDF	10 mg	IV	J9000
Adrucil	500 mg	IV	J9190
Advate	per IU		J7192
Afamelanotide implant	1 mg	IV	**J7352** ◀
Aflibercept	1 mg	OTH	**J0178**
Agalsidase beta	1 mg	IV	**J0180**
Aggrastat	0.25 mg	IM, IV	J3246
A-hydrocort	up to 50 mg	IV, IM, SC	J1710
	up to 100 mg		J1720
Akineton	per 5 mg	IM, IV	J0190
Akynzeo	300 mg and 0.5 mg		J8655
Alatrofloxacin mesylate, injection	100 mg	IV	**J0200**
Albumin			P9041, P9045, P9046, P9047
Albuterol	0.5 mg	INH	**J7620**
concentrated form	1 mg	INH	**J7610, J7611**
unit dose form	1 mg	INH	**J7609, J7613**
Aldesleukin	per single use vial	IM, IV	**J9015**
Aldomet	up to 250 mg	IV	J0210
Aldurazyme	0.1 mg		J1931
Alefacept	0.5 mg	IM, IV	**J0215**
Alemtuzumab	1 mg		J0202
Alferon N	250,000 IU	IM	J9215
Alglucerase	per 10 units	IV	**J0205**
Alglucosidase alfa	10 mg	IV	**J0220, J0221**
Alimta	10 mg		J9305
Alkaban-AQ	1 mg	IV	J9360
Alkeran	2 mg	ORAL	J8600
	50 mg	IV	J9245

◀ New ⮐ Revised ✔ Reinstated ~~deleted~~ Deleted

DRUG NAME	DOSAGE	METHOD OF ADMINISTRATION	HCPCS CODE
AlloDerm	per square centimeter		Q4116
AlloSkin	per square centimeter		Q4115
Aloxi	25 mcg		J2469
Alpha 1-proteinase inhibitor, human	10 mg	IV	**J0256, J0257**
Alphanate			**J7186**
AlphaNine SD	per IU		J7193
Alprolix	per IU		J7201
Alprostadil			
injection	1.25 mcg	OTH	**J0270**
urethral suppository	each	OTH	**J0275**
Alteplase recombinant	1 mg	IV	**J2997**
Alupent	per 10 mg	INH	**J7667, J7668**
noncompounded, unit dose	10 mg	INH	J7669
unit dose	10 mg	INH	J7670
AmBisome	10 mg	IV	J0289
Amcort	per 5 mg	IM	J3302
A-methaPred	up to 40 mg	IM, IV	J2920
	up to 125 mg	IM, IV	J2930
Amgen	1 mcg	SC	J9212
Amifostine	500 mg	IV	**J0207**
Amikacin sulfate	100 mg	IM, IV	**J0278**
Aminocaproic Acid			J3490
Aminolevulinic acid HCl	unit dose (354 mg)	OTH	**J7308**
Aminolevulinic acid HCl 10% Gel	10 mg	OTH	**J7345**
Aminolevulinate	1 g	OTH	**J7309**
Aminophylline/Aminophyllin	up to 250 mg	IV	**J0280**
Amiodarone HCl	30 mg	IV	**J0282**
Amitriptyline HCl	up to 20 mg	IM	**J1320**
Amobarbital	up to 125 mg	IM, IV	**J0300**
Amphadase	1 ml		J3470
Amphocin	50 mg	IV	J0285
Amphotericin B	50 mg	IV	**J0285**
Amphotericin B, lipid complex	10 mg	IV	**J0287-J0289**
Ampicillin			
sodium	up to 500 mg	IM, IV	**J0290**
sodium/sulbactam sodium	per 1.5 g	IM, IV	**J0295**
Amygdalin			J3570
Amytal	up to 125 mg	IM, IV	J0300
Anabolin LA 100	up to 50 mg	IM	J2320
Anadulafungin	1 mg	IV	**J0348**

◀ New ⊋ Revised ✔ Reinstated ~~deleted~~ Deleted

DRUG NAME	DOSAGE	METHOD OF ADMINISTRATION	HCPCS CODE
Anascorp	up to 120 mg	IV	J0716
Anastrozole	1 mg		J8999
Ancef	500 mg	IV, IM	J0690
Andrest 90-4	1 mg	IM	J3121
Andro-Cyp	1 mg		J1071
Andro-Cyp 200	1 mg		J1071
Andro L.A. 200	1 mg	IM	J3121
Andro-Estro 90-4	1 mg	IM	J3121
Andro/Fem	1 mg		J1071
Androgyn L.A.	1 mg	IM	J3121
Androlone-50	up to 50 mg		J2320
Androlone-D 100	up to 50 mg	IM	J2320
Andronaq-50	up to 50 mg	IM	J3140
Andronaq-LA	1 mg		J1071
Andronate-100	1 mg		J1071
Andronate-200	1 mg		J1071
Andropository 100	1 mg	IM	J3121
Andryl 200	1 mg	IM	J3121
Anectine	up to 20 mg	IM, IV	J0330
Anergan 25	up to 50 mg	IM, IV	J2550
	12.5 mg	ORAL	Q0169
Anergan 50	up to 50 mg	IM, IV	J2550
	12.5 mg	ORAL	Q0169
Angiomax	1 mg		J0583
Anidulafungin	1 mg	IV	J0348
Anistreplase	30 units	IV	**J0350**
Antiflex	up to 60 mg	IM, IV	J2360
Anti-Inhibitor	per IU	IV	**J7198**
Antispas	up to 20 mg	IM	J0500
Antithrombin III (human)	per IU	IV	**J7197**
Antithrombin recombinant	50 IU	IV	**J7196**
Anzemet	10 mg	IV	J1260
	50 mg	ORAL	S0174
	100 mg	ORAL	Q0180
Apidra Solostar	per 50 units		J1817
A.P.L.	per 1,000 USP units	IM	J0725
Apligraf	per square centimeter		Q4101
Apomorphine Hydrochloride	1 mg	SC	**J0364**
Aprepitant	1 mg	IV	**J0185**
Aprepitant	5 mg	ORAL	J8501

◀ New ⤾ Revised ✔ Reinstated ~~deleted~~ Deleted

DRUG NAME	DOSAGE	METHOD OF ADMINISTRATION	HCPCS CODE
Apresoline	up to 20 mg	IV, IM	J0360
Aprotinin	10,000 kiu		**J0365**
AquaMEPHYTON	per 1 mg	IM, SC, IV	J3430
Aralast	10 mg	IV	J0256
Aralen	up to 250 mg	IM	J0390
Aramine	per 10 mg	IV, IM, SC	J0380
Aranesp			
ESRD use	1 mcg		J0882
Non-ESRD use	1 mcg		J0881
Arbutamine	1 mg	IV	**J0395**
Arcalyst	1 mg		J2793
Aredia	per 30 mg	IV	J2430
Arfonad, *see* Trimethaphan camsylate			
Arformoterol tartrate	15 mcg	INH	**J7605**
Argatroban			
(for ESRD use)	1 mg	IV	**J0884**
(for non-ESRD use)	1 mg	IV	**J0883**
Aridol	25% in 50 ml	IV	J2150
	5 mg	INH	J7665
Arimidex			J8999
Aripiprazole	0.25 mg	IM	**J0400**
Aripiprazole, extended release	1 mg	IV	**J0401**
Aripiprazole lauroxil (aristada)	1 mg	IV	**J1944**
Aripiprazole lauroxil (aristada initio)	1 mg	IV	**J1943**
Aristocort Forte	per 5 mg	IM	J3302
Aristocort Intralesional	per 5 mg	IM	J3302
Aristospan Intra-Articular	per 5 mg	VAR	J3303
Aristospan Intralesional	per 5 mg	VAR	J3303
Arixtra	per 0.5 m		J1652
Aromasin			J8999
Arranon	50 mg		J9261
Arrestin	up to 200 mg	IM	J3250
	250 mg	ORAL	Q0173
Arsenic trioxide	1 mg	IV	**J9017**
Arzerra	10 mg		J9302
Asparaginase	1,000 units	IV, IM	**J9019**
	10,000 units	IV, IM	**J9020**
Astagraf XL	0.1 mg		J7508
Astramorph PF	up to 10 mg	IM, IV, SC	J2270
Atezolizumab	10 mg	IV	**J9022**

◀ **New** ⤺ **Revised** ✔ **Reinstated** ~~deleted~~ **Deleted**

DRUG NAME	DOSAGE	METHOD OF ADMINISTRATION	HCPCS CODE
Atgam	250 mg	IV	J7504
Ativan	2 mg	IM, IV	J2060
Atropine			
concentrated form	per mg	INH	J7635
unit dose form	per mg	INH	J7636
sulfate	0.01 mg	IV, IM, SC	J0461, J7636
Atrovent	per mg	INH	J7644, J7645
ATryn	50 IU	IV	J7196
Aurothioglucose	up to 50 mg	IM	J2910
Autologous cultured chondrocytes implant		OTH	J7330
Autoplex T	per IU	IV	J7198, J7199
AUVI-Q	0.15 mg		J0171
Avastin	10 mg		J9035
Avelox	100 mg		J2280
Avelumab	10 mg	IV	J9023
Avonex	30 mcg	IM	J1826
	1 mcg	IM	Q3027
	1 mcg	SC	Q3028
Azacitidine	1 mg	SC	J9025
Azasan	50 mg		J7500
Azathioprine	50 mg	ORAL	J7500
Azathioprine, parenteral	100 mg	IV	J7501
Azithromycin, dihydrate	1 gram	ORAL	Q0144
Azithromycin, injection	500 mg	IV	J0456
B			
Baciim			J3490
Bacitracin			J3490
Baclofen	10 mg	IT	J0475
Baclofen for intrathecal trial	50 mcg	OTH	J0476
Bactocill	up to 250 mg	IM, IV	J2700
BAL in oil	per 100 mg	IM	J0470
Banflex	up to 60 mg	IV, IM	J2360
Basiliximab	20 mg	IV	J0480
BCG live intravesical instillation	1 mg	OTH	J9030
Bebulin	per IU		J7194
Beclomethasone inhalation solution, unit dose form	per mg	INH	J7622
Belatacept	1 mg	IV	J0485
Beleodaq	10 mg		J9032
Belimumab	10 mg	IV	J0490
Belinostat	10 mg	IV	J9032

◀ New ↩ Revised ✔ Reinstated ~~deleted~~ Deleted

DRUG NAME	DOSAGE	METHOD OF ADMINISTRATION	HCPCS CODE
Bena-D 10	up to 50 mg	IV, IM	J1200
Bena-D 50	up to 50 mg	IV, IM	J1200
Benadryl	up to 50 mg	IV, IM	J1200
Benahist 10	up to 50 mg	IV, IM	J1200
Benahist 50	up to 50 mg	IV, IM	J1200
Ben-Allergin-50	up to 50 mg	IV, IM	J1200
	50 mg	ORAL	Q0163
Bendamustine HCl			
Bendeka	1 mg	IV	**J9034**
Treanda	1 mg	IV	**J9033**
Bendamustine HCl (Belrapzo/bendamustine)	1 mg	IV	**J9036**
Benefix	per IU	IV	J7195
Benlysta	10 mg		J0490
Benoject-10	up to 50 mg	IV, IM	J1200
Benoject-50	up to 50 mg	IV, IM	J1200
Benralizumab	1 mg	IV	**J0517**
Bentyl	up to 20 mg	IM	J0500
Benzocaine			J3490
Benztropine mesylate	per 1 mg	IM, IV	**J0515**
Berinert	10 units		J0597
Berubigen	up to 1,000 mcg	IM, SC	J3420
Beta amyloid	per study dose	OTH	**A9599**
Betalin 12	up to 1,000 mcg	IM, SC	J3420
Betameth	per 3 mg	IM, IV	J0702
Betamethasone Acetate			J3490
Betamethasone Acetate & Betamethasone Sodium Phosphate	per 3 mg	IM	**J0702**
Betamethasone inhalation solution, unit dose form	per mg	INH	**J7624**
Betaseron	0.25 mg	SC	J1830
Bethanechol chloride	up to 5 mg	SC	**J0520**
Bethkis	300 mg		J7682
Bevacizumab	10 mg	IV	**J9035**
Bevacizumab-awwb	10 mg	IV	**Q5107**
Bevacizumab-bvzr (Zirabev)	10 mg	IV	**Q5118**
Bezlotoxumab	10 mg	IV	**J0565**
Bicillin C-R	100,000 units		J0558
Bicillin C-R 900/300	100,000 units	IM	J0558, J0561
Bicillin L-A	100,000 units	IM	J0561
BiCNU	100 mg	IV	J9050
Bimatoprost	1 microgram	IV	J7351 ◀
Biperiden lactate	per 5 mg	IM, IV	**J0190**

◀ New ⮌ Revised ✔ Reinstated ~~deleted~~ Deleted

DRUG NAME	DOSAGE	METHOD OF ADMINISTRATION	HCPCS CODE
Bitolterol mesylate			
concentrated form	per mg	INH	J7628
unit dose form	per mg	INH	J7629
Bivalirudin	1 mg	IV	J0583
Blenoxane	15 units	IM, IV, SC	J9040
Bleomycin sulfate	15 units	IM, IV, SC	J9040
Blinatumomab	1 microgram	IV	J9039
Blincyto	1 mcg		J9039
Boniva	1 mg		J1740
Bortezomib	0.1 mg	IV	J9041
Bortezomib, not otherwise specified	0.1 mg		J9044
Botox	1 unit		J0585
Bravelle	75 IU		J3355
Brentuximab Vedotin	1 mg	IV	J9042
Brethine			
concentrated form	per 1 mg	INH	J7680
unit dose	per 1 mg	INH	J7681
	up to 1 mg	SC, IV	J3105
Brexanolone	1 mg	IV	J1632 ◀
Bricanyl Subcutaneous	up to 1 mg	SC, IV	J3105
Brompheniramine maleate	per 10 mg	IM, SC, IV	J0945
Bronkephrine, *see* Ethylnorepinephrine HCl			
Bronkosol			
concentrated form	per mg	INH	J7647, J7648
unit dose form	per mg	INH	J7649, J7650
Brovana			J7605
Budesonide inhalation solution			
concentrated form	0.25 mg	INH	J7633, J7634
unit dose form	0.5 mg	INH	J7626, J7627
Bumetanide			J3490
Bupivacaine			J3490
Buprenex	0.3 mg		J0592
Buprenorphine Hydrochloride	0.1 mg	IM	J0592
Buprenorphine/Naloxone	1 mg	ORAL	J0571
	< = 3 mg	ORAL	J0572
	> 3 mg but < = 6 mg	ORAL	J0573
	> 6 mg but < = 10 mg	ORAL	J0574
	> 10 mg	ORAL	J0575
Buprenorphine extended release	< = 100 mg	ORAL	Q9991
	> 100 mg	ORAL	Q9992

◀ New ⮌ Revised ✔ Reinstated ~~deleted~~ Deleted

DRUG NAME	DOSAGE	METHOD OF ADMINISTRATION	HCPCS CODE
Burosumab-twza	1 mg	IV	J05894
Busulfan	1 mg	IV	J0594
	2 mg	ORAL	J8510
Butorphanol tartrate	1 mg		J0595
C			
C1 Esterase Inhibitor	10 units	IV	J0596-J0599
Cabazitaxel	1 mg	IV	J9043
Cabergoline	0.25 mg	ORAL	J8515
Cafcit	5 mg	IV	J0706
Caffeine citrate	5 mg	IV	J0706
Caine-1	10 mg	IV	J2001
Caine-2	10 mg	IV	J2001
Calaspargase pegol-mknl	10 units	IV	J9118
Calcijex	0.1 mcg	IM	J0636
Calcimar	up to 400 units	SC, IM	J0630
Calcitonin-salmon	up to 400 units	SC, IM	J0630
Calcitriol	0.1 mcg	IM	J0636
Calcitrol			J8499
Calcium Disodium Versenate	up to 1,000 mg	IV, SC, IM	J0600
Calcium gluconate	per 10 ml	IV	J0610
Calcium glycerophosphate and calcium lactate	per 10 ml	IM, SC	J0620
Caldolor	100 mg	IV	J1741
Calphosan	per 10 ml	IM, SC	J0620
Camptosar	20 mg	IV	J9206
Canakinumab	1 mg	SC	J0638
Cancidas	5 mg		J0637
Capecitabine	150 mg	ORAL	J8520
	500 mg	ORAL	J8521
Capsaicin patch	per sq cm	OTH	J7336
Carbidopa 5 mg/levodopa 20 mg enteral suspension		IV	J7340
Carbocaine	per 10 ml	VAR	J0670
Carbocaine with Neo-Cobefrin	per 10 ml	VAR	J0670
Carboplatin	50 mg	IV	J9045
Carfilzomib	1 mg	IV	J9047
Carimune	500 mg		J1566
Carmustine	100 mg	IV	J9050
Carnitor	per 1 g	IV	J1955
Carticel			J7330
Caspofungin acetate	5 mg	IV	J0637
Cathflo Activase	1 mg		J2997

◀ New ⮌ Revised ✔ Reinstated ~~deleted~~ Deleted

DRUG NAME	DOSAGE	METHOD OF ADMINISTRATION	HCPCS CODE
Caverject	per 1.25 mcg		J0270
Cayston	500 mg		S0073
Cefadyl	up to 1 g	IV, IM	J0710
Cefazolin sodium	500 mg	IV, IM	J0690
Cefepime hydrochloride	500 mg	IV	J0692
Cefiderocol	5 mg	IV	J0693 ◀
Cefizox	per 500 mg	IM, IV	J0715
Cefotaxime sodium	per 1 g	IV, IM	J0698
Cefotetan			J3490
Cefoxitin sodium	1 g	IV, IM	J0694
Ceftaroline fosamil	1 mg		J0712
Ceftazidime	per 500 mg	IM, IV	J0713
Ceftazidime and avibactam	0.5 g/0.125 g	IV	J0714
Ceftizoxime sodium	per 500 mg	IV, IM	J0715
Ceftolozane 50 mg and Tazobactam 25 mg		IV	J0695
Ceftriaxone sodium	per 250 mg	IV, IM	J0696
Cefuroxime sodium, sterile	per 750 mg	IM, IV	J0697
Celestone Soluspan	per 3 mg	IM	J0702
CellCept	250 mg	ORAL	J7517
Cel-U-Jec	per 4 mg	IM, IV	Q0511
Cenacort A-40	1 mg		J3300
	per 10 mg	IM	J3301
Cenacort Forte	per 5 mg	IM	J3302
Centruroides Immune F(ab)	up to 120 mg	IV	J0716
Cephalothin sodium	up to 1 g	IM, IV	J1890
Cephapirin sodium	up to 1 g	IV, IM	J0710
Ceprotin	10 IU		J2724
Ceredase	per 10 units	IV	J0205
Cerezyme	10 units		J1786
Cerliponase alfa	1 mg	IV	J0567
Certolizumab pegol	1 mg	SC	J0717
Cerubidine	10 mg	IV	J9150
Cetirizine hydrochloride	0.5 mg	IM	J1201 ◀
Cetuximab	10 mg	IV	J9055
Chealamide	per 150 mg	IV	J3520
Chirhostim	1 mcg	IV	J2850
Chloramphenicol Sodium Succinate	up to 1 g	IV	J0720
Chlordiazepoxide HCl	up to 100 mg	IM, IV	J1990
Chloromycetin Sodium Succinate	up to 1 g	IV	J0720
Chloroprocaine HCl	per 30 ml	VAR	J2400

◀ New ⤺ Revised ✔ Reinstated ~~deleted~~ Deleted

DRUG NAME	DOSAGE	METHOD OF ADMINISTRATION	HCPCS CODE
Chloroquine HCl	up to 250 mg	IM	J0390
Chlorothiazide sodium	per 500 mg	IV	J1205
Chlorpromazine	5 mg	ORAL	Q0161
Chlorpromazine HCl	up to 50 mg	IM, IV	J3230
Cholografin Meglumine	per ml		Q9961
Chorex-5	per 1,000 USP units	IM	J0725
Chorex-10	per 1,000 USP units	IM	J0725
Chorignon	per 1,000 USP units	IM	J0725
Chorionic Gonadotropin	per 1,000 USP units	IM	J0725
Choron 10	per 1,000 USP units	IM	J0725
Cidofovir	375 mg	IV	J0740
Cilastatin sodium, imipenem	per 250 mg	IV, IM	J0743
Cimzia	1 mg	SC	J0717
Cinacalcet		ORAL	J0604
Cinryze	10 units		J0598
Cipro IV	200 mg	IV	J0706
Ciprofloxacin	200 mg	IV	J0706
otic suspension	6 mg	OTH	J7342
			J3490
Cisplatin, powder or solution	per 10 mg	IV	J9060
Cladribine	per mg	IV	J9065
Claforan	per 1 gm	IM, IV	J0698
Cleocin Phosphate			J3490
Clindamycin			J3490
Clofarabine	1 mg	IV	J9027
Clolar	1 mg		J9027
Clonidine Hydrochloride	1 mg	Epidural	J0735
Coagulation factor Xa (recombinant), inactivated-zhzo (Andexxa)	10 mg		J7169 ◀
Cobex	up to 1,000 mcg	IM, SC	J3420
Codeine phosphate	per 30 mg	IM, IV, SC	J0745
Codimal-A	per 10 mg	IM, SC, IV	J0945
Cogentin	per 1 mg	IM, IV	J0515
Colistimethate sodium	up to 150 mg	IM, IV	J0770
Collagenase, Clostridium Histolyticum	0.01 mg	OTH	J0775
Coly-Mycin M	up to 150 mg	IM, IV	J0770
Compa-Z	up to 10 mg	IM, IV	J0780
Copanlisib	1 mg	IV	J9057
Compazine	up to 10 mg	IM, IV	J0780
	5 mg	ORAL	Q0164
			J8498

◀ New ⮌ Revised ✔ Reinstated ~~deleted~~ Deleted

DRUG NAME	DOSAGE	METHOD OF ADMINISTRATION	HCPCS CODE
Compounded drug, not otherwise classified			J7999
Compro			J8498
Conray	per ml		Q9961
Conray 30	per ml		Q9958
Conray 43	per ml		Q9960
Copaxone	20 mg		J1595
Cophene-B	per 10 mg	IM, SC, IV	J0945
Copper contraceptive, intrauterine		OTH	J7300
Cordarone	30 mg	IV	J0282
Corgonject-5	per 1,000 USP units	IM	J0725
Corifact	1 IU		J7180
Corticorelin ovine triflutate	1 mcg		J0795
Corticotropin	up to 40 units	IV, IM, SC	J0800
Cortisone Acetate Micronized			J3490
Cortrosyn	per 0.25 mg	IM, IV	J0835
Corvert	1 mg		J1742
Cosmegen	0.5 mg	IV	J9120
Cosyntropin	per 0.25 mg	IM, IV	J0833, J0834
Cotranzine	up to 10 mg	IM, IV	J0780
Crizanlizumab-tmca		IV	J0791 ◀
Crofab	up to 1 gram		J0840
Cromolyn Sodium			J8499
Cromolyn sodium, unit dose form	per 10 mg	INH	J7631, J7632
Crotalidae immune f(ab')2 (equine)	120 mg	IV	J0841
Crotalidae Polyvalent Immune Fab	up to 1 gram	IV	J0840
Crysticillin 600 A.S.	up to 600,000 units	IM, IV	J2510
Cubicin	1 mg		J0878
Cuvitru			J7799
Cyclophosphamide	100 mg	IV	J9070
oral	25 mg	ORAL	J8530
Cyclosporine	25 mg	ORAL	J7515
	100 mg	ORAL	J7502
parenteral	250 mg	IV	J7516
Cymetra	1 cc		Q4112
Cyramza	5 mg		J9308
Cysto-Conray II	per ml		Q9958
Cystografin	per ml		Q9958
Cytarabine	100 mg	SC, IV	J9100
Cytarabine liposome	10 mg	IT	J9098
CytoGam	per vial		J0850

◀ New ⤻ Revised ✔ Reinstated ~~deleted~~ Deleted

DRUG NAME	DOSAGE	METHOD OF ADMINISTRATION	HCPCS CODE
Cytomegalovirus immune globulin intravenous (human)	per vial	IV	**J0850**
Cytosar-U	100 mg	SC, IV	J9100
Cytovene	500 mg	IV	J1570
Cytoxan	100 mg	IV	J8530, J9070
D			
D-5-W, infusion	1000 cc	IV	**J7070**
Dacarbazine	100 mg	IV	**J9130**
Daclizumab	25 mg	IV	**J7513**
Dacogen	1 mg		J0894
Dactinomycin	0.5 mg	IV	**J9120**
Dalalone	1 mg	IM, IV, OTH	J1100
Dalalone L.A.	1 mg	IM	J1094
Dalbavancin	5 mg	IV	**J0875**
Dalteparin sodium	per 2500 IU	SC	**J1645**
Daptomycin	1 mg	IV	**J0878**
Daratumumab	10 mg	IV	**J9145**
Darbepoetin Alfa	1 mcg	IV, SC	**J0881, J0882**
Darzalex	10 mg		J9145
Daunorubicin citrate, liposomal formulation	10 mg	IV	**J9151**
Daunorubicin HCl	10 mg	IV	**J9150**
Daunoxome	10 mg	IV	J9151
DDAVP	1 mcg	IV, SC	J2597
Decadron	1 mg	IM, IV, OTH	J1100
	0.25 mg		J8540
Decadron Phosphate	1 mg	IM, IV, OTH	J1100
Decadron-LA	1 mg	IM	J1094
Deca-Durabolin	up to 50 mg	IM	J2320
Decaject	1 mg	IM, IV, OTH	J1100
Decaject-L.A.	1 mg	IM	J1094
Decitabine	1 mg	IV	**J0894**
Decolone-50	up to 50 mg	IM	J2320
Decolone-100	up to 50 mg	IM	J2320
De-Comberol	1 mg		J1071
Deferoxamine mesylate	500 mg	IM, SC, IV	**J0895**
Definity	per ml		J3490, Q9957
Degarelix	1 mg	SC	**J9155**
Dehist	per 10 mg	IM, SC, IV	J0945
Deladumone	1 mg	IM	J3121
Deladumone OB	1 mg	IM	J3121
Delatest	1 mg	IM	J3121
Delatestadiol	1 mg	IM	J3121

◀ New ⤺ Revised ✔ Reinstated ~~deleted~~ Deleted

DRUG NAME	DOSAGE	METHOD OF ADMINISTRATION	HCPCS CODE
Delatestryl	1 mg	IM	J3121
Delestrogen	up to 10 mg	IM	J1380
Delta-Cortef	5 mg	ORAL	J7510
Demadex	10 mg/ml	IV	J3265
Demerol HCl	per 100 mg	IM, IV, SC	J2175
Denileukin diftitox	300 mcg	IV	**J9160**
Denosumab	1 mg	SC	**J0897**
Deoxycholic acid	1 mg	IM	J0591 ◀
DepAndro 100	1 mg		J1071
DepAndro 200	1 mg		J1071
DepAndrogyn	1 mg		J1071
DepGynogen	up to 5 mg	IM	J1000
DepMedalone 40	20 mg	IM	J1020
	40 mg	IM	J1030
	80 mg	IM	J1040
DepMedalone 80	20 mg	IM	J1020
	40 mg	IM	J1030
	80 mg	IM	J1040
DepoCyt	10 mg		J9098
Depo-estradiol cypionate	up to 5 mg	IM	**J1000**
Depogen	up to 5 mg	IM	J1000
Depoject	20 mg	IM	J1020
	40 mg	IM	J1030
	80 mg	IM	J1040
Depo-Medrol	20 mg	IM	J1020
	40 mg	IM	J1030
	80 mg	IM	J1040
Depopred-40	20 mg	IM	J1020
	40 mg	IM	J1030
	80 mg	IM	J1040
Depopred-80	20 mg	IM	J1020
	40 mg	IM	J1030
	80 mg	IM	J1040
Depo-Provera Contraceptive	1 mg		J1050
Depotest	1 mg		J1071
Depo-Testadiol	1 mg		J1071
Depo-Testosterone	1 mg		J1071
Depotestrogen	1 mg		J1071
Dermagraft	per square centimeter		Q4106
Desferal Mesylate	500 mg	IM, SC, IV	J0895
Desmopressin acetate	1 mcg	IV, SC	**J2597**

◀ **New** ↩ **Revised** ✔ **Reinstated** ~~deleted~~ **Deleted**

DRUG NAME	DOSAGE	METHOD OF ADMINISTRATION	HCPCS CODE
Dexacen-4	1 mg	IM, IV, OTH	J1100
Dexacen LA-8	1 mg	IM	J1094
Dexamethasone			
concentrated form	per mg	INH	**J7637**
intravitreal implant	0.1 mg	OTH	**J7312**
lacrimal ophthalmic insert	0.1 mg	OTH	**J1096**
unit form	per mg	INH	**J7638**
oral	0.25 mg	ORAL	**J8540**
acetate	1 mg	IM	**J1094**
sodium phosphate	1 mg	IM, IV, OTH	**J1100**
Dexasone	1 mg	IM, IV, OTH	J1100
Dexasone L.A.	1 mg	IM	J1094
Dexferrum	50 mg		J1750
Dexone	0.25 mg	ORAL	J8540
	1 mg	IM, IV, OTH	J1100
Dexone LA	1 mg	IM	J1094
Dexpak	0.25 mg	ORAL	J8540
Dexrazoxane hydrochloride	250 mg	IV	**J1190**
Dextran 40	500 ml	IV	**J7100**
Dextran 75	500 ml	IV	**J7110**
Dextrose 5%/normal saline solution	500 ml = 1 unit	IV	**J7042**
Dextrose/water (5%)	500 ml = 1 unit	IV	**J7060**
D.H.E. 45	per 1 mg		J1110
Diamox	up to 500 mg	IM, IV	J1120
Diazepam	up to 5 mg	IM, IV	**J3360**
Diazoxide	up to 300 mg	IV	**J1730**
Dibent	up to 20 mg	IM	J0500
Diclofenac sodium	37.5	IV	**J1130**
Dicyclomine HCl	up to 20 mg	IM	**J0500**
Didronel	per 300 mg	IV	J1436
Diethylstilbestrol diphosphate	250 mg	IV	**J9165**
Diflucan	200 mg	IV	J1450
DigiFab	per vial		J1162
Digoxin	up to 0.5 mg	IM, IV	**J1160**
Digoxin immune fab (ovine)	per vial		**J1162**
Dihydrex	up to 50 mg	IV, IM	J1200
	50 mg	ORAL	Q0163
Dihydroergotamine mesylate	per 1 mg	IM, IV	**J1110**
Dilantin	per 50 mg	IM, IV	J1165

◀ New ⊋ Revised ✔ Reinstated ~~deleted~~ Deleted

DRUG NAME	DOSAGE	METHOD OF ADMINISTRATION	HCPCS CODE
Dilaudid	up to 4 mg	SC, IM, IV	J1170
	250 mg	OTH	S0092
Dilocaine	10 mg	IV	J2001
Dilomine	up to 20 mg	IM	J0500
Dilor	up to 500 mg	IM	J1180
Dimenhydrinate	up to 50 mg	IM, IV	**J1240**
Dimercaprol	per 100 mg	IM	**J0470**
Dimethyl sulfoxide	50%, 50 ml	OTH	J1212
Dinate	up to 50 mg	IM, IV	J1240
Dioval	up to 10 mg	IM	J1380
Dioval 40	up to 10 mg	IM	J1380
Dioval XX	up to 10 mg	IM	J1380
Diphenacen-50	up to 50 mg	IV, IM	J1200
	50 mg	ORAL	Q0163
Diphenhydramine HCl			
injection	up to 50 mg	IV, IM	**J1200**
oral	50 mg	ORAL	**Q0163**
Diprivan	10 mg		J2704
			J3490
Dipyridamole	per 10 mg	IV	**J1245**
Disotate	per 150 mg	IV	J3520
Di-Spaz	up to 20 mg	IM	J0500
Ditate-DS	1 mg	IM	J3121
Diuril Sodium	per 500 mg	IV	J1205
D-Med 80	20 mg	IM	J1020
	40 mg	IM	J1030
	80 mg	IM	J1040
DMSO, Dimethyl sulfoxide 50%	50 ml	OTH	**J1212**
Dobutamine HCl	per 250 mg	IV	**J1250**
Dobutrex	per 250 mg	IV	J1250
Docefrez	1 mg		J9171
Docetaxel	20 mg	IV	**J9170**
Dolasetron mesylate			
injection	10 mg	IV	**J1260**
tablets	100 mg	ORAL	**Q0180**
Dolophine HCl	up to 10 mg	IM, SC	J1230
Dommanate	up to 50 mg	IM, IV	J1240
Donbax	10 mg		J1267
Dopamine	40 mg		**J1265**

◀ New ↩ Revised ✔ Reinstated ~~deleted~~ Deleted

DRUG NAME	DOSAGE	METHOD OF ADMINISTRATION	HCPCS CODE
Dopamine HCl	40 mg		J1265
Doribax	10 mg		J1267
Doripenem	10 mg	IV	J1267
Dornase alpha, unit dose form	per mg	INH	J7639
Dotarem	0.1 ml		A9575
Doxercalciferol	1 mcg	IV	J1270
Doxil	10 mg	IV	J9000, Q2050
Doxorubicin HCL	10 mg	IV	J9000
Doxy	100 mg		J3490
Dramamine	up to 50 mg	IM, IV	J1240
Dramanate	up to 50 mg	IM, IV	J1240
Dramilin	up to 50 mg	IM, IV	J1240
Dramocen	up to 50 mg	IM, IV	J1240
Dramoject	up to 50 mg	IM, IV	J1240
Dronabinol	2.5 mg	ORAL	Q0167
Droperidol	up to 5 mg	IM, IV	J1790
Droperidol and fentanyl citrate	up to 2 ml ampule	IM, IV	J1810
Droxia		ORAL	J8999
Drug administered through a metered dose inhaler		INH	J3535
DTIC-Dome	100 mg	IV	J9130
Dua-Gen L.A.	1 mg	IM	J3121
DuoNeb	up to 2.5 mg		J7620
Duopa	20 ml		J7340
Duoval P.A.	1 mg	IM	J3121
Durabolin	up to 50 mg	IM	J2320
Duracillin A.S.	up to 600,000 units	IM, IV	J2510
Duraclon	1 mg	Epidural	J0735
Dura-Estrin	up to 5 mg	IM	J1000
Duragen-10	up to 10 mg	IM	J1380
Duragen-20	up to 10 mg	IM	J1380
Duragen-40	up to 10 mg	IM	J1380
Duralone-40	20 mg	IM	J1020
	40 mg	IM	J1030
	80 mg	IM	J1040
Duralone-80	20 mg	IM	J1020
	40 mg	IM	J1030
	80 mg	IM	J1040
Duralutin, *see* Hydroxyprogesterone Caproate			
Duramorph	up to 10 mg	IM, IV, SC	J2270, J2274
Duratest-100	1 mg		J1071

◀ New ⮐ Revised ✔ Reinstated ~~deleted~~ Deleted

DRUG NAME	DOSAGE	METHOD OF ADMINISTRATION	HCPCS CODE
Duratest-200	1 mg		J1071
Duratestrin	1 mg		J1071
Durathate-200	1 mg	IM	J3121
Durvalumab	10 mg	IV	**J9173**
Dymenate	up to 50 mg	IM, IV	J1240
Dyphylline	up to 500 mg	IM	**J1180**
Dysport	5 units		J0586
Dalvance	5 mg		J0875
E			
Ecallantide	1 mg	SC	**J1290**
Eculizumab	10 mg	IV	**J1300**
Edaravone	1 mg	IV	**J1301**
Edetate calcium disodium	up to 1,000 mg	IV, SC, IM	**J0600**
Edetate disodium	per 150 mg	IV	**J3520**
Elaprase	1 mg		J1743
Elavil	up to 20 mg	IM	J1320
Elelyso	10 units		J3060
Eligard	7.5 mg		J9217
Elitek	0.5 mg		J2783
Ellence	2 mg		J9178
Elliotts B solution	1 ml	OTH	**J9175**
Eloctate	per IU		J7205
Elosulfase alfa	1 mg	IV	**J1322**
Elotuzumab	1 mg	IV	**J9176**
Eloxatin	0.5 mg		J9263
Elspar	10,000 units	IV, IM	J9020
Emapalunab-lzsg	1 mg	IV	**J9210**
Emend			J1453, J8501
Emete-Con, *see* Benzquinamide			
Eminase	30 units	IV	J0350
Empliciti	1 mg		J9176
Enbrel	25 mg	IM, IV	J1438
Endrate ethylenediamine-tetra-acetic acid	per 150 mg	IV	J3520
Enfortumab vedotin-ejfv	0.25 mg	IM	J9177 ◀
Enfuvirtide	1 mg	SC	**J1324**
Engerix-B			J3490
Enovil	up to 20 mg	IM	J1320
Enoxaparin sodium	10 mg	SC	**J1650**
Entyvio			J3380
Eovist	1 ml		A9581

◀ New ↩ Revised ✔ Reinstated ~~deleted~~ Deleted

DRUG NAME	DOSAGE	METHOD OF ADMINISTRATION	HCPCS CODE
Epinephrine			J7799
Epinephrine, adrenalin	0.1 mg	SC, IM	**J0171**
Epirubicin hydrochloride	2 mg		**J9178**
Epoetin alfa	100 units	IV, SC	**Q4081**
Epoetin alfa, non-ESRD use	1000 units	IV	**J0885**
Epoetin alfa, ESRD use	100 mg	IV, SC	**Q5105**
Epoetin alfa, non-ESRD use	1000 units	IV	**Q5106**
Epoetin alfa-epbx (Retacrit) non-ESRD use	1000 units	IV	**Q5106**
Epoetin alfa-epbx (Retacrit) for-ESRD use	100 units	IV	**Q5105**
Epoetin beta, ESRD use	1 mcg	IV	**J0887**
Epoetin beta, non-ESRD use	1 mcg	IV	**J0888**
Epogen	1,000 units		J0885
			Q4081
Epoprostenol	0.5 mg	IV	**J1325**
Eptifibatide, injection	5 mg	IM, IV	**J1327**
Eptinezumab-jjmr	1 mg	IV	J3032 ◀
Eravacycline	1 mg	IV	**J0122**
Eraxis	1 mg	IV	J0348
Erbitux	10 mg		J9055
Ergonovine maleate	up to 0.2 mg	IM, IV	**J1330**
Eribulin mesylate	0.1 mg	IV	**J9179**
Erivedge	150 mg		J8999
Ertapenem sodium	500 mg	IM, IV	**J1335**
Erwinase	1,000 units	IV, IM	J9019
	10,000 units	IV, IM	J9020
Erythromycin lactobionate	500 mg	IV	**J1364**
Estra-D	up to 5 mg	IM	J1000
Estradiol			
L.A.	up to 10 mg	IM	J1380
L.A. 20	up to 10 mg	IM	J1380
L.A. 40	up to 10 mg	IM	J1380
Estradiol cypionate	up to 5 mg	IM	J1000
Estradiol valerate	up to 10 mg	IM	**J1380**
Estra-L 20	up to 10 mg	IM	J1380
Estra-L 40	up to 10 mg	IM	J1380
Estra-Testrin	1 mg	IM	J3121
Estro-Cyp	up to 5 mg	IM	J1000
Estrogen, conjugated	per 25 mg	IV, IM	**J1410**
Estroject L.A.	up to 5 mg	IM	J1000
Estrone	per 1 mg	IM	**J1435**

◀ New ⟲ Revised ✔ Reinstated ~~deleted~~ Deleted

DRUG NAME	DOSAGE	METHOD OF ADMINISTRATION	HCPCS CODE
Estrone 5	per 1 mg	IM	J1435
Estrone Aqueous	per 1 mg	IM	J1435
Estronol	per 1 mg	IM	J1435
Estronol-L.A.	up to 5 mg	IM	J1000
Etanercept, injection	25 mg	IM, IV	**J1438**
Etelcalcetide	0.1 mg	IV	**Q4078**
Eteplirsen	10 mg	IV	**J1428**
Ethamolin	100 mg		J1430
Ethanolamine	100 mg		**J1430**, J3490
Ethyol	500 mg	IV	J0207
Etidronate disodium	per 300 mg	IV	**J1436**
Etonogestrel implant			**J7307**
Etopophos	10 mg	IV	J9181
Etoposide	10 mg	IV	**J9181**
oral	50 mg	ORAL	**J8560**
Euflexxa	per dose	OTH	**J7323**
Everolimus	0.25 mg	ORAL	**J7527**
Everone	1 mg	IM	J3121
Evomela	50 mg		J9245
Eylea	1 mg	OTH	J0178
F			
Fabrazyme	1 mg	IV	J0180
Factor IX			
anti-hemophilic factor, purified, non-recombinant	per IU	IV	**J7193**
anti-hemophilic factor, recombinant	per IU	IV	**J7195, J7200-J7202**
complex	per IU	IV	**J7194**
Factor VIIa (coagulation factor, recombinant)	1 mcg	IV	**J7189, J7212** ⮌
Factor VIII (anti-hemophilic factor)	per IU	IV	**J7208**
human	per IU	IV	**J7190**
porcine	per IU	IV	**J7191**
recombinant	per IU	IV	**J7182, J7185, J7192, J7188**
Factor VIII (anti-hemophilic factor, recombinant)			
(Afstyla)	per IU	IV	**J7210**
(Kovaltry)	per IU	IV	**J7211**
Factor VIII, anti-hemophilic factor (recombinant)(esperoct)	per IU	IV	J7204 ◀
Factor VIII Fc fusion (recombinant)	per IU	IV	**J7205, J7207, J7209**
Factor X (human)	per IU	IV	**J7175**
Factor XIII A-subunit (recombinant)	per IU	IV	**J7181**

◀ New ⮌ Revised ✔ Reinstated ~~deleted~~ Deleted

DRUG NAME	DOSAGE	METHOD OF ADMINISTRATION	HCPCS CODE
Factors, other hemophilia clotting	per IU	IV	J7196
Factrel	per 100 mcg	SC, IV	J1620
Fam-trastuzumab deruxtecan-nxki	1 mg	IM	J9358 ◀
Famotidine			J3490
Faslodex	25 mg		J9395
Feiba NF			J7198
Feiba VH Immuno	per IU	IV	J7196
Fentanyl citrate	0.1 mg	IM, IV	J3010
Feraheme	1 mg		Q0138, Q0139
Ferric carboxymaltose	1 mg	IV	J1439
Ferric pyrophosphate citrate powder	0.1 mg of iron	IV	J1444
Ferric pyrophosphate citrate solution	0.1 mg of iron	IV	J1443
Ferrlecit	12.5 mg		J2916
Ferumoxytol	1 mg		Q0138, Q0139
Filgrastim-aafi	1 mcg	IV	Q5110
Filgrastim			
(G-CSF)	1 mcg	SC, IV	J1442, Q5101
(TBO)	1 mcg	IV	J1447
Firazyr	1 mg	SC	J1744
Firmagon	1 mg		J9155
Flebogamma	500 mg	IV	J1572
	1 cc		J1460
Flexoject	up to 60 mg	IV, IM	J2360
Flexon	up to 60 mg	IV, IM	J2360
Flolan	0.5 mg	IV	J1325
Flo-Pred	5 mg		J7510
Florbetaben f18, diagnostic	per study dose	IV	Q9983
Floxuridine	500 mg	IV	J9200
Fluconazole	200 mg	IV	J1450
Fludara	1 mg	ORAL	J8562
	50 mg	IV	J9185
Fludarabine phosphate	1 mg	ORAL	J8562
	50 mg	IV	J9185
Flunisolide inhalation solution, unit dose form	per mg	INH	J7641
Fluocinolone		OTH	J7311, J7313
Fluocinolone acetonide (Yutiq)	0.01 mg	OTH	J7314
Fluorouracil	500 mg	IV	J9190
Fluphenazine decanoate	up to 25 mg		J2680
Flutamide			J8999
Flutemetamol f18, diagnostic	per study dose	IV	Q9982

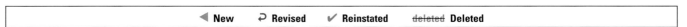

◀ New ⮌ Revised ✔ Reinstated ~~deleted~~ Deleted

DRUG NAME	DOSAGE	METHOD OF ADMINISTRATION	HCPCS CODE
Folex	5 mg	IA, IM, IT, IV	J9250
	50 mg	IA, IM, IT, IV	J9260
Folex PFS	5 mg	IA, IM, IT, IV	J9250
	50 mg	IA, IM, IT, IV	J9260
Follutein	per 1,000 USP units	IM	J0725
Folotyn	1 mg		J9307
Fomepizole	15 mg		J1451
Fomivirsen sodium	1.65 mg	Intraocular	J1452
Fondaparinux sodium	0.5 mg	SC	J1652
Formoterol	12 mcg	INH	J7640
Formoterol fumarate	20 mcg	INH	J7606
Fortaz	per 500 mg	IM, IV	J0713
Fosaprepitant	1 mg	IV	J1453
Foscarnet sodium	per 1,000 mg	IV	J1455
Foscavir	per 1,000 mg	IV	J1455
Fosnetupitant 235 mg and palonosetron 0.25 mg		IV	J1454
Fosphenytoin	50 mg	IV	Q2009
Fragmin	per 2,500 IU		J1645
Fremanezumab-vfrm	1 mg	IV	J3031
FUDR	500 mg	IV	J9200
Fulvestrant	25 mg	IM	J9395
Fungizone intravenous	50 mg	IV	J0285
Furomide M.D.	up to 20 mg	IM, IV	J1940
Furosemide	up to 20 mg	IM, IV	J1940
G			
Gablofen	10 mg		J0475
	50 mcg		J0476
Gadavist	0.1 ml		A9585
Gadoxetate disodium	1 ml	IV	A9581
Gallium nitrate	1 mg	IV	J1457
Galsulfase	1 mg	IV	J1458
Gamastan	1 cc	IM	J1460
	over 10 cc	IM	J1560
Gamma globulin	1 cc	IM	J1460
	over 10 cc	IM	J1560
Gammagard Liquid	500 mg	IV	J1569
Gammagard S/D			J1566
GammaGraft	per square centimeter		Q4111
Gammaplex	500 mg	IV	J1557

◀ New ⤾ Revised ✔ Reinstated ~~deleted~~ Deleted

DRUG NAME	DOSAGE	METHOD OF ADMINISTRATION	HCPCS CODE
Gammar	1 cc	IM	J1460
	over 10 cc	IM	J1560
Gammar-IV, *see* Immune globin intravenous (human)			
Gamulin RH			
immune globulin, human	100 IU		J2791
	1 dose package, 300 mcg	IM	J2790
immune globulin, human, solvent detergent	100 IU	IV	J2792
Gamunex	500 mg	IV	**J1561**
Ganciclovir, implant	4.5 mg	OTH	**J7310**
Ganciclovir sodium	500 mg	IV	**J1570**
Ganirelix			J3490
Garamycin, gentamicin	up to 80 mg	IM, IV	**J1580**
Gastrografin	per ml		Q9963
Gatifloxacin	10 mg	IV	**J1590**
Gazyva	10 mg		J9301
Gefitinib	250 mg	ORAL	**J8565**
Gel-One	per dose	OTH	**J7326**
Gemcitabine HCl	200 mg	IV	**J9201**
Gemcitabine HCl, not otherwise specified	200 mg	IV	**J9201**
Gemcitabine HCl (Infugem)	100 mg	IV	**J9198** ↩
Gemsar	200 mg	IV	J9201
Gemtuzumab ozogamicin	5 mg	IV	**J9300**
Gengraf	100 mg		J7502
	25 mg	ORAL	J7515
Genotropin	1 mg		J2941
Gentamicin Sulfate	up to 80 mg	IM, IV	J1580, J7699
Gentran	500 ml	IV	J7100
Gentran 75	500 ml	IV	J7110
Geodon	10 mg		J3486
Gesterol 50	per 50 mg		J2675
Givosiran	0.5 mg	IM	J0223 ◀
Glassia	10 mg	IV	**J0257**
Glatiramer Acetate	20 mg	SC	**J1595**
Gleevec (Film-Coated)	400 mg		J8999
GlucaGen	per 1 mg		J1610
Glucagon HCl	per 1 mg	SC, IM, IV	**J1610**
Glukor	per 1,000 USP units	IM	J0725
Glycopyrrolate			
concentrated form	per 1 mg	INH	**J7642**
unit dose form	per 1 mg	INH	**J7643**

◀ New ↩ Revised ✔ Reinstated ~~deleted~~ Deleted

DRUG NAME	DOSAGE	METHOD OF ADMINISTRATION	HCPCS CODE
Gold sodium thiomalate	up to 50 mg	IM	**J1600**
Golimumab	1 mg	IV	**J1602**
Golodirsen	10 mg	IM	J1429 ◀
Gonadorelin HCl	per 100 mcg	SC, IV	**J1620**
Gonal-F			J3490
Gonic	per 1,000 USP units	IM	J0725
Goserelin acetate implant	per 3.6 mg	SC	**J9202**
Graftjacket	per square centimeter		Q4107
Graftjacket Xpress	1 cc		Q4113
Granisetron HCl			
extended release	0.1 mg	IV	**J1627**
injection	100 mcg	IV	**J1626**
oral	1 mg	ORAL	**Q0166**
Guselkumab	1 mg	IV	**J1628**
Gynogen L.A. A10	up to 10 mg	IM	J1380
Gynogen L.A. A20	up to 10 mg	IM	J1380
Gynogen L.A. A40	up to 10 mg	IM	J1380
H			
Halaven	0.1 mg		J9179
Haldol	up to 5 mg	IM, IV	J1630
Haloperidol	up to 5 mg	IM, IV	**J1630**
Haloperidol decanoate	per 50 mg	IM	**J1631**
Haloperidol Lactate	up to 5 mg		J1630
Hectoral	1 mcg	IV	J1270
Helixate FS	per IU		J7192
Hemin	1 mg		**J1640**
Hemofil M	per IU	IV	J7190
Hemophilia clotting factors (e.g., anti-inhibitors)	per IU	IV	**J7198**
NOC	per IU	IV	**J7199**
Hepagam B	0.5 ml	IM	**J1571**
	0.5 ml	IV	**J1573**
Heparin sodium	1,000 units	IV, SC	**J1644**
Heparin sodium (heparin lock flush)	10 units	IV	**J1642**
Heparin Sodium (Procine)	per 1,000 units		J1644
Hep-Lock	10 units	IV	J1642
Hep-Lock U/P	10 units	IV	J1642
Herceptin	10 mg	IV	J9355
Hexabrix 320	per ml		Q9967
Hexadrol Phosphate	1 mg	IM, IV, OTH	J1100
Hexaminolevulinate hydrochloride	100 mg	IV	**A9589**

◀ **New** ⮌ **Revised** ✔ **Reinstated** ~~deleted~~ **Deleted**

DRUG NAME	DOSAGE	METHOD OF ADMINISTRATION	HCPCS CODE
Histaject	per 10 mg	IM, SC, IV	J0945
Histerone 50	up to 50 mg	IM	J3140
Histerone 100	up to 50 mg	IM	J3140
Histrelin			
acetate	10 mcg		**J1675**
implant	50 mg	OTH	**J9225**, J9226
Hizentra, *see* Immune globulin			
Humalog	per 5 units		J1815
	per 50 units		J1817
Human fibrinogen concentrate	100 mg	IV	**J7178**
Human fibrinogen concentrate (fibryga)	1 mg	IV	**J7177**
Humate-P	per IU		J7187
Humatrope	1 mg		J2941
Humira	20 mg		J0135
Humulin	per 5 units		J1815
	per 50 units		J1817
Hyalgan, Spurtaz or VISCO-3		IA	**J7321**
Hyaluronan or derivative	per dose	IV	**J7327**
Durolane	1 mg	IA	**J7318**
Gel-Syn	0.1 mg	IA	**J7328**
Gelsyn-3	0.1 mg	IV	**J7328**
Gen Visc 850	1 mg	IA	**J7320**
Hyalgan or supartz	per dose	IA	J7321 ◄
Hymovis	1 mg	IA	**J7322**
Synojoynt	1 mg	VAR	**J7331**
Triluron	1 mg	IV	**J7332**
Trivisc	1 mg	IV	**J7329**
Visco-3	per dose	IA	J7333 ◄
Hyaluronic Acid			J3490
Hyaluronidase	up to 150 units	SC, IV	**J3470**
Hyaluronidase			
ovine	up to 999 units	VAR	**J3471**
ovine	per 1000 units	VAR	**J3472**
recombinant	1 usp	SC	**J3473**
Hyate:C	per IU	IV	J7191
Hybolin Decanoate	up to 50 mg	IM	J2320
Hybolin Improved, *see* Nandrolone phenpropionate			
Hycamtin	0.25 mg	ORAL	J8705
	4 mg	IV	J9351
Hydralazine HCl	up to 20 mg	IV, IM	**J0360**
Hydrate	up to 50 mg	IM, IV	J1240

◄ **New** ↩ **Revised** ✔ **Reinstated** ~~deleted~~ **Deleted**

DRUG NAME	DOSAGE	METHOD OF ADMINISTRATION	HCPCS CODE
Hydrea			J8999
Hydrocortisone acetate	up to 25 mg	IV, IM, SC	**J1700**
Hydrocortisone sodium phosphate	up to 50 mg	IV, IM, SC	**J1710**
Hydrocortisone succinate sodium	up to 100 mg	IV, IM, SC	**J1720**
Hydrocortone Acetate	up to 25 mg	IV, IM, SC	J1700
Hydrocortone Phosphate	up to 50 mg	IM, IV, SC	J1710
Hydromorphone HCl	up to 4 mg	SC, IM, IV	**J1170**
Hydroxyprogesterone Caproate	1 mg	IM	**J1725**
(Makena)	10 mg	IV	**J1726**
NOS	10 mg	IV	**J1729**
Hydroxyurea			J8999
Hydroxyzine HCl	up to 25 mg	IM	**J3410**
Hydroxyzine Pamoate	25 mg	ORAL	**Q0177**
Hylan G-F 20		OTH	**J7322**
Hylenex	1 USP unit		J3473
Hyoscyamine sulfate	up to 0.25 mg	SC, IM, IV	**J1980**
Hyperrho S/D	300 mcg		J2790
	100 IU		J2792
Hyperstat IV	up to 300 mg	IV	J1730
Hyper-Tet	up to 250 units	IM	J1670
HypRho-D	300 mcg	IM	J2790
			J2791
	50 mcg		J2788
Hyrexin-50	up to 50 mg	IV, IM	J1200
Hyzine-50	up to 25 mg	IM	J3410
I			
Ibalizumab-uiyk	10 mg	IV	**J1746**
Ibandronate sodium	1 mg	IV	**J1740**
Ibuprofen	100 mg	IV	**J1741**
Ibutilide fumarate	1 mg	IV	**J1742**
Icatibant	1 mg	SC	**J1744**
Idamycin	5 mg	IV	J9211
Idarubicin HCl	5 mg	IV	**J9211**
Idursulfase	1 mg	IV	**J1743**
Ifex	1 g	IV	J9208
Ifosfamide	1 g	IV	**J9208**
Ilaris	1 mg		**J0638**
Iloprost	20 mcg	INH	**Q4074**
Ilotycin, *see* Erythromycin gluceptate			
Iluvien	0.01 mg		J7313
Imferon	50 mg		J1750

◀ **New** ⮌ **Revised** ✔ **Reinstated** ~~deleted~~ **Deleted**

DRUG NAME	DOSAGE	METHOD OF ADMINISTRATION	HCPCS CODE
Imiglucerase	10 units	IV	**J1786**
Imipenem 4 mg, cilistatin 4 mg, relebactam ◀	2 mg		J0742
Imitrex	6 mg	SC	J3030
Imlygic	per 1 million plaque forming units		J9325, J9999
Immune globulin			
Bivigam	500 mg	IV	**J1556**
Cuvitru	100 mg	IV	**J1555**
Flebogamma	500 mg	IV	**J1572**
Gammagard Liquid	500 mg	IV	**J1569**
Gammaplex	500 mg	IV	**J1557**
Gamunex	500 mg	IV	**J1561**
HepaGam B	0.5 ml	IM	**J1571**
	0.5 ml	IV	**J1573**
Hizentra	100 mg	SC	**J1559**
Hyaluronidase, (HYQVIA)	100 mg	IV	**J1575**
NOS	500 mg	IV	**J1566, J1599**
Octagam	500 mg	IV	**J1568**
Privigen	500 mg	IV	**J1459**
Rhophylac	100 IU	IM	**J2791**
Subcutaneous	100 mg	SC	**J1562**
Xembify ◀	100 mg	IM	J1558
Immunosuppressive drug, not otherwise classified			**J7599**
Imuran	50 mg	ORAL	J7500
	100 mg	IV	J7501
Inapsine	up to 5 mg	IM, IV	J1790
Incobotulinumtoxin type A	1 unit	IM	**J0588**
Increlex	1 mg		J2170
Inderal	up to 1 mg	IV	J1800
Inebilizumab-cdon ◀	1 mg	IV	**J1823**
Infed	50 mg		J1750
Infergen	1 mcg	SC	J9212
Inflectra			Q5102
Infliximab			
dyyb	10 mg	IM, IV	**Q5103**
abda	10 mg	IM, IV	**Q5104**
axxq, biosimilar, (AVSOLA) ◀	10 mg	IM, IV	Q5121
qbtx	10 mg	IM, IV	**Q5109**
Infumorph	10 mg		J2274
Injectafer	1 mg		J1439
Injection factor ix, glycopegylated	1 iu	IV	**J7203**

◀ New ⮌ Revised ✔ Reinstated ~~deleted~~ Deleted

DRUG NAME	DOSAGE	METHOD OF ADMINISTRATION	HCPCS CODE
Injection sulfur hexafluoride lipid microspheres	per ml	IV	Q9950
Innohep	1,000 iu	SC	J1655
Innovar	up to 2 ml ampule	IM, IV	J1810
Inotuzumab orogamicin	0.1 mg	IV	J9229
Insulin	5 units	SC	J1815
Insulin-Humalog	per 50 units		J1817
Insulin lispro	50 units	SC	J1817
Intal	per 10 mg	INH	J7631, J7632
Integra			
Bilayer Matrix Wound Dressing (BMWD)	per square centimeter		Q4104
Dermal Regeneration Template (DRT)	per square centimeter		Q4105
Flowable Wound Matrix	1 cc		Q4114
Matrix	per square centimeter		Q4108
Integrilin	5 mg	IM, IV	J1327
Interferon alfa-2a, recombinant	3 million units	SC, IM	J9213
Interferon alfa-2b, recombinant	1 million units	SC, IM	J9214
Interferon alfa-n3 (human leukocyte derived)	250,000 IU	IM	J9215
Interferon alphacon-1, recombinant	1 mcg	SC	J9212
Interferon beta-1a	30 mcg	IM	J1826
	1 mcg	IM	Q3027
	1 mcg	SC	Q3028
Interferon beta-1b	0.25 mg	SC	J1830
Interferon gamma-1b	3 million units	SC	J9216
Intrauterine copper contraceptive		OTH	J7300
Intron-A	1 million units		J9214
Invanz	500 mg		J1335
Invega Sustenna	1 mg		J2426
Ipilimumab	1 mg	IV	J9228
Ipratropium bromide, unit dose form	per mg	INH	J3535, J7620, J7644, J7645
Iressa	250 mg		J8565
Irinotecan	20 mg	IV	J9206, J9205
Iron dextran	50 mg	IV, IM	J1750
Iron sucrose	1 mg	IV	J1756
Irrigation solution for Tx of bladder calculi	per 50 ml	OTH	Q2004
Isatuximab-irfc	10 mg	IV	J9227 ◀
Isavuconazonium	1 mg	IV	J1833
Isocaine HCl	per 10 ml	VAR	J0670
Isoetharine HCl			
concentrated form	per mg	INH	J7647, J7648
unit dose form	per mg	INH	J7649, J7650

◀ New ⤼ Revised ✔ Reinstated ~~deleted~~ Deleted

DRUG NAME	DOSAGE	METHOD OF ADMINISTRATION	HCPCS CODE
Isoproterenol HCl			
concentrated form	per mg	INH	**J7657, J7658**
unit dose form	per mg	INH	**J7659, J7660**
Isovue	per ml		Q9966, Q9967
Istodax	1 mg		J9315
Isuprel			
concentrated form	per mg	INH	J7657, J7658
unit dose form	per mg	INH	J7659, J7660
Itraconazole	50 mg	IV	**J1835**
Ixabepilone	1 mg	IV	**J9207**
Ixempra	1 mg		J9207
J			
Jenamicin	up to 80 mg	IM, IV	J1580
Jetrea	0.125 mg		J7316
Jevtana	1 mg		J9043
K			
Kabikinase	per 250,000 IU	IV	J2995
Kadcyla	1 mg		J9354
Kalbitor	1 mg		J1290
Kaleinate	per 10 ml	IV	J0610
Kanamycin sulfate	up to 75 mg	IM, IV	**J1850**
	up to 500 mg	IM, IV	**J1840**
Kantrex	up to 75 mg	IM, IV	J1850
	up to 500 mg	IM, IV	J1840
Keflin	up to 1 g	IM, IV	J1890
Kefurox	per 750 mg		J0697
Kefzol	500 mg	IV, IM	J0690
Kenaject-40	1 mg		J3300
	per 10 mg	IM	J3301
Kenalog-10	1 mg		J3300
	per 10 mg	IM	J3301
Kenalog-40	1 mg		J3300
	per 10 mg	IM	J3301
Kepivance	50 mcg		J2425
Keppra	10 mg		J1953
Keroxx	1 cc	IV	**Q4202**
Kestrone 5	per 1 mg	IM	J1435
Ketorolac tromethamine	per 15 mg	IM, IV	**J1885**
Key-Pred 25	up to 1 ml	IM	J2650
Key-Pred 50	up to 1 ml	IM	J2650

◀ New ⮌ Revised ✔ Reinstated ~~deleted~~ Deleted

DRUG NAME	DOSAGE	METHOD OF ADMINISTRATION	HCPCS CODE
Key-Pred-SP, *see* Prednisolone sodium phosphate			
Keytruda	1 mg		J9271
K-Flex	up to 60 mg	IV, IM	J2360
Khapzory	0.5 mg	IV	**J0642**
Kinevac	5 mcg	IV	J2805
Kitabis PAK	per 300 mg		J7682
Klebcil	up to 75 mg	IM, IV	J1850
	up to 500 mg	IM, IV	J1840
Koate-HP (anti-hemophilic factor)			
human	per IU	IV	J7190
porcine	per IU	IV	J7191
recombinant	per IU	IV	J7192
Kogenate			
human	per IU	IV	J7190
porcine	per IU	IV	J7191
recombinant	per IU	IV	J7192
Konakion	per 1 mg	IM, SC, IV	J3430
Konyne-80	per IU	IV	J7194
Krystexxa	1 mg		J2507
Kyleena	19.5 mg	OTH	J7296
Kyprolis	1 mg		J9047
Kytril	1 mg	ORAL	Q0166
	1 mg	IV	S0091
	100 mcg	IV	J1626
L			
L.A.E. 20	up to 10 mg	IM	J1380
Laetrile, Amygdalin, vitamin B-17			**J3570**
Lanadelumab-flyo	1 mg	IV	**J0593**
Lanoxin	up to 0.5 mg	IM, IV	J1160
Lanreotide	1 mg	SC	**J1930**
Lantus	per 5 units		J1815
Largon, *see* Propiomazine HCl			
Laronidase	0.1 mg	IV	**J1931**
Lasix	up to 20 mg	IM, IV	J1940
L-Caine	10 mg	IV	J2001
Lefamulin ◀	1 mg		**J0691**
Lemtrada	1 mg		J0202
Lepirudin	50 mg		**J1945**
Leucovorin calcium	per 50 mg	IM, IV	**J0640**
Leukeran			J8999

◀ New ↩ Revised ✔ Reinstated ~~deleted~~ Deleted

DRUG NAME	DOSAGE	METHOD OF ADMINISTRATION	HCPCS CODE
Leukine	50 mcg	IV	J2820
Leuprolide acetate	per 1 mg	IM	**J9218**
Leuprolide acetate (for depot suspension)	per 3.75 mg	IM	**J1950**
	7.5 mg	IM	**J9217**
Leuprolide acetate implant	65 mg	OTH	**J9219**
Leustatin	per mg	IV	J9065
Levalbuterol HCl			
concentrated form	0.5 mg	INH	**J7607, J7612**
unit dose form	0.5 mg	INH	**J7614, J7615**
Levaquin I.U.	250 mg	IV	J1956
Levetiracetam	10 mg	IV	**J1953**
Levocarnitine	per 1 gm	IV	**J1955**
Levo-Dromoran	up to 2 mg	SC, IV	J1960
Levofloxacin	250 mg	IV	**J1956**
Levoleucovorin NOS	0.5 mg	IV	**J0641**
Levonorgestrel implant		OTH	**J7306**
Levonorgestrel-releasing intrauterine contraceptive system	52 mg	OTH	**J7297, J7298**
Kyleena	19.5 mg	OTH	**J7296**
Levorphanol tartrate	up to 2 mg	SC, IV	**J1960**
Levsin	up to 0.25 mg	SC, IM, IV	J1980
Levulan Kerastick	unit dose (354 mg)	OTH	J7308
Lexiscan	0.1 mg		J2785
Librium	up to 100 mg	IM, IV	J1990
Lidocaine HCl	10 mg	IV	**J2001**
Lidoject-1	10 mg	IV	J2001
Lidoject-2	10 mg	IV	J2001
Liletta	52 mg	OTH	J7297
Lincocin	up to 300 mg	IV	J2010
Lincomycin HCl	up to 300 mg	IV	**J2010**
Linezolid	200 mg	IV	**J2020**
Lioresal	10 mg	IT	J0475
			J0476
Liposomal			
Cytarabine	2.27 mg	IV	**J9153**
Daunorubicin	1 mg	IV	**J9153**
Liquaemin Sodium	1,000 units	IV, SC	J1644
LMD (10%)	500 ml	IV	J7100
Locort	1.5 mg		J8540
Lorazepam	2 mg	IM, IV	**J2060**
Lovenox	10 mg	SC	J1650

◀ New ⮐ Revised ✔ Reinstated ~~deleted~~ Deleted

DRUG NAME	DOSAGE	METHOD OF ADMINISTRATION	HCPCS CODE
Loxapine	1 mg	OTH	**J2062**
Lucentis	0.1 mg		J2778
Lufyllin	up to 500 mg	IM	J1180
Lumason	per ml		Q9950
Luminal Sodium	up to 120 mg	IM, IV	J2560
Lumizyme	10 mg		J0221
Lupon Depot	7.5 mg		J9217
	3.75 mg		J1950
Lupron	per 1 mg	IM	J9218
	per 3.75 mg	IM	J1950
	7.5 mg	IM	J9217
Lurbinectedin	0.1 mg	IV	J9223 ◀
Luspatercept-aamt	0.25 mg	IM	J0896 ◀
Lyophilized, *see* Cyclophosphamide, lyophilized			
M			
Macugen	0.3 mg		J2503
Magnesium sulfate	500 mg		**J3475**
Magnevist	per ml		A9579
Makena	1 mg		J1725
Mannitol	25% in 50 ml	IV	**J2150**
	5 mg	INH	**J7665**
Marcaine			J3490
Marinol	2.5 mg	ORAL	Q0167
Marmine	up to 50 mg	IM, IV	J1240
Matulane	50 mg		J8999
Maxipime	500 mg	IV	J0692
MD-76R	per ml		Q9963
MD Gastroview	per ml		Q9963
Mecasermin	1 mg	SC	**J2170**
Mechlorethamine HCl (nitrogen mustard), HN2	10 mg	IV	**J9230**
Medralone 40	20 mg	IM	J1020
	40 mg	IM	J1030
	80 mg	IM	J1040
Medralone 80	20 mg	IM	J1020
	40 mg	IM	J1030
	80 mg	IM	J1040
Medrol	per 4 mg	ORAL	J7509
Medroxyprogesterone acetate	1 mg	IM	**J1050**
Mefoxin	1 g	IV, IM	J0694
Megestrol Acetate			J8999

◀ **New** ↩ **Revised** ✔ **Reinstated** ~~deleted~~ **Deleted**

DRUG NAME	DOSAGE	METHOD OF ADMINISTRATION	HCPCS CODE
Meloxicam	1 mg	IV	J1738 ◀
Melphalan (evomela)	1 mg	IV	J9246 ◀
Melphalan HCl	50 mg	IV	J9245
Melphalan, oral	2 mg	ORAL	J8600
Menoject LA	1 mg		J1071
Mepergan injection	up to 50 mg	IM, IV	J2180
Meperidine and promethazine HCl	up to 50 mg	IM, IV	J2180
Meperidine HCl	per 100 mg	IM, IV, SC	J2175
Mepivacaine HCl	per 10 ml	VAR	J0670
Mepolizumab	1 mg	IV	J2182
Mercaptopurine			J8999
Meropenem	100 mg	IV	J2185
Merrem	100 mg		J2185
Mesna	200 mg	IV	J9209
Mesnex	200 mg	IV	J9209
Metaprel			
concentrated form	per 10 mg	INH	J7667, J7668
unit dose form	per 10 mg	INH	J7669, J7670
Metaproterenol sulfate			
concentrated form	per 10 mg	INH	J7667, J7668
unit dose form	per 10 mg	INH	J7669, J7670
Metaraminol bitartrate	per 10 mg	IV, IM, SC	J0380
Metastron	per millicurie		A9600
Methacholine chloride	1 mg	INH	J7674
Methadone HCl	up to 10 mg	IM, SC	J1230
Methergine	up to 0.2 mg		J2210
Methocarbamol	up to 10 ml	IV, IM	J2800
Methotrexate LPF	5 mg	IV, IM, IT, IA	J9250
	50 mg	IV, IM, IT, IA	J9260
Methotrexate, oral	2.5 mg	ORAL	J8610
Methotrexate sodium	5 mg	IV, IM, IT, IA	J9250
	50 mg	IV, IM, IT, IA	J9260
Methyldopate HCl	up to 250 mg	IV	J0210
Methylergonovine maleate	up to 0.2 mg		J2210
Methylnaltrexone	0.1 mg	SC	J2212
Methylprednisolone acetate	20 mg	IM	J1020
	40 mg	IM	J1030
	80 mg	IM	J1040
Methylprednisolone, oral	per 4 mg	ORAL	J7509

◀ New ⊋ Revised ✔ Reinstated ~~deleted~~ Deleted

DRUG NAME	DOSAGE	METHOD OF ADMINISTRATION	HCPCS CODE
Methylprednisolone sodium succinate	up to 40 mg	IM, IV	J2920
	up to 125 mg	IM, IV	J2930
Metoclopramide HCl	up to 10 mg	IV	J2765
Metrodin	75 IU		J3355
Metronidazole			J3490
Metvixia	1 g	OTH	J7309
Miacalcin	up to 400 units	SC, IM	J0630
Micafungin sodium	1 mg		J2248
MicRhoGAM	50 mcg		J2788
Midazolam HCl	per 1 mg	IM, IV	J2250
Milrinone lactate	5 mg	IV	J2260
Minocine	1 mg		J2265
Minocycline Hydrochloride	1 mg	IV	J2265
Mircera	1 mcg		J0887, J0888
Mirena	52 mg	OTH	J7297, J7298
Mithracin	2,500 mcg	IV	J9270
Mitomycin	0.2 mg	Ophthalmic	J7315
	5 mg	IV	J9280
Mitosol	0.2 mg	Ophthalmic	J7315
	5 mg	IV	J9280
Mitoxantrone HCl	per 5 mg	IV	J9293
Mogamulizumab-kpkc	1 mg	IV	J9204
Monocid, *see* Cefonicic sodium			
Monoclate-P			
human	per IU	IV	J7190
porcine	per IU	IV	J7191
Monoclonal antibodies, parenteral	5 mg	IV	J7505
Mononine	per IU	IV	J7193
Monovisc			J7327
Morphine sulfate	up to 10 mg	IM, IV, SC	J2270
preservative-free	10 mg	SC, IM, IV	J2274
Moxetumomab Pasudotox-tdfk	0.01 mg	IV	J9313
Moxifloxacin	100 mg	IV	J2280
Mozobil	1 mg		J2562
M-Prednisol-40	20 mg	IM	J1020
	40 mg	IM	J1030
	80 mg	IM	J1040
M-Prednisol-80	20 mg	IM	J1020
	40 mg	IM	J1030
	80 mg	IM	J1040

◀ New ⤾ Revised ✔ Reinstated ~~deleted~~ Deleted

DRUG NAME	DOSAGE	METHOD OF ADMINISTRATION	HCPCS CODE
Mucomyst			
unit dose form	per gram	INH	J7604, J7608
Mucosol			
injection	100 mg	IV	J0132
unit dose	per gram	INH	J7604, J7608
MultiHance	per ml		A9577
MultiHance Multipack	per ml		A9578
Muromonab-CD3	5 mg	IV	J7505
Muse		OTH	J0275
	1.25 mcg	OTH	J0270
Mustargen	10 mg	IV	J9230
Mutamycin			
	0.2 mg	Ophthalmic	J7315
	5 mg	IV	J9280
Mycamine	1 mg		J2248
Mycophenolate Mofetil	250 mg	ORAL	J7517
Mycophenolic acid	180 mg	ORAL	J7518
Myfortic	180 mg		J7518
Myleran	1 mg		J0594
	2 mg	ORAL	J8510
Mylotarg	5 mg	IV	J9300
Myobloc	per 100 units	IM	J0587
Myochrysine	up to 50 mg	IM	J1600
Myolin	up to 60 mg	IV, IM	J2360
N			
Nabilone	1 mg	ORAL	J8650
Nafcillin			J3490
Naglazyme	1 mg		J1458
Nalbuphine HCl	per 10 mg	IM, IV, SC	J2300
Naloxone HCl	per 1 mg	IM, IV, SC	J2310, J3490
Naltrexone			J3490
Naltrexone, depot form	1 mg	IM	J2315
Nandrobolic L.A.	up to 50 mg	IM	J2320
Nandrolone decanoate	up to 50 mg	IM	J2320
Narcan	1 mg	IM, IV, SC	J2310
Naropin	1 mg		J2795
Nasahist B	per 10 mg	IM, SC, IV	J0945
Nasal vaccine inhalation		INH	J3530
Natalizumab	1 mg	IV	J2323
Natrecor	0.1 mg		J2325

◀ New ⤾ Revised ✔ Reinstated ~~deleted~~ Deleted

DRUG NAME	DOSAGE	METHOD OF ADMINISTRATION	HCPCS CODE
Navane, *see* Thiothixene			
Navelbine	per 10 mg	IV	J9390
ND Stat	per 10 mg	IM, SC, IV	J0945
Nebcin	up to 80 mg	IM, IV	J3260
NebuPent	per 300 mg	INH	J2545, J7676
Necitumumab	1 mg	IV	**J9295**
Nelarabine	50 mg	IV	**J9261**
Nembutal Sodium Solution	per 50 mg	IM, IV, OTH	J2515
Neocyten	up to 60 mg	IV, IM	J2360
Neo-Durabolic	up to 50 mg	IM	J2320
Neoquess	up to 20 mg	IM	J0500
Neoral	100 mg		J7502
	25 mg		J7515
Neosar	100 mg	IV	J9070
Neostigmine methylsulfate	up to 0.5 mg	IM, IV, SC	**J2710**
Neo-Synephrine	up to 1 ml	SC, IM, IV	J2370
Nervocaine 1%	10 mg	IV	J2001
Nervocaine 2%	10 mg	IV	J2001
Nesacaine	per 30 ml	VAR	J2400
Nesacaine-MPF	per 30 ml	VAR	J2400
Nesiritide	0.1 mg	IV	**J2325**
Netupitant 300 mg and palonosetron 0.5 mg		ORAL	**J8655**
Neulasta	6 mg		J2505
Neumega	5 mg	SC	J2355
Neupogen			
(G-CSF)	1 mcg	SC, IV	J1442
Neutrexin	per 25 mg	IV	J3305
Nipent	per 10 mg	IV	J9268
Nivolumab	1 mg	IV	**J9299**
Nolvadex			J8999
Nordryl	up to 50 mg	IV, IM	J1200
	50 mg	ORAL	Q0163
Norflex	up to 60 mg	IV, IM	J2360
Norzine	up to 10 mg	IM	J3280
Not otherwise classified drugs			**J3490**
other than inhalation solution administered through DME			**J7799**
inhalation solution administered through DME			**J7699**
anti-neoplastic			**J9999**
chemotherapeutic		ORAL	**J8999**
immunosuppressive			**J7599**
nonchemotherapeutic		ORAL	**J8499**

◀ New ↩ Revised ✔ Reinstated ~~deleted~~ Deleted

DRUG NAME	DOSAGE	METHOD OF ADMINISTRATION	HCPCS CODE
Novantrone	per 5 mg	IV	J9293
Novarel	per 1,000 USP Units		J0725
Novolin	per 5 units		J1815
	per 50 units		J1817
Novolog	per 5 units		J1815
	per 50 units		J1817
Novo Seven	1 mcg	IV	J7189
Novoeight			J7182
NPH	5 units	SC	J1815
Nplate	100 units		J0587
	10 mcg		J2796
Nubain	per 10 mg	IM, IV, SC	J2300
Nulecit	12.5 mg		J2916
Nulicaine	10 mg	IV	J2001
Nulojix	1 mg	IV	J0485
Numorphan	up to 1 mg	IV, SC, IM	J2410
Numorphan H.P.	up to 1 mg	IV, SC, IM	J2410
Nusinersen	0.1 mg	IV	J2326
Nutropin	1 mg		J2941
O			
Oasis Burn Matrix	per square centimeter		Q4103
Oasis Wound Matrix	per square centimeter		Q4102
Obinutuzumab	10 mg		J9301
Ocriplasmin	0.125 mg	IV	J7316
Ocrelizumab	1 mg	IV	J2350
Octagam	500 mg	IV	J1568
Octreotide Acetate, injection	1 mg	IM	J2353
	25 mcg	IV, SQ	J2354
Oculinum	per unit	IM	J0585
Ofatumumab	10 mg	IV	J9302
Ofev			J8499
Ofirmev	10 mg	IV	J0131
O-Flex	up to 60 mg	IV, IM	J2360
Oforta	10 mg		J8562
Olanzapine	1 mg	IM	J2358
Olaratumab	10 mg	IV	J9285
Omadacycline	1 mg	IV	J0121
Omacetaxine Mepesuccinate	0.01 mg	IV	J9262
Omalizumab	5 mg	SC	J2357

◀ New ⟲ Revised ✔ Reinstated ~~deleted~~ Deleted

DRUG NAME	DOSAGE	METHOD OF ADMINISTRATION	HCPCS CODE
Omnipaque	per ml		Q9965, Q9966, Q9967
Omnipen-N	up to 500 mg	IM, IV	J0290
	per 1.5 gm	IM, IV	J0295
Omniscan	per ml		A9579
Omnitrope	1 mg		J2941
Omontys	0.1 mg	IV, SC	J0890
OnabotulinumtoxinA	1 unit	IM	**J0585**
Onasemnogene abeparvovec-xioi, per treatment, vector genomes	up to 5x10 15	IM	J3399 ◀
Oncaspar	per single dose vial	IM, IV	J9266
Oncovin	1 mg	IV	J9370
Ondansetron HCl	1 mg	IV	**J2405**
	1 mg	ORAL	**Q0162**
Onivyde	1 mg		J9205
Opana	up to 1 mg		J2410
Opdivo	1 mg		J9299
Oprelvekin	5 mg	SC	**J2355**
Optimark	per ml		A9579
Optiray	per ml		Q9966, Q9967
Optison	per ml		Q9956
Oraminic II	per 10 mg	IM, SC, IV	J0945
Orapred	per 5 mg	ORAL	J7510
Orbactiv	10 mg		J2407
Orencia	10 mg		J0129
Oritavancin	10 mg	IV	**J2407**
Ormazine	up to 50 mg	IM, IV	J3230
Orphenadrine citrate	up to 60 mg	IV, IM	**J2360**
Orphenate	up to 60 mg	IV, IM	J2360
Orthovisc		OTH	**J7324**
Or-Tyl	up to 20 mg	IM	**J0500**
Osmitrol			J7799
Ovidrel			J3490
Oxacillin sodium	up to 250 mg	IM, IV	**J2700**
Oxaliplatin	0.5 mg	IV	**J9263**
Oxilan	per ml		Q9967
Oxymorphone HCl	up to 1 mg	IV, SC, IM	**J2410**
Oxytetracycline HCl	up to 50 mg	IM	**J2460**
Oxytocin	up to 10 units	IV, IM	**J2590**
Ozurdex	0.1 mg		J7312

◀ **New** ⮌ **Revised** ✔ **Reinstated** ~~deleted~~ **Deleted**

DRUG NAME	DOSAGE	METHOD OF ADMINISTRATION	HCPCS CODE
P			
Paclitaxel	1 mg	IV	J9267
Paclitaxel protein-bound particles	1 mg	IV	J9264
Palifermin	50 mcg	IV	J2425
Paliperidone palmitate	1 mg	IM	J2426
Palonosetron HCl	25 mcg	IV	J2469
Netupitant 300 mg and palonosetron 0.5 mg		ORAL	J8655
Pamidronate disodium	per 30 mg	IV	J2430
Panhematin	1 mg		J1640
Panitumumab	10 mg	IV	J9303
Papaverine HCl	up to 60 mg	IV, IM	J2440
Paragard T 380 A		OTH	J7300
Paraplatin	50 mg	IV	J9045
Paricalcitol, injection	1 mcg	IV, IM	J2501
Pasireotide, long acting	1 mg	IV	J2502
Pathogen(s) test for platelets		OTH	P9100
Patisiran	0.1 mg	IV	J0222
Peforomist	20 mcg		J7606
Pegademase bovine	25 IU		J2504
Pegaptinib	0.3 mg	OTH	J2503
Pegaspargase	per single dose vial	IM, IV	J9266
Pegasys			J3490
Pegfilgrastim	0.5 mg	SC	J2505
Pegfilgrastim-bmez, biosimilar, (ziextenzo)	0.5 mg	IM	Q5120 ◀
Pegfilgrastim-jmdb	0.5 mg	SC	Q5108
Peginesatide	0.1 mg	IV, SC	J0890
Peg-Intron			J3490
Pegloticase	1 mg	IV	J2507
Pembrolizumab	1 mg	IV	J9271
Pemetrexed	10 mg	IV	J9305
Pemetrexed (Pemfexy)	10 mg	IV	J9304 ◀
Penicillin G Benzathine	100,000 units	IM	J0561
Penicillin G Benzathine and Penicillin G Procaine	100,000 units	IM	J0558
Penicillin G potassium	up to 600,000 units	IM, IV	J2540
Penicillin G procaine, aqueous	up to 600,000 units	IM, IV	J2510
Penicillin G Sodium			J3490
Pentam	per 300 mg		J7676
Pentamidine isethionate	per 300 mg	INH, IM	J2545, J7676
Pentastarch, 10%	100 ml		J2513
Pentazocine HCl	30 mg	IM, SC, IV	J3070

◀ New ⮌ Revised ✓ Reinstated ~~deleted~~ Deleted

DRUG NAME	DOSAGE	METHOD OF ADMINISTRATION	HCPCS CODE
Pentobarbital sodium	per 50 mg	IM, IV, OTH	**J2515**
Pentostatin	per 10 mg	IV	**J9268**
Peramivir	1 mg	IV	**J2547**
Perjeta	1 mg		J9306
Permapen	up to 600,000	IM	J0561
Perphenazine			
injection	up to 5 mg	IM, IV	**J3310**
tablets	4 mg	ORAL	**Q0175**
Persantine IV	per 10 mg	IV	J1245
Pertuzumab	1 mg	IV	**J9306**
Pet Imaging			
Fluciclovine F-18, diagnostic	1 millcurie	IV	**A9588**
Gallium Ga-68, dotatate, diagnostic	0.1 millicurie	IV	**A9587**
Pfizerpen	up to 600,000 units	IM, IV	J2540
Pfizerpen A.S.	up to 600,000 units	IM, IV	J2510
Phenadoz			J8498
Phenazine 25	up to 50 mg	IM, IV	J2550
	12.5 mg	ORAL	Q0169
Phenazine 50	up to 50 mg	IM, IV	J2550
	12.5 mg	ORAL	Q0169
Phenergan	12.5 mg	ORAL	Q0169
	up to 50 mg	IM, IV	J2550
			J8498
Phenobarbital sodium	up to 120 mg	IM, IV	**J2560**
Phentolamine mesylate	up to 5 mg	IM, IV	**J2760**
Phenylephrine HCl	up to 1 ml	SC, IM, IV	**J2370**, J7799
Phenylephrine 10.16 mg/Ketorolac 2.88	1 ml	VAR	**J1097**
Phenytoin sodium	per 50 mg	IM, IV	**J1165**
Photofrin	75 mg	IV	J9600
Phytonadione (Vitamin K)	per 1 mg	IM, SC, IV	**J3430**
Piperacillin/Tazobactam Sodium, injection	1.125 g	IV	**J2543**
Pitocin	up to 10 units	IV, IM	J2590
Plantinol AQ	10 mg	IV	J9060
Plasma			
cryoprecipitate reduced	each unit	IV	**P9044**
pooled multiple donor, frozen	each unit	IV	**P9023, P9070**
(single donor), pathogen reduced, frozen	each unit	IV	**P9071**
Plas+SD	each unit	IV	P9023
Platelets, pheresis, pathogen reduced	each unit	IV	**P9073**
Pathogen(s) test for platelets		OTH	**P9100**

◀ New ↩ Revised ✔ Reinstated ~~deleted~~ Deleted

DRUG NAME	DOSAGE	METHOD OF ADMINISTRATION	HCPCS CODE
Platinol	10 mg	IV, IM	J9060
Plazomicin	5 mg	IV	J0291
Plerixafor	1 mg	SC	J2562
Plicamycin	2,500 mcg	IV	J9270
Polatuzumab vedotin	1 mg	IV	J9309
Polocaine	per 10 ml	VAR	J0670
Polycillin-N	up to 500 mg	IM, IV	J0290
	per 1.5 gm	IM, IV	J0295
Polygam	500 mg		J1566
Porfimer Sodium	75 mg	IV	J9600
Portrazza	1 mg		J9295
Positron emission tomography radiopharmaceutical, diagnostic			
for non-tumor identification, NOC		IV	A9598
for tumor identification, NOC		IV	A9597
Potassium chloride	per 2 mEq	IV	J3480
Potassium Chloride	up to 1,000 cc		J7120
Pralatrexate	1 mg	IV	J9307
Pralidoxime chloride	up to 1 g	IV, IM, SC	J2730
Predalone-50	up to 1 ml	IM	J2650
Predcor-25	up to 1 ml	IM	J2650
Predcor-50	up to 1 ml	IM	J2650
Predicort-50	up to 1 ml	IM	J2650
Prednisolone acetate	up to 1 ml	IM	J2650
Prednisolone, oral	5 mg	ORAL	J7510
Prednisone, immediate release or delayed release	1 mg	ORAL	J7512
Predoject-50	up to 1 ml	IM	J2650
Pregnyl	per 1,000 USP units	IM	J0725
Premarin Intravenous	per 25 mg	IV, IM	J1410
Prescription, chemotherapeutic, not otherwise specified		ORAL	J8999
Prescription, nonchemotherapeutic, not otherwise specified		ORAL	J8499
Prialt	1 mcg		J2278
Primacor	5 mg	IV	J2260
Primatrix	per square centimeter		Q4110
Primaxin	per 250 mg	IV, IM	J0743
Priscoline HCl	up to 25 mg	IV	J2670
Privigen	500 mg	IV	J1459
Probuphine System Kit			J0570
Procainamide HCl	up to 1 g	IM, IV	J2690
Prochlorperazine	up to 10 mg	IM, IV	J0780
			J8498

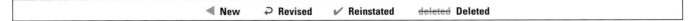
New
Revised
Reinstated
deleted Deleted

DRUG NAME	DOSAGE	METHOD OF ADMINISTRATION	HCPCS CODE
Prochlorperazine maleate	5 mg	ORAL	**Q0164**
	5 mg		S0183
Procrit			J0885
			Q4081
Pro-Depo, *see* Hydroxyprogesterone Caproate			
Profasi HP	per 1,000 USP units	IM	J0725
Profilnine Heat-Treated			
non-recombinant	per IU	IV	J7193
recombinant	per IU	IU	J7195, J7200-J7202
complex	per IU	IV	J7194
Profonol	10 mg/ml		J3490
Progestaject	per 50 mg		J2675
Progesterone	per 50 mg	IM	**J2675**
Prograf			
oral	1 mg	ORAL	J7507
parenteral	5 mg		J7525
Prohance Multipack	per ml		A9576
Prokine	50 mcg	IV	J2820
Prolastin	10 mg	IV	J0256
Proleukin	per single use vial	IM, IV	J9015
Prolia	1 mg		J0897
Prolixin Decanoate	up to 25 mg	IM, SC	J2680
Promazine HCl	up to 25 mg	IM	**J2950**
Promethazine			J8498
Promethazine HCl			
injection	up to 50 mg	IM, IV	**J2550**
oral	12.5 mg	ORAL	**Q0169**
Promethegan			J8498
Pronestyl	up to 1 g	IM, IV	J2690
Proplex SX-T			
non-recombinant	per IU	IV	J7193
recombinant	per IU		J7195, J7200-J7202
complex	per IU	IV	J7194
Proplex T			
non-recombinant	per IU	IV	J7193
recombinant	per IU		J7195, J7200-J7202
complex	per IU	IV	J7194
Propofol	10 mg	IV	**J2704**
Propranolol HCl	up to 1 mg	IV	**J1800**

◀ New ↩ Revised ✔ Reinstated ~~deleted~~ Deleted

DRUG NAME	DOSAGE	METHOD OF ADMINISTRATION	HCPCS CODE
Prorex-25			
	up to 50 mg	IM, IV	J2550
	12.5 mg	ORAL	Q0169
Prorex-50	up to 50 mg	IM, IV	J2550
	12.5 mg	ORAL	Q0169
Prostaglandin E1	per 1.25 mcg		J0270
Prostaphlin	up to 1 g	IM, IV	J2690
Prostigmin	up to 0.5 mg	IM, IV, SC	J2710
Prostin VR Pediatric	0.5 mg		J0270
Protamine sulfate	per 10 mg	IV	J2720
Protein C Concentrate	10 IU	IV	J2724
Prothazine	up to 50 mg	IM, IV	J2550
	12.5 mg	ORAL	Q0169
Protirelin	per 250 mcg	IV	J2725
Protonix			J3490
Protopam Chloride	up to 1 g	IV, IM, SC	J2730
Provenge			Q2043
Proventil			
concentrated form	1 mg	INH	J7610, J7611
unit dose form	1 mg	INH	J7609, J7613
Provocholine	per 1 mg		J7674
Prozine-50	up to 25 mg	IM	J2950
Pulmicort Respules			
concentrated form	0.25 mg	INH	J7633, J7634
unit dose	0.5 mg	INH	J7626, J7627
Pulmozyme	per mg		J7639
Pyridoxine HCl	100 mg		J3415
Q			
Quelicin	up to 20 mg	IV, IM	J0330
Quinupristin/dalfopristin	500 mg (150/350)	IV	J2770
Qutenza	per square cm		J7336
R			
Ramucirumab	5 mg	IV	J9308
Ranibizumab	0.1 mg	OTH	J2778
Ranitidine HCl, injection	25 mg	IV, IM	J2780
Rapamune	1 mg	ORAL	J7520
Rasburicase	0.5 mg	IV	J2783
Ravulizumab-cwvz	10 mg	IV	J1303
Rebif	11 mcg		Q3026
Reclast	1 mg		J3489

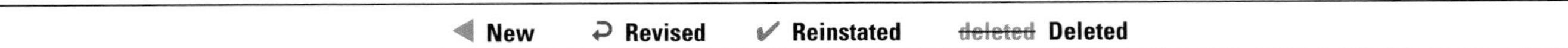
New
Revised
Reinstated
deleted Deleted

DRUG NAME	DOSAGE	METHOD OF ADMINISTRATION	HCPCS CODE
Recombinate			
human	per IU	IV	J7190
porcine	per IU	IV	J7191
recombinant	per IU	IV	J7192
Recombivax			J3490
Redisol	up to 1,000 mcg	IM, SC	J3420
Regadenoson	0.1 mg	IV	**J2785**
Regitine	up to 5 mg	IM, IV	J2760
Reglan	up to 10 mg	IV	J2765
Regular	5 units	SC	J1815
Relefact TRH	per 250 mcg	IV	J2725
Relistor	0.1 mg	SC	J2212
Remicade	10 mg	IM, IV	J1745
Remodulin	1 mg		J3285
Renflexis			Q5102
ReoPro	10 mg	IV	J0130
Rep-Pred 40	20 mg	IM	J1020
	40 mg	IM	J1030
	80 mg	IM	J1040
Rep-Pred 80	20 mg	IM	J1020
	40 mg	IM	J1030
	80 mg	IM	J1040
Resectisol			J7799
Reslizumab	1 mg	IV	**J2786**
Retavase	18.1 mg	IV	J2993
Reteplase	18.8 mg	IV	**J2993**
Retisert			J7311
Retrovir	10 mg	IV	J3485
Revefenacin inhalation solution	—	INH	**J7677**
Rheomacrodex	500 ml	IV	J7100
Rhesonativ	300 mcg	IM	J2790
	50 mg		J2788
Rheumatrex Dose Pack	2.5 mg	ORAL	J8610
Rho(D)			
immune globulin		IM, IV	**J2791**
immune globulin, human	1 dose package/ 300 mcg	IM	**J2790**
	50 mg	IM	**J2788**
immune globulin, human, solvent detergent	100	IV, IU	**J2792**
RhoGAM	300 mcg	IM	J2790
	50 mg		J2788

◀ New ↩ Revised ✔ Reinstated ~~deleted~~ Deleted

DRUG NAME	DOSAGE	METHOD OF ADMINISTRATION	HCPCS CODE
Rhophylac	100 IU	IM, IV	**J2791**
Riastap	100 mg		J7178
Rifadin			J3490
Rifampin			J3490
Rilonacept	1 mg	SC	**J2793**
RimabotulinumtoxinB	100 units	IM	**J0587**
Rimso-50	50 ml		J1212
Ringers lactate infusion	up to 1,000 cc	IV	**J7120, J7121**
Risperdal Consta	0.5 mg		J2794
Risperidone	0.5 mg	IM	**J2794**
Risperidone (perseris)	0.5 mg	IV	**J2798**
Rituxan	100 mg	IV	J9310
Rituximab	100 mg	IV	**J9310**
Rituximab-abbs	10 mg	IV	**Q5115**
Rituximab-pvvr, biosimilar, (Ruxience)	10 mg	IV	Q5119 ◀
Rixubis			J7200
Robaxin	up to 10 ml	IV, IM	J2800
Rocephin	per 250 mg	IV, IM	J0696
Roferon-A	3 million units	SC, IM	J9213
Rolapitant	0.5 mg	IV	**J2797**
Rolapitant, oral, 1 mg	1 mg	ORAL	**J8670**
Romidepsin	1 mg	IV	**J9315**
Romiplostim	10 mcg	SC	**J2796**
Romosozumab-aqqg	1 mg	IV	**J3111**
Ropivacaine Hydrochloride	1 mg	OTH	**J2795**
Rubex	10 mg	IV	J9000
Rubramin PC	up to 1,000 mcg	IM, SC	J3420
S			
Saizen	1 mg		J2941
Saline solution	10 ml		A4216
5% dextrose	500 ml	IV	**J7042**
infusion	250 cc	IV	**J7050**
	1,000 cc	IV	**J7030**
sterile	500 ml = 1 unit	IV, OTH	**J7040**
Sandimmune	25 mg	ORAL	J7515
	100 mg	ORAL	J7502
	250 mg	OTH	J7516
Sandoglobulin, *see* Immune globulin intravenous (human)			
Sandostatin, Lar Depot	25 mcg		J2354
	1 mg	IM	J2353

◀ New ⤻ Revised ✔ Reinstated ~~deleted~~ Deleted

DRUG NAME	DOSAGE	METHOD OF ADMINISTRATION	HCPCS CODE
Sargramostim (GM-CSF)	50 mcg	IV	**J2820**
Sculptra	0.5 mg	IV	**Q2028**
Sebelelipase alfa	1 mg	IV	**J2840**
Selestoject	per 4 mg	IM, IV	J0702
Sermorelin acetate	1 mcg	SC	**Q0515**
Serostim	1 mg		J2941
Signifor LAR	20 ml		J2502
Siltuximab	10 mg	IV	**J2860**
Simponi Aria	1 mg		J1602
Simulect	20 mg		J0480
Sincalide	5 mcg	IV	**J2805**
Sinografin	per ml		Q9963
Sinusol-B	per 10 mg	IM, SC, IV	J0945
Sirolimus	1 mg	ORAL	**J7520**
Sivextro	1 mg		J3090
Skyla	13.5 mg	OTH	**J7301**
Smz-TMP			J3490
Sodium Chloride	1,000 cc		J7030
	500 ml = 1 unit		J7040
	500 ml		A4217
	250 cc		J7050
Bacteriostatic	10 ml		A4216
Sodium Chloride Concentrate			J7799
Sodium ferricgluconate in sucrose	12.5 mg		**J2916**
Sodium Hyaluronate			J3490
Euflexxa			**J7323**
Hyalgan			**J7321**
Orthovisc			**J7324**
Solganal	up to 50 mg	IM	J2910
Soliris	10 mg		J1300
Solu-Cortef	up to 50 mg	IV, IM, SC	J1710
	100 mg		J1720
Solu-Medrol	up to 40 mg	IM, IV	J2920
	up to 125 mg	IM, IV	J2930
Solurex	1 mg	IM, IV, OTH	J1100
Solurex LA	1 mg	IM	J1094
Somatrem	1 mg	SC	**J2940**
Somatropin	1 mg	SC	**J2941**
Somatulin Depot	1 mg		J1930
Sparine	up to 25 mg	IM	J2950

◀ New ⤾ Revised ✔ Reinstated ~~deleted~~ Deleted

DRUG NAME	DOSAGE	METHOD OF ADMINISTRATION	HCPCS CODE
Spasmoject	up to 20 mg	IM	J0500
Spectinomycin HCl	up to 2 g	IM	J3320
Sporanox	50 mg	IV	J1835
Staphcillin, *see* Methicillin sodium			
Stelara	1 mg		J3357
Stilphostrol	250 mg	IV	J9165
Streptase	250,000 IU	IV	J2995
Streptokinase	per 250,000	IU, IV	J2995
Streptomycin	up to 1 g	IM	J3000
Streptomycin Sulfate	up to 1 g	IM	J3000
Streptozocin	1 gm	IV	J9320
Strontium-89 chloride	per millicurie		A9600
Sublimaze	0.1 mg	IM, IV	J3010
Succinylcholine chloride	up to 20 mg	IV, IM	J0330
Sufentanil Citrate			J3490
Sumarel Dosepro	6 mg		J3030
Sumatriptan succinate	6 mg	SC	J3030
Supartz		OTH	J7321
Supprelin LA	50 mg		J9226
Surostrin	up to 20 mg	IV, IM	J0330
Sus-Phrine	up to 1 ml ampule	SC, IM	J0171
Synercid	500 mg (150/350)	IV	J2770
Synkavite	per 1 mg	IM, SC, IV	J3430
Synribo	0.01 mg		J9262
Syntocinon	up to 10 units	IV, IM	J2590
Synvisc and Synvisc-One	1 mg	OTH	J7325
Syrex	10 ml		A4216
Sytobex	1,000 mcg	IM, SC	J3420
T			
Tacrolimus			
(Envarsus XR)	0.25 mg	ORAL	J7503
oral, extended release	0.1 mg	ORAL	J7508
oral, immediate release	1 mg	ORAL	J7507
parenteral	5 mg	IV	J7525
Tagraxofusp-erzs	10 mcg	IV	J9269
Taliglucerase Alfa	10 units	IV	J3060
Talimogene laherparepvec	per 1 million plaque forming units	IV	J9325
Talwin	30 mg	IM, SC, IV	J3070
Tamoxifen Citrate			J8999

◀ New ↻ Revised ✔ Reinstated ~~deleted~~ Deleted

DRUG NAME	DOSAGE	METHOD OF ADMINISTRATION	HCPCS CODE
Taractan, *see* Chlorprothixene			
Taxol	1 mg	IV	J9267
Taxotere	20 mg	IV	J9171
Tazicef	per 500 mg		J0713
Tazidime, *see* Ceftazidime Technetium TC Sestambi	per dose		**A9500**
			J0713
Tedizolid phosphate	1 mg	IV	**J3090**
TEEV	1 mg	IM	J3121
Teflaro	1 mg		J0712
Telavancin	10 mg	IV	**J3095**
Temodar	5 mg	ORAL	J8700, J9328
Temozolomide	1 mg	IV	**J9328**
	5 mg	ORAL	**J8700**
Temsirolimus	1 mg	IV	**J9330**
Tenecteplase	1 mg	IV	**J3101**
Teniposide	50 mg		**Q2017**
Tepadina	15 mg		J9340
Teprotumumab-trbw	10 mg	IV	J3241
Tequin	10 mg	IV	J1590
Terbutaline sulfate	up to 1 mg	SC, IV	**J3105**
concentrated form	per 1 mg	INH	**J7680**
unit dose form	per 1 mg	INH	**J7681**
Teriparatide	10 mcg	SC	**J3110**
Terramycin IM	up to 50 mg	IM	J2460
Testa-C	1 mg		J1071
Testadiate	1 mg	IM	J3121
Testadiate-Depo	1 mg		J1071
Testaject-LA	1 mg		J1071
Testaqua	up to 50 mg	IM	J3140
Test-Estro Cypionates	1 mg		J1071
Test-Estro-C	1 mg		J1071
Testex	up to 100 mg	IM	J3150
Testo AQ	up to 50 mg		J3140
Testoject-50	up to 50 mg	IM	J3140
Testoject-LA	1 mg		J1071
Testone			
LA 100	1 mg	IM	J3121
LA 200	1 mg	IM	J3121
Testopel Pellets			J3490
Testosterone Aqueous	up to 50 mg	IM	J3140

◄ **New** ⤾ **Revised** ✔ **Reinstated** ~~deleted~~ **Deleted**

DRUG NAME	DOSAGE	METHOD OF ADMINISTRATION	HCPCS CODE
Testosterone cypionate	1 mg	IM	**J1071**
Testosterone enanthate	1 mg	IM	**J3121**
Testosterone undecanoate	1 mg	IM	**J3145**
Testradiol 90/4	1 mg	IM	J3121
Testrin PA	1 mg	IM	J3121
Testro AQ	up to 50 mg		J3140
Tetanus immune globulin, human	up to 250 units	IM	**J1670**
Tetracycline	up to 250 mg	IM, IV	**J0120**
Thallous Chloride TI-201	per MCI		**A9505**
Theelin Aqueous	per 1 mg	IM	J1435
Theophylline	per 40 mg	IV	**J2810**
Thiamine HCl	100 mg		**J3411**
Thiethylperazine maleate			
injection	up to 10 mg	IM	**J3280**
oral	10 mg	ORAL	**Q0174**
Thiotepa	15 mg	IV	**J9340**
Thorazine	up to 50 mg	IM, IV	J3230
Thrombate III	per IU		J7197
Thymoglobulin (*see also* Immune globulin)			
anti-thymocyte globulin, equine	250 mg	IV	**J7504**
anti-thymocyte globulin, rabbit	25 mg	IV	**J7511**
Thypinone	per 250 mcg	IV	J2725
Thyrogen	0.9 mg	IM, SC	J3240
Thyrotropin Alfa, injection	0.9 mg	IM, SC	**J3240**
Ticon			
injection	up to 200 mg	IM	J3250
oral	250 mg	ORAL	Q0173
Tigan			
injection	up to 200 mg	IM	J3250
oral	250 mg	ORAL	Q0173
Tigecycline	1 mg	IV	**J3243**
Tiject-20			
injection	up to 200 mg	IM	J3250
oral	250 mg	ORAL	Q0173
Tinzaparin	1,000 IU	SC	**J1655**
Tirofiban Hydrochloride, injection	0.25 mg	IM, IV	**J3246**
TNKase	1 mg	IV	J3101
Tobi	300 mg	INH	J7682, J7685
Tobramycin, inhalation solution	300 mg	INH	**J7682, J7685**

◀ New ⤺ Revised ✔ Reinstated ~~deleted~~ Deleted

DRUG NAME	DOSAGE	METHOD OF ADMINISTRATION	HCPCS CODE
Tobramycin sulfate	up to 80 mg	IM, IV	J3260
Tocilizumab	1 mg	IV	J3262
Tofranil, *see* Imipramine HCl			
Tolazoline HCl	up to 25 mg	IV	J2670
Toposar	10 mg		J9181
Topotecan	0.25 mg	ORAL	J8705
	0.1 mg	IV	J9351
Toradol	per 15 mg	IM, IV	J1885
Torecan			
injection	up to 10 mg	IM	J3280
oral	10 mg	ORAL	Q0174
Torisel	1 mg		J9330
Tornalate			
concentrated form	per mg	INH	J7628
unit dose	per mg	INH	J7629
Torsemide	10 mg/ml	IV	J3265
Totacillin-N	up to 500 mg	IM, IV	J0290
	per 1.5 gm	IM, IV	J0295
Trabectedin	0.1 mg	IV	J9352
Trastuzumab	10 mg	IV	J9355
Trastuzumab-anns (kanjinti)	10 mg	IV	Q5117
Trastuzumab-dkst	10 mg	IV	Q5114
Trastuzumab-dttb	10 mg	IV	Q5112
Trastuzumab-pkrb	10 mg	IV	Q5113
Trastuzumab-qyyp (trazimera)	10 mg	IV	Q5116
Trastuzumab and Hyaluronidase	10 mg	IV	J9356
Treanda	1 mg	IV	J3490, J9033
Trelstar	3.75 mg		J3315
Treprostinil	1 mg		J3285, J7686
Trexall	2.5 mg	ORAL	J8610
Triam-A	1 mg		J3300
	per 10 mg	IM	J3301
Triamcinolone			
concentrated form	per 1 mg	INH	J7683
unit dose	per 1 mg	INH	J7684
Triamcinolone acetonide	1 mg		J3300
	per 10 mg	IM	J3301
Triamcinolone acetonide XR	1 mg	IM	J3304
Triamcinolone diacetate	per 5 mg	IM	J3302

◀ New ↩ Revised ✔ Reinstated ~~deleted~~ Deleted

DRUG NAME	DOSAGE	METHOD OF ADMINISTRATION	HCPCS CODE
Triamcinolone hexacetonide	per 5 mg	VAR	**J3303**
Triesence	1 mg		J3300
	per 10 mg	IM	J3301
Triethylene thio-Phosphoramide/T	15 mg		J9340
Triflupromazine HCl	up to 20 mg	IM, IV	**J3400**
Tri-Kort	1 mg		J3300
	per 10 mg	IM	J3301
Trilafon	4 mg	ORAL	Q0175
	up to 5 mg	IM, IV	J3310
Trilog	1 mg		J3300
	per 10 mg	IM	J3301
Trilone	per 5 mg		J3302
Trimethobenzamide HCl			
injection	up to 200 mg	IM	**J3250**
oral	250 mg	ORAL	**Q0173**
Trimetrexate glucuronate	per 25 mg	IV	**J3305**
Triptorelin Pamoate	3.75 mg	SC	**J3315**
Triptorelin XR	3.75 mg	SC	**J3316**
Trisenox	1 mg	IV	J9017
Trobicin	up to 2 g	IM	J3320
Trovan	100 mg	IV	J0200
Tysabri	1 mg		J2323
Tyvaso	1.74 mg		J7686
U			
Ultravist 240	per ml		Q9966
Ultravist 300	per ml		Q9967
Ultravist 370	per ml		Q9967
Ultrazine-10	up to 10 mg	IM, IV	J0780
Unasyn	per 1.5 gm	IM, IV	J0295
Unclassified drugs (*see also* Not elsewhere classified)			**J3490**
Unclassified drugs or biological used for ESRD on dialysis		IV	**J3591**
Unspecified oral antiemetic			**Q0181**
Urea	up to 40 g	IV	**J3350**
Ureaphil	up to 40 g	IV	J3350
Urecholine	up to 5 mg	SC	J0520
Urofollitropin	75 IU		**J3355**
Urokinase	5,000 IU vial	IV	**J3364**
	250,000 IU vial	IV	**J3365**
Ustekinumab	1 mg	SC	**J3357**
	1 mg	IV	**J3358**

◀ New ⤾ Revised ✔ Reinstated ~~deleted~~ Deleted

DRUG NAME	DOSAGE	METHOD OF ADMINISTRATION	HCPCS CODE
V			
Valcyte			J3490
Valergen 10	10 mg	IM	J1380
Valergen 20	10 mg	IM	J1380
Valergen 40	up to 10 mg	IM	J1380
Valertest No. 1	1 mg	IM	J3121
Valertest No. 2	1 mg	IM	J3121
Valganciclovir HCL			J8499
Valium	up to 5 mg	IM, IV	J3360
Valrubicin, intravesical	200 mg	OTH	**J9357**
Valstar	200 mg	OTH	J9357
Vancocin	500 mg	IV, IM	J3370
Vancoled	500 mg	IV, IM	J3370
Vancomycin HCl	500 mg	IV, IM	**J3370**
Vantas	50 mg		J9226, J9225
Varubi	90 mg		J8670
Vasceze	per 10 mg		J1642
Vasoxyl, *see* Methoxamine HCl			
Vectibix	10 mg		J9303
Vedolizumab	1 mg	IV	**J3380**
Velaglucerase alfa	100 units	IV	**J3385**
Velban	1 mg	IV	J9360
Velcade	0.1 mg		J9041
Veletri	0.5 mg		J1325
Velsar	1 mg	IV	J9360
Venofer	1 mg	IV	J1756
Ventavis	20 mcg		Q4074
Ventolin	0.5 mg	INH	J7620
concentrated form	1 mg	INH	J7610, J7611
unit dose form	1 mg	INH	J7609, J7613
VePesid	50 mg	ORAL	J8560
Veritas Collagen Matrix			J3490
Versed	per 1 mg	IM, IV	J2250
Verteporfin	0.1 mg	IV	**J3396**
Vesprin	up to 20 mg	IM, IV	J3400
Vestronidase alfa-vjbk	1 mg	IV	**J3397**
VFEND IV	10 mg	IV	J3465
V-Gan 25	up to 50 mg	IM, IV	J2550
	12.5 mg	ORAL	Q0169

◀ New ⤾ Revised ✔ Reinstated ~~deleted~~ Deleted

DRUG NAME	DOSAGE	METHOD OF ADMINISTRATION	HCPCS CODE
V-Gan 50	up to 50 mg	IM, IV	J2550
	12.5 mg	ORAL	Q0169
Viadur	65 mg	OTH	J9219
Vibativ	10 mg		J3095
Vinblastine sulfate	1 mg	IV	**J9360**
Vincasar PFS	1 mg	IV	J9370
Vincristine sulfate	1 mg	IV	**J9370**
Vincristine sulfate liposome	1 mg	IV	**J9371**
Vinorelbine tartrate	per 10 mg	IV	**J9390**
Vispaque	per ml		Q9966, Q9967
Vistaject-25	up to 25 mg	IM	J3410
Vistaril	up to 25 mg	IM	J3410
	25 mg	ORAL	Q0177
Vistide	375 mg	IV	J0740
Visudyne	0.1 mg	IV	J3396
Vitamin B-12 cyanocobalamin	up to 1,000 mcg	IM, SC	**J3420**
Vitamin K, phytonadione, menadione, menadiol sodium diphosphate	per 1 mg	IM, SC, IV	**J3430**
Vitrase	per 1 USP unit		J3471
Vivaglobin	100 mg		J1562
Vivitrol	1 mg		J2315
Von Willebrand Factor Complex, human	per IU VWF:RCo	IV	**J7187**
Wilate	per IU VWF	IV	**J7183**
Vonvendi	per IU VWF	IV	**J7179**
Voretigene neparvovec-rzyl	1 billion vector genomes	IV	**J3398**
Voriconazole	10 mg	IV	**J3465**
Vpriv	100 units		J3385
W			
Wehamine	up to 50 mg	IM, IV	J1240
Wehdryl	up to 50 mg	IM, IV	J1200
	50 mg	ORAL	Q0163
Wellcovorin	per 50 mg	IM, IV	J0640
Wilate	per IU	IV	J7183
Win Rho SD	100 IU	IV	J2792
Wyamine Sulfate, *see* Mephentermine sulfate			
Wycillin	up to 600,000 units	IM, IV	J2510
Wydase	up to 150 units	SC, IV	J3470
X			
Xeloda	150 mg	ORAL	J8520
	500 mg	ORAL	J8521

◀ New ⤼ Revised ✔ Reinstated ~~deleted~~ Deleted

DRUG NAME	DOSAGE	METHOD OF ADMINISTRATION	HCPCS CODE
Xeomin	1 unit		J0588
Xgera	1 mg		J0987
Xgeva	1 mg		J0897
Xiaflex	0.01 mg		J0775
Xolair	5 mg		J2357
Xopenex	0.5 mg	INH	J7620
concentrated form	1 mg	INH	J7610, J7611, J7612
unit dose form	1 mg	INH	J7609, J7613, J7614
Xylocaine HCl	10 mg	IV	J2001
Xyntha	per IU	IV	J7185, J7192, J7182, J7188
Y			
Yervoy, *see* Ipilimumab			
Yondelis	0.1 mg		J9352, J9999
Z			
Zaltrap	1 mg		J9400
Zanosar	1 g	IV	J9320
Zantac	25 mg	IV, IM	J2780
Zarxio	1 mcg		Q5101
Zemaira	10 mg	IV	J0256
Zemplar	1 mcg	IM, IV	J2501
Zenapax	25 mg	IV	J7513
Zerbaxa	1 gm		J0695
Zetran	up to 5 mg	IM, IV	J3360
Ziconotide	1 mcg	OTH	**J2278**
Zidovudine	10 mg	IV	**J3485**
Zinacef	per 750 mg	IM, IV	J0697
Zinecard	per 250 mg		J1190
Ziprasidone Mesylate	10 mg	IM	**J3486**
Zithromax	1 gm	ORAL	Q0144
injection	500 mg	IV	J0456
Ziv-Aflibercept	1 mg	IV	**J9400**
Zmax	1 g		Q0144
Zofran	1 mg	IV	J2405
	1 mg	ORAL	Q0162
Zoladex	per 3.6 mg	SC	J9202
Zoledronic Acid	1 mg	IV	**J3489**
Zolicef	500 mg	IV, IM	J0690
Zometra	1 mg		J3489

◀ **New** ⤾ **Revised** ✔ **Reinstated** ~~deleted~~ **Deleted**

DRUG NAME	DOSAGE	METHOD OF ADMINISTRATION	HCPCS CODE
Zorbtive	1 mg		J2941
Zortress	0.25 mg	ORAL	J7527
Zosyn	1.125 g	IV	J2543
Zovirax	5 mg		J8499
Zyprexa Relprevv	1 mg		J2358
Zyvox	200 mg	IV	J2020

◀ New ↩ Revised ✔ Reinstated ~~deleted~~ Deleted

HCPCS 2021

LEVEL II NATIONAL CODES

2021 HCPCS quarterly updates available on the companion website at: http://www.codingupdates.com

DISCLAIMER

Every effort has been made to make this text complete and accurate, but no guarantee, warranty, or representation is made for its accuracy or completeness. This text is based on the Centers for Medicare and Medicaid Services Healthcare Common Procedure Coding System (HCPCS).

Do not report HCPCS modifiers with MIPS CPT Category II codes, rather, use Performance Measurement Modifiers 1P, 2P, 3P, and 8P, as instructed in the CPT guidelines for Category II codes under 'Modifiers'.

LEVEL II NATIONAL MODIFIERS

- * **A1** Dressing for one wound
- * **A2** Dressing for two wounds
- * **A3** Dressing for three wounds
- * **A4** Dressing for four wounds
- * **A5** Dressing for five wounds
- * **A6** Dressing for six wounds
- * **A7** Dressing for seven wounds
- * **A8** Dressing for eight wounds
- * **A9** Dressing for nine or more wounds
- ◌ **AA** Anesthesia services performed personally by anesthesiologist
  IOM: 100-04, 12, 90.4
- ◌ **AD** Medical supervision by a physician: more than four concurrent anesthesia procedures
  IOM: 100-04, 12, 90.4
- * **AE** Registered dietician
- * **AF** Specialty physician
- * **AG** Primary physician
- ◌ **AH** Clinical psychologist
  IOM: 100-04, 12, 170
- * **AI** Principal physician of record
- ◌ **AJ** Clinical social worker
  IOM: 100-04, 12, 170; 100-04, 12, 150
- * **AK** Nonparticipating physician
- ◌ **AM** Physician, team member service
  Not assigned for Medicare
  Cross Reference QM
- * **AO** Alternate payment method declined by provider of service
- * **AP** Determination of refractive state was not performed in the course of diagnostic ophthalmological examination
- * **AQ** Physician providing a service in an unlisted health professional shortage area (HPSA)
- * **AR** Physician provider services in a physician scarcity area
- * **AS** Physician assistant, nurse practitioner, or clinical nurse specialist services for assistant at surgery
- * **AT** Acute treatment (this modifier should be used when reporting service 98940, 98941, 98942)
- * **AU** Item furnished in conjunction with a urological, ostomy, or tracheostomy supply
- * **AV** Item furnished in conjunction with a prosthetic device, prosthetic or orthotic
- * **AW** Item furnished in conjunction with a surgical dressing
- * **AX** Item furnished in conjunction with dialysis services
- * **AY** Item or service furnished to an ESRD patient that is not for the treatment of ESRD
- ⊘ **AZ** Physician providing a service in a dental health professional shortage area for the purpose of an electronic health record incentive payment
- * **BA** Item furnished in conjunction with parenteral enteral nutrition (PEN) services
- * **BL** Special acquisition of blood and blood products
- * **BO** Orally administered nutrition, not by feeding tube
- * **BP** The beneficiary has been informed of the purchase and rental options and has elected to purchase the item
- * **BR** The beneficiary has been informed of the purchase and rental options and has elected to rent the item
- * **BU** The beneficiary has been informed of the purchase and rental options and after 30 days has not informed the supplier of his/her decision
- * **CA** Procedure payable only in the inpatient setting when performed emergently on an outpatient who expires prior to admission
- * **CB** Service ordered by a renal dialysis facility (RDF) physician as part of the ESRD beneficiary's dialysis benefit, is not part of the composite rate, and is separately reimbursable
- * **CC** Procedure code change (Use CC when the procedure code submitted was changed either for administrative reasons or because an incorrect code was filed)
- ◌ **CD** AMCC test has been ordered by an ESRD facility or MCP physician that is part of the composite rate and is not separately billable

▶ New ⮌ Revised ✔ Reinstated ~~deleted~~ Deleted ⊘ Not covered or valid by Medicare
◌ Special coverage instructions * Carrier discretion Ⓑ Bill Part B MAC Ⓑ Bill DME MAC

CE AMCC test has been ordered by an ESRD facility or MCP physician that is a composite rate test but is beyond the normal frequency covered under the rate and is separately reimbursable based on medical necessity

CF AMCC test has been ordered by an ESRD facility or MCP physician that is not part of the composite rate and is separately billable

* **CG** Policy criteria applied

CH 0 percent impaired, limited or restricted

CI At least 1 percent but less than 20 percent impaired, limited or restricted

CJ At least 20 percent but less than 40 percent impaired, limited or restricted

CK At least 40 percent but less than 60 percent impaired, limited or restricted

CL At least 60 percent but less than 80 percent impaired, limited or restricted

CM At least 80 percent but less than 100 percent impaired, limited or restricted

CN 100 percent impaired, limited or restricted

* **CO** Outpatient occupational therapy services furnished in whole or in part by an occupational therapy assistant

* **CR** Catastrophe/Disaster related

* **CS** Cost-sharing waived for specified covid-19 testing-related services that result in and order for or administration of a covid-19 test and/or used for cost-sharing waived preventive services furnished via telehealth in rural health clinics and federally qualified health centers during the covid-19 public health emergency

* **CT** Computed tomography services furnished using equipment that does not meet each of the attributes of the national electrical manufacturers association (NEMA) XR-29-2013 standard

Coding Clinic: 2017, Q1, P6

* **CQ** Outpatient physical therapy services furnished in whole or in part by a physical therapist assistant

* **DA** Oral health assessment by a licensed health professional other than a dentist

* **E1** Upper left, eyelid

Coding Clinic: 2016, Q3, P3

* **E2** Lower left, eyelid

Coding Clinic: 2016, Q3, P3

* **E3** Upper right, eyelid

Coding Clinic: 2011, Q3, P6

* **E4** Lower right, eyelid

EA Erythropoetic stimulating agent (ESA) administered to treat anemia due to anti-cancer chemotherapy

CMS requires claims for non-ESRD ESAs (J0881 and J0885) to include one of three modifiers: EA, EB, EC.

EB Erythropoetic stimulating agent (ESA) administered to treat anemia due to anti-cancer radiotherapy

CMS requires claims for non-ESRD ESAs (J0881 and J0885) to include one of three modifiers: EA, EB, EC.

EC Erythropoetic stimulating agent (ESA) administered to treat anemia not due to anti-cancer radiotherapy or anti-cancer chemotherapy

CMS requires claims for non-ESRD ESAs (J0881 and J0885) to include one of three modifiers: EA, EB, EC.

ED Hematocrit level has exceeded 39% (or hemoglobin level has exceeded 13.0 g/dl) for 3 or more consecutive billing cycles immediately prior to and including the current cycle

EE Hematocrit level has not exceeded 39% (or hemoglobin level has not exceeded 13.0 g/dl) for 3 or more consecutive billing cycles immediately prior to and including the current cycle

EJ Subsequent claims for a defined course of therapy, e.g., EPO, sodium hyaluronate, infliximab

EM Emergency reserve supply (for ESRD benefit only)

* **EP** Service provided as part of Medicaid early periodic screening diagnosis and treatment (EPSDT) program

* **ER** Items and services furnished by a provider-based, off-campus emergency department

* **ET** Emergency services

* **EX** Expatriate beneficiary

* **EY** No physician or other licensed health care provider order for this item or service

Items billed before a signed and dated order has been received by the supplier must be submitted with an EY modifier added to each related HCPCS code.

MIPS | Qp Quantity Physician | Qh Quantity Hospital | ♀ Female only | ♂ Male only | A Age | DMEPOS | A2-Z3 ASC Payment Indicator | A-Y ASC Status Indicator | Coding Clinic

✻ **F1** Left hand, second digit

✻ **F2** Left hand, third digit

✻ **F3** Left hand, fourth digit

✻ **F4** Left hand, fifth digit

✻ **F5** Right hand, thumb

✻ **F6** Right hand, second digit

✻ **F7** Right hand, third digit

✻ **F8** Right hand, fourth digit

✻ **F9** Right hand, fifth digit

✻ **FA** Left hand, thumb

⊘ **FB** Item provided without cost to provider, supplier or practitioner, or full credit received for replaced device (examples, but not limited to, covered under warranty, replaced due to defect, free samples)

◌ **FC** Partial credit received for replaced device

✻ **FP** Service provided as part of family planning program

✻ **FX** X-ray taken using film

Coding Clinic: 2017, Q1, P6

✻ **FY** X-ray taken using computed radiography technology/cassette-based imaging

✻ **G0** Telehealth services for diagnosis, evaluation, or treatment, of symptoms of an acute stroke

✻ **G1** Most recent URR reading of less than 60

IOM: 100-04, 8, 50.9

✻ **G2** Most recent URR reading of 60 to 64.9

IOM: 100-04, 8, 50.9

✻ **G3** Most recent URR reading of 65 to 69.9

IOM: 100-04, 8, 50.9

✻ **G4** Most recent URR reading of 70 to 74.9

IOM: 100-04, 8, 50.9

✻ **G5** Most recent URR reading of 75 or greater

IOM: 100-04, 8, 50.9

✻ **G6** ESRD patient for whom less than six dialysis sessions have been provided in a month

IOM: 100-04, 8, 50.9

◌ **G7** Pregnancy resulted from rape or incest or pregnancy certified by physician as life threatening

IOM: 100-02, 15, 20.1; 100-03, 3, 170.3

✻ **G8** Monitored anesthesia care (MAC) for deep complex, complicated, or markedly invasive surgical procedure

✻ **G9** Monitored anesthesia care for patient who has history of severe cardiopulmonary condition

✻ **GA** Waiver of liability statement issued as required by payer policy, individual case

An item/service is expected to be denied as not reasonable and necessary and an ABN is on file. Modifier GA can be used on either a specific or a miscellaneous HCPCS code. Modifiers GA and GY should never be reported together on the same line for the same HCPCS code.

✻ **GB** Claim being resubmitted for payment because it is no longer covered under a global payment demonstration

◌ **GC** This service has been performed in part by a resident under the direction of a teaching physician

IOM: 100-04, 12, 90.4, 100

◌ **GE** This service has been performed by a resident without the presence of a teaching physician under the primary care exception

✻ **GF** Non-physician (e.g., nurse practitioner (NP), certified registered nurse anesthetist (CRNA), certified registered nurse (CRN), clinical nurse specialist (CNS), physician assistant (PA)) services in a critical access hospital

✻ **GG** Performance and payment of a screening mammogram and diagnostic mammogram on the same patient, same day

✻ **GH** Diagnostic mammogram converted from screening mammogram on same day

✻ **GJ** "Opt out" physician or practitioner emergency or urgent service

✻ **GK** Reasonable and necessary item/service associated with a GA or GZ modifier

An upgrade is defined as an item that goes beyond what is medically necessary under Medicare's coverage requirements. An item can be considered an upgrade even if the physician has signed an order for it. When suppliers know that an item will not be paid in full because it does not meet the coverage criteria stated in the LCD, the supplier can still obtain partial payment at the time of initial determination if the claim is billed using one of the upgrade modifiers (GK or GL). (https://www.cms.gov/manuals/downloads/clm104c01.pdf)

✻ **GL**	Medically unnecessary upgrade provided instead of non-upgraded item, no charge, no Advance Beneficiary Notice (ABN)
✻ **GM**	Multiple patients on one ambulance trip
✻ **GN**	Services delivered under an outpatient speech language pathology plan of care
✻ **GO**	Services delivered under an outpatient occupational therapy plan of care
✻ **GP**	Services delivered under an outpatient physical therapy plan of care
✻ **GQ**	Via asynchronous telecommunications system
✻ **GR**	This service was performed in whole or in part by a resident in a Department of Veterans Affairs medical center or clinic, supervised in accordance with VA policy
GS	Dosage of erythropoietin-stimulating agent has been reduced and maintained in response to hematocrit or hemoglobin level
GT	Via interactive audio and video telecommunication systems
✻ **GU**	Waiver of liability statement issued as required by payer policy, routine notice
GV	Attending physician not employed or paid under arrangement by the patient's hospice provider
GW	Service not related to the hospice patient's terminal condition
✻ **GX**	Notice of liability issued, voluntary under payer policy GX modifier must be submitted with non-covered charges only. This modifier differentiates from the required uses in conjunction with ABN. (https://www.cms.gov/manuals/downloads/clm104c01.pdf)
⃠ **GY**	Item or service statutorily excluded, does not meet the definition of any Medicare benefit or, for non-Medicare insurers, is not a contract benefit Examples of "statutorily excluded" include: Infusion drug not administered using a durable infusion pump, a wheelchair that is for use for mobility outside the home or hearing aids. GA and GY should never be coded together on the same line for the same HCPCS code. (https://www.cms.gov/manuals/downloads/clm104c01.pdf)
⃠ **GZ**	Item or service expected to be denied as not reasonable or necessary Used when an ABN is not on file and can be used on either a specific or a miscellaneous HCPCS code. It would never be correct to place any combination of GY, GZ or GA modifiers on the same claim line and will result in rejected or denied claim for invalid coding. (https://www.cms.gov/manuals/downloads/clm104c01.pdf)
⃠ **H9**	Court-ordered
⃠ **HA**	Child/adolescent program
⃠ **HB**	Adult program, nongeriatric
⃠ **HC**	Adult program, geriatric
⃠ **HD**	Pregnant/parenting women's program
⃠ **HE**	Mental health program
⃠ **HF**	Substance abuse program
⃠ **HG**	Opioid addiction treatment program
⃠ **HH**	Integrated mental health/substance abuse program
⃠ **HI**	Integrated mental health and intellectual disability/developmental disabilities program
⃠ **HJ**	Employee assistance program
⃠ **HK**	Specialized mental health programs for high-risk populations
⃠ **HL**	Intern
⃠ **HM**	Less than bachelors degree level
⃠ **HN**	Bachelors degree level
⃠ **HO**	Masters degree level
⃠ **HP**	Doctoral level
⃠ **HQ**	Group setting
⃠ **HR**	Family/couple with client present
⃠ **HS**	Family/couple without client present
⃠ **HT**	Multi-disciplinary team
⃠ **HU**	Funded by child welfare agency
⃠ **HV**	Funded by state addictions agency
⃠ **HW**	Funded by state mental health agency
⃠ **HX**	Funded by county/local agency
⃠ **HY**	Funded by juvenile justice agency
⃠ **HZ**	Funded by criminal justice agency
✻ **J1**	Competitive acquisition program no-pay submission for a prescription number
✻ **J2**	Competitive acquisition program, restocking of emergency drugs after emergency administration

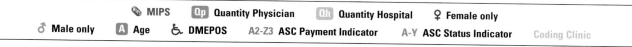

* J3 Competitive acquisition program (CAP), drug not available through CAP as written, reimbursed under average sales price methodology
* J4 DMEPOS item subject to DMEPOS competitive bidding program that is furnished by a hospital upon discharge
▶* J5 Off-the-shelf orthotic subject to dmepos competitive bidding program that is furnished as part of a physical therapist or occupational therapist professional service
* JA Administered intravenously

  This modifier is informational only (not a payment modifier) and may be submitted with all injection codes. According to Medicare, reporting this modifier is voluntary. (CMS Pub. 100-04, chapter 8, section 60.2.3.1 and Pub. 100-04, chapter 17, section 80.11)
* JB Administered subcutaneously
* JC Skin substitute used as a graft
* JD Skin substitute not used as a graft
* JE Administered via dialysate
* JG Drug or biological acquired with 340B drug pricing program discount
* JW Drug amount discarded/not administered to any patient

  Use JW to identify unused drugs or biologicals from single use vial/package that are appropriately discarded. Bill on separate line for payment of discarded drug/biological.

  IOM: 100-4, 17, 40

  Coding Clinic: 2016, Q4, P4-7; 2010, Q3, P10
* K0 Lower extremity prosthesis functional Level 0 - does not have the ability or potential to ambulate or transfer safely with or without assistance and a prosthesis does not enhance their quality of life or mobility.
* K1 Lower extremity prosthesis functional Level 1 - has the ability or potential to use a prosthesis for transfers or ambulation on level surfaces at fixed cadence. Typical of the limited and unlimited household ambulator.
* K2 Lower extremity prosthesis functional Level 2 - has the ability or potential for ambulation with the ability to traverse low level environmental barriers such as curbs, stairs or uneven surfaces. Typical of the limited community ambulator.
* K3 Lower extremity prosthesis functional Level 3 - has the ability or potential for ambulation with variable cadence. Typical of the community ambulator who has the ability to traverse most environmental barriers and may have vocational, therapeutic, or exercise activity that demands prosthetic utilization beyond simple locomotion.
* K4 Lower extremity prosthesis functional Level 4 - has the ability or potential for prosthetic ambulation that exceeds the basic ambulation skills, exhibiting high impact, stress, or energy levels, typical of the prosthetic demands of the child, active adult, or athlete.
* KA Add on option/accessory for wheelchair
* KB Beneficiary requested upgrade for ABN, more than 4 modifiers identified on claim
* KC Replacement of special power wheelchair interface
* KD Drug or biological infused through DME
* KE Bid under round one of the DMEPOS competitive bidding program for use with non-competitive bid base equipment
* KF Item designated by FDA as Class III device
* KG DMEPOS item subject to DMEPOS competitive bidding program number 1
* KH DMEPOS item, initial claim, purchase or first month rental
* KI DMEPOS item, second or third month rental
* KJ DMEPOS item, parenteral enteral nutrition (PEN) pump or capped rental, months four to fifteen
* KK DMEPOS item subject to DMEPOS competitive bidding program number 2
* KL DMEPOS item delivered via mail
* KM Replacement of facial prosthesis including new impression/moulage
* KN Replacement of facial prosthesis using previous master model
* KO Single drug unit dose formulation
* KP First drug of a multiple drug unit dose formulation
* KQ Second or subsequent drug of a multiple drug unit dose formulation
* KR Rental item, billing for partial month

◌ KS Glucose monitor supply for diabetic beneficiary not treated with insulin

▶ New ⤾ Revised ✔ Reinstated ~~deleted~~ Deleted ⊘ Not covered or valid by Medicare
◌ Special coverage instructions * Carrier discretion Ⓑ Bill Part B MAC Ⓔ Bill DME MAC

*	**KT**	Beneficiary resides in a competitive bidding area and travels outside that competitive bidding area and receives a competitive bid item
*	**KU**	DMEPOS item subject to DMEPOS competitive bidding program number 3
*	**KV**	DMEPOS item subject to DMEPOS competitive bidding program that is furnished as part of a professional service
*	**KW**	DMEPOS item subject to DMEPOS competitive bidding program number 4
*	**KX**	Requirements specified in the medical policy have been met Used for physical, occupational, or speech-language therapy to request an exception to therapy payment caps and indicate the services are reasonable and necessary and that there is documentation of medical necessity in the patient's medical record. (Pub 100-04 Attachment - Business Requirements Centers for Medicare and Medicaid Services, Transmittal 2457, April 27, 2012) Medicare requires modifier KX for implanted permanent cardiac pacemakers, single chamber or duel chamber, for one of the following CPT codes: 33206, 33207, 33208.
*	**KY**	DMEPOS item subject to DMEPOS competitive bidding program number 5
*	**KZ**	New coverage not implemented by managed care
*	**LC**	Left circumflex coronary artery
*	**LD**	Left anterior descending coronary artery
*	**LL**	Lease/rental (use the LL modifier when DME equipment rental is to be applied against the purchase price)
*	**LM**	Left main coronary artery
*	**LR**	Laboratory round trip
◎	**LS**	FDA-monitored intraocular lens implant
*	**LT**	Left side (used to identify procedures performed on the left side of the body) Modifiers LT and RT identify procedures which can be performed on paired organs. Used for procedures performed on one side only. Should also be used when the procedures are similar but not identical and are performed on paired body parts. Coding Clinic: 2016, Q3, P5
*	**M2**	Medicare secondary payer (MSP)
*	**MA**	Ordering professional is not required to consult a clinical decision support mechanism due to service being rendered to a patient with a suspected or confirmed emergency medical condition
*	**MB**	Ordering professional is not required to consult a clinical decision support mechanism due to the significant hardship exception of insufficient internet access
*	**MC**	Ordering professional is not required to consult a clinical decision support mechanism due to the significant hardship exception of electronic health record or clinical decision support mechanism vendor issues
*	**MD**	Ordering professional is not required to consult a clinical decision support mechanism due to the significant hardship exception of extreme and uncontrollable circumstances
*	**ME**	The order for this service adheres to appropriate use criteria in the clinical decision support mechanism consulted by the ordering professional
*	**MF**	The order for this service does not adhere to the appropriate use criteria in the clinical decision support mechanism consulted by the ordering professional
*	**MG**	The order for this service does not have applicable appropriate use criteria in the qualified clinical decision support mechanism consulted by the ordering professional
*	**MH**	Unknown if ordering professional consulted a clinical decision support mechanism for this service, related information was not provided to the furnishing professional or provider
*	**MS**	Six month maintenance and servicing fee for reasonable and necessary parts and labor which are not covered under any manufacturer or supplier warranty
*	**NB**	Nebulizer system, any type, FDA-cleared for use with specific drug
*	**NR**	New when rented (use the NR modifier when DME which was new at the time of rental is subsequently purchased)
*	**NU**	New equipment
*	**P1**	A normal healthy patient
*	**P2**	A patient with mild systemic disease
*	**P3**	A patient with severe systemic disease

* **P4** A patient with severe systemic disease that is a constant threat to life
* **P5** A moribund patient who is not expected to survive without the operation
* **P6** A declared brain-dead patient whose organs are being removed for donor purposes
⊘ **PA** Surgical or other invasive procedure on wrong body part
⊘ **PB** Surgical or other invasive procedure on wrong patient
⊘ **PC** Wrong surgery or other invasive procedure on patient
* **PD** Diagnostic or related non diagnostic item or service provided in a wholly owned or operated entity to a patient who is admitted as an inpatient within 3 days
* **PI** Positron emission tomography (PET) or PET/computed tomography (CT) to inform the initial treatment strategy of tumors that are biopsy proven or strongly suspected of being cancerous based on other diagnostic testing
* **PL** Progressive addition lenses
* **PM** Post mortem
* **PN** Non-excepted service provided at an off-campus, outpatient, provider-based department of a hospital
* **PO** Expected services provided at off-campus, outpatient, provider-based department of a hospital
* **PS** Positron emission tomography (PET) or PET/computed tomography (CT) to inform the subsequent treatment strategy of cancerous tumors when the beneficiary's treating physician determines that the PET study is needed to inform subsequent anti-tumor strategy
* **PT** Colorectal cancer screening test; converted to diagnostic text or other procedure

  Assign this modifier with the appropriate CPT procedure code for colonoscopy, flexible sigmoidoscopy, or barium enema when the service is initiated as a colorectal cancer screening service but then becomes a diagnostic service. MLN Matters article MM7012 (PDF, 75 KB) Reference Medicare Transmittal 3232 April 3, 2015.

  Coding Clinic: 2011, Q1, P10

Q0 Investigational clinical service provided in a clinical research study that is in an approved clinical research study

Q1 Routine clinical service provided in a clinical research study that is in an approved clinical research study

* **Q2** Demonstration procedure/service
* **Q3** Live kidney donor surgery and related services
* **Q4** Service for ordering/referring physician qualifies as a service exemption

Q5 Service furnished under a reciprocal billing arrangement by a substitute physician or by a substitute physical therapist furnishing outpatient physical therapy services in a health professional shortage area, a medically underserved area, or a rural area

IOM: 100-04, 1, 30.2.10

Q6 Service furnished under a fee-for-time compensation arrangement by a substitute physician or by a substitute physical therapist furnishing outpatient physical therapy services in a health professional shortage area, a medically underserved area, or a rural area

IOM: 100-04, 1, 30.2.11

* **Q7** One Class A finding
* **Q8** Two Class B findings
* **Q9** One Class B and two Class C findings
* **QA** Prescribed amounts of stationary oxygen for daytime use while at rest and nighttime use differ and the average of the two amounts is less than 1 liter per minute (lpm)
* **QB** Prescribed amounts of stationary oxygen for daytime use while at rest and nighttime use differ and the average of the two amounts exceeds 4 liters per minute (lpm) and portable oxygen is prescribed
* **QC** Single channel monitoring
* **QD** Recording and storage in solid state memory by a digital recorder
* **QE** Prescribed amount of stationary oxygen while at rest is less than 1 liter per minute (LPM)
* **QF** Prescribed amount of stationary oxygen while at rest exceeds 4 liters per minute (LPM) and portable oxygen is prescribed

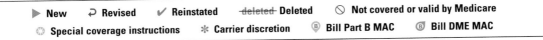

▶ New ↻ Revised ✓ Reinstated ~~deleted~~ Deleted ⊘ Not covered or valid by Medicare
Special coverage instructions * Carrier discretion Bill Part B MAC Bill DME MAC

* **QG** Prescribed amount of stationary oxygen while at rest is greater than 4 liters per minute (LPM)

* **QH** Oxygen conserving device is being used with an oxygen delivery system

QJ Services/items provided to a prisoner or patient in state or local custody, however, the state or local government, as applicable, meets the requirements in 42 CFR 411.4 (B)

QK Medical direction of two, three, or four concurrent anesthesia procedures involving qualified individuals

IOM: 100-04, 12, 50K, 90

* **QL** Patient pronounced dead after ambulance called

* **QM** Ambulance service provided under arrangement by a provider of services

* **QN** Ambulance service furnished directly by a provider of services

QP Documentation is on file showing that the laboratory test(s) was ordered individually or ordered as a CPT-recognized panel other than automated profile codes 80002-80019, G0058, G0059, and G0060

* **QQ** Ordering professional consulted a qualified clinical decision support mechanism for this service and the related data was provided to the furnishing professional

* **QR** Prescribed amounts of stationary oxygen for daytime use while at rest and nighttime use differ and the average of the two amounts is greater than 4 liters per minute (lpm)

QS Monitored anesthesia care service

IOM: 100-04, 12, 30.6, 501

* **QT** Recording and storage on tape by an analog tape recorder

* **QW** CLIA-waived test

* **QX** CRNA service: with medical direction by a physician

QY Medical direction of one certified registered nurse anesthetist (CRNA) by an anesthesiologist

IOM: 100-04, 12, 50K, 90

* **QZ** CRNA service: without medical direction by a physician

* **RA** Replacement of a DME, orthotic or prosthetic item

Contractors will deny claims for replacement parts when furnished in conjunction with the repair of a capped rental item and billed with modifier RB, including claims for parts submitted using code E1399, that are billed during the capped rental period (i.e., the last day of the 13th month of continuous use or before). Repair includes all maintenance, servicing, and repair of capped rental DME because it is included in the allowed rental payment amounts. (Pub 100-20 One-Time Notification Centers for Medicare & Medicaid Services, Transmittal: 901, May 13, 2011)

* **RB** Replacement of a part of a DME, orthotic or prosthetic item furnished as part of a repair

* **RC** Right coronary artery

* **RD** Drug provided to beneficiary, but not administered "incident-to"

* **RE** Furnished in full compliance with FDA-mandated risk evaluation and mitigation strategy (REMS)

* **RI** Ramus intermedius coronary artery

* **RR** Rental (use the 'RR' modifier when DME is to be rented)

* **RT** Right side (used to identify procedures performed on the right side of the body)

Modifiers LT and RT identify procedures which can be performed on paired organs. Used for procedures performed on one side only. Should also be used when the procedures are similar but not identical and are performed on paired body parts.

Coding Clinic: 2016, Q3, P5

⊘ **SA** Nurse practitioner rendering service in collaboration with a physician

⊘ **SB** Nurse midwife

* **SC** Medically necessary service or supply

⊘ **SD** Services provided by registered nurse with specialized, highly technical home infusion training

⊘ **SE** State and/or federally funded programs/services

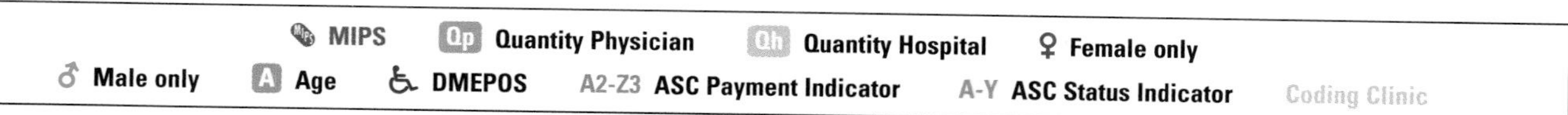
MIPS
Qp Quantity Physician
Qh Quantity Hospital
Female only
Male only
A Age
DMEPOS
A2-Z3 ASC Payment Indicator
A-Y ASC Status Indicator
Coding Clinic

✻	**SF**	Second opinion ordered by a professional review organization (PRO) per Section 9401, P.L. 99-272 (100% reimbursement – no Medicare deductible or coinsurance)
✻	**SG**	Ambulatory surgical center (ASC) facility service Only valid for surgical codes. After 1/1/08 not required for ASC facility charges.
⃠	**SH**	Second concurrently administered infusion therapy
⃠	**SJ**	Third or more concurrently administered infusion therapy
⃠	**SK**	Member of high risk population (use only with codes for immunization)
⃠	**SL**	State supplied vaccine
⃠	**SM**	Second surgical opinion
⃠	**SN**	Third surgical opinion
⃠	**SQ**	Item ordered by home health
⃠	**SS**	Home infusion services provided in the infusion suite of the IV therapy provider
⃠	**ST**	Related to trauma or injury
⃠	**SU**	Procedure performed in physician's office (to denote use of facility and equipment)
⃠	**SV**	Pharmaceuticals delivered to patient's home but not utilized
✻	**SW**	Services provided by a certified diabetic educator
⃠	**SY**	Persons who are in close contact with member of high-risk population (use only with codes for immunization)
✻	**T1**	Left foot, second digit
✻	**T2**	Left foot, third digit
✻	**T3**	Left foot, fourth digit
✻	**T4**	Left foot, fifth digit
✻	**T5**	Right foot, great toe
✻	**T6**	Right foot, second digit
✻	**T7**	Right foot, third digit
✻	**T8**	Right foot, fourth digit
✻	**T9**	Right foot, fifth digit
✻	**TA**	Left foot, great toe
✻	**TB**	Drug or biological acquired with 340B drug pricing program discount, reported for informational purposes
✻	**TC**	Technical component; under certain circumstances, a charge may be made for the technical component alone; under those circumstances the technical component charge is identified by adding modifier TC to the usual procedure number; technical component charges are institutional charges and not billed separately by physicians; however, portable x-ray suppliers only bill for technical component and should utilize modifier TC; the charge data from portable x-ray suppliers will then be used to build customary and prevailing profiles.
⃠	**TD**	RN
⃠	**TE**	LPN/LVN
⃠	**TF**	Intermediate level of care
⃠	**TG**	Complex/high tech level of care
⃠	**TH**	Obstetrical treatment/services, prenatal or postpartum
⃠	**TJ**	Program group, child and/or adolescent
⃠	**TK**	Extra patient or passenger, non-ambulance
⃠	**TL**	Early intervention/individualized family service plan (IFSP)
⃠	**TM**	Individualized education program (IEP)
⃠	**TN**	Rural/outside providers' customary service area
⃠	**TP**	Medical transport, unloaded vehicle
⃠	**TQ**	Basic life support transport by a volunteer ambulance provider
⃠	**TR**	School-based individual education program (IEP) services provided outside the public school district responsible for the student
✻	**TS**	Follow-up service
⃠	**TT**	Individualized service provided to more than one patient in same setting
⃠	**TU**	Special payment rate, overtime
⃠	**TV**	Special payment rates, holidays/ weekends
⃠	**TW**	Back-up equipment
⃠	**U1**	Medicaid Level of Care 1, as defined by each State
⃠	**U2**	Medicaid Level of Care 2, as defined by each State
⃠	**U3**	Medicaid Level of Care 3, as defined by each State

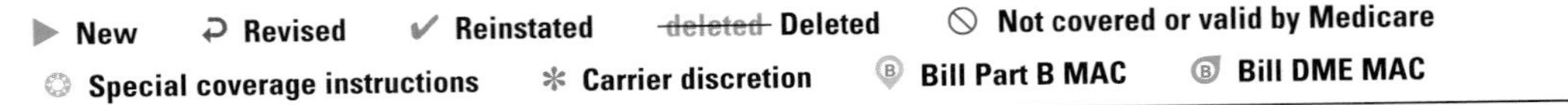

▶ New
Revised
✓ Reinstated
~~deleted~~ Deleted
⃠ Not covered or valid by Medicare
Special coverage instructions
✻ Carrier discretion
Bill Part B MAC
Bill DME MAC

⊘ **U4** Medicaid Level of Care 4, as defined by each State

⊘ **U5** Medicaid Level of Care 5, as defined by each State

⊘ **U6** Medicaid Level of Care 6, as defined by each State

⊘ **U7** Medicaid Level of Care 7, as defined by each State

⊘ **U8** Medicaid Level of Care 8, as defined by each State

⊘ **U9** Medicaid Level of Care 9, as defined by each State

⊘ **UA** Medicaid Level of Care 10, as defined by each State

⊘ **UB** Medicaid Level of Care 11, as defined by each State

⊘ **UC** Medicaid Level of Care 12, as defined by each State

⊘ **UD** Medicaid Level of Care 13, as defined by each State

* **UE** Used durable medical equipment

⊘ **UF** Services provided in the morning

⊘ **UG** Services provided in the afternoon

⊘ **UH** Services provided in the evening

* **UJ** Services provided at night

⊘ **UK** Services provided on behalf of the client to someone other than the client (collateral relationship)

* **UN** Two patients served

* **UP** Three patients served

* **UQ** Four patients served

* **UR** Five patients served

* **US** Six or more patients served

* **V1** Demonstration Modifier 1

* **V2** Demonstration Modifier 2

* **V3** Demonstration Modifier 3

► * **V4** Demonstration modifier 4

* **V5** Vascular catheter (alone or with any other vascular access)

* **V6** Arteriovenous graft (or other vascular access not including a vascular catheter)

* **V7** Arteriovenous fistula only (in use with two needles)

* **VM** Medicare diabetes prevention program (MDPP) virtual make-up session

* **VP** Aphakic patient

* **X1** Continuous/broad services: for reporting services by clinicians, who provide the principal care for a patient, with no planned endpoint of the relationship; services in this category represent comprehensive care, dealing with the entire scope of patient problems, either directly or in a care coordination role; reporting clinician service examples include, but are not limited to: primary care, and clinicians providing comprehensive care to patients in addition to specialty care

* **X2** Continuous/focused services: for reporting services by clinicians whose expertise is needed for the ongoing management of a chronic disease or a condition that needs to be managed and followed with no planned endpoint to the relationship; reporting clinician service examples include but are not limited to: a rheumatologist taking care of the patient's rheumatoid arthritis longitudinally but not providing general primary care services

* **X3** Episodic/broad services: for reporting services by clinicians who have broad responsibility for the comprehensive needs of the patient that is limited to a defined period and circumstance such as a hospitalization; reporting clinician service examples include but are not limited to the hospitalist's services rendered providing comprehensive and general care to a patient while admitted to the hospital

* **X4** Episodic/focused services: for reporting services by clinicians who provide focused care on particular types of treatment limited to a defined period and circumstance; the patient has a problem, acute or chronic, that will be treated with surgery, radiation, or some other type of generally time-limited intervention; reporting clinician service examples include but are not limited to, the orthopedic surgeon performing a knee replacement and seeing the patient through the postoperative period

* **X5** Diagnostic services requested by another clinician: for reporting services by a clinician who furnishes care to the patient only as requested by another clinician or subsequent and related services requested by another clinician; this modifier is reported for patient relationships that may not be adequately captured by the above alternative categories; reporting clinician service examples include but are not limited to, the radiologist's interpretation of an imaging study requested by another clinician

* **XE** Separate encounter, a service that is distinct because it occurred during a separate encounter

* **XP** Separate practitioner, a service that is distinct because it was performed by a different practitioner

* **XS** Separate structure, a service that is distinct because it was performed on a separate organ/structure

* **XU** Unusual non-overlapping service, the use of a service that is distinct because it does not overlap usual components of the main service

Ambulance Modifiers

Modifiers that are used on claims for ambulance services are created by combining two alpha characters. Each alpha character, with the exception of X, represents an origin (source) code or a destination code. The pair of alpha codes creates one modifier. The first position alpha-code = origin; the second position alpha-code = destination. On form CMS-1491, used to report ambulance services, Item 12 should contain the origin code and Item 13 should contain the destination code. Origin and destination codes and their descriptions are as follows:

D	Diagnostic or therapeutic site other than P or H when these are used as origin codes
E	Residential, domiciliary, custodial facility (other than an 1819 facility)
G	Hospital-based ESRD facility
H	Hospital
I	Site of transfer (e.g., airport or helicopter pad) between modes of ambulance transport
J	Freestanding ESRD facility
N	Skilled nursing facility
P	Physician's office
R	Residence
S	Scene of accident or acute event
X	Intermediate stop at physician's office on way to hospital (destination code only)

TRANSPORT SERVICES INCLUDING AMBULANCE (A0000-A0999)

⃠ **A0021** Ambulance service, outside state per mile, transport (Medicaid only) Ⓑ Qp Qh E1

Cross Reference A0030

⃠ **A0080** Non-emergency transportation, per mile - vehicle provided by volunteer (individual or organization), with no vested interest Ⓑ Qp Qh E1

⃠ **A0090** Non-emergency transportation, per mile - vehicle provided by individual (family member, self, neighbor) with vested interest Ⓑ Qp Qh E1

⃠ **A0100** Non-emergency transportation; taxi Ⓑ Qp Qh E1

⃠ **A0110** Non-emergency transportation and bus, intra- or interstate carrier Ⓑ Qp Qh E1

⃠ **A0120** Non-emergency transportation: mini-bus, mountain area transports, or other transportation systems Ⓑ Qp Qh E1

⃠ **A0130** Non-emergency transportation: wheelchair van Ⓑ Qp Qh E1

⃠ **A0140** Non-emergency transportation and air travel (private or commercial), intra- or interstate Ⓑ Qp Qh E1

⃠ **A0160** Non-emergency transportation: per mile - caseworker or social worker Ⓑ Qp Qh E1

⃠ **A0170** Transportation: ancillary: parking fees, tolls, other Ⓑ Qp Qh E1

⃠ **A0180** Non-emergency transportation: ancillary: lodging - recipient Ⓑ Qp Qh E1

⃠ **A0190** Non-emergency transportation: ancillary: meals - recipient Ⓑ Qp Qh E1

⃠ **A0200** Non-emergency transportation: ancillary: lodging - escort Ⓑ Qp Qh E1

⃠ **A0210** Non-emergency transportation: ancillary: meals - escort Ⓑ Qp Qh E1

⃠ **A0225** Ambulance service, neonatal transport, base rate, emergency transport, one way Ⓑ Qp Qh E1

⃠ **A0380** BLS mileage (per mile) Ⓑ Qp Qh E1

Cross Reference A0425

⃠ **A0382** BLS routine disposable supplies Ⓑ Qp Qh E1

⃠ **A0384** BLS specialized service disposable supplies; defibrillation (used by ALS ambulances and BLS ambulances in jurisdictions where defibrillation is permitted in BLS ambulances) Ⓑ Qp Qh E1

⃠ **A0390** ALS mileage (per mile) Ⓑ Qp Qh E1

Cross Reference A0425

⃠ **A0392** ALS specialized service disposable supplies; defibrillation (to be used only in jurisdictions where defibrillation cannot be performed in BLS ambulances) Ⓑ Qp Qh E1

⃠ **A0394** ALS specialized service disposable supplies; IV drug therapy Ⓑ Qp Qh E1

⃠ **A0396** ALS specialized service disposable supplies; esophageal intubation Ⓑ Qp Qh E1

⃠ **A0398** ALS routine disposable supplies Ⓑ Qp Qh E1

⃠ **A0420** Ambulance waiting time (ALS or BLS), one half (½) hour increments Ⓑ Qp Qh E1

Waiting Time Table

UNITS	TIME	UNITS	TIME
1	½ to 1 hr.	6	3 to 3½ hrs.
2	1 to 1½ hrs.	7	3½ to 4 hrs.
3	1½ to 2 hrs.	8	4 to 4½ hrs.
4	2 to 2½ hrs.	9	4½ to 5 hrs.
5	2½ to 3 hrs.	10	5 to 5½ hrs.

⃠ **A0422** Ambulance (ALS or BLS) oxygen and oxygen supplies, life sustaining situation Ⓑ Qp Qh E1

⃠ **A0424** Extra ambulance attendant, ground (ALS or BLS) or air (fixed or rotary winged); (requires medical review) Ⓑ Qp Qh E1

* **A0425** Ground mileage, per statute mile Ⓑ Qp Qh A

* **A0426** Ambulance service, advanced life support, non-emergency transport, Level 1 (ALS 1) Ⓑ Qp Qh A

* **A0427** Ambulance service, advanced life support, emergency transport, Level 1 (ALS 1-Emergency) Ⓑ Qp Qh A

* **A0428** Ambulance service, basic life support, non-emergency transport (BLS) Ⓑ Qp Qh A

* **A0429** Ambulance service, basic life support, emergency transport (BLS-Emergency) Ⓑ Qp Qh A

MIPS | Qp Quantity Physician | Qh Quantity Hospital | ♀ Female only
♂ Male only | A Age | DMEPOS | A2-Z3 ASC Payment Indicator | A-Y ASC Status Indicator | Coding Clinic

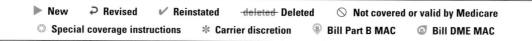

* **A0430** Ambulance service, conventional air services, transport, one way (fixed wing) Qp Qh — A

* **A0431** Ambulance service, conventional air services, transport, one way (rotary wing) Qp Qh — A

* **A0432** Paramedic intercept (PI), rural area, transport furnished by a volunteer ambulance company, which is prohibited by state law from billing third party payers Qp Qh — A

* **A0433** Advanced life support, Level 2 (ALS2) Qp Qh — A

* **A0434** Specialty care transport (SCT) Qp Qh — A

* **A0435** Fixed wing air mileage, per statute mile Qp Qh — A

* **A0436** Rotary wing air mileage, per statute mile Qp Qh — A

⊘ **A0888** Noncovered ambulance mileage, per mile (e.g., for miles traveled beyond closest appropriate facility) Qp Qh — E1

MCM: 2125

⊘ **A0998** Ambulance response and treatment, no transport Qp Qh — E1

IOM: 100-02, 10, 20

A0999 Unlisted ambulance service — A

IOM: 100-02, 10, 20

MEDICAL AND SURGICAL SUPPLIES (A4000-A8004)

Injection and Infusion

* **A4206** Syringe with needle, sterile 1 cc or less, each — N

* **A4207** Syringe with needle, sterile 2 cc, each — N

* **A4208** Syringe with needle, sterile 3 cc, each — N

* **A4209** Syringe with needle, sterile 5 cc or greater, each — N

⊘ **A4210** Needle-free injection device, each Qp Qh — E1

IOM: 100-03, 4, 280.1

A4211 Supplies for self-administered injections Qp Qh — N

IOM: 100-02, 15, 50

* **A4212** Non-coring needle or stylet with or without catheter Qp Qh — N

* **A4213** Syringe, sterile, 20 cc or greater, each — N

* **A4215** Needle, sterile, any size, each — N

A4216 Sterile water, saline and/or dextrose diluent/flush, 10 ml — N

Other: Sodium Chloride, Bacteriostatic, Syrex

IOM: 100-02, 15, 50

A4217 Sterile water/saline, 500 ml — N

Other: Sodium Chloride

IOM: 100-02, 15, 50

A4218 Sterile saline or water, metered dose dispenser, 10 ml — N

Other: Sodium Chloride

A4220 Refill kit for implantable infusion pump Qp Qh — N

Do not report with 95990 or 95991 since Medicare payment for these codes includes the refill kit.

IOM: 100-03, 4, 280.1

* **A4221** Supplies for maintenance of non-insulin drug infusion catheter, per week (list drugs separately) Qp Qh — N

Includes dressings for catheter site and flush solutions not directly related to drug infusion.

* **A4222** Infusion supplies for external drug infusion pump, per cassette or bag (list drug separately) Qp Qh — N

Includes cassette or bag, diluting solutions, tubing and/or administration supplies, port cap changes, compounding charges, and preparation charges.

* **A4223** Infusion supplies not used with external infusion pump, per cassette or bag (list drugs separately) — N

IOM: 100-03, 4, 280.1

* **A4224** Supplies for maintenance of insulin infusion catheter, per week Qp Qh — N

A4225 Supplies for external insulin infusion pump, syringe type cartridge, sterile, each Qp Qh — N

IOM: 100-03, 1, 50.3

* **A4226** Supplies for maintenance of insulin infusion pump with dosage rate adjustment using therapeutic continuous glucose sensing, per week — N

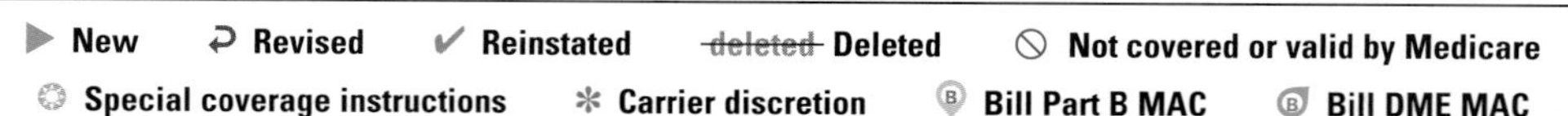
New
Revised
Reinstated
deleted Deleted
Not covered or valid by Medicare
Special coverage instructions
Carrier discretion
Bill Part B MAC
Bill DME MAC

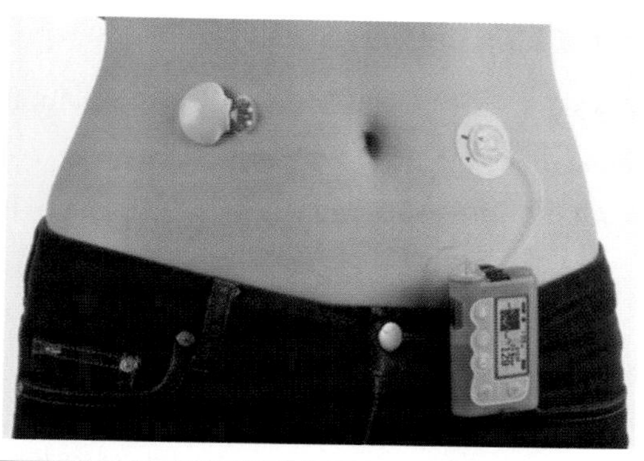

Figure 1 Insulin pump.

A4230 Infusion set for external insulin pump, non-needle cannula type N

Requires prior authorization and copy of invoice.

IOM: 100-03, 4, 280.1

A4231 Infusion set for external insulin pump, needle type N

Requires prior authorization and copy of invoice.

IOM: 100-03, 4, 280.1

A4232 Syringe with needle for external insulin pump, sterile, 3 cc Qp Qh E1

Reports insulin reservoir for use with external insulin infusion pump (E0784); may be glass or plastic; includes needle for drawing up insulin. Does not include insulin for use in reservoir.

IOM: 100-03, 4, 280.1

Replacement Batteries

* **A4233** Replacement battery, alkaline (other than J cell), for use with medically necessary home blood glucose monitor owned by patient, each Qh ♿ E1
* **A4234** Replacement battery, alkaline, J cell, for use with medically necessary home blood glucose monitor owned by patient, each Qh ♿ E1
* **A4235** Replacement battery, lithium, for use with medically necessary home blood glucose monitor owned by patient, each Qp Qh ♿ E1
* **A4236** Replacement battery, silver oxide, for use with medically necessary home blood glucose monitor owned by patient, each Qh ♿ E1

Miscellaneous Supplies

* **A4244** Alcohol or peroxide, per pint N
* **A4245** Alcohol wipes, per box N
* **A4246** Betadine or Phisohex solution, per pint N
* **A4247** Betadine or iodine swabs/wipes, per box N
* **A4248** Chlorhexidine containing antiseptic, 1 ml N

A4250 Urine test or reagent strips or tablets (100 tablets or strips) Qp Qh E1

IOM: 100-02, 15, 110

A4252 Blood ketone test or reagent strip, each Qp Qh E1

Medicare Statute 1861(n)

A4253 Blood glucose test or reagent strips for home blood glucose monitor, per 50 strips Qp Qh ♿ N

Test strips (1 unit = 50 strips); non-insulin treated (every 3 months) 100 test strips (1×/day testing), 100 lancets (1×/day testing); modifier KS

IOM: 100-03, 1, 40.2

A4255 Platforms for home blood glucose monitor, 50 per box Qp Qh ♿ N

IOM: 100-03, 1, 40.2

A4256 Normal, low and high calibrator solution/chips Qp Qh ♿ N

IOM: 100-03, 1, 40.2

* **A4257** Replacement lens shield cartridge for use with laser skin piercing device, each Qp Qh ♿ E1

A4258 Spring-powered device for lancet, each Qp Qh ♿ N

IOM: 100-03, 1, 40.2

A4259 Lancets, per box of 100 Qp Qh ♿ N

IOM: 100-03, 1, 40.2

A4261 Cervical cap for contraceptive use Qp Qh ♀ E1

Medicare Statute 1862A1

A4262 Temporary, absorbable lacrimal duct implant, each Qp Qh N

IOM: 100-04, 12, 20.3, 30.4

A4263 Permanent, long term, non-dissolvable lacrimal duct implant, each Qp Qh N

Bundled with insertion if performed in physician office.

IOM: 100-04, 12, 30.4

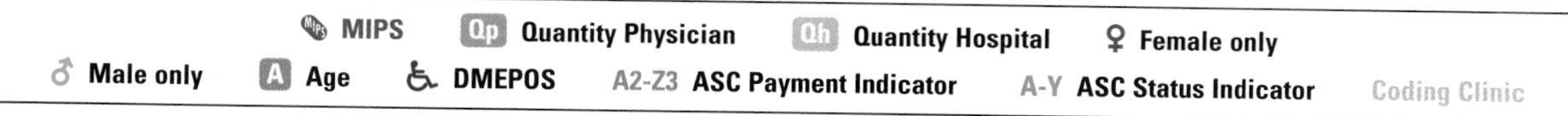

⦸ **A4264** Permanent implantable contraceptive intratubal occlusion device(s) and delivery system Ⓑ Qp Qh ♀ E1

Reports the Essure device.

A4265 Paraffin, per pound Ⓑ Ⓓ Qp Qh ♿ N

IOM: 100-03, 4, 280.1

⦸ **A4266** Diaphragm for contraceptive use Ⓑ Qp Qh ♀ E1

⦸ **A4267** Contraceptive supply, condom, male, each Ⓑ Qp Qh ♂ E1

⦸ **A4268** Contraceptive supply, condom, female, each Ⓑ Qp Qh ♀ E1

⦸ **A4269** Contraceptive supply, spermicide (e.g., foam, gel), each Ⓑ Qp Qh E1

* **A4270** Disposable endoscope sheath, each Ⓑ Qp Qh N

* **A4280** Adhesive skin support attachment for use with external breast prosthesis, each Ⓓ Qh ♀ ♿ N

* **A4281** Tubing for breast pump, replacement Ⓓ ♀ E1

* **A4282** Adapter for breast pump, replacement Ⓓ ♀ E1

* **A4283** Cap for breast pump bottle, replacement Ⓓ ♀ E1

* **A4284** Breast shield and splash protector for use with breast pump, replacement Ⓓ ♀ E1

* **A4285** Polycarbonate bottle for use with breast pump, replacement Ⓓ ♀ E1

* **A4286** Locking ring for breast pump, replacement Ⓓ ♀ E1

* **A4290** Sacral nerve stimulation test lead, each Ⓑ N

Service not separately priced by Part B (e.g., services not covered, bundled, used by Part A only)

Implantable Catheters

A4300 Implantable access catheter, (e.g., venous, arterial, epidural subarachnoid, or peritoneal, etc.) external access Ⓑ Qp Qh N

IOM: 100-02, 15, 120

* **A4301** Implantable access total; catheter, port/reservoir (e.g., venous, arterial, epidural, subarachnoid, peritoneal, etc.) Ⓑ Qp Qh N

Disposable Drug Delivery System

* **A4305** Disposable drug delivery system, flow rate of 50 ml or greater per hour Ⓑ Ⓓ Qp Qh N

* **A4306** Disposable drug delivery system, flow rate of less than 50 ml per hour Ⓑ Ⓓ Qp Qh N

Incontinence Appliances and Care Supplies

A4310 Insertion tray without drainage bag and without catheter (accessories only) Ⓑ Ⓓ Qp Qh ♿ N

IOM: 100-02, 15, 120

A4311 Insertion tray without drainage bag with indwelling catheter, Foley type, two-way latex with coating (Teflon, silicone, silicone elastomer, or hydrophilic, etc.) Ⓑ Ⓓ Qp Qh ♿ N

IOM: 100-02, 15, 120

A4312 Insertion tray without drainage bag with indwelling catheter, Foley type, two-way, all silicone Ⓑ Ⓓ Qp Qh ♿ N

Must meet criteria for indwelling catheter and medical record must justify need for:

- Recurrent encrustation
- Inability to pass a straight catheter
- Sensitivity to latex

Must be medically necessary.

IOM: 100-02, 15, 120

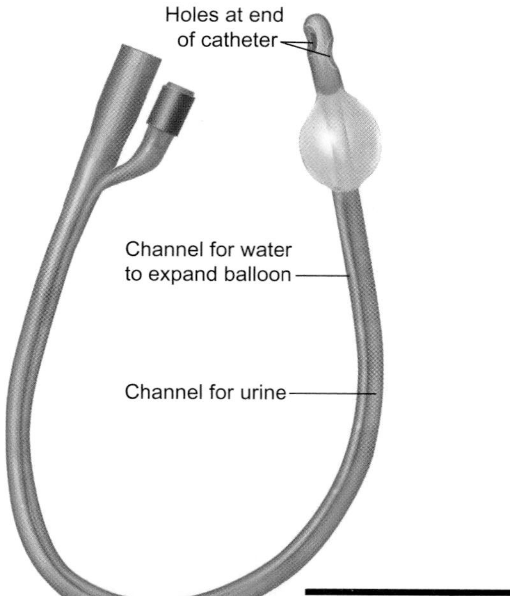
Holes at end of catheter
Channel for water to expand balloon
Channel for urine

Figure 2 Foley catheter.

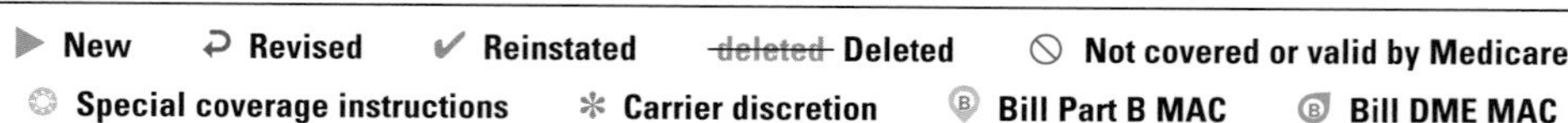
▶ New ↻ Revised ✔ Reinstated ~~deleted~~ Deleted ⦸ Not covered or valid by Medicare
Special coverage instructions * Carrier discretion Ⓑ Bill Part B MAC Ⓓ Bill DME MAC

A4313 Insertion tray without drainage bag with indwelling catheter, Foley type, three-way, for continuous irrigation Qp Qh N

Must meet criteria for indwelling catheter and medical record must justify need for:

- Recurrent encrustation
- Inability to pass a straight catheter
- Sensitivity to latex

Must be medically necessary.

IOM: 100-02, 15, 120

A4314 Insertion tray with drainage bag with indwelling catheter, Foley type, two-way latex with coating (Teflon, silicone, silicone elastomer or hydrophilic, etc.) Qp Qh N

IOM: 100-02, 15, 120

A4315 Insertion tray with drainage bag with indwelling catheter, Foley type, two-way, all silicone Qp Qh N

IOM: 100-02, 15, 120

A4316 Insertion tray with drainage bag with indwelling catheter, Foley type, three-way, for continuous irrigation Qp Qh N

IOM: 100-02, 15, 120

A4320 Irrigation tray with bulb or piston syringe, any purpose Qp Qh N

IOM: 100-02, 15, 120

A4321 Therapeutic agent for urinary catheter irrigation N

IOM: 100-02, 15, 120

A4322 Irrigation syringe, bulb, or piston, each Qp Qh N

IOM: 100-02, 15, 120

A4326 Male external catheter with integral collection chamber, any type, each Qp Qh ♂ N

IOM: 100-02, 15, 120

A4327 Female external urinary collection device; meatal cup, each Qp Qh ♀ N

IOM: 100-02, 15, 120

A4328 Female external urinary collection device; pouch, each Qp Qh ♀ N

IOM: 100-02, 15, 120

A4330 Perianal fecal collection pouch with adhesive, each Qp Qh N

IOM: 100-02, 15, 120

A4331 Extension drainage tubing, any type, any length, with connector/adaptor, for use with urinary leg bag or urostomy pouch, each Qh N

IOM: 100-02, 15, 120

A4332 Lubricant, individual sterile packet, each Qp Qh N

IOM: 100-02, 15, 120

A4333 Urinary catheter anchoring device, adhesive skin attachment, each N

IOM: 100-02, 15, 120

A4334 Urinary catheter anchoring device, leg strap, each N

IOM: 100-02, 15, 120

A4335 Incontinence supply; miscellaneous Qp Qh N

IOM: 100-02, 15, 120

A4336 Incontinence supply, urethral insert, any type, each N

IOM: 100-02, 15, 120

A4337 Incontinence supply, rectal insert, any type, each Qp Qh N

IOM: 100-02, 15, 120

A4338 Indwelling catheter; Foley type, two-way latex with coating (Teflon, silicone, silicone elastomer, or hydrophilic, etc.), each Qp Qh N

IOM: 100-02, 15, 120

A4340 Indwelling catheter; specialty type (e.g., coude, mushroom, wing, etc.), each Qp Qh N

Must meet criteria for indwelling catheter and medical record must justify need for:

- Recurrent encrustation
- Inability to pass a straight catheter
- Sensitivity to latex

Must be medically necessary.

IOM: 100-02, 15, 120

A4344 Indwelling catheter, Foley type, two-way, all silicone, each Qp Qh N

Must meet criteria for indwelling catheter and medical record must justify need for:

- Recurrent encrustation
- Inability to pass a straight catheter
- Sensitivity to latex

Must be medically necessary.

IOM: 100-02, 15, 120

MIPS | Qp Quantity Physician | Qh Quantity Hospital | ♀ Female only
♂ Male only | A Age | DMEPOS | A2-Z3 ASC Payment Indicator | A-Y ASC Status Indicator | Coding Clinic

A4346 Indwelling catheter; Foley type, three way for continuous irrigation, each N

IOM: 100-02, 15, 120

A4349 Male external catheter, with or without adhesive, disposable, each N

IOM: 100-02, 15, 120

A4351 Intermittent urinary catheter; straight tip, with or without coating (Teflon, silicone, silicone elastomer, or hydrophilic, etc.), each N

IOM: 100-02, 15, 120

A4352 Intermittent urinary catheter; coude (curved) tip, with or without coating (Teflon, silicone, silicone elastomeric, or hydrophilic, etc.), each N

IOM: 100-02, 15, 120

A4353 Intermittent urinary catheter, with insertion supplies N

IOM: 100-02, 15, 120

A4354 Insertion tray with drainage bag but without catheter N

IOM: 100-02, 15, 120

A4355 Irrigation tubing set for continuous bladder irrigation through a three-way indwelling Foley catheter, each N

IOM: 100-02, 15, 120

External Urinary Supplies

A4356 External urethral clamp or compression device (not to be used for catheter clamp), each N

IOM: 100-02, 15, 120

A4357 Bedside drainage bag, day or night, with or without anti-reflux device, with or without tube, each N

IOM: 100-02, 15, 120

A4358 Urinary drainage bag, leg or abdomen, vinyl, with or without tube, with straps, each N

IOM: 100-02, 15, 120

A4360 Disposable external urethral clamp or compression device, with pad and/or pouch, each N

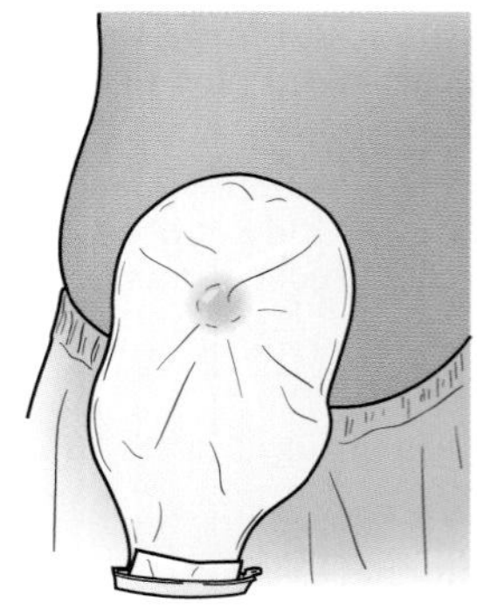

Figure 3 Ostomy pouch.

Ostomy Supplies

A4361 Ostomy faceplate, each N

IOM: 100-02, 15, 120

A4362 Skin barrier; solid, 4 × 4 or equivalent; each N

IOM: 100-02, 15, 120

A4363 Ostomy clamp, any type, replacement only, each E1

A4364 Adhesive, liquid or equal, any type, per oz N

Fee schedule category: Ostomy, tracheostomy, and urologicals items.

IOM: 100-02, 15, 120

* **A4366** Ostomy vent, any type, each N

A4367 Ostomy belt, each N

IOM: 100-02, 15, 120

* **A4368** Ostomy filter, any type, each N

A4369 Ostomy skin barrier, liquid (spray, brush, etc.), per oz N

IOM: 100-02, 15, 120

A4371 Ostomy skin barrier, powder, per oz N

IOM: 100-02, 15, 120

A4372 Ostomy skin barrier, solid 4 × 4 or equivalent, standard wear, with built-in convexity, each N

IOM: 100-02, 15, 120

A4373 Ostomy skin barrier, with flange (solid, flexible, or accordion), with built-in convexity, any size, each N

IOM: 100-02, 15, 120

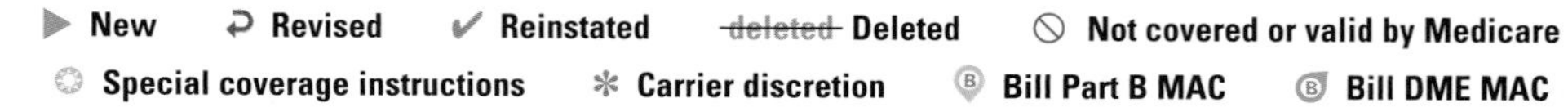

▶ New ↩ Revised ✔ Reinstated ~~deleted~~ Deleted ⊘ Not covered or valid by Medicare
Special coverage instructions * Carrier discretion Ⓑ Bill Part B MAC Ⓑ Bill DME MAC

A4375 Ostomy pouch, drainable, with faceplate attached, plastic, each Qp Qh N
IOM: 100-02, 15, 120

A4376 Ostomy pouch, drainable, with faceplate attached, rubber, each Qp Qh N
IOM: 100-02, 15, 120

A4377 Ostomy pouch, drainable, for use on faceplate, plastic, each Qp Qh N
IOM: 100-02, 15, 120

A4378 Ostomy pouch, drainable, for use on faceplate, rubber, each Qp Qh N
IOM: 100-02, 15, 120

A4379 Ostomy pouch, urinary, with faceplate attached, plastic, each Qp Qh N
IOM: 100-02, 15, 120

A4380 Ostomy pouch, urinary, with faceplate attached, rubber, each Qp Qh N
IOM: 100-02, 15, 120

A4381 Ostomy pouch, urinary, for use on faceplate, plastic, each Qp Qh N
IOM: 100-02, 15, 120

A4382 Ostomy pouch, urinary, for use on faceplate, heavy plastic, each Qp Qh N
IOM: 100-02, 15, 120

A4383 Ostomy pouch, urinary, for use on faceplate, rubber, each Qp Qh N
IOM: 100-02, 15, 120

A4384 Ostomy faceplate equivalent, silicone ring, each Qp Qh N
IOM: 100-02, 15, 120

A4385 Ostomy skin barrier, solid 4 × 4 or equivalent, extended wear, without built-in convexity, each Qp Qh N
IOM: 100-02, 15, 120

A4387 Ostomy pouch closed, with barrier attached, with built-in convexity (1 piece), each Qh N
IOM: 100-02, 15, 120

A4388 Ostomy pouch, drainable, with extended wear barrier attached (1 piece), each Qh N
IOM: 100-02, 15, 120

A4389 Ostomy pouch, drainable, with barrier attached, with built-in convexity (1 piece), each Qp Qh N
IOM: 100-02, 15, 120

A4390 Ostomy pouch, drainable, with extended wear barrier attached, with built-in convexity (1 piece), each Qh N
IOM: 100-02, 15, 120

A4391 Ostomy pouch, urinary, with extended wear barrier attached (1 piece), each Qh N
IOM: 100-02, 15, 120

A4392 Ostomy pouch, urinary, with standard wear barrier attached, with built-in convexity (1 piece), each Qp Qh N
IOM: 100-02, 15, 120

A4393 Ostomy pouch, urinary, with extended wear barrier attached, with built-in convexity (1 piece), each Qh N
IOM: 100-02, 15, 120

A4394 Ostomy deodorant, with or without lubricant, for use in ostomy pouch, per fluid ounce N
IOM: 100-02, 15, 20

A4395 Ostomy deodorant for use in ostomy pouch, solid, per tablet N
IOM: 100-02, 15, 20

A4396 Ostomy belt with peristomal hernia support Qh N
IOM: 100-02, 15, 120

A4397 Irrigation supply; sleeve, each Qp Qh N
IOM: 100-02, 15, 120

A4398 Ostomy irrigation supply; bag, each Qp Qh N
IOM: 100-02, 15, 120

A4399 Ostomy irrigation supply; cone/catheter, with or without brush Qp Qh N
IOM: 100-02, 15, 120

A4400 Ostomy irrigation set Qp Qh N
IOM: 100-02, 15, 120

A4402 Lubricant, per ounce Qp Qh N
IOM: 100-02, 15, 120

A4404 Ostomy ring, each Qp Qh N
IOM: 100-02, 15, 120

A4405 Ostomy skin barrier, non-pectin based, paste, per ounce N
IOM: 100-02, 15, 120

⊙ **A4406** Ostomy skin barrier, pectin-based, paste, per ounce Ⓑ Ⓓ ♿ N

IOM: 100-02, 15, 120

⊙ **A4407** Ostomy skin barrier, with flange (solid, flexible, or accordion), extended wear, with built-in convexity, 4 × 4 inches or smaller, each Ⓑ Ⓓ Qp Qh ♿ N

IOM: 100-02, 15, 120

⊙ **A4408** Ostomy skin barrier, with flange (solid, flexible, or accordion), extended wear, with built-in convexity, larger than 4 × 4 inches, each Ⓑ Ⓓ Qh ♿ N

IOM: 100-02, 15, 120

⊙ **A4409** Ostomy skin barrier, with flange (solid, flexible, or accordion), extended wear, without built-in convexity, 4 × 4 inches or smaller, each Ⓑ Ⓓ Qh ♿ N

IOM: 100-02, 15, 120

⊙ **A4410** Ostomy skin barrier, with flange (solid, flexible, or accordion), extended wear, without built-in convexity, larger than 4 × 4 inches, each Ⓑ Ⓓ Qp Qh ♿ N

IOM: 100-02, 15, 120

⊙ **A4411** Ostomy skin barrier, solid 4 × 4 or equivalent, extended wear, with built-in convexity, each Ⓑ Ⓓ Qh ♿ N

⊙ **A4412** Ostomy pouch, drainable, high output, for use on a barrier with flange (2 piece system), without filter, each Ⓑ Ⓓ Qh ♿ N

IOM: 100-02, 15, 120

⊙ **A4413** Ostomy pouch, drainable, high output, for use on a barrier with flange (2 piece system), with filter, each Ⓑ Ⓓ Qp Qh ♿ N

IOM: 100-02, 15, 120

⊙ **A4414** Ostomy skin barrier, with flange (solid, flexible, or accordion), without built-in convexity, 4 × 4 inches or smaller, each Ⓑ Ⓓ Qh ♿ N

IOM: 100-02, 15, 120

⊙ **A4415** Ostomy skin barrier, with flange (solid, flexible, or accordion), without built-in convexity, larger than 4 × 4 inches, each Ⓑ Ⓓ Qh ♿ N

IOM: 100-02, 15, 120

* **A4416** Ostomy pouch, closed, with barrier attached, with filter (1 piece), each Ⓑ Ⓓ Qp Qh ♿ N

* **A4417** Ostomy pouch, closed, with barrier attached, with built-in convexity, with filter (1 piece), each Ⓑ Ⓓ Qh ♿ N

* **A4418** Ostomy pouch, closed; without barrier attached, with filter (1 piece), each Ⓑ Ⓓ Qh ♿ N

* **A4419** Ostomy pouch, closed; for use on barrier with non-locking flange, with filter (2 piece), each Ⓑ Ⓓ Qp Qh ♿ N

* **A4420** Ostomy pouch, closed; for use on barrier with locking flange (2 piece), each Ⓑ Ⓓ Qh ♿ N

* **A4421** Ostomy supply; miscellaneous Ⓑ Ⓓ N

⊙ **A4422** Ostomy absorbent material (sheet/pad/crystal packet) for use in ostomy pouch to thicken liquid stomal output, each Ⓑ Ⓓ ♿ N

IOM: 100-02, 15, 120

* **A4423** Ostomy pouch, closed; for use on barrier with locking flange, with filter (2 piece), each Ⓑ Ⓓ Qp Qh ♿ N

* **A4424** Ostomy pouch, drainable, with barrier attached, with filter (1 piece), each Ⓑ Ⓓ Qh ♿ N

* **A4425** Ostomy pouch, drainable; for use on barrier with non-locking flange, with filter (2 piece system), each Ⓑ Ⓓ Qh ♿ N

* **A4426** Ostomy pouch, drainable; for use on barrier with locking flange (2 piece system), each Ⓑ Ⓓ Qp Qh ♿ N

* **A4427** Ostomy pouch, drainable; for use on barrier with locking flange, with filter (2 piece system), each Ⓑ Ⓓ Qh ♿ N

* **A4428** Ostomy pouch, urinary, with extended wear barrier attached, with faucet-type tap with valve (1 piece), each Ⓑ Ⓓ Qh ♿ N

* **A4429** Ostomy pouch, urinary, with barrier attached, with built-in convexity, with faucet-type tap with valve (1 piece), each Ⓑ Ⓓ Qp Qh ♿ N

* **A4430** Ostomy pouch, urinary, with extended wear barrier attached, with built-in convexity, with faucet-type tap with valve (1 piece), each Ⓑ Ⓓ Qh ♿ N

* **A4431** Ostomy pouch, urinary; with barrier attached, with faucet-type tap with valve (1 piece), each Ⓑ Ⓓ Qh ♿ N

* **A4432** Ostomy pouch, urinary; for use on barrier with non-locking flange, with faucet-type tap with valve (2 piece), each Ⓑ Ⓓ Qp Qh ♿ N

* **A4433** Ostomy pouch, urinary; for use on barrier with locking flange (2 piece), each Ⓑ Ⓓ Qh ♿ N

* A4434 Ostomy pouch, urinary; for use on barrier with locking flange, with faucet-type tap with valve (2 piece), each Qh N

* A4435 Ostomy pouch, drainable, high output, with extended wear barrier (one-piece system), with or without filter, each Qp Qh N

Miscellaneous Supplies

A4450 Tape, non-waterproof, per 18 square inches N

If used with surgical dressings, billed with AW modifier (in addition to appropriate A1-A9 modifier).

IOM: 100-02, 15, 120

A4452 Tape, waterproof, per 18 square inches N

If used with surgical dressings, billed with AW modifier (in addition to appropriate A1-A9 modifier).

IOM: 100-02, 15, 120

A4455 Adhesive remover or solvent (for tape, cement or other adhesive), per ounce Qp Qh N

IOM: 100-02, 15, 120

A4456 Adhesive remover, wipes, any type, each N

May be reimbursed for male or female clients to home health DME providers and DME medical suppliers in the home setting.

IOM: 100-02, 15, 120

* A4458 Enema bag with tubing, reusable N

* A4459 Manual pump-operated enema system, includes balloon, catheter and all accessories, reusable, any type Qp Qh N

* A4461 Surgical dressing holder, non-reusable, each Qp Qh N

* A4463 Surgical dressing holder, reusable, each Qh N

* A4465 Non-elastic binder for extremity Qp Qh N

A4467 Belt, strap, sleeve, garment, or covering, any type Qp Qh E1

A4470 Gravlee jet washer Qp Qh N

Symptoms suggestive of endometrial disease must be present for this disposable diagnostic tool to be covered.

IOM: 100-02, 16, 90; 100-03, 4, 230.5

A4480 VABRA aspirator Qp Qh N

Symptoms suggestive of endometrial disease must be present for this disposable diagnostic tool to be covered.

IOM: 100-02, 16, 90; 100-03, 4, 230.6

A4481 Tracheostoma filter, any type, any size, each Qh N

IOM: 100-02, 15, 120

A4483 Moisture exchanger, disposable, for use with invasive mechanical ventilation N

IOM: 100-02, 15, 120

A4490 Surgical stockings above knee length, each Qp Qh E1

IOM: 100-02, 15, 100; 100-02, 15, 110; 100-03, 4, 280.1

A4495 Surgical stockings thigh length, each Qp Qh E1

IOM: 100-02, 15, 100; 100-02, 15, 110; 100-03, 4, 280.1

A4500 Surgical stockings below knee length, each Qp Qh E1

IOM: 100-02, 15, 100; 100-02, 15, 110; 100-03, 4, 280.1

A4510 Surgical stockings full length, each Qp Qh E1

IOM: 100-02, 15, 100; 100-02, 15, 110; 100-03, 4, 280.1

A4520 Incontinence garment, any type (e.g., brief, diaper), each Qp Qh E1

IOM: 100-03, 4, 280.1

A4550 Surgical trays Qp Qh B

No longer payable by Medicare; included in practice expense for procedures. Some private payers may pay, most private payers follow Medicare guidelines.

IOM: 100-04, 12, 20.3, 30.4

A4553 Non-disposable underpads, all sizes Qp Qh E1

IOM: 100-03, 4, 280.1

A4554 Disposable underpads, all sizes Qp Qh E1

IOM: 100-03, 4, 280.1

A4555 Electrode/transducer for use with electrical stimulation device used for cancer treatment, replacement only Qp Qh E1

* A4556 Electrodes (e.g., apnea monitor), per pair Qp Qh N

✻ **A4557** Lead wires (e.g., apnea monitor), per pair N

✻ **A4558** Conductive gel or paste, for use with electrical device (e.g., TENS, NMES), per oz N

✻ **A4559** Coupling gel or paste, for use with ultrasound device, per oz N

✻ **A4561** Pessary, rubber, any type N

✻ **A4562** Pessary, non-rubber, any type N

✻ **A4563** Rectal control system for vaginal insertion, for long term use, includes pump and all supplies and accessories, any type each N

✻ **A4565** Slings N

⊘ **A4566** Shoulder sling or vest design, abduction restrainer, with or without swathe control, prefabricated, includes fitting and adjustment E1

⊘ **A4570** Splint E1

IOM: 100-02, 6, 10; 100-02, 15, 100; 100-04, 4, 240

✻ **A4575** Topical hyperbaric oxygen chamber, disposable A

⊘ **A4580** Cast supplies (e.g., plaster) E1

IOM: 100-02, 6, 10; 100-02, 15, 100; 100-04, 4, 240

⊘ **A4590** Special casting material (e.g., fiberglass) E1

IOM: 100-02, 6, 10; 100-02, 15, 100; 100-04, 4, 240

A4595 Electrical stimulator supplies, 2 lead, per month (e.g., TENS, NMES) N

IOM: 100-03, 2, 160.13

✻ **A4600** Sleeve for intermittent limb compression device, replacement only, each E1

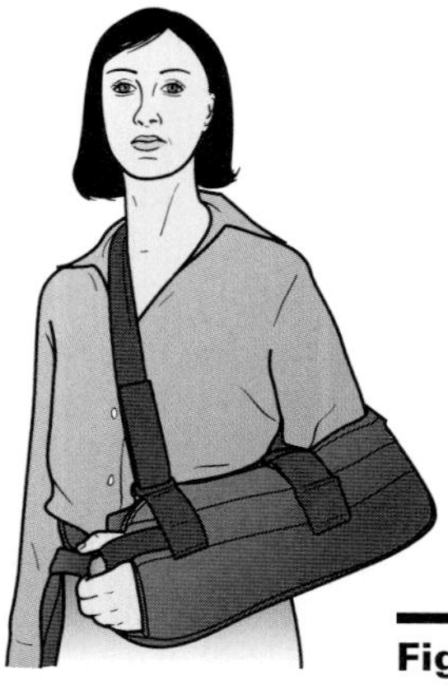

Figure 4 Arm sling.

✻ **A4601** Lithium ion battery, rechargeable, for non-prosthetic use, replacement E1

✻ **A4602** Replacement battery for external infusion pump owned by patient, lithium, 1.5 volt, each N

✻ **A4604** Tubing with integrated heating element for use with positive airway pressure device N

✻ **A4605** Tracheal suction catheter, closed system, each N

✻ **A4606** Oxygen probe for use with oximeter device, replacement N

✻ **A4608** Transtracheal oxygen catheter, each N

Supplies for Respiratory and Oxygen Equipment

⊘ **A4611** Battery, heavy duty; replacement for patient owned ventilator E1

Medicare Statute 1834(a)(3)(a)

⊘ **A4612** Battery cables; replacement for patient-owned ventilator E1

Medicare Statute 1834(a)(3)(a)

⊘ **A4613** Battery charger; replacement for patient-owned ventilator E1

Medicare Statute 1834(a)(3)(a)

✻ **A4614** Peak expiratory flow rate meter, hand held N

A4615 Cannula, nasal N

IOM: 100-03, 2, 160.6; 100-04, 20, 100.2

A4616 Tubing (oxygen), per foot N

IOM: 100-03, 2, 160.6; 100-04, 20, 100.2

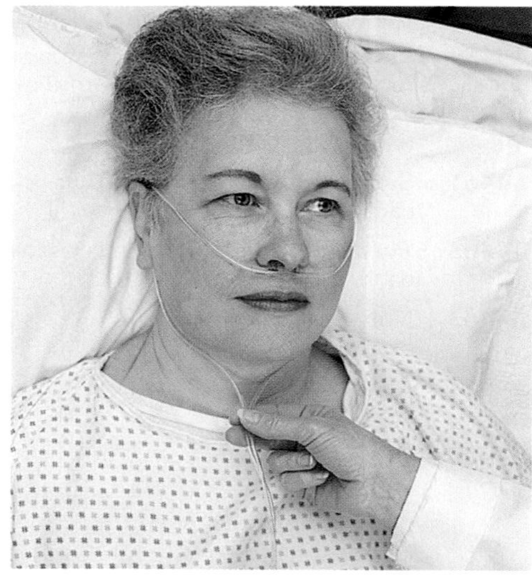

Figure 5 Nasal cannula.

A4617 Mouth piece N

IOM: 100-03, 2, 160.6; 100-04, 20, 100.2

A4618 Breathing circuits Qp Qh N

IOM: 100-03, 2, 160.6; 100-04, 20, 100.2

A4619 Face tent N

IOM: 100-03, 2, 160.6; 100-04, 20, 100.2

A4620 Variable concentration mask N

IOM: 100-03, 2, 160.6; 100-04, 20, 100.2

A4623 Tracheostomy, inner cannula Qh N

IOM: 100-02, 15, 120; 100-03, 1, 20.9

* **A4624** Tracheal suction catheter, any type, other than closed system, each Qh N

Sterile suction catheters are medically necessary only for tracheostomy suctioning. Limitations include three suction catheters per day when covered for medically necessary tracheostomy suctioning. Assign DX V44.0 or V55.0 on the claim form. (CMS Manual System, Pub. 100-3, NCD manual, Chapter 1, Section 280-1)

A4625 Tracheostomy care kit for new tracheostomy Qp Qh N

Dressings used with tracheostomies are included in the allowance for the code. This starter kit is covered after a surgical tracheostomy. (https://www.noridianmedicare.com/dme/coverage/docs/lcds/current_lcds/tracheostomy_care_supplies.htm)

IOM: 100-02, 15, 120

A4626 Tracheostomy cleaning brush, each N

IOM: 100-02, 15, 120

⊘ **A4627** Spacer, bag, or reservoir, with or without mask, for use with metered dose inhaler Qp Qh E1

IOM: 100-02, 15, 110

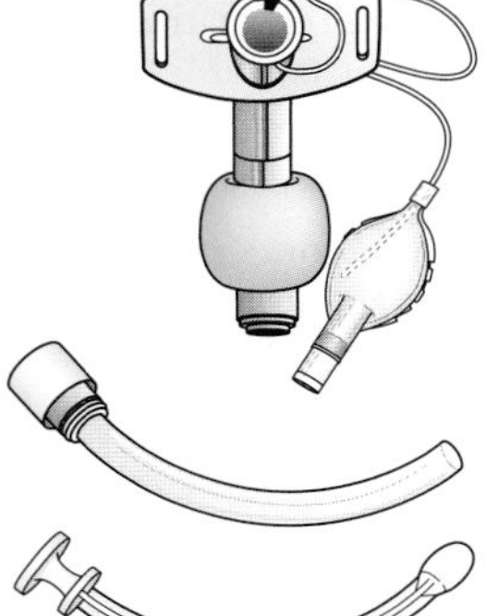

Figure 6 Tracheostomy cannula.

* **A4628** Oropharyngeal suction catheter, each Qh N

No more than three catheters per week are covered for medically necessary oropharyngeal suctioning because the catheters can be reused if cleansed and disinfected. (MS Manual System, Pub. 100-3, NCD manual, Chapter 1, Section 280-1)

A4629 Tracheostomy care kit for established tracheostomy Qh N

IOM: 100-02, 15, 120

Replacement Parts

A4630 Replacement batteries, medically necessary, transcutaneous electrical stimulator, owned by patient E1

IOM: 100-03, 3, 160.7

* **A4633** Replacement bulb/lamp for ultraviolet light therapy system, each Qp Qh E1

* **A4634** Replacement bulb for therapeutic light box, tabletop model N

A4635 Underarm pad, crutch, replacement, each Qp Qh E1

IOM: 100-03, 4, 280.1

A4636 Replacement, handgrip, cane, crutch, or walker, each Qh E1

IOM: 100-03, 4, 280.1

A4637 Replacement, tip, cane, crutch, walker, each Qh E1

IOM: 100-03, 4, 280.1

* **A4638** Replacement battery for patient-owned ear pulse generator, each Qp Qh E1

* **A4639** Replacement pad for infrared heating pad system, each E1

A4640 Replacement pad for use with medically necessary alternating pressure pad owned by patient Qp Qh E1

IOM: 100-03, 4, 280.1; 100-08, 5, 5.2.3

Supplies for Radiological Procedures

* **A4641** Radiopharmaceutical, diagnostic, not otherwise classified N

Is not an applicable tracer for PET scans

* **A4642** Indium In-111 satumomab pendetide, diagnostic, per study dose, up to 6 millicuries Qp Qh N

Miscellaneous Supplies

* **A4648** Tissue marker, implantable, any type, each Qp Qh — N
  Coding Clinic: 2018, Q2, P4,5; 2013, Q3, P9
* **A4649** Surgical supply miscellaneous Qp — N
* **A4650** Implantable radiation dosimeter, each Qp Qh — N
* **A4651** Calibrated microcapillary tube, each — N
  IOM: 100-04, 3, 40.3
* **A4652** Microcapillary tube sealant — N
  IOM: 100-04, 3, 40.3

Supplies for Dialysis

* **A4653** Peritoneal dialysis catheter anchoring device, belt, each Qp Qh — N
* **A4657** Syringe, with or without needle, each Qp Qh — N
  IOM: 100-04, 8, 90.3.2
* **A4660** Sphygmomanometer/blood pressure apparatus with cuff and stethoscope Qp Qh — N
  IOM: 100-04, 8, 90.3.2
* **A4663** Blood pressure cuff only Qp Qh — N
  IOM: 100-04, 8, 90.3.2
* **A4670** Automatic blood pressure monitor Qp Qh — E1
  IOM: 100-04, 8, 90.3.2
* **A4671** Disposable cycler set used with cycler dialysis machine, each Qp Qh — B
  IOM: 100-04, 8, 90.3.2
* **A4672** Drainage extension line, sterile, for dialysis, each Qp Qh — B
  IOM: 100-04, 8, 90.3.2
* **A4673** Extension line with easy lock connectors, used with dialysis Qp Qh — B
  IOM: 100-04, 8, 90.3.2
* **A4674** Chemicals/antiseptics solution used to clean/sterilize dialysis equipment, per 8 oz Qp Qh — B
  IOM: 100-04, 8, 90.3.2
* **A4680** Activated carbon filters for hemodialysis, each Qp Qh — N
  IOM: 100-04, 8, 90.3.2
* **A4690** Dialyzers (artificial kidneys), all types, all sizes, for hemodialysis, each Qp Qh — N
  IOM: 100-04, 8, 90.3.2
* **A4706** Bicarbonate concentrate, solution, for hemodialysis, per gallon Qp Qh — N
  IOM: 100-04, 8, 90.3.2
* **A4707** Bicarbonate concentrate, powder, for hemodialysis, per packet Qp Qh — N
  IOM: 100-04, 8, 90.3.2
* **A4708** Acetate concentrate solution, for hemodialysis, per gallon Qp Qh — N
  IOM: 100-04, 8, 90.3.2
* **A4709** Acid concentrate, solution, for hemodialysis, per gallon Qp Qh — N
  IOM: 100-04, 8, 90.3.2
* **A4714** Treated water (deionized, distilled, or reverse osmosis) for peritoneal dialysis, per gallon Qp Qh — N
  IOM: 100-03, 4, 230.7; 100-04, 3, 40.3
* **A4719** "Y set" tubing for peritoneal dialysis Qp Qh — N
  IOM: 100-04, 8, 90.3.2
* **A4720** Dialysate solution, any concentration of dextrose, fluid volume greater than 249 cc, but less than or equal to 999 cc, for peritoneal dialysis Qp Qh — N
  Do not use AX modifier.
  IOM: 100-04, 8, 90.3.2
* **A4721** Dialysate solution, any concentration of dextrose, fluid volume greater than 999 cc but less than or equal to 1999 cc, for peritoneal dialysis Qp Qh — N
  IOM: 100-04, 8, 90.3.2
* **A4722** Dialysate solution, any concentration of dextrose, fluid volume greater than 1999 cc but less than or equal to 2999 cc, for peritoneal dialysis Qp Qh — N
  IOM: 100-04, 8, 90.3.2
* **A4723** Dialysate solution, any concentration of dextrose, fluid volume greater than 2999 cc but less than or equal to 3999 cc, for peritoneal dialysis Qp Qh — N
  IOM: 100-04, 8, 90.3.2
* **A4724** Dialysate solution, any concentration of dextrose, fluid volume greater than 3999 cc but less than or equal to 4999 cc for peritoneal dialysis Qp Qh — N
  IOM: 100-04, 8, 90.3.2

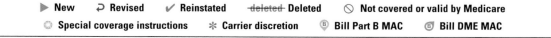
New
Revised
Reinstated
deleted Deleted
Not covered or valid by Medicare
Special coverage instructions
Carrier discretion
Bill Part B MAC
Bill DME MAC

A4725 Dialysate solution, any concentration of dextrose, fluid volume greater than 4999 cc but less than or equal to 5999 cc, for peritoneal dialysis Qp Qh N

IOM: 100-04, 8, 90.3.2

A4726 Dialysate solution, any concentration of dextrose, fluid volume greater than 5999 cc, for peritoneal dialysis Qp Qh N

IOM: 100-04, 8, 90.3.2

* **A4728** Dialysate solution, non-dextrose containing, 500 ml Qp Qh B

A4730 Fistula cannulation set for hemodialysis, each Qp Qh N

IOM: 100-04, 8, 90.3.2

A4736 Topical anesthetic, for dialysis, per gram Qp Qh N

IOM: 100-04, 8, 90.3.2

A4737 Injectable anesthetic, for dialysis, per 10 ml Qp Qh N

IOM: 100-04, 8, 90.3.2

A4740 Shunt accessory, for hemodialysis, any type, each Qp Qh N

IOM: 100-04, 8, 90.3.2

A4750 Blood tubing, arterial or venous, for hemodialysis, each Qp Qh N

IOM: 100-04, 8, 90.3.2

A4755 Blood tubing, arterial and venous combined, for hemodialysis, each Qp Qh N

IOM: 100-04, 8, 90.3.2

A4760 Dialysate solution test kit, for peritoneal dialysis, any type, each Qp Qh N

IOM: 100-04, 8, 90.3.2

A4765 Dialysate concentrate, powder, additive for peritoneal dialysis, per packet Qp Qh N

IOM: 100-04, 8, 90.3.2

A4766 Dialysate concentrate, solution, additive for peritoneal dialysis, per 10 ml Qp Qh N

IOM: 100-04, 8, 90.3.2

A4770 Blood collection tube, vacuum, for dialysis, per 50 Qp Qh N

IOM: 100-04, 8, 90.3.2

A4771 Serum clotting time tube, for dialysis, per 50 Qp Qh N

IOM: 100-04, 8, 90.3.2

A4772 Blood glucose test strips, for dialysis, per 50 Qp Qh N

IOM: 100-04, 8, 90.3.2

A4773 Occult blood test strips, for dialysis, per 50 Qp Qh N

IOM: 100-04, 8, 90.3.2

A4774 Ammonia test strips, for dialysis, per 50 Qp Qh N

IOM: 100-04, 8, 90.3.2

A4802 Protamine sulfate, for hemodialysis, per 50 mg Qp Qh N

IOM: 100-04, 8, 90.3.2

A4860 Disposable catheter tips for peritoneal dialysis, per 10 Qp Qh N

IOM: 100-04, 8, 90.3.2

A4870 Plumbing and/or electrical work for home hemodialysis equipment Qp Qh N

IOM: 100-04, 8, 90.3.2

A4890 Contracts, repair and maintenance, for hemodialysis equipment Qp Qh N

IOM: 100-02, 15, 110.2

A4911 Drain bag/bottle, for dialysis, each Qp Qh N

A4913 Miscellaneous dialysis supplies, not otherwise specified Qp Qh N

Items not related to dialysis must not be billed with the miscellaneous codes A4913 or E1699.

A4918 Venous pressure clamp, for hemodialysis, each Qp Qh N

A4927 Gloves, non-sterile, per 100 Qp Qh N

A4928 Surgical mask, per 20 Qp Qh N

A4929 Tourniquet for dialysis, each Qp Qh N

A4930 Gloves, sterile, per pair Qp Qh N

* **A4931** Oral thermometer, reusable, any type, each Qp Qh N

* **A4932** Rectal thermometer, reusable, any type, each Qp Qh N

Additional Ostomy Supplies

A5051 Ostomy pouch, closed; with barrier attached (1 piece), each Qp Qh & N

IOM: 100-02, 15, 120

A5052 Ostomy pouch, closed; without barrier attached (1 piece), each Qp Qh & N

IOM: 100-02, 15, 120

MIPS | Qp Quantity Physician | Qh Quantity Hospital | ♀ Female only | ♂ Male only | A Age | & DMEPOS | A2-Z3 ASC Payment Indicator | A-Y ASC Status Indicator | Coding Clinic

A5053 Ostomy pouch, closed; for use on faceplate, each Qp Qh N

IOM: 100-02, 15, 120

A5054 Ostomy pouch, closed; for use on barrier with flange (2 piece), each Qp N

IOM: 100-02, 15, 120

A5055 Stoma cap Qp Qh N

IOM: 100-02, 15, 120

A5056 Ostomy pouch, drainable, with extended wear barrier attached, with filter (1 piece), each Qp Qh N

IOM: 100-02, 15, 120

A5057 Ostomy pouch, drainable, with extended wear barrier attached, with built in convexity, with filter (1 piece), each Qp Qh N

IOM: 100-02, 15, 120

* **A5061** Ostomy pouch, drainable; with barrier attached (1 piece), each Qp Qh N

IOM: 100-02, 15, 120

A5062 Ostomy pouch, drainable; without barrier attached (1 piece), each Qp Qh N

IOM: 100-02, 15, 120

A5063 Ostomy pouch, drainable; for use on barrier with flange (2 piece system), each Qp Qh N

IOM: 100-02, 15, 120

A5071 Ostomy pouch, urinary; with barrier attached (1 piece), each Qp Qh N

IOM: 100-02, 15, 120

A5072 Ostomy pouch, urinary; without barrier attached (1 piece), each Qp Qh N

IOM: 100-02, 15, 120

A5073 Ostomy pouch, urinary; for use on barrier with flange (2 piece), each Qp Qh N

IOM: 100-02, 15, 120

A5081 Stoma plug or seal, any type Qp Qh N

IOM: 100-02, 15, 120

A5082 Continent device; catheter for continent stoma Qp Qh N

IOM: 100-02, 15, 120

* **A5083** Continent device, stoma absorptive cover for continent stoma Qh N

A5093 Ostomy accessory; convex insert Qp Qh N

IOM: 100-02, 15, 120

Additional Incontinence and Ostomy Supplies

A5102 Bedside drainage bottle with or without tubing, rigid or expandable, each Qp Qh N

IOM: 100-02, 15, 120

A5105 Urinary suspensory, with leg bag, with or without tube, each Qp Qh N

IOM: 100-02, 15, 120

A5112 Urinary drainage bag, leg bag, leg or abdomen, latex, with or without tube, with straps, each Qp Qh N

IOM: 100-02, 15, 120

A5113 Leg strap; latex, replacement only, per set Qp Qh E1

IOM: 100-02, 15, 120

A5114 Leg strap; foam or fabric, replacement only, per set Qp Qh E1

IOM: 100-02, 15, 120

A5120 Skin barrier, wipes or swabs, each Qp Qh N

IOM: 100-02, 15, 120

A5121 Skin barrier; solid, 6 × 6 or equivalent, each Qp Qh N

IOM: 100-02, 15, 120

A5122 Skin barrier; solid, 8 × 8 or equivalent, each Qp Qh N

IOM: 100-02, 15, 120

A5126 Adhesive or non-adhesive; disk or foam pad Qp Qh N

IOM: 100-02, 15, 120

A5131 Appliance cleaner, incontinence and ostomy appliances, per 16 oz Qp Qh N

IOM: 100-02, 15, 120

A5200 Percutaneous catheter/tube anchoring device, adhesive skin attachment Qh N

IOM: 100-02, 15, 120

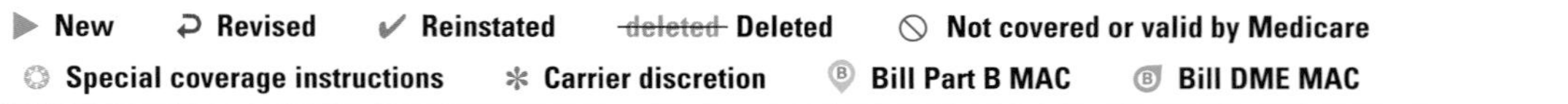
New
Revised
Reinstated
deleted Deleted
Not covered or valid by Medicare
Special coverage instructions
Carrier discretion
Bill Part B MAC
Bill DME MAC

Diabetic Shoes, Fitting, and Modifications

A5500 For diabetics only, fitting (including follow-up), custom preparation and supply of off-the-shelf depth-inlay shoe manufactured to accommodate multi-density insert(s), per shoe Qp Qh Y

IOM: 100-02, 15, 140

A5501 For diabetics only, fitting (including follow-up), custom preparation and supply of shoe molded from cast(s) of patient's foot (custom-molded shoe), per shoe Qp Qh Y

The diabetic patient must have at least one of the following conditions: peripheral neuropathy with evidence of callus formation, pre-ulcerative calluses, previous ulceration, foot deformity, previous amputation or poor circulation.

IOM: 100-02, 15, 140

A5503 For diabetics only, modification (including fitting) of off-the-shelf depth-inlay shoe or custom-molded shoe with roller or rigid rocker bottom, per shoe Qp Qh Y

IOM: 100-02, 15, 140

A5504 For diabetics only, modification (including fitting) of off-the-shelf depth-inlay shoe or custom-molded shoe with wedge(s), per shoe Qp Qh Y

IOM: 100-02, 15, 140

A5505 For diabetics only, modification (including fitting) of off-the-shelf depth-inlay shoe or custom-molded shoe with metatarsal bar, per shoe Qp Qh Y

IOM: 100-02, 15, 140

A5506 For diabetics only, modification (including fitting) of off-the-shelf depth-inlay shoe or custom-molded shoe with off-set heel(s), per shoe Qp Qh Y

IOM: 100-02, 15, 140

A5507 For diabetics only, not otherwise specified modification (including fitting) of off-the-shelf depth-inlay shoe or custom-molded shoe, per shoe Qp Qh Y

Only used for not otherwise specified therapeutic modifications to shoe or for repairs to a diabetic shoe(s)

IOM: 100-02, 15, 140

A5508 For diabetics only, deluxe feature of off-the-shelf depth-inlay shoe or custom-molded shoe, per shoe Qp Qh Y

IOM: 100-02, 15, 40

A5510 For diabetics only, direct formed, compression molded to patient's foot without external heat source, multiple-density insert(s) prefabricated, per shoe Qp Qh N

IOM: 100-02, 15, 140

* **A5512** For diabetics only, multiple density insert, direct formed, molded to foot after external heat source of 230 degrees Fahrenheit or higher, total contact with patient's foot, including arch, base layer minimum of 1/4 inch material of shore a 35 durometer or 3/16 inch material of shore a 40 durometer (or higher), prefabricated, each Qp Qh Y

* **A5513** For diabetics only, multiple density insert, custom molded from model of patient's foot, total contact with patient's foot, including arch, base layer minimum of 3/16 inch material of shore a 35 durometer (or higher), includes arch filler and other shaping material, custom fabricated, each Qp Qh Y

A5514 For diabetics only, multiple density insert, made by direct carving with cam technology from a rectified CAD model created from a digitized scan of the patient, total contact with patient's foot, including arch, base layer minimum of 3/16 inch material of shore a 35 durometer (or higher), includes arch filler and other shaping material, custom fabricated, each Y

Dressings

A6000 Non-contact wound warming wound cover for use with the non-contact wound warming device and warming card Qp Qh E1

IOM: 100-02, 16, 20

A6010 Collagen based wound filler, dry form, sterile, per gram of collagen N

IOM: 100-02, 15, 100

A6011 Collagen based wound filler, gel/paste, per gram of collagen N

IOM: 100-02, 15, 100

A6021 Collagen dressing, sterile, size 16 sq. in. or less, each N

IOM: 100-02, 15, 100

A6022 Collagen dressing, sterile, size more than 16 sq. in. but less than or equal to 48 sq. in., each Qp N

IOM: 100-02, 15, 100

MIPS | Qp Quantity Physician | Qh Quantity Hospital | ♀ Female only | ♂ Male only | A Age | DMEPOS | A2-Z3 ASC Payment Indicator | A-Y ASC Status Indicator | Coding Clinic

A6023 Collagen dressing, sterile, size more than 48 sq. in., each N

IOM: 100-02, 15, 100

A6024 Collagen dressing wound filler, sterile, per 6 inches N

IOM: 100-02, 15, 100

* **A6025** Gel sheet for dermal or epidermal application (e.g., silicone, hydrogel, other), each N

If used for the treatment of keloids or other scars, a silicone gel sheet will not meet the definition of the surgical dressing benefit and will be denied as noncovered.

A6154 Wound pouch, each Qp Qh N

Waterproof collection device with drainable port that adheres to skin around wound. Usual dressing change is up to 3 times per week.

IOM: 100-02, 15, 100

A6196 Alginate or other fiber gelling dressing, wound cover, sterile, pad size 16 sq. in. or less, each dressing Qp N

IOM: 100-02, 15, 100

A6197 Alginate or other fiber gelling dressing, wound cover, sterile, pad size more than 16 sq. in., but less than or equal to 48 sq. in., each dressing Qp N

IOM: 100-02, 15, 100

A6198 Alginate or other fiber gelling dressing, wound cover, sterile, pad size more than 48 sq. in., each dressing Qp N

IOM: 100-02, 15, 100

A6199 Alginate or other fiber gelling dressing, wound filler, sterile, per 6 inches Qp N

IOM: 100-02, 15, 100

A6203 Composite dressing, sterile, pad size 16 sq. in. or less, with any size adhesive border, each dressing Qp N

Usual composite dressing change is up to 3 times per week, one wound cover per dressing change.

IOM: 100-02, 15, 100

A6204 Composite dressing, sterile, pad size more than 16 sq. in. but less than or equal to 48 sq. in., with any size adhesive border, each dressing Qp N

Usual composite dressing change is up to 3 times per week, one wound cover per dressing change.

IOM: 100-02, 15, 100

A6205 Composite dressing, sterile, pad size more than 48 sq. in., with any size adhesive border, each dressing Qp Qh N

Usual composite dressing change is up to 3 times per week, one wound cover per dressing change.

IOM: 100-02, 15, 100

A6206 Contact layer, sterile, 16 sq. in. or less, each dressing Qp N

Contact layers are porous to allow wound fluid to pass through for absorption by separate overlying dressing and are not intended to be changed with each dressing change. Usual dressing change is up to once per week.

IOM: 100-02, 15, 100

A6207 Contact layer, sterile, more than 16 sq. in. but less than or equal to 48 sq. in., each dressing Qp N

Contact layer dressings are used to line the entire wound; they are not intended to be changed with each dressing change. Usual dressing change is up to once per week.

IOM: 100-02, 15, 100

A6208 Contact layer, sterile, more than 48 sq. in., each dressing Qp N

Contact layer dressings are used to line the entire wound; they are not intended to be changed with each dressing change. Usual dressing change is up to once per week.

IOM: 100-02, 15, 100

A6209 Foam dressing, wound cover, sterile, pad size 16 sq. in. or less, without adhesive border, each dressing Qp N

Made of open cell, medical grade expanded polymer; with nonadherent property over wound site.

IOM: 100-02, 15, 100

A6210 Foam dressing, wound cover, sterile, pad size more than 16 sq. in. but less than or equal to 48 sq. in., without adhesive border, each dressing Qp N

Foam dressings are covered items when used on full thickness wounds (e.g., stage III or IV ulcers) with moderate to heavy exudates. Usual dressing change for a foam wound cover when used as primary dressing is up to 3 times per week. When foam wound cover is used as a secondary dressing for wounds with very heavy exudates, dressing change may be up to 3 times per week. Usual dressing change for foam wound fillers is up to once per day (A6209-A6215).

IOM: 100-02, 15, 100

A6211 Foam dressing, wound cover, sterile, pad size more than 48 sq. in., without adhesive border, each dressing Qp N

IOM: 100-02, 15, 100

A6212 Foam dressing, wound cover, sterile, pad size 16 sq. in. or less, with any size adhesive border, each dressing Qp N

IOM: 100-02, 15, 100

A6213 Foam dressing, wound cover, sterile, pad size more than 16 sq. in. but less than or equal to 48 sq. in., with any size adhesive border, each dressing Qp N

IOM: 100-02, 15, 100

A6214 Foam dressing, wound cover, sterile, pad size more than 48 sq. in., with any size adhesive border, each dressing Qp N

IOM: 100-02, 15, 100

A6215 Foam dressing, wound filler, sterile, per gram Qp N

IOM: 100-02, 15, 100

A6216 Gauze, non-impregnated, non-sterile, pad size 16 sq. in. or less, without adhesive border, each dressing Qp N

IOM: 100-02, 15, 100

A6217 Gauze, non-impregnated, non-sterile, pad size more than 16 sq. in. but less than or equal to 48 sq. in., without adhesive border, each dressing Qp N

IOM: 100-02, 15, 100

A6218 Gauze, non-impregnated, non-sterile, pad size more than 48 sq. in., without adhesive border, each dressing Qp N

IOM: 100-02, 15, 100

A6219 Gauze, non-impregnated, sterile, pad size 16 sq. in. or less, with any size adhesive border, each dressing Qp N

IOM: 100-02, 15, 100

A6220 Gauze, non-impregnated, sterile, pad size more than 16 sq. in. but less than or equal to 48 sq. in., with any size adhesive border, each dressing Qp N

IOM: 100-02, 15, 100

A6221 Gauze, non-impregnated, sterile, pad size more than 48 sq. in., with any size adhesive border, each dressing N

IOM: 100-02, 15, 100

A6222 Gauze, impregnated with other than water, normal saline, or hydrogel, sterile, pad size 16 sq. in. or less, without adhesive border, each dressing Qp N

Substances may have been incorporated into dressing material (i.e., iodinated agents, petrolatum, zinc paste, crystalline sodium chloride, chlorhexadine gluconate [CHG], bismuth tribromophenate [BTP], water, aqueous saline, hydrogel, or agents).

IOM: 100-02, 15, 100

A6223 Gauze, impregnated with other than water, normal saline, or hydrogel, sterile, pad size more than 16 sq. in. but less than or equal to 48 sq. in., without adhesive border, each dressing Qp N

IOM: 100-02, 15, 100

A6224 Gauze, impregnated with other than water, normal saline, or hydrogel, sterile, pad size more than 48 sq. in., without adhesive border, each dressing Qp N

IOM: 100-02, 15, 100

A6228 Gauze, impregnated, water or normal saline, sterile, pad size 16 sq. in. or less, without adhesive border, each dressing Qp Qh N

IOM: 100-02, 15, 100

A6229 Gauze, impregnated, water or normal saline, sterile, pad size more than 16 sq. in. but less than or equal to 48 sq. in., without adhesive border, each dressing Qp N

IOM: 100-02, 15, 100

A6230 Gauze, impregnated, water or normal saline, sterile, pad size more than 48 sq. in., without adhesive border, each dressing Qp Qh N

IOM: 100-02, 15, 100

A6231 Gauze, impregnated, hydrogel, for direct wound contact, sterile, pad size 16 sq. in. or less, each dressing Qp N

IOM: 100-02, 15, 100

A6232 Gauze, impregnated, hydrogel, for direct wound contact, sterile, pad size greater than 16 sq. in., but less than or equal to 48 sq. in., each dressing N

IOM: 100-02, 15, 100

A6233 Gauze, impregnated, hydrogel, for direct wound contact, sterile, pad size more than 48 sq. in., each dressing N

IOM: 100-02, 15, 100

A6234 Hydrocolloid dressing, wound cover, sterile, pad size 16 sq. in. or less, without adhesive border, each dressing Qp N

This type of dressing is usually used on wounds with light to moderate exudate with an average of three dressing changes per week.

IOM: 100-02, 15, 100

A6235 Hydrocolloid dressing, wound cover, sterile, pad size more than 16 sq. in. but less than or equal to 48 sq. in., without adhesive border, each dressing Qp N

IOM: 100-02, 15, 100

A6236 Hydrocolloid dressing, wound cover, sterile, pad size more than 48 sq. in., without adhesive border, each dressing Qp Qh N

IOM: 100-02, 15, 100

A6237 Hydrocolloid dressing, wound cover, sterile, pad size 16 sq. in. or less, with any size adhesive border, each dressing Qp N

IOM: 100-02, 15, 100

A6238 Hydrocolloid dressing, wound cover, sterile, pad size more than 16 sq. in. but less than or equal to 48 sq. in., with any size adhesive border, each dressing Qp Qh N

IOM: 100-02, 15, 100

A6239 Hydrocolloid dressing, wound cover, sterile, pad size more than 48 sq. in., with any size adhesive border, each dressing Qp Qh N

IOM: 100-02, 15, 100

A6240 Hydrocolloid dressing, wound filler, paste, sterile, per ounce Qp Qh N

IOM: 100-02, 15, 100

A6241 Hydrocolloid dressing, wound filler, dry form, sterile, per gram Qp Qh N

IOM: 100-02, 15, 100

A6242 Hydrogel dressing, wound cover, sterile, pad size 16 sq. in. or less, without adhesive border, each dressing Qp N

Considered medically necessary when used on full thickness wounds with minimal or no exudate (e.g., stage III or IV ulcers).

Usually up to one dressing change per day is considered medically necessary, but if well documented and medically necessary, the payer may allow more frequent dressing changes.

IOM: 100-02, 15, 100

A6243 Hydrogel dressing, wound cover, sterile, pad size more than 16 sq. in. but less than or equal to 48 sq. in., without adhesive border, each dressing Qp N

IOM: 100-02, 15, 100

A6244 Hydrogel dressing, wound cover, sterile, pad size more than 48 sq. in., without adhesive border, each dressing Qp Qh N

IOM: 100-02, 15, 100

A6245 Hydrogel dressing, wound cover, sterile, pad size 16 sq. in. or less, with any size adhesive border, each dressing Qp N

Coverage of a non-elastic gradient compression wrap is limited to one per 6 months per leg.

IOM: 100-02, 15, 100

New | Revised | Reinstated | ~~deleted~~ Deleted | Not covered or valid by Medicare
Special coverage instructions | Carrier discretion | Bill Part B MAC | Bill DME MAC

A6246 Hydrogel dressing, wound cover, sterile, pad size more than 16 sq. in. but less than or equal to 48 sq. in., with any size adhesive border, each dressing Qp Qh N

IOM: 100-02, 15, 100

A6247 Hydrogel dressing, wound cover, sterile, pad size more than 48 sq. in., with any size adhesive border, each dressing Qp Qh N

IOM: 100-02, 15, 100

A6248 Hydrogel dressing, wound filler, gel, per fluid ounce Qp N

IOM: 100-02, 15, 100

A6250 Skin sealants, protectants, moisturizers, ointments, any type, any size Qp Qh N

IOM: 100-02, 15, 100

A6251 Specialty absorptive dressing, wound cover, sterile, pad size 16 sq. in. or less, without adhesive border, each dressing Qp N

IOM: 100-02, 15, 100

A6252 Specialty absorptive dressing, wound cover, sterile, pad size more than 16 sq. in. but less than or equal to 48 sq. in., without adhesive border, each dressing Qp N

IOM: 100-02, 15, 100

A6253 Specialty absorptive dressing, wound cover, sterile, pad size more than 48 sq. in., without adhesive border, each dressing Qp N

IOM: 100-02, 15, 100

A6254 Specialty absorptive dressing, wound cover, sterile, pad size 16 sq. in. or less, with any size adhesive border, each dressing Qp N

IOM: 100-02, 15, 100

A6255 Specialty absorptive dressing, wound cover, sterile, pad size more than 16 sq. in. but less than or equal to 48 sq. in., with any size adhesive border, each dressing Qp N

IOM: 100-02, 15, 100

A6256 Specialty absorptive dressing, wound cover, sterile, pad size more than 48 sq. in., with any size adhesive border, each dressing Qp Qh N

Considered medically necessary when used for moderately or highly exudative wounds (e.g., stage III or IV ulcers).

IOM: 100-02, 15, 100

A6257 Transparent film, sterile, 16 sq. in. or less, each dressing Qp N

Considered medically necessary when used on open partial thickness wounds with minimal exudate or closed wounds.

IOM: 100-02, 15, 100

A6258 Transparent film, sterile, more than 16 sq. in. but less than or equal to 48 sq. in., each dressing Qp N

IOM: 100-02, 15, 100

A6259 Transparent film, sterile, more than 48 sq. in., each dressing Qp Qh N

IOM: 100-02, 15, 100

A6260 Wound cleansers, any type, any size Qp N

IOM: 100-02, 15, 100

A6261 Wound filler, gel/paste, per fluid ounce, not otherwise specified Qp Qh N

Units of service for wound fillers are 1 gram, 1 fluid ounce, 6 inch length, or 1 yard depending on product.

IOM: 100-02, 15, 100

A6262 Wound filler, dry form, per gram, not otherwise specified Qp Qh N

Dry forms (e.g., powder, granules, beads) are used to eliminate dead space in an open wound.

IOM: 100-02, 15, 100

A6266 Gauze, impregnated, other than water, normal saline, or zinc paste, sterile, any width, per linear yard Qp N

IOM: 100-02, 15, 100

A6402 Gauze, non-impregnated, sterile, pad size 16 sq. in. or less, without adhesive border, each dressing Qp N

IOM: 100-02, 15, 100

A6403 Gauze, non-impregnated, sterile, pad size more than 16 sq. in., less than or equal to 48 sq. in., without adhesive border, each dressing Qp N

IOM: 100-02, 15, 100

A6404 Gauze, non-impregnated, sterile, pad size more than 48 sq. in., without adhesive border, each dressing Qp Qh N

IOM: 100-02, 15, 100

* **A6407** Packing strips, non-impregnated, sterile, up to 2 inches in width, per linear yard N

IOM: 100-02, 15, 100

A6410 Eye pad, sterile, each Qp Qh N

IOM: 100-02, 15, 100

A6411 Eye pad, non-sterile, each N

IOM: 100-02, 15, 100

✻ **A6412** Eye patch, occlusive, each N

Bandages

⃠ **A6413** Adhesive bandage, first-aid type, any size, each E1

First aid type bandage is a wound cover with a pad size of less than 4 sq. in. Does not meet the definition of the surgical dressing benefit and will be denied as non-covered.

Medicare Statute 1861(s)(5)

✻ **A6441** Padding bandage, non-elastic, non-woven/non-knitted, width greater than or equal to three inches and less than five inches, per yard N

✻ **A6442** Conforming bandage, non-elastic, knitted/woven, non-sterile, width less than three inches, per yard N

Non-elastic, moderate or high compression that is typically sustained for one week

✻ **A6443** Conforming bandage, non-elastic, knitted/woven, non-sterile, width greater than or equal to three inches and less than five inches, per yard N

✻ **A6444** Conforming bandage, non-elastic, knitted/woven, non-sterile, width greater than or equal to five inches, per yard N

✻ **A6445** Conforming bandage, non-elastic, knitted/woven, sterile, width less than three inches, per yard N

✻ **A6446** Conforming bandage, non-elastic, knitted/woven, sterile, width greater than or equal to three inches and less than five inches, per yard N

✻ **A6447** Conforming bandage, non-elastic, knitted/woven, sterile, width greater than or equal to five inches, per yard N

✻ **A6448** Light compression bandage, elastic, knitted/woven, width less than three inches, per yard N

Used to hold wound cover dressings in place over a wound. Example is an ACE type elastic bandage.

✻ **A6449** Light compression bandage, elastic, knitted/woven, width greater than or equal to three inches and less than five inches, per yard N

✻ **A6450** Light compression bandage, elastic, knitted/woven, width greater than or equal to five inches, per yard N

✻ **A6451** Moderate compression bandage, elastic, knitted/woven, load resistance of 1.25 to 1.34 foot pounds at 50% maximum stretch, width greater than or equal to three inches and less than five inches, per yard N

Elastic bandages that produce moderate compression that is typically sustained for one week

Medicare considers coverage if part of a multi-layer compression bandage system for the treatment of a venous stasis ulcer. Do not assign for strains or sprains.

✻ **A6452** High compression bandage, elastic, knitted/woven, load resistance greater than or equal to 1.35 foot pounds at 50% maximum stretch, width greater than or equal to three inches and less than five inches, per yard N

Elastic bandages that produce high compression that is typically sustained for one week

✻ **A6453** Self-adherent bandage, elastic, non-knitted/non-woven, width less than three inches, per yard N

✻ **A6454** Self-adherent bandage, elastic, non-knitted/non-woven, width greater than or equal to three inches and less than five inches, per yard N

✻ **A6455** Self-adherent bandage, elastic, non-knitted/non-woven, width greater than or equal to five inches, per yard N

✻ **A6456** Zinc paste impregnated bandage, non-elastic, knitted/woven, width greater than or equal to three inches and less than five inches, per yard N

✻ **A6457** Tubular dressing with or without elastic, any width, per linear yard N

✻ **A6460** Synthetic resorbable wound dressing, sterile, pad size 16 sq. in. or less, without adhesive border, each dressing N

✻ **A6461** Synthetic resorbable wound dressing, sterile, pad size more than 16 sq. in. but less than or equal to 48 sq. in., without adhesive border, each dressing N

Compression Garments

A6501 Compression burn garment, bodysuit (head to foot), custom fabricated Qp Qh N

Garments used to reduce hypertrophic scarring and joint contractures following burn injury

IOM: 100-02, 15, 100

A6502 Compression burn garment, chin strap, custom fabricated Qp Qh N

IOM: 100-02, 15, 100

A6503 Compression burn garment, facial hood, custom fabricated Qp Qh N

IOM: 100-02, 15, 100

A6504 Compression burn garment, glove to wrist, custom fabricated Qp Qh N

IOM: 100-02, 15, 100

A6505 Compression burn garment, glove to elbow, custom fabricated Qp Qh N

IOM: 100-02, 15, 100

A6506 Compression burn garment, glove to axilla, custom fabricated Qp Qh N

IOM: 100-02, 15, 100

A6507 Compression burn garment, foot to knee length, custom fabricated Qp Qh N

IOM: 100-02, 15, 100

A6508 Compression burn garment, foot to thigh length, custom fabricated Qp Qh N

IOM: 100-02, 15, 100

A6509 Compression burn garment, upper trunk to waist including arm openings (vest), custom fabricated Qp Qh N

IOM: 100-02, 15, 100

A6510 Compression burn garment, trunk, including arms down to leg openings (leotard), custom fabricated Qp Qh N

IOM: 100-02, 15, 100

A6511 Compression burn garment, lower trunk including leg openings (panty), custom fabricated Qp Qh N

IOM: 100-02, 15, 100

A6512 Compression burn garment, not otherwise classified N

IOM: 100-02, 15, 100

* **A6513** Compression burn mask, face and/or neck, plastic or equal, custom fabricated Qp Qh B

A6530 Gradient compression stocking, below knee, 18-30 mmHg, each Qp Qh E1

IOM: 100-03, 4, 280.1

A6531 Gradient compression stocking, below knee, 30-40 mmHg, each Qp Qh N

Covered when used in treatment of open venous stasis ulcer. Modifiers A1-A9 are not assigned. Must be billed with AW, RT, or LT.

IOM: 100-02, 15, 100

A6532 Gradient compression stocking, below knee, 40-50 mmHg, each Qp Qh N

Covered when used in treatment of open venous stasis ulcer. Modifiers A1-A9 are not assigned. Must be billed with AW, RT, or LT.

IOM: 100-02, 15, 100

A6533 Gradient compression stocking, thigh length, 18-30 mmHg, each Qp Qh E1

IOM: 100-02, 15, 130; 100-03, 4, 280.1

A6534 Gradient compression stocking, thigh length, 30-40 mmHg, each Qp Qh E1

IOM: 100-02, 15, 130; 100-03, 4, 280.1

A6535 Gradient compression stocking, thigh length, 40-50 mmHg, each Qp Qh E1

IOM: 100-02, 15, 130; 100-03, 4, 280.1

A6536 Gradient compression stocking, full length/chap style, 18-30 mmHg, each Qp Qh E1

IOM: 100-02, 15, 130; 100-03, 4, 280.1

A6537 Gradient compression stocking, full length/chap style, 30-40 mmHg, each Qp Qh E1

IOM: 100-02, 15, 130; 100-03, 4, 280.1

A6538 Gradient compression stocking, full length/chap style, 40-50 mmHg, each Qp Qh E1

IOM: 100-02, 15, 130; 100-03, 4, 280.1

A6539 Gradient compression stocking, waist length, 18-30 mmHg, each Qp Qh E1

IOM: 100-02, 15, 130; 100-03, 4, 280.1

A6540 Gradient compression stocking, waist length, 30-40 mmHg, each Qp Qh E1

IOM: 100-02, 15, 130; 100-03, 4, 280.1

⃠ **A6541** Gradient compression stocking, waist length, 40-50 mmHg, each Ⓑ Qp Qh E1

IOM: 100-02, 15, 130; 100-03, 4, 280.1

⃠ **A6544** Gradient compression stocking, garter belt Ⓑ Qp Qh E1

IOM: 100-02, 15, 130; 100-03, 4, 280.1

A6545 Gradient compression wrap, non-elastic, below knee, 30-50 mm hg, each Ⓑ Qp Qh ♿ N

Modifiers RT and/or LT must be appended. When assigned for bilateral items (left/right) on the same date of service, bill both items on the same claim line using RT/LT modifiers and 2 units of service.

IOM: 10-02, 15, 100

⃠ **A6549** Gradient compression stocking/sleeve, not otherwise specified Ⓑ Qp Qh E1

IOM: 100-02, 15, 130; 100-03, 4, 280.1

Wound Care

* **A6550** Wound care set, for negative pressure wound therapy electrical pump, includes all supplies and accessories Ⓑ Qh ♿ N

Respiratory Supplies

* **A7000** Canister, disposable, used with suction pump, each Ⓑ Qp Qh ♿ Y

* **A7001** Canister, non-disposable, used with suction pump, each Ⓑ Qh ♿ Y

* **A7002** Tubing, used with suction pump, each Ⓑ Qh ♿ Y

* **A7003** Administration set, with small volume nonfiltered pneumatic nebulizer, disposable Ⓑ Qp Qh ♿ Y

* **A7004** Small volume nonfiltered pneumatic nebulizer, disposable Ⓑ Qh ♿ Y

* **A7005** Administration set, with small volume nonfiltered pneumatic nebulizer, non-disposable Ⓑ Qp Qh ♿ Y

* **A7006** Administration set, with small volume filtered pneumatic nebulizer Ⓑ Qp Qh ♿ Y

* **A7007** Large volume nebulizer, disposable, unfilled, used with aerosol compressor Ⓑ Qh ♿ Y

* **A7008** Large volume nebulizer, disposable, prefilled, used with aerosol compressor Ⓑ ♿ Y

* **A7009** Reservoir bottle, nondisposable, used with large volume ultrasonic nebulizer Ⓑ ♿ Y

* **A7010** Corrugated tubing, disposable, used with large volume nebulizer, 100 feet Ⓑ Qh ♿ Y

* **A7012** Water collection device, used with large volume nebulizer Ⓑ Qh ♿ Y

* **A7013** Filter, disposable, used with aerosol compressor or ultrasonic generator Ⓑ Qp Qh ♿ Y

* **A7014** Filter, non-disposable, used with aerosol compressor or ultrasonic generator Ⓑ Qp Qh ♿ Y

* **A7015** Aerosol mask, used with DME nebulizer Ⓑ Qh ♿ Y

* **A7016** Dome and mouthpiece, used with small volume ultrasonic nebulizer Ⓑ Qp Qh ♿ Y

A7017 Nebulizer, durable, glass or autoclavable plastic, bottle type, not used with oxygen Ⓑ Qp Qh ♿ Y

IOM: 100-03, 4, 280.1

* **A7018** Water, distilled, used with large volume nebulizer, 1000 ml Ⓑ Qh ♿ Y

* **A7020** Interface for cough stimulating device, includes all components, replacement only Ⓑ Qp Qh ♿ Y

* **A7025** High frequency chest wall oscillation system vest, replacement for use with patient owned equipment, each Ⓑ Qp Qh ♿ N

* **A7026** High frequency chest wall oscillation system hose, replacement for use with patient owned equipment, each Ⓑ Qp Qh ♿ Y

* **A7027** Combination oral/nasal mask, used with continuous positive airway pressure device, each Ⓑ Qp Qh ♿ Y

* **A7028** Oral cushion for combination oral/nasal mask, replacement only, each Ⓑ Qp Qh ♿ Y

* **A7029** Nasal pillows for combination oral/nasal mask, replacement only, pair Ⓑ Qp Qh ♿ Y

* **A7030** Full face mask used with positive airway pressure device, each Ⓑ Qh ♿ Y

* **A7031** Face mask interface, replacement for full face mask, each Ⓑ Qh ♿ Y

* **A7032** Cushion for use on nasal mask interface, replacement only, each Ⓑ Qp Qh ♿ Y

* **A7033** Pillow for use on nasal cannula type interface, replacement only, pair Qh Y

* **A7034** Nasal interface (mask or cannula type) used with positive airway pressure device, with or without head strap Qh Y

* **A7035** Headgear used with positive airway pressure device Qp Qh Y

* **A7036** Chinstrap used with positive airway pressure device Qp Qh Y

* **A7037** Tubing used with positive airway pressure device Qp Qh Y

* **A7038** Filter, disposable, used with positive airway pressure device Qh Y

* **A7039** Filter, non disposable, used with positive airway pressure device Qp Qh Y

* **A7040** One way chest drain valve Qp Qh N

* **A7041** Water seal drainage container and tubing for use with implanted chest tube Qp Qh N

* **A7044** Oral interface used with positive airway pressure device, each Qp Qh Y

A7045 Exhalation port with or without swivel used with accessories for positive airway devices, replacement only Qh Y

IOM: 100-03, 4, 230.17

A7046 Water chamber for humidifier, used with positive airway pressure device, replacement, each Qh Y

IOM: 100-03, 4, 230.17

* **A7047** Oral interface used with respiratory suction pump, each Qp Qh N

* **A7048** Vacuum drainage collection unit and tubing kit, including all supplies needed for collection unit change, for use with implanted catheter, each Qp Qh N

Tracheostomy Supplies

A7501 Tracheostoma valve, including diaphragm, each Qp Qh N

IOM: 100-02, 15, 120

A7502 Replacement diaphragm/faceplate for tracheostoma valve, each Qh N

IOM: 100-02, 15, 120

A7503 Filter holder or filter cap, reusable, for use in a tracheostoma heat and moisture exchange system, each Qh N

IOM: 100-02, 15, 120

A7504 Filter for use in a tracheostoma heat and moisture exchange system, each Qp Qh N

IOM: 100-02, 15, 120

A7505 Housing, reusable without adhesive, for use in a heat and moisture exchange system and/or with a tracheostoma valve, each Qh N

IOM: 100-02, 15, 120

A7506 Adhesive disc for use in a heat and moisture exchange system and/or with tracheostoma valve, any type, each Qh N

IOM: 100-02, 15, 120

A7507 Filter holder and integrated filter without adhesive, for use in a tracheostoma heat and moisture exchange system, each Qp Qh N

IOM: 100-02, 15, 120

A7508 Housing and integrated adhesive, for use in a tracheostoma heat and moisture exchange system and/or with a tracheostoma valve, each Qh N

IOM: 100-02, 15, 120

A7509 Filter holder and integrated filter housing, and adhesive, for use as a tracheostoma heat and moisture exchange system, each Qh N

IOM: 100-02, 15, 120

* **A7520** Tracheostomy/laryngectomy tube, non-cuffed, polyvinylchloride (PVC), silicone or equal, each Qp Qh N

* **A7521** Tracheostomy/laryngectomy tube, cuffed, polyvinylchloride (PVC), silicone or equal, each Qh N

* **A7522** Tracheostomy/laryngectomy tube, stainless steel or equal (sterilizable and reusable), each Qh N

* **A7523** Tracheostomy shower protector, each N

* **A7524** Tracheostoma stent/stud/button, each Qp Qh N

* **A7525** Tracheostomy mask, each Qh N

* **A7526** Tracheostomy tube collar/holder, each Qh N

* **A7527** Tracheostomy/laryngectomy tube plug/stop, each Qp Qh N

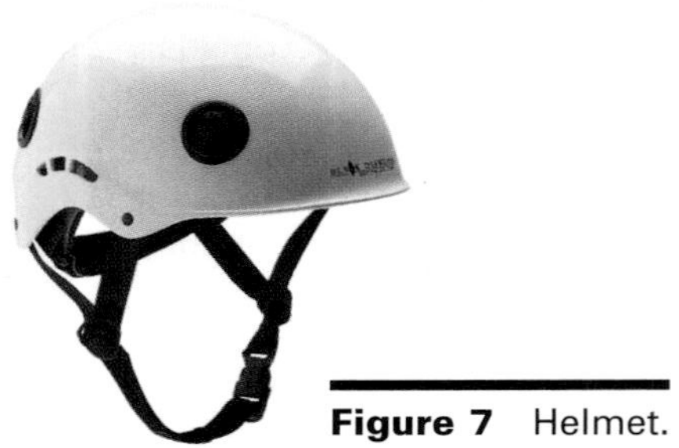

Figure 7 Helmet.

Helmets

	Code	Description	
✻	**A8000**	Helmet, protective, soft, prefabricated, includes all components and accessories Ⓓ ♿	Y
✻	**A8001**	Helmet, protective, hard, prefabricated, includes all components and accessories Ⓓ ♿	Y
✻	**A8002**	Helmet, protective, soft, custom fabricated, includes all components and accessories Ⓓ ♿	Y
✻	**A8003**	Helmet, protective, hard, custom fabricated, includes all components and accessories Ⓓ ♿	Y
✻	**A8004**	Soft interface for helmet, replacement only Ⓓ ♿	Y

ADMINISTRATIVE, MISCELLANEOUS, AND INVESTIGATIONAL (A9000-A9999)

Note: The following codes do not imply that codes in other sections are necessarily covered.

Miscellaneous Supplies

	Code	Description	
◌	**A9150**	Non-prescription drugs Ⓑ *IOM: 100-02, 15, 50*	B
⃠	**A9152**	Single vitamin/mineral/trace element, oral, per dose, not otherwise specified Ⓑ Qp Qh	E1
⃠	**A9153**	Multiple vitamins, with or without minerals and trace elements, oral, per dose, not otherwise specified Ⓑ Qp Qh	E1
✻	**A9155**	Artificial saliva, 30 ml Ⓑ Qp Qh	B
⃠	**A9180**	Pediculosis (lice infestation) treatment, topical, for administration by patient/caretaker Ⓑ Qp Qh	E1
⃠	**A9270**	Non-covered item or service Ⓓ Qp Qh *IOM: 100-02, 16, 20*	E1
⃠	**A9272**	Wound suction, disposable, includes dressing, all accessories and components, any type, each Ⓓ Qp Qh *Medicare Statute 1861(n)*	E1
⃠	**A9273**	Cold or hot water bottle, ice cap or collar, heat and/or cold wrap, any type Ⓓ Qp Qh	E1
⃠	**A9274**	External ambulatory insulin delivery system, disposable, each, includes all supplies and accessories Ⓓ Qp Qh *Medicare Statute 1861(n)*	E1
⃠	**A9275**	Home glucose disposable monitor, includes test strips Ⓓ Qp Qh	E1
⃠	**A9276**	Sensor; invasive (e.g., subcutaneous), disposable, for use with interstitial continuous glucose monitoring system, one unit = 1 day supply Ⓓ Qp Qh *Medicare Statute 1861(n)*	E1
⃠	**A9277**	Transmitter; external, for use with interstitial continuous glucose monitoring system Ⓓ Qp Qh *Medicare Statute 1861(n)*	E1
⃠	**A9278**	Receiver (monitor); external, for use with interstitial continuous glucose monitoring system Ⓓ Qp Qh *Medicare Statute 1861(n)*	E1
⃠	**A9279**	Monitoring feature/device, stand-alone or integrated, any type, includes all accessories, components and electronics, not otherwise classified Ⓓ Qp Qh *Medicare Statute 1861(n)*	E1
⃠	**A9280**	Alert or alarm device, not otherwise classified Ⓓ Qp Qh *Medicare Statute 1861*	E1
⃠	**A9281**	Reaching/grabbing device, any type, any length, each Ⓓ Qp Qh *Medicare Statute 1862 SSA*	E1
⃠	**A9282**	Wig, any type, each Ⓓ Qp Qh *Medicare Statute 1862 SSA*	E1
⃠	**A9283**	Foot pressure off loading/supportive device, any type, each Ⓓ Qp Qh *Medicare Statute 1862A(i)13*	E1
◌	**A9284**	Spirometer, non-electronic, includes all accessories Ⓓ Qp Qh	N
✻	**A9285**	Inversion/eversion correction device Ⓓ Qp Qh	A
⃠	**A9286**	Hygienic item or device, disposable or non-disposable, any type, each Ⓓ Qp Qh *Medicare Statute 1834*	E1

▶ New ↩ Revised ✔ Reinstated ~~deleted~~ Deleted ⃠ Not covered or valid by Medicare
◌ Special coverage instructions ✻ Carrier discretion Ⓑ Bill Part B MAC Ⓓ Bill DME MAC

⊘ **A9300** Exercise equipment Qp Qh E1
IOM: 100-02, 15, 110.1; 100-03, 4, 280.1

Supplies for Radiology Procedures (Radiopharmaceuticals)

* **A9500** Technetium Tc-99m sestamibi, diagnostic, per study dose Qp Qh N1 N
  Should be filed on same claim as procedure code reporting radiopharmaceutical. Verify with payer definition of a "study."
  Coding Clinic: 2006, Q2, P5
* **A9501** Technetium Tc-99m teboroxime, diagnostic, per study dose Qp Qh N1 N
* **A9502** Technetium Tc-99m tetrofosmin, diagnostic, per study dose Qp Qh N1 N
  Coding Clinic: 2006, Q2, P5
* **A9503** Technetium Tc-99m medronate, diagnostic, per study dose, up to 30 millicuries Qp Qh N1 N
* **A9504** Technetium Tc-99m apcitide, diagnostic, per study dose, up to 20 millicuries Qp Qh N1 N
* **A9505** Thallium Tl-201 thallous chloride, diagnostic, per millicurie Qp Qh N1 N
* **A9507** Indium In-111 capromab pendetide, diagnostic, per study dose, up to 10 millicuries Qp Qh N1 N
* **A9508** Iodine I-131 iobenguane sulfate, diagnostic, per 0.5 millicurie Qp Qh N1 N
* **A9509** Iodine I-123 sodium iodide, diagnostic, per millicurie Qp Qh N1 N
* **A9510** Technetium Tc-99m disofenin, diagnostic, per study dose, up to 15 millicuries Qp Qh N1 N
* **A9512** Technetium Tc-99m pertechnetate, diagnostic, per millicurie Qp Qh N1 N
* **A9513** Lutetium lu 177, dotatate, therapeutic, 1 millicurie G
* **A9515** Choline C-11, diagnostic, per study dose up to 20 millicuries Qp Qh K2 G
* **A9516** Iodine I-123 sodium iodide, diagnostic, per 100 microcuries, up to 999 microcuries Qp Qh N1 N
* **A9517** Iodine I-131 sodium iodide capsule(s), therapeutic, per millicurie Qp Qh K
* **A9520** Technetium Tc-99m tilmanocept, diagnostic, up to 0.5 millicuries Qp Qh N1 N
* **A9521** Technetium Tc-99m exametazime, diagnostic, per study dose, up to 25 millicuries Qp Qh N1 N
* **A9524** Iodine I-131 iodinated serum albumin, diagnostic, per 5 microcuries Qp Qh N1 N
* **A9526** Nitrogen N-13 ammonia, diagnostic, per study dose, up to 40 millicuries Qp Qh N1 N
* **A9527** Iodine I-125, sodium iodide solution, therapeutic, per millicurie Qp Qh H2 U
* **A9528** Iodine I-131 sodium iodide capsule(s), diagnostic, per millicurie Qp Qh N1 N
* **A9529** Iodine I-131 sodium iodide solution, diagnostic, per millicurie Qp Qh N1 N
* **A9530** Iodine I-131 sodium iodide solution, therapeutic, per millicurie Qp Qh K
* **A9531** Iodine I-131 sodium iodide, diagnostic, per microcurie (up to 100 microcuries) Qp Qh N1 N
* **A9532** Iodine I-125 serum albumin, diagnostic, per 5 microcuries Qp Qh N1 N
* **A9536** Technetium Tc-99m depreotide, diagnostic, per study dose, up to 35 millicuries Qp Qh N1 N
* **A9537** Technetium Tc-99m mebrofenin, diagnostic, per study dose, up to 15 millicuries Qp Qh N1 N
* **A9538** Technetium Tc-99m pyrophosphate, diagnostic, per study dose, up to 25 millicuries Qp Qh N1 N
* **A9539** Technetium Tc-99m pentetate, diagnostic, per study dose, up to 25 millicuries Qp Qh N1 N
* **A9540** Technetium Tc-99m macroaggregated albumin, diagnostic, per study dose, up to 10 millicuries Qp Qh N1 N
* **A9541** Technetium Tc-99m sulfur colloid, diagnostic, per study dose, up to 20 millicuries Qp Qh N1 N
* **A9542** Indium In-111 ibritumomab tiuxetan, diagnostic, per study dose, up to 5 millicuries Qp Qh N1 N
  Specifically for diagnostic use.
* **A9543** Yttrium Y-90 ibritumomab tiuxetan, therapeutic, per treatment dose, up to 40 millicuries Qp Qh K
  Specifically for therapeutic use.

* **A9546** Cobalt Co-57/58, cyanocobalamin, diagnostic, per study dose, up to 1 microcurie Ⓑ Qp Qh N1 N

* **A9547** Indium In-111 oxyquinoline, diagnostic, per 0.5 millicurie Ⓑ Qp Qh N1 N

* **A9548** Indium In-111 pentetate, diagnostic, per 0.5 millicurie Ⓑ Qp Qh N1 N

* **A9550** Technetium Tc-99m sodium gluceptate, diagnostic, per study dose, up to 25 millicuries Ⓑ Qp Qh N1 N

* **A9551** Technetium Tc-99m succimer, diagnostic, per study dose, up to 10 millicuries Ⓑ Qp Qh N1 N

* **A9552** Fluorodeoxyglucose F-18 FDG, diagnostic, per study dose, up to 45 millicuries Ⓑ Qp Qh N1 N

  Coding Clinic: 2008, Q3, P7

* **A9553** Chromium Cr-51 sodium chromate, diagnostic, per study dose, up to 250 microcuries Ⓑ Qp Qh N1 N

* **A9554** Iodine I-125 sodium Iothalamate, diagnostic, per study dose, up to 10 microcuries Ⓑ Qp Qh N1 N

* **A9555** Rubidium Rb-82, diagnostic, per study dose, up to 60 millicuries Ⓑ Qp Qh N1 N

* **A9556** Gallium Ga-67 citrate, diagnostic, per millicurie Ⓑ Qp Qh N1 N

* **A9557** Technetium Tc-99m bicisate, diagnostic, per study dose, up to 25 millicuries Ⓑ Qp Qh N1 N

* **A9558** Xenon Xe-133 gas, diagnostic, per 10 millicuries Ⓑ Qp Qh N1 N

* **A9559** Cobalt Co-57 cyanocobalamin, oral, diagnostic, per study dose, up to 1 microcurie Ⓑ Qp Qh N1 N

* **A9560** Technetium Tc-99m labeled red blood cells, diagnostic, per study dose, up to 30 millicuries Ⓑ Qp Qh N1 N

  Coding Clinic: 2008, Q3, P7

* **A9561** Technetium Tc-99m oxidronate, diagnostic, per study dose, up to 30 millicuries Ⓑ Qp Qh N1 N

* **A9562** Technetium Tc-99m mertiatide, diagnostic, per study dose, up to 15 millicuries Ⓑ Qp Qh N1 N

* **A9563** Sodium phosphate P-32, therapeutic, per millicurie Ⓑ Qp Qh K

* **A9564** Chromic phosphate P-32 suspension, therapeutic, per millicurie Ⓑ Qp Qh E1

* **A9566** Technetium Tc-99m fanolesomab, diagnostic, per study dose, up to 25 millicuries Ⓑ Qp Qh N1 N

* **A9567** Technetium Tc-99m pentetate, diagnostic, aerosol, per study dose, up to 75 millicuries Ⓑ Qp Qh N1 N

* **A9568** Technetium TC-99m arcitumomab, diagnostic, per study dose, up to 45 millicuries Ⓑ Qp Qh N1 N

* **A9569** Technetium Tc-99m exametazime labeled autologous white blood cells, diagnostic, per study dose Ⓑ Qp Qh N1 N

* **A9570** Indium In-111 labeled autologous white blood cells, diagnostic, per study dose Ⓑ Qp Qh N1 N

* **A9571** Indium In-111 labeled autologous platelets, diagnostic, per study dose Ⓑ Qp Qh N1 N

* **A9572** Indium In-111 pentetreotide, diagnostic, per study dose, up to 6 millicuries Ⓑ Qp Qh N1 N

* **A9575** Injection, gadoterate meglumine, 0.1 ml Ⓑ Qp Qh N1 N

  Other: Dotarem

* **A9576** Injection, gadoteridol, (ProHance Multipack), per ml Ⓑ Qp Qh N1 N

* **A9577** Injection, gadobenate dimeglumine (MultiHance), per ml Ⓑ Qp Qh N1 N

* **A9578** Injection, gadobenate dimeglumine (MultiHance Multipack), per ml Ⓑ Qp Qh N1 N

* **A9579** Injection, gadolinium-based magnetic resonance contrast agent, not otherwise specified (NOS), per ml Ⓑ Qp Qh N1 N

  Other: Magnevist, Omniscan, Optimark, Prohance

* **A9580** Sodium fluoride F-18, diagnostic, per study dose, up to 30 millicuries Ⓑ Qp Qh N1 N

* **A9581** Injection, gadoxetate disodium, 1 ml Ⓑ Qp Qh N1 N

  Local Medicare contractors may require the use of modifier JW to identify unused product from single-dose vials that are appropriately discarded.

  Other: Eovist

* **A9582** Iodine I-123 iobenguane, diagnostic, per study dose, up to 15 millicuries Ⓑ Qp Qh N1 N

  Molecular imaging agent that assists in the identification of rare neuroendocrine tumors.

▶ New ↩ Revised ✔ Reinstated ~~deleted~~ Deleted ⊘ Not covered or valid by Medicare
Special coverage instructions * Carrier discretion Ⓑ Bill Part B MAC Ⓓ Bill DME MAC

* **A9583** Injection, gadofosveset trisodium, 1 ml Qp Qh N1 N

* **A9584** Iodine 1-123 ioflupane, diagnostic, per study dose, up to 5 millicuries Qp Qh N1 N

Coding Clinic: 2012, Q1, P9

* **A9585** Injection, gadobutrol, 0.1 ml Qp Qh N1 N

Other: Gadavist

Coding Clinic: 2012, Q1, P8

A9586 Florbetapir F18, diagnostic, per study dose, up to 10 millicuries Qp Qh N1 N

* **A9587** Gallium Ga-68, dotatate, diagnostic, 0.1 millicurie Qp Qh K2 G

Coding Clinic: 2017, Q1, P9

* **A9589** Instillation, hexaminolevulinate hydrochloride, 100 mg N1 N

* **A9588** Fluciclovine F-18, diagnostic, 1 millicurie Qp Qh K2 G

Coding Clinic: 2017, Q1, P9

* **A9590** Iodine I-131, iobenguane, 1 millicurie N

▶ * **A9591** Fluoroestradiol F 18, diagnostic, 1 millicurie K2 G

* **A9597** Positron emission tomography radiopharmaceutical, diagnostic, for tumor identification, not otherwise classified N1 N

Coding Clinic: 2017, Q1, P8-9

* **A9598** Positron emission tomography radiopharmaceutical, diagnostic, for non-tumor identification, not otherwise classified N1 N

Coding Clinic: 2017, Q1, P8-9

* **A9600** Strontium Sr-89 chloride, therapeutic, per millicurie Qp Qh K

* **A9604** Samarium SM-153 lexidronam, therapeutic, per treatment dose, up to 150 millicuries Qp Qh K

* **A9606** Radium Ra-223 dichloride, therapeutic, per microcurie Qp Qh K

A9698 Non-radioactive contrast imaging material, not otherwise classified, per study N1 N

IOM: 100-04, 12, 70; 100-04, 13, 20

Coding Clinic: 2017, Q1, P8

* **A9699** Radiopharmaceutical, therapeutic, not otherwise classified N

A9700 Supply of injectable contrast material for use in echocardiography, per study Qp Qh N1 N

IOM: 100-04, 12, 30.4

Coding Clinic: 2017, Q1, P8

Miscellaneous Service Component

* **A9900** Miscellaneous DME supply, accessory, and/or service component of another HCPCS code Y

On DMEPOS fee schedule as a payable replacement for miscellaneous implanted or non-implanted items.

* **A9901** DME delivery, set up, and/or dispensing service component of another HCPCS code A

* **A9999** Miscellaneous DME supply or accessory, not otherwise specified Y

On DMEPOS fee schedule as a payable replacement for miscellaneous implanted or non-implanted items.

ENTERAL AND PARENTERAL THERAPY (B4000-B9999)

Enteral Feeding Supplies

B4034 Enteral feeding supply kit; syringe fed, per day, includes but not limited to feeding/flushing syringe, administration set tubing, dressings, tape Qh Y

Dressings used with gastrostomy tubes for enteral nutrition (covered under the prosthetic device benefit) are included in the payment.

IOM: 100-02, 15, 120; 100-03, 3, 180.2; 100-04, 20, 100.2.2

PEN: On Fee Schedule

B4035 Enteral feeding supply kit; pump fed, per day, includes but not limited to feeding/flushing syringe, administration set tubing, dressings, tape Qh Y

IOM: 100-02, 15, 120; 100-03, 3, 180.2; 100-04, 20, 100.2.2

PEN: On Fee Schedule

B4036 Enteral feeding supply kit; gravity fed, per day, includes but not limited to feeding/flushing syringe, administration set tubing, dressings, tape Qh Y

IOM: 100-02, 15, 120; 100-03, 3, 180.2; 100-04, 20, 100.2.2

PEN: On Fee Schedule

B4081 Nasogastric tubing with stylet Qp Qh Y

More than 3 nasogastric tubes (B4081-B4083), or 1 gastrostomy/jejunostomy tube (B4087-B4088) every three months is rarely medically necessary.

IOM: 100-02, 15, 120; 100-03, 3, 180.2; 100-04, 20, 100.2.2

PEN: On Fee Schedule

B4082 Nasogastric tubing without stylet Qp Qh Y

IOM: 100-02, 15, 120; 100-03, 3, 180.2; 100-04, 20, 100.2.2

PEN: On Fee Schedule

B4083 Stomach tube - Levine type Qp Qh Y

IOM: 100-02, 15, 120; 100-03, 3, 180.2; 100-04, 20, 100.2.2

PEN: On Fee Schedule

* **B4087** Gastrostomy/jejunostomy tube, standard, any material, any type, each Qp Qh A

PEN: On Fee Schedule

* **B4088** Gastrostomy/jejunostomy tube, low-profile, any material, any type, each Qp Qh A

PEN: On Fee Schedule

Enteral Formulas and Additives

B4100 Food thickener, administered orally, per ounce E1

B4102 Enteral formula, for adults, used to replace fluids and electrolytes (e.g., clear liquids), 500 ml = 1 unit A Y

IOM: 100-03, 3, 180.2

B4103 Enteral formula, for pediatrics, used to replace fluids and electrolytes (e.g., clear liquids), 500 ml = 1 unit A Y

IOM: 100-03, 3, 180.2

B4104 Additive for enteral formula (e.g., fiber) E1

IOM: 100-03, 3, 180.2

B4105 In-line cartridge containing digestive enzyme(s) for enteral feeding, each Y

Cross Reference Q9994

B4149 Enteral formula, manufactured blenderized natural foods with intact nutrients, includes proteins, fats, carbohydrates, vitamins and minerals, may include fiber, administered through an enteral feeding tube, 100 calories = 1 unit Qp Qh Y

Produced to meet unique nutrient needs for specific disease conditions; medical record must document specific condition and need for special nutrient.

IOM: 100-02, 15, 120; 100-03, 3, 180.2; 100-04, 20, 100.2.2

PEN: On Fee Schedule

B4150 Enteral formulae, nutritionally complete with intact nutrients, includes proteins, fats, carbohydrates, vitamins, and minerals, may include fiber, administered through an enteral feeding tube, 100 calories = 1 unit Qh Y

IOM: 100-02, 15, 120; 100-03, 3, 180.2; 100-04, 20, 100.2.2

PEN: On Fee Schedule

B4152 Enteral formula, nutritionally complete, calorically dense (equal to or greater than 1.5 kcal/ml) with intact nutrients, includes proteins, fats, carbohydrates, vitamins and minerals, may include fiber, administered through an enteral feeding tube, 100 calories = 1 unit Qh Y

IOM: 100-02, 15, 120; 100-03, 3, 180.2; 100-04, 20, 100.2.2

PEN: On Fee Schedule

B4153 Enteral formula, nutritionally complete, hydrolyzed proteins (amino acids and peptide chain), includes fats, carbohydrates, vitamins and minerals, may include fiber, administered through an enteral feeding tube, 100 calories = 1 unit Qp Qh Y

If 2 enteral nutrition products described by same HCPCS code and provided at same time billed on single claim line with units of service reflecting total calories of both nutrients

IOM: 100-02, 15, 120; 100-03, 3, 180.2; 100-04, 20, 100.2.2

PEN: On Fee Schedule

B4154 Enteral formula, nutritionally complete, for special metabolic needs, excludes inherited disease of metabolism, includes altered composition of proteins, fats, carbohydrates, vitamins and/or minerals, may include fiber, administered through an enteral feeding tube, 100 calories = 1 unit Qh Y

IOM: 100-02, 15, 120; 100-03, 3, 180.2; 100-04, 20, 100.2.2

PEN: On Fee Schedule

B4155 Enteral formula, nutritionally incomplete/modular nutrients, includes specific nutrients, carbohydrates (e.g., glucose polymers), proteins/amino acids (e.g., glutamine, arginine), fat (e.g., medium chain triglycerides) or combination, administered through an enteral feeding tube, 100 calories = 1 unit Qh Y

IOM: 100-02, 15, 120; 100-03, 3, 180.2; 100-04, 20, 100.2.2

PEN: On Fee Schedule

B4157 Enteral formula, nutritionally complete, for special metabolic needs for inherited disease of metabolism, includes proteins, fats, carbohydrates, vitamins and minerals, may include fiber, administered through an enteral feeding tube, 100 calories = 1 unit Qp Qh Y

IOM: 100-03, 3, 180.2

B4158 Enteral formula, for pediatrics, nutritionally complete with intact nutrients, includes proteins, fats, carbohydrates, vitamins and minerals, may include fiber and/or iron, administered through an enteral feeding tube, 100 calories = 1 unit Qh A Y

IOM: 100-03, 3, 180.2

B4159 Enteral formula, for pediatrics, nutritionally complete soy based with intact nutrients, includes proteins, fats, carbohydrates, vitamins and minerals, may include fiber and/or iron, administered through an enteral feeding tube, 100 calories = 1 unit Qh A Y

IOM: 100-03, 3, 180.2

B4160 Enteral formula, for pediatrics, nutritionally complete calorically dense (equal to or greater than 0.7 kcal/ml) with intact nutrients, includes proteins, fats, carbohydrates, vitamins and minerals, may include fiber, administered through an enteral feeding tube, 100 calories = 1 unit Qp Qh A Y

IOM: 100-03, 3, 180.2

B4161 Enteral formula, for pediatrics, hydrolyzed/amino acids and peptide chain proteins, includes fats, carbohydrates, vitamins and minerals, may include fiber, administered through an enteral feeding tube, 100 calories = 1 unit Qh A Y

IOM: 100-03, 3, 180.2

B4162 Enteral formula, for pediatrics, special metabolic needs for inherited disease of metabolism, includes proteins, fats, carbohydrates, vitamins and minerals, may include fiber, administered through an enteral feeding tube, 100 calories = 1 unit Qh A Y

IOM: 100-03, 3, 180.2

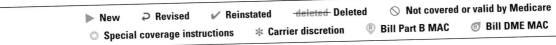

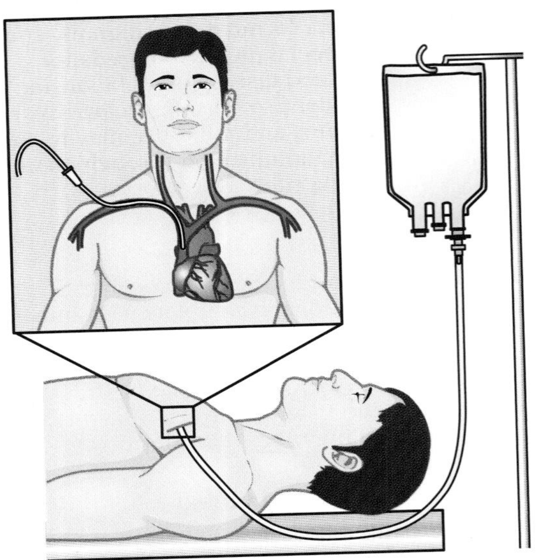

Figure 8 Total Parenteral Nutrition (TPN) involves percutaneous placement of central venous catheter into vena cava or right atrium.

Parenteral Nutritional Solutions and Supplies

B4164 Parenteral nutrition solution: carbohydrates (dextrose), 50% or less (500 ml = 1 unit) - home mix Qp Qh Y

IOM: 100-02, 15, 120; 100-03, 3, 180.2; 100-04, 20, 100.2.2

PEN: On Fee Schedule

B4168 Parenteral nutrition solution; amino acid, 3.5%, (500 ml = 1 unit) - home mix Qp Qh Y

IOM: 100-02, 15, 120; 100-03, 3, 180.2; 100-04, 20, 100.2.2

PEN: On Fee Schedule

B4172 Parenteral nutrition solution; amino acid, 5.5% through 7%, (500 ml = 1 unit) - home mix Qp Qh Y

IOM: 100-02, 15, 120; 100-03, 3, 180.2; 100-04, 20, 100.2.2

B4176 Parenteral nutrition solution; amino acid, 7% through 8.5%, (500 ml = 1 unit) - home mix Qp Qh Y

IOM: 100-02, 15, 120; 100-03, 3, 180.2; 100-04, 20, 100.2.2

PEN: On Fee Schedule

B4178 Parenteral nutrition solution: amino acid, greater than 8.5% (500 ml = 1 unit) - home mix Qp Qh Y

IOM: 100-02, 15, 120; 100-03, 3, 180.2; 100-04, 20, 100.2.2

PEN: On Fee Schedule

B4180 Parenteral nutrition solution; carbohydrates (dextrose), greater than 50% (500 ml = 1 unit) - home mix Qp Qh Y

IOM: 100-02, 15, 120; 100-03, 3, 180.2; 100-04, 20, 100.2.2

PEN: On Fee Schedule

B4185 Parenteral nutrition solution, not otherwise specified, 10 grams lipids B

PEN: On Fee Schedule

B4187 Omegaven, 10 grams lipids Y

B4189 Parenteral nutrition solution; compounded amino acid and carbohydrates with electrolytes, trace elements, and vitamins, including preparation, any strength, 10 to 51 grams of protein - premix Qp Qh Y

IOM: 100-02, 15, 120; 100-03, 3, 180.2; 100-04, 20, 100.2.2

PEN: On Fee Schedule

B4193 Parenteral nutrition solution; compounded amino acid and carbohydrates with electrolytes, trace elements, and vitamins, including preparation, any strength, 52 to 73 grams of protein - premix Qh Y

IOM: 100-02, 15, 120; 100-03, 3, 180.2; 100-04, 20, 100.2.2

PEN: On Fee Schedule

B4197 Parenteral nutrition solution; compounded amino acid and carbohydrates with electrolytes, trace elements and vitamins, including preparation, any strength, 74 to 100 grams of protein - premix Qh Y

IOM: 100-02, 15, 120; 100-03, 3, 180.2; 100-04, 20, 100.2.2

PEN: On Fee Schedule

B4199 Parenteral nutrition solution; compounded amino acid and carbohydrates with electrolytes, trace elements and vitamins, including preparation, any strength, over 100 grams of protein - premix Qp Qh Y

IOM: 100-02, 15, 120; 100-03, 3, 180.2; 100-04, 20, 100.2.2

PEN: On Fee Schedule

B4216 Parenteral nutrition; additives (vitamins, trace elements, heparin, electrolytes) home mix per day Ⓑ Qh Y

IOM: 100-02, 15, 120; 100-03, 3, 180.2; 100-04, 20, 100.2.2

PEN: On Fee Schedule

B4220 Parenteral nutrition supply kit; premix, per day Ⓑ Qh Y

IOM: 100-02, 15, 120; 100-03, 3, 180.2; 100-04, 20, 100.2.2

PEN: On Fee Schedule

B4222 Parenteral nutrition supply kit; home mix, per day Ⓑ Qh Y

IOM: 100-02, 15, 120; 100-03, 3, 180.2; 100-04, 20, 100.2.2

PEN: On Fee Schedule

B4224 Parenteral nutrition administration kit, per day Ⓑ Qh Y

Dressings used with parenteral nutrition (covered under the prosthetic device benefit) are included in the payment. (www.cms.gov/medicare-coverage-database/)

IOM: 100-02, 15, 120; 100-03, 3, 180.2; 100-04, 20, 100.2.2

PEN: On Fee Schedule

B5000 Parenteral nutrition solution compounded amino acid and carbohydrates with electrolytes, trace elements, and vitamins, including preparation, any strength, renal - Aminosyn-RF, NephrAmine, RenAmine - premix Ⓑ Qp Qh Y

IOM: 100-02, 15, 120; 100-03, 3, 180.2; 100-04, 20, 100.2.2

PEN: On Fee Schedule

B5100 Parenteral nutrition solution compounded amino acid and carbohydrates with electrolytes, trace elements, and vitamins, including preparation, any strength, hepatic, HepatAmine - premix Ⓑ Qp Qh Y

IOM: 100-02, 15, 120; 100-03, 3, 180.2; 100-04, 20, 100.2.2

PEN: On Fee Schedule

B5200 Parenteral nutrition solution compounded amino acid and carbohydrates with electrolytes, trace elements, and vitamins, including preparation, any strength, stress-branch chain amino acids-FreAmine-HBC - premix Ⓑ Qp Qh Y

IOM: 100-02, 15, 120; 100-03, 3, 180.2; 100-04, 20, 100.2.2

Enteral and Parenteral Pumps

B9002 Enteral nutrition infusion pump, any type Ⓑ Qh Y

IOM: 100-02, 15, 120; 100-03, 3, 180.2; 100-04, 20, 100.2.2

PEN: On Fee Schedule

B9004 Parenteral nutrition infusion pump, portable Ⓑ Qh Y

IOM: 100-02, 15, 120; 100-03, 3, 180.2; 100-04, 20, 100.2.2

PEN: On Fee Schedule

B9006 Parenteral nutrition infusion pump, stationary Ⓑ Qh Y

IOM: 100-02, 15, 120; 100-03, 3, 180.2; 100-04, 20, 100.2.2

PEN: On Fee Schedule

B9998 NOC for enteral supplies Ⓑ Y

IOM: 100-02, 15, 120; 100-03, 3, 180.2; 100-04, 20, 100.2.2

B9999 NOC for parenteral supplies Ⓑ Y

Determine if an alternative HCPCS Level II or a CPT code better describes the service being reported. This code should be reported only if a more specific code is unavailable.

IOM: 100-02, 15, 120; 100-03, 3, 180.2; 100-04, 20, 100.2.2

CMS HOSPITAL OUTPATIENT PAYMENT SYSTEM (C1000-C9999)

Note: C-codes are used on Medicare Ambulatory Surgical Center (ASC) and Hospital Outpatient Prospective Payment System (OPPS) claims, but may also be recognized on claims from other providers or by other payment systems. As of 10/01/2006, the following non-OPPS providers have been able to bill Medicare using the C-codes, or an appropriate CPT code on Types of Bill (TOBs) 12X, 13X, or 85X:

- Critical Access Hospitals (CAHs);
- Indian Health Service Hospitals (IHS);
- Hospitals located in American Samoa, Guam, Saipan or the Virgin Islands; and
- Maryland waiver hospitals.

The billing of C-codes by Method I and Method II Critical Access Hospitals (CAHs) is limited to the billing for facility (technical) services. The C-codes shall not be billed by Method II CAHs for professional services with revenue codes (RCs) 96X, 97X, or 98X.

C codes are updated quarterly by the Centers for Medicare and Medicaid Services (CMS).

Devices and Supplies

▶ **C1052** Hemostatic agent, gastrointestinal, topical J7 H

▶ **C1062** Intravertebral body fracture augmentation with implant (e.g., metal, polymer) J7 H

C1713 Anchor/Screw for opposing bone-to-bone or soft tissue-to-bone (implantable) Qh N1 N

Medicare Statute 1833(t)

Coding Clinic: 2020, Q4, P7-8; 2018, Q2, P5; Q1, P4; 2016, Q3, P16; 2015, Q3, P2; 2010, Q2, P3

C1714 Catheter, transluminal atherectomy, directional Qh N1 N

Medicare Statute 1833(t)

C1715 Brachytherapy needle Qh N1 N

Medicare Statute 1833(t)

Brachytherapy Sources

C1716 Brachytherapy source, non-stranded, gold-198, per source Qp Qh H2 U

Medicare Statute 1833(t)

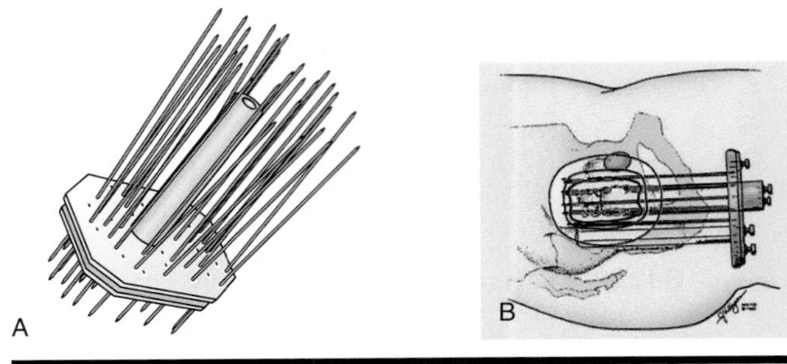
A
B

Figure 9 (A) Brachytherapy device, (B) Brachytherapy device inserted.

C1717 Brachytherapy source, non-stranded, high dose rate iridium 192, per source Qp Qh H2 U

Medicare Statute 1833(t)

C1719 Brachytherapy source, non-stranded, non-high dose rate iridium-192, per source Qp Qh H2 U

Medicare Statute 1833(t)

Cardioverter-Defibrilators

C1721 Cardioverter-defibrillator, dual chamber (implantable) Qp Qh N1 N

Related CPT codes: 33224, 33240, 33249.

Medicare Statute 1833(t)

C1722 Cardioverter-defibrillator, single chamber (implantable) Qp Qh N1 N

Related CPT codes: 33240, 33249.

Medicare Statute 1833(t)

Coding Clinic: 2017, Q2, P5; 2006, Q2, P9

Catheters

C1724 Catheter, transluminal atherectomy, rotational Qh N1 N

Medicare Statute 1833(t)

Coding Clinic: 2016, Q3, P9

C1725 Catheter, transluminal angioplasty, non-laser (may include guidance, infusion/perfusion capability) Qh N1 N

Medicare Statute 1833(t)

Coding Clinic: 2016, Q3, P16, P19

C1726 Catheter, balloon dilatation, non-vascular Qh N1 N

Medicare Statute 1833(t)

Coding Clinic: 2016, Q3, P16, P19

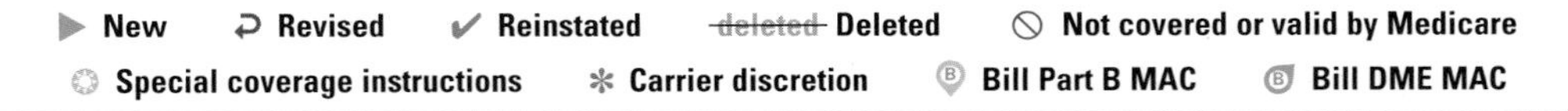
▶ New ↩ Revised ✔ Reinstated ~~deleted~~ Deleted ⊘ Not covered or valid by Medicare
Special coverage instructions ✱ Carrier discretion Bill Part B MAC Bill DME MAC

C1727 Catheter, balloon tissue dissector, non-vascular (insertable) Qh N1 N
Medicare Statute 1833(t)
Coding Clinic: 2016, Q3, P16

C1728 Catheter, brachytherapy seed administration Qh N1 N
Medicare Statute 1833(t)

C1729 Catheter, drainage Qh N1 N
Medicare Statute 1833(t)
Coding Clinic: 2016, Q3, P17

C1730 Catheter, electrophysiology, diagnostic, other than 3D mapping (19 or fewer electrodes) Qp Qh N1 N
Medicare Statute 1833(t)
Coding Clinic: 2016, Q3, P17

C1731 Catheter, electrophysiology, diagnostic, other than 3D mapping (20 or more electrodes) Qp Qh N1 N
Medicare Statute 1833(t)
Coding Clinic: 2016, Q3, P17

C1732 Catheter, electrophysiology, diagnostic/ablation, 3D or vector mapping Qp Qh N1 N
Medicare Statute 1833(t)
Coding Clinic: 2016, Q3, P15, P17, P19

C1733 Catheter, electrophysiology, diagnostic/ablation, other than 3D or vector mapping, other than cool-tip Qp Qh N1 N
Medicare Statute 1833(t)
Coding Clinic: 2016, Q3, P17

C1734 Orthopedic/device/drug matrix for opposing bone-to-bone or soft tissue-to-bone (implantable) N1

▶ **C1748** Endoscope, single-use (i.e. disposable), upper gi, imaging/illumination device (insertable) J7 H

C1749 Endoscope, retrograde imaging/illumination colonoscope device (implantable) Qp Qh N1 N
Medicare Statute 1833(t)

C1750 Catheter, hemodialysis/peritoneal, long-term Qh N1 N
Medicare Statute 1833(t)
Coding Clinic: 2015, Q4, P6

C1751 Catheter, infusion, inserted peripherally, centrally, or midline (other than hemodialysis) Qh N1 N
Medicare Statute 1833(t)

C1752 Catheter, hemodialysis/peritoneal, short-term Qh N1 N
Medicare Statute 1833(t)

C1753 Catheter, intravascular ultrasound Qh N1 N
Medicare Statute 1833(t)

C1754 Catheter, intradiscal Qh N1 N
Medicare Statute 1833(t)

C1755 Catheter, instraspinal Qh N1 N
Medicare Statute 1833(t)

C1756 Catheter, pacing, transesophageal Qh N1 N
Medicare Statute 1833(t)

C1757 Catheter, thrombectomy/embolectomy Qh N1 N
Medicare Statute 1833(t)

C1758 Catheter, ureteral Qh N1 N
Medicare Statute 1833(t)

C1759 Catheter, intracardiac echocardiography Qh N1 N
Medicare Statute 1833(t)

Devices

C1760 Closure device, vascular (implantable/insertable) Qh N1 N
Medicare Statute 1833(t)
Coding Clinic: 2016, Q3, P19

C1762 Connective tissue, human (includes fascia lata) Qh N1 N
Medicare Statute 1833(t)
Coding Clinic: 2016, Q3, P9, P16, P19; 2015, Q3, P2; 2003, Q3, P12

C1763 Connective tissue, non-human (includes synthetic) Qh N1 N
Medicare Statute 1833(t)
Coding Clinic: 2016, Q3, P9, P17, P19; 2010, Q4, P3; Q2, P3; 2003, Q3, P12

C1764 Event recorder, cardiac (implantable) Qp Qh N1 N
Medicare Statute 1833(t)
Coding Clinic: 2015, Q2, P8

C1765 Adhesion barrier Qh N1 N
Medicare Statute 1833(t)
Coding Clinic: 2016, Q3, P16

C1766 Introducer/sheath, guiding, intracardiac electrophysiological, steerable, other than peel-away Qh N1 N
Medicare Statute 1833(t)

C1767 Generator, neurostimulator (implantable), nonrechargeable Qp Qh N1 N

Related CPT codes: 61885, 61886, 63685, 64590.

Medicare Statute 1833(t)

Coding Clinic: 2007, Q1, P8

C1768 Graft, vascular Qh N1 N

Medicare Statute 1833(t)

C1769 Guide wire Qh N1 N

Medicare Statute 1833(t)

Coding Clinic: 2019, Q3, P10; 2016, Q3, P3; 2007, Q2, P7-8

C1770 Imaging coil, magnetic reasonance (insertable) Qh N1 N

Medicare Statute 1833(t)

C1771 Repair device, urinary, incontinence, with sling graft Qp Qh N1 N

Medicare Statute 1833(t)

Coding Clinic: 2016, Q3, P19; 2008, Q3, P7

C1772 Infusion pump, programmable (implantable) Qp Qh N1 N

Medicare Statute 1833(t)

C1773 Retrieval device, insertable (used to retrieve fractured medical devices) Qh N1 N

Medicare Statute 1833(t)

Coding Clinic: 2016, Q3, P19

C1776 Joint device (implantable) Qp Qh N1 N

Medicare Statute 1833(t)

Coding Clinic: 2020, Q1, P16; 2018, Q3, P6; 2016, Q3, P3, P18; 2010, Q3, P6; 2008, Q4, P10

C1777 Lead, cardioverter-defibrillator, endocardial single coil (implantable) Qh N1 N

Related CPT codes: 33216, 33217, 33249.

Medicare Statute 1833(t)

Coding Clinic: 2017, Q2, P5; 2006, Q2, P9

C1778 Lead, neurostimulator (implantable) Qp Qh N1 N

Related CPT codes: 43647, 63650, 63655, 63663, 63664, 64553, 64555, 64560, 64561, 64565, 64573, 64575, 64577, 64580, 64581.

Medicare Statute 1833(t)

Coding Clinic: 2019, Q1, P5; 2007, Q1, P8

C1779 Lead, pacemaker, trasvenous VDD single pass Qh N1 N

Related CPT codes: 33206, 33207, 33208, 33210, 33211, 33214, 33216, 33217, 33249.

Medicare Statute 1833(t)

Coding Clinic: 2016, Q3, P19

C1780 Lens, intraocular (new technology) Qh N1 N

Medicare Statute 1833(t)

Coding Clinic: 2016, Q3, P18

C1781 Mesh (implantable) Qh N1 N

Medicare Statute 1833(t)

Coding Clinic: 2019, Q1, P5; 2016, Q3, P18-19; 2012, Q2, P3; 2010, Q2, P2-3

C1782 Morcellator Qp Qh N1 N

Medicare Statute 1833(t)

Coding Clinic: 2016, Q3, P18

C1783 Ocular implant, aqueous drainage assist device Qh N1 N

Medicare Statute 1833(t)

Coding Clinic: 2017, Q1, P5

C1784 Ocular device, intraoperative, detached retina Qh N1 N

Medicare Statute 1833(t)

Coding Clinic: 2016, Q3, P18

C1785 Pacemaker, dual chamber, rate-responsive (implantable) Qp Qh N1 N

Related CPT codes: 33206, 33207, 33208, 33213, 33214, 33224.

Medicare Statute 1833(t)

Pacemaker lead in the right atrium
(+)
Pulse generator
A
Pacemaker leads in the right atrium and right ventricle
(+)
Pulse generator
B
Biventricular pacemaker
= Electrical impulse
(+)
Pulse generator
Leads
C

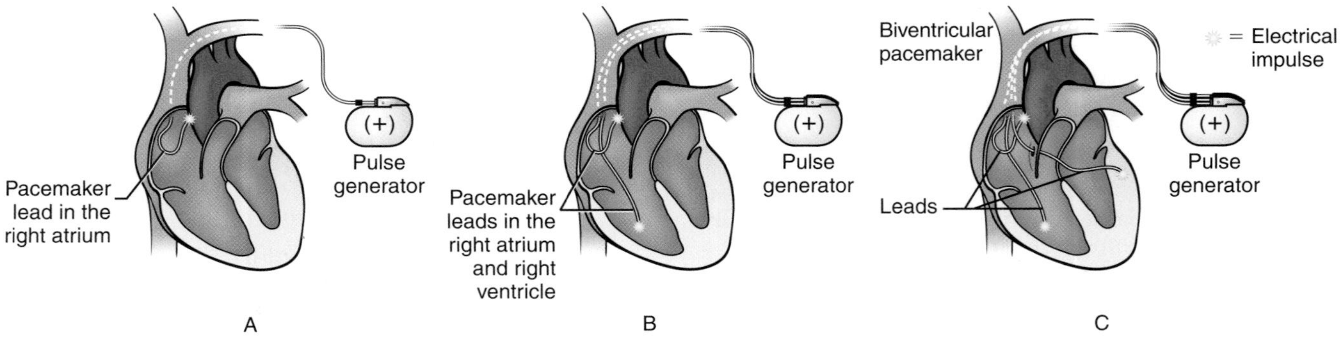

Figure 10 (A) Single pacemaker, (B) Dual pacemaker, (C) Biventricular pacemaker.

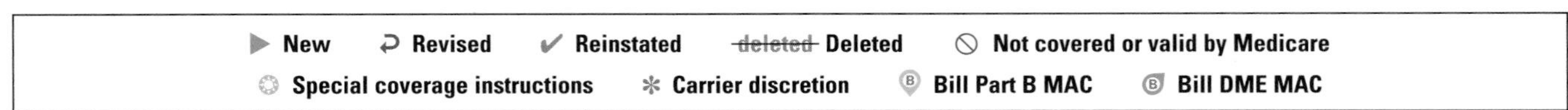
New
Revised
Reinstated
deleted Deleted
Not covered or valid by Medicare
Special coverage instructions
Carrier discretion
Bill Part B MAC
Bill DME MAC

C1786 Pacemaker, single chamber, rate-responsive (implantable) Qp Qh N1 N
Related CPT codes: 33206, 33207, 33212.
Medicare Statute 1833(t)

C1787 Patient programmer, neurostimulator Qh N1 N
Medicare Statute 1833(t)
Coding Clinic: 2016, Q3, P19

C1788 Port, indwelling (implantable) Qh N1 N
Medicare Statute 1833(t)

C1789 Prosthesis, breast (implantable) Qh N1 N
Medicare Statute 1833(t)

C1813 Prosthesis, penile, inflatable Qp Qh ♂ N1 N
Medicare Statute 1833(t)

C1814 Retinal tamponade device, silicone oil Qh N1 N
Medicare Statute 1833(t)
Coding Clinic: 2016, Q3, P19; 2006, Q2, P9

C1815 Prosthesis, urinary sphincter (implantable) Qp Qh N1 N
Medicare Statute 1833(t)

C1816 Receiver and/or transmitter, neurostimulator (implantable) Qh N1 N
Medicare Statute 1833(t)

C1817 Septal defect implant system, intracardiac Qp Qh N1 N
Medicare Statute 1833(t)
Coding Clinic: 2016, Q3, P19

C1818 Integrated keratoprosthesic Qh N1 N
Medicare Statute 1833(t)
Coding Clinic: 2016, Q3, P18

C1819 Surgical tissue localization and excision device (implantable) Qh N1 N
Medicare Statute 1833(t)

C1820 Generator, neurostimulator (implantable), with rechargeable battery and charging system Qp Qh N1 N
Related CPT codes: 61885, 61886, 63685, 64590.
Medicare Statute 1833(t)
Coding Clinic: 2016, Q2, P7

C1821 Interspinous process distraction device (implantable) Qh N1 N
Medicare Statute 1833(t)

C1822 Generator, neurostimulator (implantable), high frequency, with rechargeable battery and charging system Qp Qh N1 N
Medicare Statute 1833(T)
Coding Clinic: 2016, Q2, P7

C1823 Generator, neurostimulator (implantable), non-rechargeable, with transvenous sensing and stimulation leads H
Medicare Statute 1833(t)

C1824 Generator, cardiac contractility modulation (implantable) N1

▶ **C1825** Generator, neurostimulator (implantable), non-rechargeable with carotid sinus baroreceptor stimulation lead(s) J7 H

C1830 Powered bone marrow biopsy needle Qp Qh N1 N
Medicare Statute 1833(t)

C1839 Iris prosthesis N1

C1840 Lens, intraocular (telescopic) Qp Qh N1 N
Medicare Statute 1833(t)
Coding Clinic: 2012, Q3, P10

C1841 Retinal prosthesis, includes all internal and external components Qp Qh J7 N
Medicare Statute 1833(t)

C1842 Retinal prosthesis, includes all internal and external components; add-on to C1841 Qp Qh J7 E1
Medicare Statute 1833(t)
Coding Clinic: 2017, Q1, P6

▶ **C1849** Skin substitute, synthetic, resorbable, per square centimeter N1 N

C1874 Stent, coated/covered, with delivery system Qh N1 N
Medicare Statute 1833(t)
Coding Clinic: 2016, Q3, P16-17, P19

C1875 Stent, coated/covered, without delivery system Qh N1 N
Medicare Statute 1833(t)
Coding Clinic: 2020, Q2, P9; 2016, Q3, P16-17

C1876 Stent, non-coated/non-covered, with delivery system Qh N1 N
Medicare Statute 1833(t)
Coding Clinic: 2016, Q3, P19

C1877 Stent, non-coated/non-covered, without delivery system Qh N1 N
Medicare Statute 1833(t)

C1878 Material for vocal cord medialization, synthetic (implantable) Qh N1 N
Medicare Statute 1833(t)
Coding Clinic: 2016, Q3, P18

C1880 Vena cava filter Qh N1 N
Medicare Statute 1833(t)

C1881 Dialysis access system (implantable) Qh N1 N
Medicare Statute 1833(t)

C1882 Cardioverter-defibrillator, other than single or dual chamber (implantable) Qp Qh N1 N
Related CPT codes: 33224, 33240, 33249.
Medicare Statute 1833(t)
Coding Clinic: 2016, Q3, P16; 2012, Q2, P9; 2006, Q2, P9

C1883 Adapter/Extension, pacing lead or neurostimulator lead (implantable) Qh N1 N
Medicare Statute 1833(t)
Coding Clinic: 2016, Q3, P15, P17; 2007, Q1, P8

C1884 Embolization protective system Qh N1 N
Medicare Statute 1833(t)
Coding Clinic: 2016, Q3, P17

C1885 Catheter, transluminal angioplasty, laser Qh N1 N
Medicare Statute 1833(t)
Coding Clinic: 2016, Q3, p16, Q1, P5

C1886 Catheter, extravascular tissue ablation, any modality (insertable) Qp Qh N1 N
Medicare Statute 1833(t)

C1887 Catheter, guiding (may include infusion/perfusion capability) Qh N1 N
Medicare Statute 1833(t)
Coding Clinic: 2016, Q3, P17

C1888 Catheter, ablation, non-cardiac, endovascular (implantable) Qh N1 N
Medicare Statute 1833(t)
Coding Clinic: 2016, Q3, P16

C1889 Implantable/insertable device, not otherwise classified N1 N
Medicare Statute 1833(T)

C1891 Infusion pump, non-programmable, permanent (implantable) Qp Qh N1 N
Medicare Statute 1833(t)

C1892 Introducer/sheath, guiding, intracardiac electrophysiological, fixed-curve, peel-away Qh N1 N
Medicare Statute 1833(t)
Coding Clinic: 2016, Q3, P19

C1893 Introducer/sheath, guiding, intracardiac electrophysiological, fixed-curve, other than peel-away Qh N1 N
Medicare Statute 1833(t)

C1894 Introducer/sheath, other than guiding, other than intracardiac electrophysiological, non-laser Qh N1 N
Medicare Statute 1833(t)

C1895 Lead, cardioverter-defibrillator, endocardial dual coil (implantable) Qh N1 N
Related CPT codes: 33216, 33217, 33249.
Medicare Statute 1833(t)
Coding Clinic: 2006, Q2, P9

C1896 Lead, cardioverter-defibrillator, other than endocardial single or dual coil (implantable) Qh N1 N
Related CPT codes: 33216, 33217, 33249.
Medicare Statute 1833(t)

C1897 Lead, neurostimulator test kit (implantable) Qh N1 N
Related CPT codes: 43647, 63650, 63655, 63663, 63664, 64553, 64555, 64560, 64561, 64565, 64575, 64577, 64580, 64581.
Medicare Statute 1833(t)
Coding Clinic: 2007, Q1, P8

C1898 Lead, pacemaker, other than transvenous VDD single pass Qh N1 N
Related CPT codes: 33206, 33207, 33208, 33210, 33211, 33214, 33216, 33217, 33249.
Medicare Statute 1833(t)
Coding Clinic: 2002, Q3, P8

C1899 Lead, pacemaker/cardioverter-defibrillator combination (implantable) Qh N1 N
Related CPT codes: 33216, 33217, 33249.
Medicare Statute 1833(t)

C1900 Lead, left ventricular coronary venous system Qp Qh N1 N
Related CPT codes: 33224, 33225.
Medicare Statute 1833(t)
Coding Clinic: 2016, Q3, P18

C1982 Catheter, pressure-generating, one-way valve, intermittently occlusive N1

C2596 Probe, image-guided, robotic, waterjet ablation N1 H

C2613 Lung biopsy plug with delivery system Qp Qh N1 H
Medicare Statute 1833(t)
Coding Clinic: 2015, Q2, P11

C2614 Probe, percutaneous lumbar discectomy Qh N1 N
Medicare Statute 1833(t)

C2615 Sealant, pulmonary, liquid Qh N1 N
Medicare Statute 1833(t)
Coding Clinic: 2016, Q3, P18

Brachytherapy Source

C2616 Brachytherapy source, non-stranded, yttrium-90, per source Qp Qh H2 U
Medicare Statute 1833(t)

Cardiovascular and Genitourinary Devices

C2617 Stent, non-coronary, temporary, without delivery system Qh N1 N
Medicare Statute 1833(t)
Coding Clinic: 2018, Q1, P4; 2016, Q3, P3, P19

C2618 Probe/needle, cryoablation Qh N1 N
Medicare Statute 1833(t)

C2619 Pacemaker, dual chamber, non rate-responsive (implantable) Qp Qh N1 N
Related CPT codes: 33206, 33207, 33208, 33213, 33214, 33224.
Medicare Statute 1833(t)

C2620 Pacemaker, single chamber, non rate-responsive (implantable) Qp Qh N1 N
Related CPT codes: 33206, 33207, 33212, 33224.
Medicare Statute 1833(t)

C2621 Pacemaker, other than single or dual chamber (implantable) Qp Qh N1 N
Related CPT codes: 33206, 33207, 33208, 33212, 33213, 33214, 33224.
Medicare Statute 1833(t)
Coding Clinic: 2016, Q3, P18; 2002, Q3, P8

C2622 Prosthesis, penile, non-inflatable Qp Qh ♂ N1 N
Medicare Statute 1833(t)

C2623 Catheter, transluminal angioplasty, drug-coated, non-laser Qp Qh N1 N
Medicare Statute 1833(t)

C2624 Implantable wireless pulmonary artery pressure sensor with delivery catheter, including all system components Qp Qh N1 N
Medicare Statute 1833(t)
Coding Clinic: 2015, Q3, P2

C2625 Stent, non-coronary, temporary, with delivery system Qh N1 N
Medicare Statute 1833(t)
Coding Clinic: 2016, Q3, P19; 2015, Q2, P9

C2626 Infusion pump, non-programmable, temporary (implantable) Qp Qh N1 N
Medicare Statute 1833(t)
Coding Clinic: 2016, Q3, P18

C2627 Catheter, suprapubic/cystoscopic Qh N1 N
Medicare Statute 1833(t)

C2628 Catheter, occlusion Qh N1 N
Medicare Statute 1833(t)

C2629 Introducer/Sheath, other than guiding, other than intracardiac electrophysiological, laser Qh N1 N
Medicare Statute 1833(t)

C2630 Catheter, electrophysiology, diagnostic/ablation, other than 3D or vector mapping, cool-tip Qp Qh N1 N
Medicare Statute 1833(t)
Coding Clinic: 2016, Q3, P17

C2631 Repair device, urinary, incontinence, without sling graft Qp Qh N1 N
Medicare Statute 1833(t)

Brachytherapy Sources

C2634 Brachytherapy source, non-stranded, high activity, iodine-125, greater than 1.01 mci (NIST), per source Qp Qh H2 U
Medicare Statute 1833(t)

C2635 Brachytherapy source, non-stranded, high activity, palladium-103, greater than 2.2 mci (NIST), per source Qp Qh H2 U
Medicare Statute 1833(t)

C2636 Brachytherapy linear source, non-stranded, palladium-103, per 1 mm Qp Qh H2 U

C2637 Brachytherapy source, non-stranded, Ytterbium-169, per source Qp Qh B
Medicare Statute 1833(t)

C2638 Brachytherapy source, stranded, iodine-125, per source Qp Qh H2 U
Medicare Statute 1833(t)(2)

C2639 Brachytherapy source, non-stranded, iodine-125, per source Qp Qh H2 U
Medicare Statute 1833(t)(2)

MIPS | Qp Quantity Physician | Qh Quantity Hospital | ♀ Female only
♂ Male only | A Age | DMEPOS | A2-Z3 ASC Payment Indicator | A-Y ASC Status Indicator | Coding Clinic

C2640 Brachytherapy source, stranded, palladium-103, per source Qp Qh H2 U

Medicare Statute 1833(t)(2)

C2641 Brachytherapy source, non-stranded, palladium-103, per source Qp Qh H2 U

Medicare Statute 1833(t)(2)

C2642 Brachytherapy source, stranded, cesium-131, per source Qp Qh H2 U

Medicare Statute 1833(t)(2)

C2643 Brachytherapy source, non-stranded, cesium-131, per source Qp Qh H2 U

Medicare Statute 1833(t)(2)

C2644 Brachytherapy source, Cesium-131 chloride solution, per millicurie Qp Qh H2 U

Medicare Statute 1833(t)

C2645 Brachytherapy planar source, palladium-103, per square millimeter Qp Qh H2 U

Medicare Statute 1833(T)

C2698 Brachytherapy source, stranded, not otherwise specified, per source H2 U

Medicare Statute 1833(t)(2)

C2699 Brachytherapy source, non-stranded, not otherwise specified, per source H2 U

Medicare Statute 1833(t)(2)

Skin Substitute Graft Application

C5271 Application of low cost skin substitute graft to trunk, arms, legs, total wound surface area up to 100 sq cm; first 25 sq cm or less wound surface area Qp Qh T

Medicare Statute 1833(t)

C5272 Application of low cost skin substitute graft to trunk, arms, legs, total wound surface area up to 100 sq cm; each additional 25 sq cm wound surface area, or part thereof (list separately in addition to code for primary procedure) Qp Qh N

Medicare Statute 1833(t)

C5273 Application of low cost skin substitute graft to trunk, arms, legs, total wound surface area greater than or equal to 100 sq cm; first 100 sq cm wound surface area, or 1% of body area of infants and children Qp Qh A T

Medicare Statute 1833(t)

C5274 Application of low cost skin substitute graft to trunk, arms, legs, total wound surface area greater than or equal to 100 sq cm; each additional 100 sq cm wound surface area, or part thereof, or each additional 1% of body area of infants and children, or part thereof (list separately in addition to code for primary procedure) Qp Qh A N

Medicare Statute 1833(t)

C5275 Application of low cost skin substitute graft to face, scalp, eyelids, mouth, neck, ears, orbits, genitalia, hands, feet, and/or multiple digits, total wound surface area up to 100 sq cm; first 25 sq cm or less wound surface area Qp Qh T

Medicare Statute 1833(t)

C5276 Application of low cost skin substitute graft to face, scalp, eyelids, mouth, neck, ears, orbits, genitalia, hands, feet, and/or multiple digits, total wound surface area up to 100 sq cm; each additional 25 sq cm wound surface area, or part thereof (list separately in addition to code for primary procedure) Qp Qh N

Medicare Statute 1833(t)

C5277 Application of low cost skin substitute graft to face, scalp, eyelids, mouth, neck, ears, orbits, genitalia, hands, feet, and/or multiple digits, total wound surface area greater than or equal to 100 sq cm; first 100 sq cm wound surface area, or 1% of body area of infants and children Qp Qh A T

Medicare Statute 1833(t)

C5278 Application of low cost skin substitute graft to face, scalp, eyelids, mouth, neck, ears, orbits, genitalia, hands, feet, and/or multiple digits, total wound surface area greater than or equal to 100 sq cm; each additional 100 sq cm wound surface area, or part thereof, or each additional 1% of body area of infants and children, or part thereof (list separately in addition to code for primary procedure) Qp Qh A N

Medicare Statute 1833(t)

Magnetic Resonance Angiography: Trunk and Lower Extremities

C8900 Magnetic resonance angiography with contrast, abdomen Qp Qh Z2 Q3

Medicare Statute 1833(t)(2)

C8901 Magnetic resonance angiography without contrast, abdomen Qp Qh Z2 Q3

Medicare Statute 1833(t)(2)

C8902 Magnetic resonance angiography without contrast followed by with contrast, abdomen Qp Qh Z2 Q3

Medicare Statute 1833(t)(2)

C8903 Magnetic resonance imaging with contrast, breast; unilateral Qp Qh Z2 Q3

Medicare Statute 1833(t)(2)

C8905 Magnetic resonance imaging without contrast followed by with contrast, breast; unilateral Qp Qh Z2 Q3

Medicare Statute 1833(t)(2)

C8906 Magnetic resonance imaging with contrast, breast; bilateral Qp Qh Z2 Q3

Medicare Statute 1833(t)(2)

C8908 Magnetic resonance imaging without contrast followed by with contrast, breast; bilateral Qp Qh Z2 Q3

Medicare Statute 1833(t)(2)

C8909 Magnetic resonance angiography with contrast, chest (excluding myocardium) Qp Qh Z2 Q3

Medicare Statute 1833(t)(2)

C8910 Magnetic resonance angiography without contrast, chest (excluding myocardium) Qp Qh Z2 Q3

Medicare Statute 1833(t)(2)

C8911 Magnetic resonance angiography without contrast followed by with contrast, chest (excluding myocardium) Qp Qh Z2 Q3

Medicare Statute 1833(t)(2)

C8912 Magnetic resonance angiography with contrast, lower extremity Qp Qh Z2 Q3

Medicare Statute 1833(t)(2)

C8913 Magnetic resonance angiography without contrast, lower extremity Qp Qh Z2 Q3

Medicare Statute 1833(t)(2)

C8914 Magnetic resonance angiography without contrast followed by with contrast, lower extremity Qp Qh Z2 Q3

Medicare Statute 1833(t)(2)

C8918 Magnetic resonance angiography with contrast, pelvis Qp Qh Z2 Q3

Medicare Statute 1833(t)(2)

C8919 Magnetic resonance angiography without contrast, pelvis Qp Qh Z2 Q3

Medicare Statute 1833(t)(2)

C8920 Magnetic resonance angiography without contrast followed by with contrast, pelvis Qp Qh Z2 Q3

Medicare Statute 1833(t)(2)

Transthoracic and Transesophageal Echocardiography

C8921 Transthoracic echocardiography with contrast, or without contrast followed by with contrast, for congenital cardiac anomalies; complete Qp Qh S

Medicare Statute 1833(t)(2)

Coding Clinic: 2012, Q3, P8

C8922 Transthoracic echocardiography with contrast, or without contrast followed by with contrast, for congenital cardiac anomalies; follow-up or limited study Qp Qh S

Medicare Statute 1833(t)(2)

Coding Clinic: 2012, Q3, P8

C8923 Transthoracic echocardiography with contrast, or without contrast followed by with contrast, real-time with image documentation (2D), includes M-mode recording, when performed, complete, without spectral or color Doppler echocardiography Qp Qh S

Medicare Statute 1833(t)(2)

Coding Clinic: 2012, Q3, P8

C8924 Transthoracic echocardiography with contrast, or without contrast followed by with contrast, real-time with image documentation (2D), includes M-mode recording, when performed, follow-up or limited study Qp Qh S

Medicare Statute 1833(t)(2)

Coding Clinic: 2012, Q3, P8

C8925 Transesophageal echocardiography (TEE) with contrast, or without contrast followed by with contrast, real time with image documentation (2D) (with or without M-mode recording); including probe placement, image acquisition, interpretation and report Qp Qh S

Medicare Statute 1833(t)(2)

Coding Clinic: 2012, Q3, P8

C8926 Transesophageal echocardiography (TEE) with contrast, or without contrast followed by with contrast, for congenital cardiac anomalies; including probe placement, image acquisition, interpretation and report Qp Qh S

Medicare Statute 1833(t)(2)

Coding Clinic: 2012, Q3, P8

C8927 Transesophageal echocardiography (TEE) with contrast, or without contrast followed by with contrast, for monitoring purposes, including probe placement, real time 2-dimensional image acquisition and interpretation leading to ongoing (continuous) assessment of (dynamically changing) cardiac pumping function and to therapeutic measures on an immediate time basis Qp Qh S

Medicare Statute 1833(t)(2)

Coding Clinic: 2012, Q3, P8

C8928 Transthoracic echocardiography with contrast, or without contrast followed by with contrast, real-time with image documentation (2D), includes M-mode recording, when performed, during rest and cardiovascular stress test using treadmill, bicycle exercise and/or pharmacologically induced stress, with interpretation and report Qp Qh S

Medicare Statute 1833(t)(2)

Coding Clinic: 2012, Q3, P8

C8929 Transthoracic echocardiography with contrast, or without contrast followed by with contrast, real-time with image documentation (2D), includes M-mode recording, when performed, complete, with spectral Doppler echocardiography, and with color flow Doppler echocardiography Qp Qh S

Medicare Statute 1833(t)(2)

Coding Clinic: 2012, Q3, P8

C8930 Transthoracic echocardiography, with contrast, or without contrast followed by with contrast, real-time with image documentation (2D), includes M-mode recording, when performed, during rest and cardiovascular stress test using treadmill, bicycle exercise and/or pharmacologically induced stress, with interpretation and report; including performance of continuous electrocardiographic monitoring, with physician supervision Qp Qh S

Medicare Statute 1833(t)(2)

Coding Clinic: 2012, Q3, P8

Magnetic Resonance Angiography: Spine and Upper Extremities

C8931 Magnetic resonance angiography with contrast, spinal canal and contents Qp Qh Z2 Q3

Medicare Statute 1833(t)

C8932 Magnetic resonance angiography without contrast, spinal canal and contents Qp Qh Z2 Q3

Medicare Statute 1833(t)

C8933 Magnetic resonance angiography without contrast followed by with contrast, spinal canal and contents Qp Qh Z2 Q3

Medicare Statute 1833(t)

C8934 Magnetic resonance angiography with contrast, upper extremity Qh Z2 Q3

Medicare Statute 1833(t)

C8935 Magnetic resonance angiography without contrast, upper extremity Qh Z2 Q3

Medicare Statute 1833(t)

C8936 Magnetic resonance angiography without contrast followed by with contrast, upper extremity Qh Z2 Q3

Medicare Statute 1833(t)

C8937 Computer-aided detection, including computer algorithm analysis of breast MRI image data for lesion detection/characterization, pharmacokinetic analysis, with further physician review for interpretation (list separately in addition to code for primary procedure) N

Medicare Statute 1833(t)

Drugs and Biologicals

C8957 Intravenous infusion for therapy/diagnosis; initiation of prolonged infusion (more than 8 hours), requiring use of portable or implantable pump Qp Qh S

Medicare Statute 1833(t)

Coding Clinic: 2008, Q3, P8

C9034 Injection, dexamethasone 9%, intraocular, 1 mcg G

Medicare Statute 1833(t)

~~C9041 Injection, coagulation factor Xa (recombinant), inactivated (Andexxa), 10 mg~~ ✖

C9046 Cocaine hydrochloride nasal solution for topical administration, 1 mg K2 G

C9047 Injection, caplacizumab-yhdp, 1 mg K2 G

~~C9054 Injection, lefamulin (Xenleta), 1 mg~~ ✖

~~C9055 Injection, brexanolone, 1mg~~ ✖

▶ C9061 Injection, teprotumumab-trbw, 10 mg

▶ C9063 Injection, eptinezumab-jjmr, 1 mg

▶ New ↩ Revised ✔ Reinstated ~~deleted~~ Deleted ⊘ Not covered or valid by Medicare
Special coverage instructions ✻ Carrier discretion Ⓑ Bill Part B MAC Ⓔ Bill DME MAC

▶ **C9065** Injection, romidepsin, non-lypohilized (e.g. liquid), 1 m K2 G

▶ **C9067** Gallium ga-68, dotatoc, diagnostic, 0.01 mci K2 G

▶ **C9068** Copper cu-64, dotatate, diagnostic, 1 millicurie K2 G

▶ **C9069** Injection, belantamab mafodontin-blmf, 0.5 mg K2 G

▶ **C9070** Injection, tafasitamab-cxix, 2 mg K2 G

▶ **C9071** Injection, viltolarsen, 10 mg K2 G

▶ **C9072** Injection, immune globulin (ASCENIV), 500 mg K2 G

▶ **C9073** Brexucabtagene autoleucel, up to 200 million autologous anti-cd19 car positive viable T cells, including leukapheresis and dose preparation procedures, per therapeutic dose K2 G

C9113 Injection, pantoprazole sodium, per vial Qp Qh N1 N

Medicare Statute 1833(t)

▶ **C9122** Mometasone furoate sinus implant, 10 micrograms (sinuva) K2 G

C9132 Prothrombin complex concentrate (human), Kcentra, per i.u. of Factor IX activity Qp Qh K2 K

Medicare Statute 1833(t)

C9248 Injection, clevidipine butyrate, 1 mg Qp Qh N1 N

Medicare Statute 1833(t)

C9250 Human plasma fibrin sealant, vapor-heated, solvent-detergent (ARTISS), 2 ml Qp Qh K2 K

Example of diagnosis codes to be reported with C9250: T20.00-T25.799.

Medicare Statute 621MMA

C9254 Injection, lacosamide, 1 mg Qp Qh N1 N

Medicare Statute 621MMA

C9257 injection, bevacizumab, 0.25 mg Qp Qh K2 K

Medicare Statute 1833(t)

C9285 Lidocaine 70 mg/tetracaine 70 mg, per patch Qp Qh N1 N

Medicare Statute 1833(t)

Coding Clinic: 2011, Q3, P9

C9290 Injection, bupivacine liposome, 1 mg Qp Qh N1 N

Medicare Statute 1833(t)

C9293 Injection, glucarpidase, 10 units Qp Qh K2 K

Medicare Statute 1833(t)

C9352 Microporous collagen implantable tube (NeuraGen Nerve Guide), per centimeter length Qp Qh N1 N

Medicare Statute 621MMA

C9353 Microporous collagen implantable slit tube (NeuraWrap Nerve Protector), per centimeter length Qp Qh N1 N

Medicare Statute 621MMA

C9354 Acellular pericardial tissue matrix of non-human origin (Veritas), per square centimeter Qp Qh N1 N

Medicare Statute 621MMA

C9355 Collagen nerve cuff (NeuroMatrix), per 0.5 centimeter length Qp Qh N1 N

Medicare Statute 621MMA

C9356 Tendon, porous matrix of cross-linked collagen and glycosaminoglycan matrix (TenoGlide Tendon Protector Sheet), per square centimeter Qp Qh N1 N

Medicare Statute 621MMA

C9358 Dermal substitute, native, non-denatured collagen, fetal bovine origin (SurgiMend Collagen Matrix), per 0.5 square centimeters Qp Qh N1 N

Medicare Statute 621MMA

Coding Clinic: 2013, Q3, P9; 2012, Q2, P7

C9359 Porous purified collagen matrix bone void filler (Integra Mozaik Osteoconductive Scaffold Putty, Integra OS Osteoconductive Scaffold Putty), per 0.5 cc Qp Qh N1 N

Medicare Statute 1833(t)

Coding Clinic: 2015, Q3, P2

C9360 Dermal substitute, native, non-denatured collagen, neonatal bovine origin (SurgiMend Collagen Matrix), per 0.5 square centimeters Qp Qh N1 N

Medicare Statute 621MMA

Coding Clinic: 2012, Q2, P7

C9361 Collagen matrix nerve wrap (NeuroMend Collagen Nerve Wrap), per 0.5 centimeter length Qp Qh N1 N

Medicare Statute 621MMA

C9362 Porous purified collagen matrix bone void filler (Integra Mozaik Osteoconductive Scaffold Strip), per 0.5 cc Qp Qh N1 N

Medicare Statute 621MMA

Coding Clinic: 2010, Q2, P8

◎ **C9363** Skin substitute, Integra Meshed Bilayer Wound Matrix, per square centimeter Qp Qh N1 N
Medicare Statute 621MMA
Coding Clinic: 2012, Q2, P7; 2010, Q2, P8

◎ **C9364** Porcine implant, Permacol, per square centimeter Qp Qh N1 N
Medicare Statute 621MMA

◎ **C9399** Unclassified drugs or biologicals K7 A
Medicare Statute 621MMA
Coding Clinic: 2017, Q1, P1-3, P8; 2016, Q4, P10; 2014, Q2, P8; 2013, Q2, P3; 2010, Q3, P8

◎ **C9460** Injection, cangrelor, 1 mg Qp Qh K2 G
Medicare Statute 1833(t)

◎ **C9462** Injection, delafloxacin, 1 mg K2 G
Medicare Statute 1833(t)

◎ **C9482** Injection, sotalol hydrochloride, 1 mg Qp Qh K2 G
Medicare Statute 1833(t)
Coding Clinic: 2016, Q4, P9

◎ **C9488** Injection, conivaptan hydrochloride, 1 mg K2 G
Medicare Statute 1833(t)

Percutaneous Transcatheter and Transluminal Coronary Procedures

◎ **C9600** Percutaneous transcatheter placement of drug-eluting intracoronary stent(s), with coronary angioplasty when performed; a single major coronary artery or branch Qp Qh J1
Medicare Statute 1833(t)

◎ **C9601** Percutaneous transcatheter placement of drug-eluting intracoronary stent(s), with coronary angioplasty when performed; each additional branch of a major coronary artery (list separately in addition to code for primary procedure) Qp Qh N
Medicare Statute 1833(t)

◎ **C9602** Percutaneous transluminal coronary atherectomy, with drug-eluting intracoronary stent, with coronary angioplasty when performed; a single major coronary artery or branch Qp Qh J1
Medicare Statute 1833(t)

◎ **C9603** Percutaneous transluminal coronary atherectomy, with drug-eluting intracoronary stent, with coronary angioplasty when performed; each additional branch of a major coronary artery (list separately in addition to code for primary procedure) Qp Qh N
Medicare Statute 1833(t)

◎ **C9604** Percutaneous transluminal revascularization of or through coronary artery bypass graft (internal mammary, free arterial, venous), any combination of drug-eluting intracoronary stent, atherectomy and angioplasty, including distal protection when performed; a single vessel Qp Qh J1

◎ **C9605** Percutaneous transluminal revascularization of or through coronary artery bypass graft (internal mammary, free arterial, venous), any combination of drug-eluting intracoronary stent, atherectomy and angioplasty, including distal protection when performed; each additional branch subtended by the bypass graft (list separately in addition to code for primary procedure) Qp Qh N
Medicare Statute 1833(t)

◎ **C9606** Percutaneous transluminal revascularization of acute total/subtotal occlusion during acute myocardial infarction, coronary artery or coronary artery bypass graft, any combination of drug-eluting intracoronary stent, atherectomy and angioplasty, including aspiration thrombectomy when performed, single vessel Qp Qh J1
Medicare Statute 1833(t)

◎ **C9607** Percutaneous transluminal revascularization of chronic total occlusion, coronary artery, coronary artery branch, or coronary artery bypass graft, any combination of drug-eluting intracoronary stent, atherectomy and angioplasty; single vessel Qp Qh J1
Medicare Statute 1833(t)

◎ **C9608** Percutaneous transluminal revascularization of chronic total occlusion, coronary artery, coronary artery branch, or coronary artery bypass graft, any combination of drug-eluting intracoronary stent, atherectomy and angioplasty; each additional coronary artery, coronary artery branch, or bypass graft (list separately in addition to code for primary procedure) Qp Qh N
Medicare Statute 1833(t)

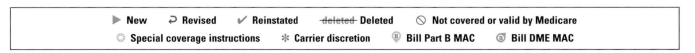

Therapeutic Services and Supplies

C9725 Placement of endorectal intracavitary applicator for high intensity brachytherapy Qp Qh T

Medicare Statute 1833(t)

C9726 Placement and removal (if performed) of applicator into breast for intraoperative radiation therapy, add-on to primary breast procedure Qh N

Medicare Statute 1833(t)

C9727 Insertion of implants into the soft palate; minimum of three implants Qp Qh T

Medicare Statute 1833(t)

C9728 Placement of interstitial device(s) for radiation therapy/surgery guidance (e.g., fiducial markers, dosimeter), for other than the following sites (any approach): abdomen, pelvis, prostate, retroperitoneum, thorax, single or multiple Qp Qh S

Medicare Statute 1833(t)

Coding Clinic: 2018, Q2, P4

C9733 Non-ophthalmic fluorescent vascular angiography Qp Qh Q2

Medicare Statute 1833(t)

Coding Clinic: 2012, Q1, P7

C9734 Focused ultrasound ablation/therapeutic intervention, other than uterine leiomyomata, with magnetic resonance (MR) guidance Qp Qh J1

Medicare Statute 1833(t)

C9738 Adjunctive blue light cystoscopy with fluorescent imaging agent (list separately in addition to code for primary procedure) N1 N

Medicare Statute 1833(t)

C9739 Cystourethroscopy, with insertion of transprostatic implant; 1 to 3 implants Qp Qh J1

Medicare Statute 1833(t)

Coding Clinic: 2014, Q2, P6

C9740 Cystourethroscopy, with insertion of transprostatic implant; 4 or more implants Qp Qh J1

Medicare Statute 1833(t)

Coding Clinic: 2014, Q2, P6

~~C9745 Nasal endoscopy, surgical; balloon dilation of eustachian tube~~ ✖

~~C9747 Ablation of prostate, transrectal, high intensity focused ultrasound (HIFU), including imaging guidance~~ ✖

~~C9749 Repair of nasal vestibular lateral wall stenosis with implant(s)~~ ✖

C9751 Bronchoscopy, rigid or flexible, transbronchial ablation of lesion(s) by microwave energy, including fluoroscopic guidance, when performed, with computed tomography acquisition(s) and 3-D rendering, computer-assisted, image-guided navigation, and endobronchial ultrasound (EBUS) guided transtracheal and/or transbronchial sampling (e.g., aspiration[s]/biopsy[ies]) and all mediastinal and/or hilar lymph node stations or structures and therapeutic intervention(s) T

Medicare Statute 1833(t)

C9752 Destruction of intraosseous basivertebral nerve, first two vertebral bodies, including imaging guidance (e.g., fluoroscopy), lumbar/sacrum J1

Medicare Statute 1833(t)

Coding Clinic: 2020, Q3, P11

C9753 Destruction of intraosseous basivertebral nerve, each additional vertebral body, including imaging guidance (e.g., fluoroscopy), lumbar/sacrum (list separately in addition to code for primary procedure) N

Medicare Statute 1833(t)

~~C9754 Creation of arteriovenous fistula, percutaneous; direct, any site, including all imaging and radiologic supervision and interpretation, when performed and secondary procedures to redirect blood flow (e.g., transluminal balloon angioplasty, coil embolization, when performed)~~ ✖

~~C9755 Creation of arteriovenous fistula, percutaneous using magnetic-guided arterial and venous catheters and radiofrequency energy, including flow-directing procedures (e.g., vascular coil embolization with radiologic supervision and interpretation, when performed) and fistulogram(s), angiography, venography, and/or ultrasound, with radiologic supervision and interpretation, when performed~~ ✖

C9756 Intraoperative near-infrared fluorescence lymphatic mapping of lymph node(s) (sentinel or tumor draining) with administration of indocyanine green (ICG) (list separately in addition to code for primary procedure) N

MIPS | Qp Quantity Physician | Qh Quantity Hospital | ♀ Female only | ♂ Male only | A Age | DMEPOS | A2-Z3 ASC Payment Indicator | A-Y ASC Status Indicator | Coding Clinic

C9757 Laminotomy (hemilaminectomy), with decompression of nerve root(s), including partial facetectomy, foraminotomy and excision of herniated intervertebral disc, and repair of annular defect with implantation of bone anchored annular closure device, including annular defect measurement, alignment and sizing assessment, and image guidance; 1 interspace, lumbar J1

C9758 Blinded procedure for NYHA class III/IV heart failure; transcatheter implantation of interatrial shunt or placebo control, including right heart catheterization, trans-esophageal echocardiography (TEE)/intracardiac echocardiography (ICE), and all imaging with or without guidance (e.g., ultrasound, fluoroscopy), performed in an approved investigational device exemption (IDE) study T

▶ **C9759** Transcatheter intraoperative blood vessel microinfusion(s) (e.g., intraluminal, vascular wall and/or perivascular) therapy, any vessel, including radiological supervision and interpretation, when performed N

▶ **C9760** Non-randomized, non-blinded procedure for NYHA class ii, iii, iv heart failure; transcatheter implantation of interatrial shunt, including right and left heart catheterization, transeptal puncture, trans-esophageal echocardiography (tee)/intracardiac echocardiography (ice), and all imaging with or without guidance (e.g., ultrasound, fluoroscopy), performed in an approved investigational device exemption (ide) study T

▶ **C9761** Cystourethroscopy, with ureteroscopy and/or pyeloscopy, with lithotripsy (ureteral catheterization is included) and vacuum aspiration of the kidney, collecting system and urethra if applicable J1

▶ **C9762** Cardiac magnetic resonance imaging for morphology and function, quantification of segmental dysfunction; with strain imaging Z2 Q3

▶ **C9763** Cardiac magnetic resonance imaging for morphology and function, quantification of segmental dysfunction; with stress imaging Z2 Q3

▶ **C9764** Revascularization, endovascular, open or percutaneous, any vessel(s); with intravascular lithotripsy, includes angioplasty within the same vessel(s), when performed J1

▶ **C9765** Revascularization, endovascular, open or percutaneous, any vessel(s); with intravascular lithotripsy, and transluminal stent placement(s), includes angioplasty within the same vessel(s), when performed J1

▶ **C9766** Revascularization, endovascular, open or percutaneous, any vessel(s); with intravascular lithotripsy and atherectomy, includes angioplasty within the same vessel(s), when performed

▶ **C9767** Revascularization, endovascular, open or percutaneous, any vessel(s); with intravascular lithotripsy and transluminal stent placement(s), and atherectomy, includes angioplasty within the same vessel(s), when performed J1

▶ **C9768** Endoscopic ultrasound-guided direct measurement of hepatic portosystemic pressure gradient by any method (list separately in addition to code for primary procedure) N

▶ **C9769** Cystourethroscopy, with insertion of temporary prostatic implant/stent with fixation/anchor and incisional struts N

▶ **C9770** Vitrectomy, mechanical, pars plana approach, with subretinal injection of pharmacologic/biologic agent T

▶ **C9771** Nasal/sinus endoscopy, cryoablation nasal tissue(s) and/or nerve(s), unilateral or bilateral J1

▶ **C9772** Revascularization, endovascular, open or percutaneous, tibial/peroneal artery(ies), with intravascular lithotripsy, includes angioplasty within the same vessel(s), when performed J1

▶ **C9973** Revascularization, endovascular, open or percutaneous, tibial/peroneal artery(ies); with intravascular lithotripsy, and transluminal stent placement(s), includes angioplasty within the same vessel(s), when performed J1

▶ New ⤺ Revised ✔ Reinstated ~~deleted~~ Deleted ⊘ Not covered or valid by Medicare
Special coverage instructions ✻ Carrier discretion Ⓑ Bill Part B MAC Ⓑ Bill DME MAC

C9774 Revascularization, endovascular, open or percutaneous, tibial/peroneal artery(ies); with intravascular lithotripsy and atherectomy, includes angioplasty within the same vessel(s), when performed J1

C9775 Revascularization, endovascular, open or percutaneous, tibial/peroneal artery(ies); with intravascular lithotripsy and transluminal stent placement(s), and atherectomy, includes angioplasty within the same vessel(s), when performed J1

C9803 Hospital outpatient clinic visit specimen collection for severe acute respiratory syndrome coronavirus 2 (SARS-CoV-2) (coronavirus disease [COVID-19]), any specimen source Q1

C9898 Radiolabeled product provided during a hospital inpatient stay Qh N

C9899 Implanted prosthetic device, payable only for inpatients who do not have inpatient coverage A

Medicare Statute 1833(t)

DENTAL PROCEDURES (D0000-D9999)

Diagnostic (D0120-D0999)

Clinical Oral Evaluations

↻ **D0120** Periodic oral evaluation - established patient Ⓑ E1

An evaluation performed on a patient of record to determine any changes in the patient's dental and medical health status since a previous comprehensive or periodic evaluation. This includes an oral cancer evaluation, periodontal screening where indicated, and may require interpretation of information acquired through additional diagnostic procedures. Report additional diagnostic procedures separately.

D0140 Limited oral evaluation - problem focused Ⓑ E1

An evaluation limited to a specific oral health problem or complaint. This may require interpretation of information acquired through additional diagnostic procedures. Report additional diagnostic procedures separately. Definitive procedures may be required on the same date as the evaluation. Typically, patients receiving this type of evaluation present with a specific problem and/or dental emergencies, trauma, acute infections, etc.

D0145 Oral evaluation for a patient under three years of age and counseling with primary caregiver Ⓑ A E1

Diagnostic services performed for a child under the age of three, preferably within the first six months of the eruption of the first primary tooth, including recording the oral and physical health history, evaluation of caries susceptibility, development of an appropriate preventive oral health regimen and communication with and counseling of the child's parent, legal guardian and/or primary caregiver.

↻ **D0150** Comprehensive oral evaluation - new or established patient Ⓑ S

Used by a general dentist and/or a specialist when evaluating a patient comprehensively. This applies to new patients; established patients who have had a significant change in health conditions or other unusual circumstances, by report, or established patients who have been absent from active treatment for three or more years. It is a thorough evaluation and recording of the extraoral and intraoral hard and soft tissues. It may require interpretation of information acquired through additional diagnostic procedures. Additional diagnostic procedures should be reported separately. This includes an evaluation for oral cancer, the evaluation and recording of the patient's dental and medical history and a general health assessment. It may include the evaluation and recording of dental caries, missing or unerupted teeth, restorations, existing prostheses, occlusal relationships, periodontal conditions (including periodontal screening and/or charting), hard and soft tissue anomalies, etc.

D0160 Detailed and extensive oral evaluation - problem focused, by report Ⓑ E1

A detailed and extensive problem focused evaluation entails extensive diagnostic and cognitive modalities based on the findings of a comprehensive oral evaluation. Integration of more extensive diagnostic modalities to develop a treatment plan for a specific problem is required. The condition requiring this type of evaluation should be described and documented. Examples of conditions requiring this type of evaluation may include dentofacial anomalies, complicated perio-prosthetic conditions, complex temporomandibular dysfunction, facial pain of unknown origin, conditions requiring multi-disciplinary consultation, etc.

▶ New ↻ Revised ✔ Reinstated ~~deleted~~ Deleted ⃠ Not covered or valid by Medicare
Special coverage instructions ✻ Carrier discretion Ⓑ Bill Part B MAC Ⓓ Bill DME MAC

D0170 Re-evaluation - limited, problem focused (established patient; not post-operative visit) Ⓑ E1

Assessing the status of a previously existing condition. For example: a traumatic injury where no treatment was rendered but patient needs follow-up monitoring; evaluation for undiagnosed continuing pain; soft tissue lesion requiring follow-up evaluation.

D0171 Re-evaluation - post-operative office visit Ⓑ E1

D0180 Comprehensive periodontal evaluation - new or established patient Ⓑ E1

This procedure is indicated for patients showing signs or symptoms of periodontal disease and for patients with risk factors such as smoking or diabetes. It includes evaluation of periodontal conditions, probing and charting, evaluation and recording of the patient's dental and medical history and general health assessment. It may include the evaluation and recording of dental caries, missing or unerupted teeth, restorations, occlusal relationships and oral cancer evaluation.

Pre-Diagnostic Services

D0190 Screening of a patient Ⓑ E1

A screening, including state or federally mandated screenings, to determine an individual's need to be seen by a dentist for diagnosis.

D0191 Assessment of a patient Ⓑ E1

A limited clinical inspection that is performed to identify possible signs of oral or systemic disease, malformation, or injury, and the potential need for referral for diagnosis and treatment.

Diagnostic Imaging

D0210 Intraoral - complete series of radiographic images Ⓑ E1

A radiographic survey of the whole mouth, usually consisting of 14-22 periapical and posterior bitewing images intended to display the crowns and roots of all teeth, periapical areas and alveolar bone.

Cross Reference 70320

D0220 Intraoral - periapical first radiographic image Ⓑ E1

Cross Reference 70300

D0230 Intraoral - periapical each additional radiographic image Ⓑ E1

Cross Reference 70310

D0240 Intraoral - occlusal radiographic image Ⓑ S

D0250 Extra-oral — 2D projection radiographic image created using a stationary radiation source, detector Ⓑ S

These images include, but are not limited to: Lateral Skull; Posterior-Anterior Skull; Submentovertex; Waters; Reverse Tomes; Oblique Mandibular Body; Lateral Ramus.

D0251 Extra-oral posterior dental radiographic image Ⓑ Q1

Image limited to exposure of complete posterior teeth in both dental arches. This is a unique image that is not derived from another image.

D0270 Bitewing - single radiographic image Ⓑ S

D0272 Bitewings - two radiographic images Ⓑ S

D0273 Bitewings - three radiographic images Ⓑ E1

D0274 Bitewings - four radiographic images Ⓑ S

D0277 Vertical bitewings - 7 to 8 radiographic images Ⓑ S

This does not constitute a full mouth intraoral radiographic series.

D0310 Sialography Ⓑ E1

Cross Reference 70390

D0320 Temporomandibular joint arthrogram, including injection Ⓑ E1

Cross Reference 70332

D0321 Other temporomandibular joint radiographic image, by report Ⓑ E1

Cross Reference 76499

D0322 Tomographic survey Ⓑ E1

D0330 Panoramic radiographic image Ⓑ E1

Cross Reference 70320

MIPS | Qp Quantity Physician | Qh Quantity Hospital | ♀ Female only
♂ Male only | A Age | DMEPOS | A2-Z3 ASC Payment Indicator | A-Y ASC Status Indicator | Coding Clinic

D0340 2D cephalometric radiographic image - acquisition, measurement and analysis Ⓑ E1

Image of the head made using a cephalostat to standardize anatomic positioning, and with reproducible x-ray beam geometry.

Cross Reference 70350

D0350 2D oral/facial photographic image obtained intra-orally or extra-orally Ⓑ E1

D0351 3D photographic image Ⓑ E1

This procedure is for dental or maxillofacial diagnostic purposes. Not applicable for a CAD-CAM procedure.

D0364 Cone beam CT capture and interpretation with limited field of view - less than one whole jaw Ⓑ E1

D0365 Cone beam CT capture and interpretation with field of view of one full dental arch - mandible Ⓑ E1

D0366 Cone beam CT capture and interpretation with field of view of one full dental arch - maxilla, with or without cranium Ⓑ E1

D0367 Cone beam CT capture and interpretation with field of view of both jaws, with or without cranium Ⓑ E1

D0368 Cone beam CT capture and interpretation for TMJ series including two or more exposures Ⓑ E1

D0369 Maxillofacial MRI capture and interpretation Ⓑ E1

D0370 Maxillofacial ultrasound capture and interpretation Ⓑ E1

D0371 Sialoendoscopy capture and interpretation Ⓑ E1

D0380 Cone beam CT image capture with limited field of view - less than one whole jaw Ⓑ E1

D0381 Cone beam CT image capture with field of view of one full dental arch - mandible Ⓑ E1

D0382 Cone beam CT image capture with field of view of one full dental arch - maxilla, with or without cranium Ⓑ E1

D0383 Cone beam CT image capture with field of view of both jaws, with or without cranium Ⓑ E1

D0384 Cone beam CT image capture for TMJ series including two or more exposures Ⓑ E1

D0385 Maxillofacial MRI image capture Ⓑ E1

D0386 Maxillofacial ultrasound image capture Ⓑ E1

D0391 Interpretation of diagnostic image by a practitioner not associated with capture of the image, including report Ⓑ E1

D0393 Treatment simulation using 3D image volume Ⓑ E1

The use of 3D image volumes for simulation of treatment including, but not limited to, dental implant placement, orthognathic surgery and orthodontic tooth movement.

D0394 Digital subtraction of two or more images or image volumes of the same modality Ⓑ E1

To demonstrate changes that have occurred over time.

D0395 Fusion of two or more 3D image volumes of one or more modalities Ⓑ E1

Tests and Examinations

D0411 HbA1c in-office point of service testing Ⓑ E1

D0412 Blood glucose level test - in-office using a glucose meter Ⓑ E1

D0414 Laboratory processing of microbial specimen to include culture and sensitivity studies, preparation and transmission of written report Ⓑ E1

D0415 Collection of microorganisms for culture and sensitivity Ⓑ E1

Cross Reference D0410

D0416 Viral culture Ⓑ B

A diagnostic test to identify viral organisms, most often herpes virus.

D0417 Collection and preparation of saliva sample for laboratory diagnostic testing Ⓑ E1

D0418 Analysis of saliva sample Ⓑ E1

Chemical or biological analysis of saliva sample for diagnostic purposes.

D0419 Assessment of salivary flow by measurement E1

D0422 Collection and preparation of genetic sample material for laboratory analysis and report Ⓑ E1

D0423 Genetic test for susceptibility to diseases - specimen analysis Ⓑ E1

Certified laboratory analysis to detect specific genetic variations associated with increased susceptibility for diseases.

D0425 Caries susceptibility tests E1

Not to be used for carious dentin staining.

D0431 Adjunctive pre-diagnostic test that aids in detection of mucosal abnormalities including premalignant and malignant lesions, not to include cytology or biopsy procedures B

D0460 Pulp vitality tests S

Includes multiple teeth and contra-lateral comparison(s), as indicated.

D0470 Diagnostic casts E1

Also known as diagnostic models or study models.

Oral Pathology Laboratory (Use Codes D0472 – D0502)

D0472 Accession of tissue, gross examination, preparation and transmission of written report B

To be used in reporting architecturally intact tissue obtained by invasive means.

D0473 Accession of tissue, gross and microscopic examination, preparation and transmission of written report B

To be used in reporting architecturally intact tissue obtained by invasive means.

D0474 Accession of tissue, gross and microscopic examination, including assessment of surgical margins for presence of disease, preparation and transmission of written report B

To be used in reporting architecturally intact tissue obtained by invasive means.

D0475 Decalcification procedure B

Procedure in which hard tissue is processed in order to allow sectioning and subsequent microscopic examination.

D0476 Special stains for microorganisms B

Procedure in which additional stains are applied to biopsy or surgical specimen in order to identify microorganisms.

D0477 Special stains, not for microorganisms B

Procedure in which additional stains are applied to a biopsy or surgical specimen in order to identify such things as melanin, mucin, iron, glycogen, etc.

D0478 Immunohistochemical stains B

A procedure in which specific antibody based reagents are applied to tissue samples in order to facilitate diagnosis.

D0479 Tissue in-situ hybridization, including interpretation B

A procedure which allows for the identification of nucleic acids, DNA and RNA, in the tissue sample in order to aid in the diagnosis of microorganisms and tumors.

D0480 Accession of exfoliative cytologic smears, microscopic examination, preparation and transmission of written report B

To be used in reporting disaggregated, non-transepithelial cell cytology sample via mild scraping of the oral mucosa.

D0481 Electron microscopy B

D0482 Direct immunofluorescence B

A technique used to identify immunoreactants which are localized to the patient's skin or mucous membranes.

D0483 Indirect immunofluorescence B

A technique used to identify circulating immunoreactants.

D0484 Consultation on slides prepared elsewhere B

A service provided in which microscopic slides of a biopsy specimen prepared at another laboratory are evaluated to aid in the diagnosis of a difficult case or to offer a consultative opinion at the patient's request. The findings are delivered by written report.

D0485 Consultation, including preparation of slides from biopsy material supplied by referring source B

A service that requires the consulting pathologist to prepare the slides as well as render a written report. The slides are evaluated to aid in the diagnosis of a difficult case or to offer a consultative opinion at the patient's request.

D0486 Laboratory accession of transepithelial cytologic sample, microscopic examination, preparation and transmission of written report E1

Analysis, and written report of findings, of cytologic sample of disaggregated transepithelial cells.

D0502 Other oral pathology procedures, by report B

Tests and Examinations

D0600 Non-ionizing diagnostic procedure capable of quantifying, monitoring, and recording changes in structure of enamel, dentin, and cementum Ⓑ S

D0601 Caries risk assessment and documentation, with a finding of low risk Ⓑ E1

Using recognized assessment tools.

D0602 Caries risk assessment and documentation, with a finding of moderate risk Ⓑ E1

Using recognized assessment tools.

D0603 Caries risk assessment and documentation, with a finding of high risk Ⓑ E1

Using recognized assessment tools.

▶ **D0604** Antigen testing for public health related pathogen, including coronavirus

▶ **D0605** Antibody testing for public health related pathogen, including coronavirus

▶ **D0701** Panoramic radiographic image – image capture only

▶ **D0702** 2-D cephalometric radiographic image – image capture only

▶ **D0703** 2-D oral/facial photographic image obtained intra-orally or extra-orally – image capture only

▶ **D0704** 3-D photographic image – image capture only

▶ **D0705** Extra-oral posterior dental radiographic image – image capture only

Image limited to exposure of complete posterior teeth in both dental arches.

This is a unique image that is not derived from another image.

▶ **D0706** Intraoral – occlusal radiographic image – image capture only

▶ **D0707** Intraoral – periapical radiographic image – image capture only

▶ **D0708** Intraoral – bitewing radiographic image – image capture only

Image axis may be horizontal or vertical.

▶ **D0709** Intraoral – complete series of radiographic images – image capture only

A radiographic survey of the whole mouth, usually consisting of 14-22 images (periapical and posterior bitewing as indicated) intended to display the crowns and roots of all teeth, periapical areas and alveolar bone.

None

D0999 Unspecified diagnostic procedure, by report Ⓑ B

Used for procedure that is not adequately described by a code. Describe procedure.

Preventative (D1110-D1999)

Dental Prophylaxis

⮌ **D1110** Prophylaxis - adult Ⓑ A E1

Removal of plaque, calculus and stains from the tooth structures and implants in the permanent and transitional dentition. It is intended to control local irritational factors.

⮌ **D1120** Prophylaxis - child Ⓑ A E1

Removal of plaque, calculus and stains from the tooth structures and implants in the primary and transitional dentition. It is intended to control local irritational factors.

Topical Fluoride Treatment (Office Procedure)

D1206 Topical application of fluoride varnish Ⓑ E1

D1208 Topical application of fluoride — excluding varnish Ⓑ E1

Other Preventative Services

D1310 Nutritional counseling for the control of dental disease Ⓑ E1

Counseling on food selection and dietary habits as a part of treatment and control of periodontal disease and caries.

▶ New ⮌ Revised ✔ Reinstated ~~deleted~~ Deleted ⦸ Not covered or valid by Medicare
Special coverage instructions ✱ Carrier discretion Ⓑ Bill Part B MAC Ⓓ Bill DME MAC

D1320 Tobacco counseling for the control and prevention of oral disease Ⓑ E1

Tobacco prevention and cessation services reduce patient risks of developing tobacco-related oral diseases and conditions and improves prognosis for certain dental therapies.

▶ **D1321** Counseling for the control and prevention of adverse oral, behavioral, and systemic health effects associated with high-risk substance use

Counseling services may include patient education about adverse oral, behavioral, and systemic effects associated with high-risk substance use and administration routes. This includes ingesting, injecting, inhaling and vaping. Substances used in a high-risk manner may include but are not limited to alcohol, opioids, nicotine, cannabis, methamphetamine and other pharmaceuticals or chemicals.

D1330 Oral hygiene instruction Ⓑ E1

This may include instructions for home care. Examples include tooth brushing technique, flossing, use of special oral hygiene aids.

D1351 Sealant - per tooth Ⓑ E1

Mechanically and/or chemically prepared enamel surface sealed to prevent decay.

D1352 Preventive resin restoration in a moderate to high caries risk patient — permanent tooth Ⓑ E1

Conservative restoration of an active cavitated lesion in a pit or fissure that does not extend into dentin; includes placement of a sealant in any radiating non-carious fissures or pits.

D1353 Sealant repair — per tooth Ⓑ E1

D1354 Interim caries arresting medicament application — per tooth Ⓑ E1

Conservative treatment of an active, non-symptomatic carious lesion by topical application of a caries arresting or inhibiting medicament and without mechanical removal of sound tooth structure.

▶ **D1355** Caries preventive medicament application – per tooth

For primary prevention or remineralization. Medicaments applied do not include topical fluorides.

Space Maintenance (Passive Appliances)

D1510 Space maintainer - fixed - unilateral - per quadrant Ⓑ S

Excludes a distal shoe space maintainer.

D1516 Space Maintainer - fixed - bilateral, maxillary Ⓑ S

D1517 Space Maintainer - fixed - bilateral, mandibular Ⓑ S

D1520 Space maintainer - removable - unilateral - per quadrant Ⓑ S

D1526 Space maintainer - removable - bilateral, maxillary Ⓑ S

D1527 Space maintainer - removable - bilateral, mandibular Ⓑ S

D1551 Re-cement or re-bond bilateral space maintainer - maxillary S

D1552 Re-cement or re-bond bilateral space maintainer - mandibular S

D1553 Re-cement or re-bond unilateral space maintainer - per quadrant S

D1556 Removal of fixed unilateral space maintainer - per quadrant E1

D1557 Removal of fixed bilateral space maintainer - maxillary E1

D1558 Removal of fixed bilateral space maintainer - mandibular E1

Space Maintainers

D1575 Distal shoe space maintainer - fixed - unilateral - per quadrant Ⓑ S

Fabrication and delivery of fixed appliance extending subgingivally and distally to guide the eruption of the first permanent molar. Does not include ongoing follow-up or adjustments, or replacement appliances, once the tooth has erupted.

None

D1999 Unspecified preventive procedure, by report Ⓑ E1

Used for procedure that is not adequately described by another CDT Code. Describe procedure.

Restorative (D2140-D2999)

Amalgam Restorations (Including Polishing)

D2140 Amalgam - one surface, primary or permanent Ⓑ E1

D2150 Amalgam - two surfaces, primary or permanent Ⓑ E1

D2160 Amalgam - three surfaces, primary or permanent Ⓑ E1

D2161 Amalgam - four or more surfaces, primary or permanent Ⓑ E1

Resin-Based Composite Restorations – Direct

D2330 Resin-based composite - one surface, anterior Ⓑ E1

D2331 Resin-based composite - two surfaces, anterior Ⓑ E1

D2332 Resin-based composite - three surfaces, anterior Ⓑ E1

D2335 Resin-based composite - four or more surfaces or involving incisal angle (anterior) Ⓑ E1

Incisal angle to be defined as one of the angles formed by the junction of the incisal and the mesial or distal surface of an anterior tooth.

D2390 Resin-based composite crown, anterior Ⓑ E1

Full resin-based composite coverage of tooth.

D2391 Resin-based composite - one surface, posterior Ⓑ E1

Used to restore a carious lesion into the dentin or a deeply eroded area into the dentin. Not a preventive procedure.

D2392 Resin-based composite - two surfaces, posterior Ⓑ E1

D2393 Resin-based composite - three surfaces, posterior Ⓑ E1

D2394 Resin-based composite - four or more surfaces, posterior Ⓑ E1

Gold Foil Restorations

D2410 Gold foil - one surface Ⓑ E1

D2420 Gold foil - two surfaces Ⓑ E1

D2430 Gold foil - three surfaces Ⓑ E1

Inlay/Onlay Restorations

D2510 Inlay - metallic - one surface Ⓑ E1

D2520 Inlay - metallic - two surfaces Ⓑ E1

D2530 Inlay - metallic - three or more surfaces Ⓑ E1

D2542 Onlay - metallic - two surfaces Ⓑ E1

D2543 Onlay - metallic - three surfaces Ⓑ E1

D2544 Onlay - metallic - four or more surfaces Ⓑ E1

D2610 Inlay - porcelain/ceramic - one surface Ⓑ E1

D2620 Inlay - porcelain/ceramic - two surfaces Ⓑ E1

D2630 Inlay - porcelain/ceramic - three or more surfaces Ⓑ E1

D2642 Onlay - porcelain/ceramic - two surfaces Ⓑ E1

D2643 Onlay - porcelain/ceramic - three surfaces Ⓑ E1

D2644 Onlay - porcelain/ceramic - four or more surfaces Ⓑ E1

D2650 Inlay - resin-based composite - one surface Ⓑ E1

D2651 Inlay - resin-based composite - two surfaces Ⓑ E1

D2652 Inlay - resin-based composite - three or more surfaces Ⓑ E1

D2662 Onlay - resin-based composite - two surfaces Ⓑ E1

D2663 Onlay - resin-based composite - three surfaces Ⓑ E1

D2664 Onlay - resin-based composite - four or more surfaces Ⓑ E1

Crowns – Single Restoration Only

D2710 Crown - resin-based composite (indirect) Ⓑ E1

D2712 Crown - 3/4 resin-based composite (indirect) Ⓑ E1

This procedure does not include facial veneers.

D2720 Crown - resin with high noble metal Ⓑ E1

D2721 Crown - resin with predominantly base metal Ⓑ E1

D2722 Crown - resin with noble metal Ⓑ E1

D2740 Crown - porcelain/ceramic Ⓑ E1

D2750 Crown - porcelain fused to high noble metal Ⓑ E1

D2751 Crown - porcelain fused to predominantly base metal Ⓑ E1

D2752 Crown - porcelain fused to noble metal Ⓑ E1

D2753 Crown - porcelain fused to titanium and titanium alloys E1

D2780 Crown - 3/4 cast high noble metal Ⓑ E1

D2781 Crown - 3/4 cast predominantly base metal Ⓑ E1

▶ New ⊋ Revised ✔ Reinstated ~~deleted~~ Deleted ⊘ Not covered or valid by Medicare
Special coverage instructions ✻ Carrier discretion Ⓑ Bill Part B MAC Ⓑ Bill DME MAC

D2782 Crown - 3/4 cast noble metal Ⓑ E1

D2783 Crown - 3/4 porcelain/ceramic Ⓑ E1

This procedure does not include facial veneers.

D2790 Crown - full cast high noble metal Ⓑ E1

D2791 Crown - full cast predominantly base metal Ⓑ E1

D2792 Crown - full cast noble metal Ⓑ E1

D2794 Crown - titanium and titanium alloys Ⓑ E1

D2799 Provisional crown - further treatment or completion of diagnosis necessary prior to final impression Ⓑ E1

Not to be used as a temporary crown for a routine prosthetic restoration.

Other Restorative Services

D2910 Re-cement or re-bond inlay, onlay, veneer or partial coverage restoration Ⓑ E1

D2915 Re-cement or re-bond indirectly fabricated cast or prefabricated post and core Ⓑ E1

D2920 Re-cement or re-bond crown Ⓑ E1

D2921 Reattachment of tooth fragment, incisal edge or cusp Ⓑ E1

▶ **D2928** Prefabricated porcelain/ceramic crown – permanent tooth

D2929 Prefabricated porcelain/ceramic crown - primary tooth Ⓑ E1

D2930 Prefabricated stainless steel crown - primary tooth Ⓑ E1

D2931 Prefabricated stainless steel crown - permanent tooth Ⓑ E1

D2932 Prefabricated resin crown Ⓑ E1

D2933 Prefabricated stainless steel crown with resin window Ⓑ E1

Open-face stainless steel crown with aesthetic resin facing or veneer.

D2934 Prefabricated esthetic coated stainless steel crown - primary tooth Ⓑ E1

Stainless steel primary crown with exterior esthetic coating.

D2940 Protective restoration Ⓑ E1

Direct placement of a restorative material to protect tooth and/or tissue form. This procedure may be used to relieve pain, promote healing, or prevent further deterioration. Not to be used for endodontic access closure, or as a base or liner under a restoration.

D2941 Interim therapeutic restoration - primary dentition Ⓑ E1

Placement of an adhesive restorative material following caries debridement by hand or other method for the management of early childhood caries. Not considered a definitive restoration.

D2949 Restorative foundation for an indirect restoration Ⓑ E1

Placement of restorative material to yield a more ideal form, including elimination of undercuts.

D2950 Core build-up, including any pins when required Ⓑ E1

Refers to building up of coronal structure when there is insufficient retention for a separate extracoronal restorative procedure. A core build-up is not a filler to eliminate any undercut, box form, or concave irregularity in a preparation.

D2951 Pin retention - per tooth, in addition to restoration Ⓑ E1

D2952 Post and core in addition to crown, indirectly fabricated Ⓑ E1

Post and core are custom fabricated as a single unit.

D2953 Each additional indirectly fabricated post - same tooth Ⓑ E1

To be used with D2952.

D2954 Prefabricated post and core in addition to crown Ⓑ E1

Core is built around a prefabricated post. This procedure includes the core material.

D2955 Post removal Ⓑ E1

D2957 Each additional prefabricated post - same tooth Ⓑ E1

To be used with D2954.

⊋ **D2960** Labial veneer (laminate) - direct Ⓑ E1

Refers to labial/facial direct resin bonded veneers.

⊋ **D2961** Labial veneer (resin laminate) - indirect Ⓑ E1

Refers to labial/facial indirect resin bonded veneers.

⊋ **D2962** Labial veneer (porcelain laminate) - indirect Ⓑ E1

Refers also to facial veneers that extend interproximally and/or cover the incisal edge. Porcelain/ceramic veneers presently include all ceramic and porcelain veneers.

D2971 Additional procedures to construct new crown under existing partial denture framework Ⓑ E1

To be reported in addition to a crown code.

D2975 Coping Ⓑ E1

A thin covering of the coronal portion of a tooth, usually devoid of anatomic contour, that can be used as a definitive restoration.

D2980 Crown repair, necessitated by restorative material failure Ⓑ E1

D2981 Inlay repair necessitated by restorative material failure Ⓑ E1

D2982 Onlay repair necessitated by restorative material failure Ⓑ E1

D2983 Veneer repair necessitated by restorative material failure Ⓑ E1

D2990 Resin infiltration of incipient smooth surface lesions Ⓑ E1

Placement of an infiltrating resin restoration for strengthening, stabilizing and/or limiting the progression of the lesion.

None

D2999 Unspecified restorative procedure, by report Ⓑ S

Use for procedure that is not adequately described by a code. Describe procedure.

Endodontics (D3110-D3999)

Pulp Capping

D3110 Pulp cap - direct (excluding final restoration) Ⓑ E1

Procedure in which the exposed pulp is covered with a dressing or cement that protects the pulp and promotes healing and repair.

D3120 Pulp cap - indirect (excluding final restoration) Ⓑ E1

Procedure in which the nearly exposed pulp is covered with a protective dressing to protect the pulp from additional injury and to promote healing and repair via formation of secondary dentin. This code is not to be used for bases and liners when all caries has been removed.

Pulpotomy

D3220 Therapeutic pulpotomy (excluding final restoration) removal of pulp coronal to the dentinocemental junction and application of medicament Ⓑ E1

Pulpotomy is the surgical removal of a portion of the pulp with the aim of maintaining the vitality of the remaining portion by means of an adequate dressing.

– To be performed on primary or permanent teeth.

– This is not to be construed as the first stage of root canal therapy.

– Not to be used for apexogenesis.

D3221 Pulpal debridement, primary and permanent teeth Ⓑ E1

Pulpal debridement for the relief of acute pain prior to conventional root canal therapy. This procedure is not to be used when endodontic treatment is completed on the same day.

D3222 Partial pulpotomy for apexogenesis - permanent tooth with incomplete root development Ⓑ E1

Removal of a portion of the pulp and application of a medicament with the aim of maintaining the vitality of the remaining portion to encourage continued physiological development and formation of the root. This procedure is not to be construed as the first stage of root canal therapy.

Endodontic Therapy on Primary Teeth

D3230 Pulpal therapy (resorbable filling) - anterior, primary tooth (excluding final restoration) Ⓑ E1

Primary incisors and cuspids.

D3240 Pulpal therapy (resorbable filling) - posterior, primary tooth (excluding final restoration) Ⓑ E1

Primary first and second molars.

Endodontic Therapy (Including Treatment Plan, Clinical Procedures and Follow-Up Care)

D3310 Endodontic therapy, anterior tooth (excluding final restoration) Ⓑ E1

D3320 Endodontic therapy, premolar tooth (excluding final restoration) Ⓑ E1

D3330 Endodontic therapy, molar (excluding final restoration) Ⓑ E1

▶ New ↩ Revised ✔ Reinstated ~~deleted~~ Deleted ⊘ Not covered or valid by Medicare
Special coverage instructions ✱ Carrier discretion Ⓑ Bill Part B MAC Ⓓ Bill DME MAC

D3331 Treatment of root canal obstruction; non-surgical access E1

In lieu of surgery, the formation of a pathway to achieve an apical seal without surgical intervention because of a non-negotiable root canal blocked by foreign bodies, including but not limited to separated instruments, broken posts or calcification of 50% or more of the length of the tooth root.

D3332 Incomplete endodontic therapy; inoperable, unrestorable or fractured tooth E1

Considerable time is necessary to determine diagnosis and/or provide initial treatment before the fracture makes the tooth unretainable.

D3333 Internal root repair of perforation defects E1

Non-surgical seal of perforation caused by resorption and/or decay but not iatrogenic by provider filing claim.

Endodontic Retreatment

D3346 Retreatment of previous root canal therapy - anterior E1

D3347 Retreatment of previous root canal therapy - premolar E1

D3348 Retreatment of previous root canal therapy - molar E1

Apexification/Recalcification

D3351 Apexification/recalcification - initial visit (apical closure/calcific repair of perforations, root resorption, etc.) E1

Includes opening tooth, preparation of canal spaces, first placement of medication and necessary radiographs. (This procedure may include first phase of complete root canal therapy.)

D3352 Apexification/recalcification - interim medication replacement (apical closure/calcific repair of perforations, root resorption, pulp space disinfection, etc.) E1

For visits in which the intra-canal medication is replaced with new medication. Includes any necessary radiographs.

D3353 Apexification/recalcification - final visit (includes completed root canal therapy - apical closure/calcific repair of perforations, root resorption, etc.) E1

Includes removal of intra-canal medication and procedures necessary to place final root canal filling material including necessary radiographs. (This procedure includes last phase of complete root canal therapy.)

Pulpal Regeneration

D3355 Pulpal regeneration - initial visit E1

Includes opening tooth, preparation of canal spaces, placement of medication.

D3356 Pulpal regeneration - interim medication replacement E1

D3357 Pulpal regeneration - completion of treatment E1

Does not include final restoration.

Apicoectomy/Periradicular Services

D3410 Apicoectomy - anterior E1

For surgery on root of anterior tooth. Does not include placement of retrograde filling material.

D3421 Apicoectomy - premolar (first root) E1

For surgery on one root of a premolar. Does not include placement of retrograde filling material. If more than one root is treated, see D3426.

D3425 Apicoectomy - molar (first root) E1

For surgery on one root of a molar tooth. Does not include placement of retrograde filling material. If more than one root is treated, see D3426.

D3426 Apicoectomy (each additional root) E1

Typically used for premolar and molar surgeries when more than one root is treated during the same procedure. This does not include retrograde filling material placement.

~~D3427 Periradicular surgery without apicoectomy~~ ✖

D3428 Bone graft in conjunction with periradicular surgery - per tooth, single site E1

Includes non-autogenous graft material.

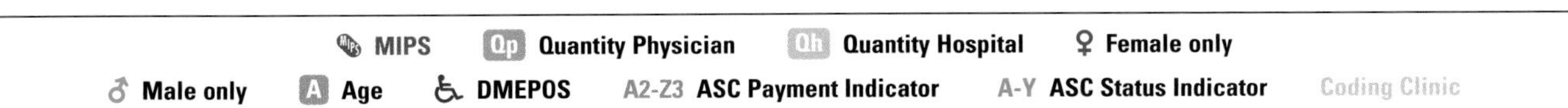
MIPS Qp Quantity Physician Qh Quantity Hospital ♀ Female only
♂ Male only A Age DMEPOS A2-Z3 ASC Payment Indicator A-Y ASC Status Indicator Coding Clinic

D3429 Bone graft in conjunction with periradicular surgery - each additional contiguous tooth in the same surgical site Ⓑ E1

Includes non-autogenous graft material.

D3430 Retrograde filling - per root Ⓑ E1

For placement of retrograde filling material during periradicular surgery procedures. If more than one filling is placed in one root - report as D3999 and describe.

D3431 Biologic materials to aid in soft and osseous tissue regeneration in conjunction with periradicular surgery Ⓑ E1

D3432 Guided tissue regeneration, resorbable barrier, per site, in conjunction with periradicular surgery Ⓑ E1

D3450 Root amputation - per root Ⓑ E1

Root resection of a multi-rooted tooth while leaving the crown. If the crown is sectioned, see D3920.

D3460 Endodontic endosseous implant Ⓑ S

Placement of implant material, which extends from a pulpal space into the bone beyond the end of the root.

D3470 Intentional replantation (including necessary splinting) Ⓑ E1

For the intentional removal, inspection and treatment of the root and replacement of a tooth into its own socket. This does not include necessary retrograde filling material placement.

▶ **D3471** Surgical repair of root resorption – anterior

For surgery on root of anterior tooth. Does not include placement of restoration.

▶ **D3472** Surgical repair of root resorption – premolar

For surgery on root of premolar tooth. Does not include placement of restoration.

▶ **D3473** Surgical repair of root resorption – molar

For surgery on root of molar tooth. Does not include placement of restoration.

▶ **D3501** Surgical exposure of root surface without apicoectomy or repair of root resorption – anterior

Exposure of root surface followed by observation and surgical closure of the exposed area. Not to be used for or in conjunction with apicoectomy or repair of root resorption.

▶ **D3502** Surgical exposure of root surface without apicoectomy or repair of root resorption – premolar

Exposure of root surface followed by observation and surgical closure of the exposed area. Not to be used for or in conjunction with apicoectomy or repair of root resorption.

▶ **D3503** Surgical exposure of root surface without apicoectomy or repair of root resorption – molar

Exposure of root surface followed by observation and surgical closure of the exposed area. Not to be used for or in conjunction with apicoectomy or repair of root resorption.

Other Endodontic Procedures

D3910 Surgical procedure for isolation of tooth with rubber dam Ⓑ E1

D3920 Hemisection (including any root removal), not including root canal therapy Ⓑ E1

Includes separation of a multi-rooted tooth into separate sections containing the root and the overlying portion of the crown. It may also include the removal of one or more of those sections.

D3950 Canal preparation and fitting of preformed dowel or post Ⓑ E1

Should not be reported in conjunction with D2952, D2953, D2954 or D2957 by the same practitioner.

None

D3999 Unspecified endodontic procedure, by report Ⓑ S

Used for procedure that is not adequately described by a code. Describe procedure.

▶ New ⤺ Revised ✔ Reinstated ~~deleted~~ Deleted ⊘ Not covered or valid by Medicare
Special coverage instructions ✻ Carrier discretion Ⓑ Bill Part B MAC Ⓔ Bill DME MAC

Periodontics (D4210-D4999)

Surgical Services (Including Usual Postoperative Care)

D4210 Gingivectomy or gingivoplasty - four or more contiguous teeth or tooth bounded spaces per quadrant Ⓑ E1

It is performed to eliminate suprabony pockets or to restore normal architecture when gingival enlargements or asymmetrical or unaesthetic topography is evident with normal bony configuration.

Cross Reference 41820

D4211 Gingivectomy or gingivoplasty - one to three contiguous teeth or tooth bounded spaces per quadrant Ⓑ E1

It is performed to eliminate suprabony pockets or to restore normal architecture when gingival enlargements or asymmetrical or unaesthetic topography is evident with normal bony configuration.

D4212 Gingivectomy or gingivoplasty to allow access for restorative procedure, per tooth Ⓑ E1

D4230 Anatomical crown exposure - four or more contiguous teeth or bounded tooth spaces per quadrant Ⓑ E1

This procedure is utilized in an otherwise periodontally healthy area to remove enlarged gingival tissue and supporting bone (ostectomy) to provide an anatomically correct gingival relationship.

D4231 Anatomical crown exposure - one to three teeth or bounded tooth spaces per quadrant Ⓑ E1

This procedure is utilized in an otherwise periodontally healthy area to remove enlarged gingival tissue and supporting bone (ostectomy) to provide an anatomically correct gingival relationship.

D4240 Gingival flap procedure, including root planing - four or more contiguous teeth or tooth bounded spaces per quadrant Ⓑ E1

A soft tissue flap is reflected or resected to allow debridement of the root surface and the removal of granulation tissue. Osseous recontouring is not accomplished in conjunction with this procedure. May include open flap curettage, reverse bevel flap surgery, modified Kirkland flap procedure, and modified Widman surgery. This procedure is performed in the presence of moderate to deep probing depths, loss of attachment, need to maintain aesthetics, need for increased access to the root surface and alveolar bone, or to determine the presence of a cracked tooth, fractured root, or external root resorption. Other procedures may be required concurrent to D4240 and should be reported separately using their own unique codes.

D4241 Gingival flap procedure, including root planing - one to three contiguous teeth or tooth bounded spaces per quadrant Ⓑ E1

A soft tissue flap is reflected or resected to allow debridement of the root surface and the removal of granulation tissue. Osseous recontouring is not accomplished in conjunction with this procedure. May include open flap curettage, reverse bevel flap surgery, modified Kirkland flap procedure, and modified Widman surgery. This procedure is performed in the presence of moderate to deep probing depths, loss of attachment, need to maintain aesthetics, need for increased access to the root surface and alveolar bone, or to determine the presence of a cracked tooth, fractured root, or external root resorption. Other procedures may be required concurrent to D4241 and should be reported separately using their own unique codes.

D4245 Apically positioned flap Ⓑ E1

Procedure is used to preserve keratinized gingiva in conjunction with osseous resection and second stage implant procedure. Procedure may also be used to preserve keratinized/attached gingiva during surgical exposure of labially impacted teeth, and may be used during treatment of peri-implantitis.

D4249 Clinical crown lengthening - hard tissue Ⓑ E1

This procedure is employed to allow a restorative procedure on a tooth with little or no tooth structure exposed to the oral cavity. Crown lengthening requires reflection of a full thickness flap and removal of bone, altering the crown to root ratio. It is performed in a healthy periodontal environment, as opposed to osseous surgery, which is performed in the presence of periodontal disease.

D4260 Osseous surgery (including elevation of a full thickness flap and closure) - four or more contiguous teeth or tooth bounded spaces per quadrant Ⓑ S

This procedure modifies the bony support of the teeth by reshaping the alveolar process to achieve a more physiologic form during the surgical procedure. This must include the removal of supporting bone (ostectomy) and/or non-supporting bone (osteoplasty). Other procedures may be required concurrent to D4260 and should be reported using their own unique codes.

D4261 Osseous surgery (including elevation of a full thickness flap and closure) - one to three contiguous teeth or tooth bounded spaces per quadrant Ⓑ E1

This procedure modifies the bony support of the teeth by reshaping the alveolar process to achieve a more physiologic form during the surgical procedure. This must include the removal of supporting bone (ostectomy) and/or non-supporting bone (osteoplasty). Other procedures may be required concurrent to D4261 and should be reported using their own unique codes.

D4263 Bone replacement graft - retained natural tooth - first site in quadrant Ⓑ S

This procedure involves the use of grafts to stimulate periodontal regeneration when the disease process has led to a deformity of the bone. This procedure does not include flap entry and closure, wound debridement, osseous contouring, or the placement of biologic materials to aid in osseous tissue regeneration or barrier membranes. Other separate procedures delivered concurrently are documented with their own codes. Not to be reported for an edentulous space or an extraction site.

D4264 Bone replacement graft - retained natural tooth - each additional site in quadrant Ⓑ S

This procedure involves the use of grafts to stimulate periodontal regeneration when the disease process has led to a deformity of the bone. This procedure does not include flap entry and closure, wound debridement, osseous contouring, or the placement of biologic materials to aid in osseous tissue regeneration or barrier membranes. This procedure is performed concurrently with one or more bone replacement grafts to document the number of sites involved. Not to be reported for an edentulous space or an extraction site.

D4265 Biologic materials to aid in soft and osseous tissue regeneration Ⓑ E1

Biologic materials may be used alone or with other regenerative substrates such as bone and barrier membranes, depending upon their formulation and the presentation of the periodontal defect. This procedure does not include surgical entry and closure, wound debridement, osseous contouring, or the placement of graft materials and/or barrier membranes. Other separate procedures may be required concurrent to D4265 and should be reported using their own unique codes.

D4266 Guided tissue regeneration - resorbable barrier, per site Ⓑ E1

This procedure does not include flap entry and closure, or, when indicated, wound debridement, osseous contouring, bone replacement grafts, and placement of biologic materials to aid in osseous regeneration. This procedure can be used for periodontal and peri-implant defects.

D4267 Guided tissue regeneration - nonresorbable barrier, per site, (includes membrane removal) Ⓑ E1

This procedure does not include flap entry and closure, or, when indicated, wound debridement, osseous contouring, bone replacement grafts, and placement of biologic materials to aid in osseous regeneration. This procedure can be used for periodontal and peri-implant defects.

D4268 Surgical revision procedure, per tooth Ⓑ S

This procedure is to refine the results of a previously provided surgical procedure. This may require a surgical procedure to modify the irregular contours of hard or soft tissue. A mucoperiosteal flap may be elevated to allow access to reshape alveolar bone. The flaps are replaced or repositioned and sutured.

D4270 Pedicle soft tissue graft procedure Ⓑ S

A pedicle flap of gingiva can be raised from an edentulous ridge, adjacent teeth, or from the existing gingiva on the tooth and moved laterally or coronally to replace alveolar mucosa as marginal tissue. The procedure can be used to cover an exposed root or to eliminate a gingival defect if the root is not too prominent in the arch.

D4273 Autogenous connective tissue graft procedure (including donor and recipient surgical sites) first tooth, implant, or edentulous tooth position in graft Ⓑ S

There are two surgical sites. The recipient site utilizes a split thickness incision, retaining the overlapping flap of gingiva and/or mucosa. The connective tissue is dissected from a separate donor site leaving an epithelialized flap for closure.

D4274 Mesial/distal wedge procedure, single tooth (when not performed in conjuction with surgical procedures in the same anatomical area) Ⓑ E1

This procedure is performed in an edentulous area adjacent to a tooth, allowing removal of a tissue wedge to gain access for debridement, permit close flap adaptation, and reduce pocket depths.

D4275 Non-autogenous connective tissue graft (including recipient site and donor material) first tooth, implant, or edentulous tooth position in graft Ⓑ E1

There is only a recipient surgical site utilizing split thickness incision, retaining the overlaying flap of gingiva and/or mucosa. A donor surgical site is not present.

D4276 Combined connective tissue and double pedicle graft, per tooth Ⓑ E1

Advanced gingival recession often cannot be corrected with a single procedure. Combined tissue grafting procedures are needed to achieve the desired outcome.

D4277 Free soft tissue graft procedure (including recipient and donor surgical sites) first tooth, implant or edentulous tooth position in graft Ⓑ E1

D4278 Free soft tissue graft procedure (including recipient and donor surgical sites) each additional contiguous tooth, implant or edentulous tooth position in same graft site Ⓑ E1

Used in conjunction with D4277.

D4283 Autogenous connective tissue graft procedure (including donor and recipient surgical sites) - each additional contiguous tooth, implant or edentulous tooth position in same graft site Ⓑ E1

Used in conjunction with D4273.

D4285 Non-autogenous connective tissue graft procedure (including recipient surgical site and donor material) - each additional contiguous tooth, implant or edentulous tooth position in same graft site Ⓑ E1

Used in conjunction with D4275.

Non-Surgical Periodontal Services

D4320 Provisional splinting - intracoronal Ⓑ E1

This is an interim stabilization of mobile teeth. A variety of methods and appliances may be employed for this purpose. Identify the teeth involved.

D4321 Provisional splinting - extracoronal Ⓑ E1

This is an interim stabilization of mobile teeth. A variety of methods and appliances may be employed for this purpose. Identify the teeth involved.

D4341 Periodontal scaling and root planing - four or more teeth per quadrant Ⓑ E1

This procedure involves instrumentation of the crown and root surfaces of the teeth to remove plaque and calculus from these surfaces. It is indicated for patients with periodontal disease and is therapeutic, not prophylactic, in nature. Root planing is the definitive procedure designed for the removal of cementum and dentin that is rough, and/or permeated by calculus or contaminated with toxins or microorganisms. Some soft tissue removal occurs. This procedure may be used as a definitive treatment in some stages of periodontal disease and/or as a part of pre-surgical procedures in others.

D4342 Periodontal scaling and root planing - one to three teeth, per quadrant Ⓑ E1

This procedure involves instrumentation of the crown and root surfaces of the teeth to remove plaque and calculus from these surfaces. It is indicated for patients with periodontal disease and is therapeutic, not prophylactic, in nature. Root planing is the definitive procedure designed for the removal of cementum and dentin that is rough, and/or permeated by calculus or contaminated with toxins or microorganisms. Some soft tissue removal occurs. This procedure may be used as a definitive treatment in some stages of periodontal disease and/or as a part of pre-surgical procedures in others.

D4346 Scaling in presence of generalized moderate or severe gingival inflammation - full mouth, after oral evaluation Ⓑ E1

The removal of plaque, calculus and stains from supra- and sub-gingival tooth surfaces when there is generalized moderate or severe gingival inflammation in the absence of periodontitis. It is indicated for patients who have swollen, inflamed gingiva, generalized suprabony pockets, and moderate to severe bleeding on probing. Should not be reported in conjunction with prophylaxis, scaling and root planing, or debridement procedures.

D4355 Full mouth debridement to enable a comprehensive oral evaluation and diagnosis on a subsequent visit Ⓑ S

Full mouth debridement involves the preliminary removal of plaque and calculus that interferes with the ability of the dentist to perform a comprehensive oral evaluation. Not to be completed on the same day as D0150, D0160, or D0180.

D4381 Localized delivery of antimicrobial agents via a controlled release vehicle into diseased crevicular tissue, per tooth Ⓑ S

FDA approved subgingival delivery devices containing antimicrobial medication(s) are inserted into periodontal pockets to suppress the pathogenic microbiota. These devices slowly release the pharmacological agents so they can remain at the intended site of action in a therapeutic concentration for a sufficient length of time.

Other Periodontal Services

D4910 Periodontal maintenance Ⓑ E1

This procedure is instituted following periodontal therapy and continues at varying intervals, determined by the clinical evaluation of the dentist, for the life of the dentition or any implant replacements. It includes removal of the bacterial plaque and calculus from supragingival and subgingival regions, site specific scaling and root planing where indicated, and polishing the teeth. If new or recurring periodontal disease appears, additional diagnostic and treatment procedures must be considered.

D4920 Unscheduled dressing change (by someone other than treating dentist or their staff) Ⓑ E1

D4921 Gingival irrigation - per quadrant Ⓑ E1

Irrigation of gingival pockets with medicinal agent. Not to be used to report use of mouth rinses or non-invasive chemical debridement.

None

D4999 Unspecified periodontal procedure, by report Ⓑ E1

Use for procedure that is not adequately described by a code. Describe procedure.

Prosthodontics (removable)

Complete Dentures (Including Routine Post-Delivery Care)

D5110 Complete denture - maxillary Ⓑ E1

D5120 Complete denture - mandibular Ⓑ E1

D5130 Immediate denture - maxillary Ⓑ E1

Includes limited follow-up care only; does not include required future rebasing/relining procedure(s).

D5140 Immediate denture - mandibular Ⓑ E1

Includes limited follow-up care only; does not include required future rebasing/relining procedure(s).

Partial Dentures (Including Routine Post-Delivery Care)

D5211 Maxillary partial denture-resin base (including retentive/clasping materials, rests and teeth) Ⓑ E1

Includes acrylic resin base denture with resin or wrought wire clasps.

D5212 Mandibular partial denture-resin base (including, retentive/clasping materials, rests and teeth) Ⓑ E1

Includes acrylic resin base denture with resin or wrought wire clasps.

D5213 Maxillary partial denture - cast metal framework with resin denture bases (including retentive/clasping materials, rests and teeth) Ⓑ E1

D5214 Mandibular partial denture - cast metal framework with resin denture bases (including retentive/clasping materials, rests and teeth) Ⓑ E1

D5221 Immediate maxillary partial denture - resin base (including retentive/clasping materials, rests and teeth) Ⓑ E1

Includes limited follow-up care only; does not include future rebasing/relining procedure(s).

D5222 Immediate mandibular partial denture - resin base (including retentive/clasping materials, rests and teeth) Ⓑ E1

Includes limited follow-up care only; does not include future rebasing/relining procedure(s).

D5223 Immediate maxillary partial denture - cast metal framework with resin denture bases (including retentive/clasping materials, rests and teeth) Ⓑ E1

Includes limited follow-up care only; does not include future rebasing/relining procedure(s).

D5224 Immediate mandibular partial denture - cast metal framework with resin denture bases (including retentive/clasping materials, rests and teeth) Ⓑ E1

Includes limited follow-up care only; does not include future rebasing/relining procedure(s).

⮐ **D5225** Maxillary partial denture - flexible base (including retentive/clasping materials, rests and teeth) Ⓑ E1

⮐ **D5226** Mandibular partial denture - flexible base (including retentive/clasping materials, rests and teeth) Ⓑ E1

⮐ **D5282** Removable unilateral partial denture - one piece cast metal (including retentive/clasping materials, and teeth), maxillary Ⓑ E1

⮐ **D5283** Removable unilateral partial denture - one piece cast metal (including retentive/clasping materials, rests, and teeth), mandibular Ⓑ E1

⮐ **D5284** Removable unilateral partial denture - one piece flexible base (including retentive/clasping materials, rests, rests, and teeth) - per quadrant E1

⮐ **D5286** Removable unilateral partial denture - one piece resin (including retentive/clasping materials, rests, and teeth) - per quadrant E1

Adjustment to Dentures

D5410 Adjust complete denture - maxillary Ⓑ E1

D5411 Adjust complete denture - mandibular Ⓑ E1

D5421 Adjust partial denture - maxillary Ⓑ E1

D5422 Adjust partial denture - mandibular Ⓑ E1

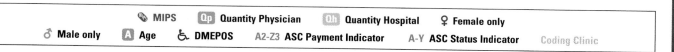

Repairs to Complete Dentures

D5511 Repair broken complete denture base, mandibular Ⓑ E1

D5512 Repair broken complete denture base, maxillary Ⓑ E1

D5520 Replace missing or broken teeth-complete denture (each tooth) Ⓑ E1

Repairs to Partial Dentures

D5611 Repair resin partial denture base, mandibular Ⓑ E1

D5612 Repair resin partial denture base, maxillary Ⓑ E1

D5621 Repair cast partial framework, mandibular Ⓑ E1

D5622 Repair cast partial framework, maxillary Ⓑ E1

D5630 Repair or replace broken, retentive clasping materials - per tooth Ⓑ E1

D5640 Replace broken teeth - per tooth Ⓑ E1

D5650 Add tooth to existing partial denture Ⓑ E1

D5660 Add clasp to existing partial denture - per tooth Ⓑ E1

D5670 Replace all teeth and acrylic on cast metal framework (maxillary) Ⓑ E1

D5671 Replace all teeth and acrylic on cast metal framework (mandibular) Ⓑ E1

Denture Rebase Procedures

D5710 Rebase complete maxillary denture Ⓑ E1

D5711 Rebase complete mandibular denture Ⓑ E1

D5720 Rebase maxillary partial denture Ⓑ E1

D5721 Rebase mandibular partial denture Ⓑ E1

Denture Reline Procedures

⮎ **D5730** Reline complete maxillary denture (direct) Ⓑ E1

⮎ **D5731** Reline lower complete mandibular denture (direct) Ⓑ E1

⮎ **D5740** Reline maxillary partial denture (direct) Ⓑ E1

⮎ **D5741** Reline mandibular partial denture (direct) Ⓑ E1

⮎ **D5750** Reline complete maxillary denture (indirect) Ⓑ E1

⮎ **D5751** Reline complete mandibular denture (indirect) Ⓑ E1

⮎ **D5760** Reline maxillary partial denture (indirect) Ⓑ E1

⮎ **D5761** Reline mandibular partial denture (indirect) Ⓑ E1

Interim Prosthesis

D5810 Interim complete denture (maxillary) Ⓑ E1

D5811 Interim complete denture (mandibular) Ⓑ E1

⮎ **D5820** Interim partial denture (including retentive/clasping materials, rests, and teeth), maxillary Ⓑ E1

~~Includes any necessary clasps and rests.~~ ✖

⮎ **D5821** Interim partial denture (including retentive/clasping materials, rests, and teeth), mandibular Ⓑ E1

~~Includes any necessary clasps and rests.~~ ✖

Other Removable Prosthetic Services

D5850 Tissue conditioning, maxillary Ⓑ E1

Treatment reline using materials designed to heal unhealthy ridges prior to more definitive final restoration.

D5851 Tissue conditioning, mandibular Ⓑ E1

Treatment reline using materials designed to heal unhealthy ridges prior to more definitive final restoration.

D5862 Precision attachment, by report Ⓑ E1

Each set of male and female components should be reported as one precision attachment. Describe the type of attachment used.

D5863 Overdenture - complete maxillary Ⓑ E1

D5864 Overdenture - partial maxillary Ⓑ E1

D5865 Overdenture - complete mandibular Ⓑ E1

D5866 Overdenture - partial mandibular Ⓑ E1

D5867 Replacement of replaceable part of semi-precision or precision attachment (male or female component) Ⓑ E1

D5875 Modification of removable prosthesis following implant surgery Ⓑ E1

Attachment assemblies are reported using separate codes.

D5876 Add metal substructure to acrylic full denture (per arch) Ⓑ E1

▶ New ⮎ Revised ✔ Reinstated ~~deleted~~ Deleted ⊘ Not covered or valid by Medicare
Special coverage instructions ✻ Carrier discretion Ⓑ Bill Part B MAC Ⓓ Bill DME MAC

None

D5899 Unspecified removable prosthodontic procedure, by report Ⓑ E1

Use for a procedure that is not adequately described by a code. Describe procedure.

Maxillofacial Prosthetics

D5911 Facial moulage (sectional) Ⓑ S

A sectional facial moulage impression is a procedure used to record the soft tissue contours of a portion of the face. Occasionally several separate sectional impressions are made, then reassembled to provide a full facial contour cast. The impression is utilized to create a partial facial moulage and generally is not reusable.

D5912 Facial moulage (complete) Ⓑ S

Synonymous terminology: facial impression, face mask impression. A complete facial moulage impression is a procedure used to record the soft tissue contours of the whole face. The impression is utilized to create a facial moulage and generally is not reusable.

D5913 Nasal prosthesis Ⓑ E1

Synonymous terminology: artificial nose. A removable prosthesis attached to the skin, which artificially restores part or all of the nose. Fabrication of a nasal prosthesis requires creation of an original mold. Additional prostheses usually can be made from the same mold, and assuming no further tissue changes occur, the same mold can be utilized for extended periods of time. When a new prosthesis is made from the existing mold, this procedure is termed a nasal prosthesis replacement.

Cross Reference 21087

D5914 Auricular prosthesis Ⓑ E1

Synonymous terminology: artificial ear, ear prosthesis. A removable prosthesis, which artificially restores part or all of the natural ear. Usually, replacement prostheses can be made from the original mold if tissue bed changes have not occurred. Creation of an auricular prosthesis requires fabrication of a mold, from which additional prostheses usually can be made, as needed later (auricular prosthesis, replacement).

Cross Reference 21086

D5915 Orbital prosthesis Ⓑ E1

A prosthesis, which artificially restores the eye, eyelids, and adjacent hard and soft tissue, lost as a result of trauma or surgery. Fabrication of an orbital prosthesis requires creation of an original mold. Additional prostheses usually can be made from the same mold, and assuming no further tissue changes occur, the same mold can be utilized for extended periods of time. When a new prosthesis is made from the existing mold, this procedure is termed an orbital prosthesis replacement.

Cross Reference L8611

D5916 Ocular prosthesis Ⓑ E1

Synonymous terminology: artificial eye, glass eye. A prosthesis, which artificially replaces an eye missing as a result of trauma, surgery or congenital absence. The prosthesis does not replace missing eyelids or adjacent skin, mucosa or muscle. Ocular prostheses require semiannual or annual cleaning and polishing. Also, occasional revisions to re-adapt the prosthesis to the tissue bed may be necessary. Glass eyes are rarely made and cannot be re-adapted.

Cross Reference V2623, V2629

D5919 Facial prosthesis Ⓑ E1

Synonymous terminology: prosthetic dressing. A removable prosthesis, which artificially replaces a portion of the face, lost due to surgery, trauma or congenital absence. Flexion of natural tissues may preclude adaptation and movement of the prosthesis to match the adjacent skin. Salivary leakage, when communicating with the oral cavity, adversely affects retention.

Cross Reference 21088

D5922 Nasal septal prosthesis Ⓑ E1

Synonymous terminology: septal plug, septal button. Removable prosthesis to occlude (obturate) a hole within the nasal septal wall. Adverse chemical degradation in this moist environment may require frequent replacement. Silicone prostheses are occasionally subject to fungal invasion.

Cross Reference 30220

D5923 Ocular prosthesis, interim Ⓑ E1

Synonymous terminology: eye shell, shell, ocular conformer, conformer. A temporary replacement generally made of clear acrylic resin for an eye lost due to surgery or trauma. No attempt is made to re-establish aesthetics. Fabrication of an interim ocular prosthesis generally implies subsequent fabrication of an aesthetic ocular prosthesis.

Cross Reference 92330

D5924 Cranial prosthesis Ⓑ E1

Synonymous terminology: skull plate, cranioplasty prosthesis, cranial implant. A biocompatible, permanently implanted replacement of a portion of the skull bones; an artificial replacement for a portion of the skull bone.

Cross Reference 62143

D5925 Facial augmentation implant prosthesis Ⓑ E1

Synonymous terminology: facial implant. An implantable biocompatible material generally onlayed upon an existing bony area beneath the skin tissue to fill in or collectively raise portions of the overlaying facial skin tissues to create acceptable contours. Although some forms of pre-made surgical implants are commercially available, the facial augmentation is usually custom made for surgical implantation for each individual patient due to the irregular or extensive nature of the facial deficit.

Cross Reference 21208

D5926 Nasal prosthesis, replacement Ⓑ E1

Synonymous terminology: replacement nose. An artificial nose produced from a previously made mold. A replacement prosthesis does not require fabrication of a new mold. Generally, several prostheses can be made from the same mold assuming no changes occur in the tissue bed due to surgery or age related topographical variations.

Cross Reference 21087

D5927 Auricular prosthesis, replacement Ⓑ E1

Synonymous terminology: replacement ear. An artificial ear produced from a previously made mold. A replacement prosthesis does not require fabrication of a new mold. Generally, several prostheses can be made from the same mold assuming no changes occur in the tissue bed due to surgery or age related topographical variations.

Cross Reference 21086

D5928 Orbital prosthesis, replacement Ⓑ E1

A replacement for a previously made orbital prosthesis. A replacement prosthesis does not require fabrication of a new mold. Generally, several prostheses can be made from the same mold assuming no changes occur in the tissue bed due to surgery or age related topographical variations.

Cross Reference 67550

D5929 Facial prosthesis, replacement Ⓑ E1

A replacement facial prosthesis made from the original mold. A replacement prosthesis does not require fabrication of a new mold. Generally, several prostheses can be made from the same mold assuming no changes occur in the tissue bed due to further surgery or age related topographical variations.

Cross Reference 21088

D5931 Obturator prosthesis, surgical Ⓑ E1

Synonymous terminology: obturator, surgical stayplate, immediate temporary obturator. A temporary prosthesis inserted during or immediately following surgical or traumatic loss of a portion or all of one or both maxillary bones and contiguous alveolar structures (e.g., gingival tissue, teeth). Frequent revisions of surgical obturators are necessary during the ensuing healing phase (approximately six months). Some dentists prefer to replace many or all teeth removed by the surgical procedure in the surgical obturator, while others do not replace any teeth. Further surgical revisions may require fabrication of another surgical obturator (e.g., an initially planned small defect may be revised and greatly enlarged after the final pathology report indicates margins are not free of tumor).

Cross Reference 21079

D5932 Obturator prosthesis, definitive Ⓑ E1

Synonymous terminology: obturator. A prosthesis, which artificially replaces part or all of the maxilla and associated teeth, lost due to surgery, trauma or congenital defects. A definitive obturator is made when it is deemed that further tissue changes or recurrence of tumor are unlikely and a more permanent prosthetic rehabilitation can be achieved; it is intended for long-term use.

Cross Reference 21080

D5933 Obturator prosthesis, modification Ⓑ E1

Synonymous terminology: adjustment, denture adjustment, temporary or office reline. Revision or alteration of an existing obturator (surgical, interim, or definitive); possible modifications include relief of the denture base due to tissue compression, augmentation of the seal or peripheral areas to affect adequate sealing or separation between the nasal and oral cavities.

Cross Reference 21080

D5934 Mandibular resection prosthesis with guide flange Ⓑ E1

Synonymous terminology: resection device, resection appliance. A prosthesis which guides the remaining portion of the mandible, left after a partial resection, into a more normal relationship with the maxilla. This allows for some tooth-to-tooth or an improved tooth contact. It may also artificially replace missing teeth and thereby increase masticatory efficiency.

Cross Reference 21081

D5935 Mandibular resection prosthesis without guide flange Ⓑ E1

A prosthesis which helps guide the partially resected mandible to a more normal relation with the maxilla allowing for increased tooth contact. It does not have a flange or ramp, however, to assist in directional closure. It may replace missing teeth and thereby increase masticatory efficiency. Dentists who treat mandibulectomy patients may prefer to replace some, all or none of the teeth in the defect area. Frequently, the defect's margins preclude even partial replacement. Use of a guide (a mandibular resection prosthesis with a guide flange) may not be possible due to anatomical limitations or poor patient tolerance. Ramps, extended occlusal arrangements and irregular occlusal positioning relative to the denture foundation frequently preclude stability of the prostheses, and thus some prostheses are poorly tolerated under such adverse circumstances.

Cross Reference 21081

D5936 Obturator/prosthesis, interim Ⓑ E1

Synonymous terminology: immediate postoperative obturator. A prosthesis which is made following completion of the initial healing after a surgical resection of a portion or all of one or both the maxillae; frequently many or all teeth in the defect area are replaced by this prosthesis. This prosthesis replaces the surgical obturator, which is usually inserted at, or immediately following the resection.

Generally, an interim obturator is made to facilitate closure of the resultant defect after initial healing has been completed. Unlike the surgical obturator, which usually is made prior to surgery and frequently revised in the operating room during surgery, the interim obturator is made when the defect margins are clearly defined and further surgical revisions are not planned. It is a provisional prosthesis, which may replace some or all lost teeth, and other lost bone and soft tissue structures. Also, it frequently must be revised (termed an obturator prosthesis modification) during subsequent dental procedures (e.g., restorations, gingival surgery) as well as to compensate for further tissue shrinkage before a definitive obturator prosthesis is made.

Cross Reference 21079

D5937 Trismus appliance (not for tm treatment) Ⓑ E1

Synonymous terminology: occlusal device for mandibular trismus, dynamic bite opener. A prosthesis, which assists the patient in increasing their oral aperture width in order to eat as well as maintain oral hygiene. Several versions and designs are possible, all intending to ease the severe lack of oral opening experienced by many patients immediately following extensive intraoral surgical procedures.

D5951 Feeding aid Ⓑ E1

Synonymous terminology: feeding prosthesis. A prosthesis, which maintains the right and left maxillary segments of an infant cleft palate patient in their proper orientation until surgery is performed to repair the cleft. It closes the oral-nasal cavity defect, thus enhancing sucking and swallowing. Used on an interim basis, this prosthesis achieves separation of the oral and nasal cavities in infants born with wide clefts necessitating delayed closure. It is eliminated if surgical closure can be affected or, alternatively, with eruption of the deciduous dentition a pediatric speech aid may be made to facilitate closure of the defect.

D5952 Speech aid prosthesis, pediatric Ⓑ A E1

Synonymous terminology: nasopharyngeal obturator, speech appliance, obturator, cleft palate appliance, prosthetic speech aid, speech bulb. A temporary or interim prosthesis used to close a defect in the hard and/ or soft palate. It may replace tissue lost due to developmental or surgical alterations. It is necessary for the production of intelligible speech. Normal lateral growth of the palatal bones necessitates occasional replacement of this prosthesis. Intermittent revisions of the obturator section can assist in maintenance of palatalpharyngeal closure (termed a speech aid prosthesis modification). Frequently, such prostheses are not fabricated before the deciduous dentition is fully erupted since clasp retention is often essential.

Cross Reference 21084

D5953 Speech aid prosthesis, adult Ⓑ A E1

Synonymous terminology: prosthetic speech appliance, speech aid, speech bulb. A definitive prosthesis, which can improve speech in adult cleft palate patients either by obturating (sealing off) a palatal cleft or fistula, or occasionally by assisting an incompetent soft palate. Both mechanisms are necessary to achieve velopharyngeal competency. Generally, this prosthesis is fabricated when no further growth is anticipated and the objective is to achieve long-term use. Hence, more precise materials and techniques are utilized. Occasionally such procedures are accomplished in conjunction with precision attachments in crown work undertaken on some or all maxillary teeth to achieve improved aesthetics.

Cross Reference 21084

D5954 Palatal augmentation prosthesis Ⓑ E1

Synonymous terminology: superimposed prosthesis, maxillary glossectomy prosthesis, maxillary speech prosthesis, palatal drop prosthesis. A removable prosthesis which alters the hard and/or soft palate's topographical form adjacent to the tongue.

Cross Reference 21082

D5955 Palatal lift prosthesis, definitive Ⓑ E1

A prosthesis which elevates the soft palate superiorly and aids in restoration of soft palate functions which may be lost due to an acquired, congenital or developmental defect. A definitive palatal lift is usually made for patients whose experience with an interim palatal lift has been successful, especially if surgical alterations are deemed unwarranted.

Cross Reference 21083

D5958 Palatal lift prosthesis, interim Ⓑ E1

Synonymous terminology: diagnostic palatal lift. A prosthesis which elevates and assists in restoring soft palate function which may be lost due to clefting, surgery, trauma or unknown paralysis. It is intended for interim use to determine its usefulness in achieving palatalpharyngeal competency or enhance swallowing reflexes. This prosthesis is intended for interim use as a diagnostic aid to assess the level of possible improvement in speech intelligibility. Some clinicians believe use of a palatal lift on an interim basis may stimulate an otherwise flaccid soft palate to increase functional activity, subsequently lessening its need.

Cross Reference 21083

D5959 Palatal lift prosthesis, modification Ⓑ E1

Synonymous terminology: revision of lift, adjustment. Alterations in the adaptation, contour, form or function of an existing palatal lift necessitated due to tissue impingement, lack of function, poor clasp adaptation or the like.

Cross Reference 21083

D5960 Speech aid prosthesis, modification Ⓑ E1

Synonymous terminology: adjustment, repair, revision. Any revision of a pediatric or adult speech aid not necessitating its replacement. Frequently, revisions of the obturating section of any speech aid is required to facilitate enhanced speech intelligibility. Such revisions or repairs do not require complete remaking of the prosthesis, thus extending its longevity.

Cross Reference 21084

D5982 Surgical stent Ⓑ E1

Synonymous terminology: periodontal stent, skin graft stent, columellar stent. Stents are utilized to apply pressure to soft tissues to facilitate healing and prevent cicatrization or collapse. A surgical stent may be required in surgical and post-surgical revisions to achieve close approximation of tissues. Usually such materials as temporary or interim soft denture liners, gutta percha, or dental modeling impression compound may be used.

Cross Reference 21085

D5983 Radiation carrier Ⓑ S

Synonymous terminology: radiotherapy prosthesis, carrier prosthesis, radiation applicator, radium carrier, intracavity carrier, intracavity applicator. A device used to administer radiation to confined areas by means of capsules, beads or needles of radiation emitting materials such as radium or cesium. Its function is to hold the radiation source securely in the same location during the entire period of treatment. Radiation oncologists occasionally request these devices to achieve close approximation and controlled application of radiation to a tumor deemed amiable to eradication.

D5984 Radiation shield Ⓑ S

Synonymous terminology: radiation stent, tongue protector, lead shield. An intraoral prosthesis designed to shield adjacent tissues from radiation during orthovoltage treatment of malignant lesions of the head and neck region.

D5985 Radiation cone locator Ⓑ S

Synonymous terminology: docking device, cone locator. A prosthesis utilized to direct and reduplicate the path of radiation to an oral tumor during a split course of irradiation.

D5986 Fluoride gel carrier Ⓑ E1

Synonymous terminology: fluoride applicator. A prosthesis, which covers the teeth in either dental arch and is used to apply topical fluoride in close proximity to tooth enamel and dentin for several minutes daily.

D5987 Commissure splint Ⓑ S

Synonymous terminology: lip splint. A device placed between the lips, which assists in achieving increased opening between the lips. Use of such devices enhances opening where surgical, chemical or electrical alterations of the lips has resulted in severe restriction or contractures.

D5988 Surgical splint Ⓑ E1

Synonymous terminology: Gunning splint, modified Gunning splint, labiolingual splint, fenestrated splint, Kingsley splint, cast metal splint. Splints are designed to utilize existing teeth and/or alveolar processes as points of anchorage to assist in stabilization and immobilization of broken bones during healing. They are used to re-establish, as much as possible, normal occlusal relationships during the process of immobilization. Frequently, existing prostheses (e.g., a patient's complete dentures) can be modified to serve as surgical splints. Frequently, surgical splints have arch bars added to facilitate intermaxillary fixation. Rubber elastics may be used to assist in this process. Circummandibular eyelet hooks can be utilized for enhanced stabilization with wiring to adjacent bone.

D5991 Vesicobullous disease medicament carrier Ⓑ E1

A custom fabricated carrier that covers the teeth and alveolar mucosa, or alveolar mucosa alone, and is used to deliver prescription medicaments for treatment of immunologically mediated vesiculobullous disease.

D5992 Adjust maxillofacial prosthetic appliance, by report Ⓑ E1

D5993 Maintenance and cleaning of a maxillofacial prosthesis (extra or intra-oral) other than required adjustments, by report Ⓑ E1

~~D5994 Periodontal medicament carrier with peripheral seal - laboratory processed~~ ✖

~~A custom fabricated, laboratory processed carrier that covers the teeth and alveolar mucosa. Used as a vehicle to deliver prescribed medicaments for sustained contact with the gingiva, alveolar mucosa, and into the periodontal sulcus or pocket.~~

▶ **D5995** Periodontal medicament carrier with peripheral seal – laboratory processed – maxillary

A custom fabricated, laboratory processed carrier for the maxillary arch that covers the teeth and alveolar mucosa. Used as a vehicle to deliver prescribed medicaments for sustained contact with the gingiva, alveolar mucosa, and into the periodontal sulcus or pocket.

▶ New ⤻ Revised ✔ Reinstated ~~deleted~~ Deleted ⊘ Not covered or valid by Medicare
Special coverage instructions ✻ Carrier discretion Ⓑ Bill Part B MAC Ⓑ Bill DME MAC

D5996 Periodontal medicament carrier with peripheral seal – laboratory processed – mandibular

A custom fabricated, laboratory processed carrier for the mandibular arch that covers the teeth and alveolar mucosa. Used as a vehicle to deliver prescribed medicaments for sustained contact with the gingiva, alveolar mucosa, and into the periodontal sulcus or pocket.

D5999 Unspecified maxillofacial prosthesis, by report E1

Used for procedure that is not adequately described by a code. Describe procedure.

Implant Services (D6010-D6199)

D6010-D6199: FPD = fixed partial denture

Surgical Services

D6010 Surgical placement of implant body: endosteal implant E1

Cross Reference 21248

D6011 Surgical access to an implant body (second stage implant surgery) E1

This procedure, also known as second stage implant surgery, involves removal of tissue that covers the implant body so that a fixture of any type can be placed, or an existing fixture be replaced with another. Examples of fixtures include but are not limited to healing caps, abutments shaped to help contour the gingival margins or the final restorative prosthesis.

D6012 Surgical placement of interim implant body for transitional prosthesis: endosteal implant E1

Includes removal during later therapy to accommodate the definitive restoration, which may include placement of other implants.

D6013 Surgical placement of mini implant E1

D6040 Surgical placement: eposteal implant E1

An eposteal (subperiosteal) framework of a biocompatible material designed and fabricated to fit on the surface of the bone of the mandible or maxilla with permucosal extensions which provide support and attachment of a prosthesis. This may be a complete arch or unilateral appliance. Eposteal implants rest upon the bone and under the periosteum.

Cross Reference 21245

D6050 Surgical placement: transosteal implant E1

A transosteal (transosseous) biocompatible device with threaded posts penetrating both the superior and inferior cortical bone plates of the mandibular symphysis and exiting through the permucosa providing support and attachment for a dental prosthesis. Transosteal implants are placed completely through the bone and into the oral cavity from extraoral or intraoral.

Cross Reference 21244

Implant Supported Prosthetics

D6051 Interim abutment - includes placement and removal E1

Includes placement and removal. A healing cap is not an interim abutment.

~~**D6052** Semi-precision attachment abutment~~ ✖

~~Includes placement of keeper assembly.~~

D6055 Connecting bar — implant supported or abutment supported E1

Utilized to stabilize and anchor a prosthesis.

D6056 Prefabricated abutment - includes modification and placement E1

Modification of a prefabricated abutment may be necessary.

D6057 Custom fabricated abutment - includes placement E1

Created by a laboratory process, specific for an individual application.

MIPS
Qp Quantity Physician
Qh Quantity Hospital
♀ Female only
♂ Male only
A Age
DMEPOS
A2-Z3 ASC Payment Indicator
A-Y ASC Status Indicator
Coding Clinic

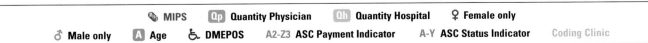

D6058 Abutment supported porcelain/ceramic crown Ⓑ E1

A single crown restoration that is retained, supported and stabilized by an abutment on an implant.

D6059 Abutment supported porcelain fused to metal crown (high noble metal) Ⓑ E1

A single metal-ceramic crown restoration that is retained, supported and stabilized by an abutment on an implant.

D6060 Abutment supported porcelain fused to metal crown (predominantly base metal) Ⓑ E1

A single metal-ceramic crown restoration that is retained, supported and stabilized by an abutment on an implant.

D6061 Abutment supported porcelain fused to metal crown (noble metal) Ⓑ E1

A single metal-ceramic crown restoration that is retained, supported and stabilized by an abutment on an implant.

D6062 Abutment supported cast metal crown (high noble metal) Ⓑ E1

A single cast metal crown restoration that is retained, supported and stabilized by an abutment on an implant.

D6063 Abutment supported cast metal crown (predominantly base metal) Ⓑ E1

A single cast metal crown restoration that is retained, supported and stabilized by an abutment on an implant.

D6064 Abutment supported cast metal crown (noble metal) Ⓑ E1

A single cast metal crown restoration that is retained, supported and stabilized by an abutment on an implant.

D6065 Implant supported porcelain/ceramic crown Ⓑ E1

A single crown restoration that is retained, supported and stabilized by an implant.

D6066 Implant supported crown - porcelain fused to high noble alloys Ⓑ E1

A single metal-ceramic crown restoration that is retained, supported and stabilized by an implant.

D6067 Implant supported crown - high noble alloys Ⓑ E1

A single cast metal or milled crown restoration that is retained, supported and stabilized by an implant.

D6068 Abutment supported retainer for porcelain/ceramic FPD Ⓑ E1

A ceramic retainer for a fixed partial denture that gains retention, support and stability from an abutment on an implant.

D6069 Abutment supported retainer for porcelain fused to metal FPD (high noble metal) Ⓑ E1

A metal-ceramic retainer for a fixed partial denture that gains retention, support and stability from an abutment on an implant.

D6070 Abutment supported retainer for porcelain fused to metal FPD (predominantly base metal) Ⓑ E1

A metal-ceramic retainer for a fixed partial denture that gains retention, support and stability from an abutment on an implant.

D6071 Abutment supported retainer for porcelain fused to metal FPD (noble metal) Ⓑ E1

A metal-ceramic retainer for a fixed partial denture that gains retention, support and stability from an abutment on an implant.

D6072 Abutment supported retainer for cast metal FPD (high noble metal) Ⓑ E1

A cast metal retainer for a fixed partial denture that gains retention, support and stability from an abutment on an implant.

D6073 Abutment supported retainer for cast metal FPD (predominantly base metal) Ⓑ E1

A cast metal retainer for a fixed partial denture that gains retention, support and stability from an abutment on an implant.

D6074 Abutment supported retainer for cast metal FPD (noble metal) Ⓑ E1

A cast metal retainer for a fixed partial denture that gains retention, support and stability from an abutment on an implant.

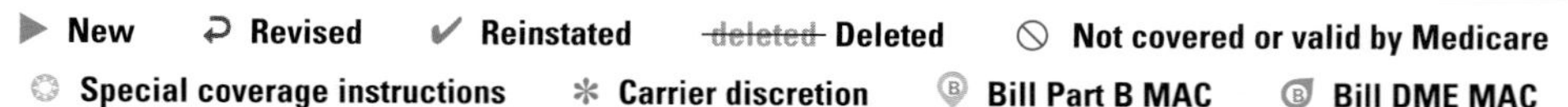

▶ New ↩ Revised ✓ Reinstated ~~deleted~~ Deleted ⊘ Not covered or valid by Medicare
Special coverage instructions ✻ Carrier discretion Ⓑ Bill Part B MAC Ⓓ Bill DME MAC

D6075 Implant supported retainer for ceramic FPD Ⓑ E1

A ceramic retainer for a fixed partial denture that gains retention, support and stability from an implant.

D6076 Implant supported retainer for FPD - porcelain fused to high noble alloys Ⓑ E1

A metal-ceramic retainer for a fixed partial denture that gains retention, support and stability from an implant.

D6077 Implant supported retainer for metal FPD - high noble alloys Ⓑ E1

A cast metal retainer for a fixed partial denture that gains retention, support and stability from an implant.

Other Implant Services

D6080 Implant maintenance procedures when prostheses are removed and reinserted, including cleansing of prostheses and abutments Ⓑ E1

This procedure includes active debriding of the implant(s) and examination of all aspects of the implant system(s), including the occlusion and stability of the superstructure. The patient is also instructed in thorough daily cleansing of the implant(s). This is not a per implant code, and is indicated for implant supported fixed prostheses.

D6081 Scaling and debridement in the presence of inflammation or mucositis of a single implant, including cleaning of the implant surfaces, without flap entry and closure Ⓑ E1

This procedure is not performed in conjunction with D1110, D4910, or D4346.

D6082 Implant supported crown - porcelain fused to predominantly base alloys E1

D6083 Implant supported crown - porcelain fused to noble alloys E1

D6084 Implant supported crown - porcelain fused to titanium and titanium alloys E1

D6085 Provisional implant crown Ⓑ E1

Used when a period of healing is necessary prior to fabrication and placement of permanent prosthetic.

D6086 Implant supported crown - predominantly base alloys E1

D6087 Implant supported crown - noble alloys E1

D6088 Implant supported crown - titanium and titanium alloys E1

D6090 Repair implant supported prosthesis by report Ⓑ E1

This procedure involves the repair or replacement of any part of the implant supported prosthesis.

Cross Reference 21299

↩ **D6091** Replacement of replaceable part of semi-precision or precision attachment (male or female component) of implant/abutment supported prosthesis, per attachment Ⓑ E1

This procedure applies to the replaceable male or female component of the attachment.

D6092 Re-cement or re-bond implant/abutment supported crown Ⓑ E1

D6093 Re-cement or re-bond implant/abutment supported fixed partial denture Ⓑ E1

D6094 Abutment supported crown - titanium and titanium alloys Ⓑ E1

A single crown restoration that is retained, supported and stabilized by an abutment on an implant. May be cast or milled.

D6095 Repair implant abutment, by report Ⓑ E1

This procedure involves the repair or replacement of any part of the implant abutment.

Cross Reference 21299

D6096 Remove broken implant retaining screw Ⓑ E1

D6097 Abutment supported crown - porcelain fused to titanium and titanium alloys E1

A single metal-ceramic crown restoration that is retained, supported, and stabilized by an abutment on an implant.

↩ **D6098** Implant supported retainer - porcelain fused to predominantly base alloys E1

A metal-ceramic retainer for a fixed partial denture that gains retention, support, and stability from an implant.

D6099 Implant supported retainer for FPD - porcelain fused to noble alloys E1

A metal-ceramic retainer for a fixed partial denture that gains retention, support, and stability from an implant.

Surgical Services

D6100 Implant removal, by report Ⓑ E1

This procedure involves the surgical removal of an implant. Describe procedure.

Cross Reference 21299

D6101 Debridement of a peri-implant defect or defects surrounding a single implant, and surface cleaning of exposed implant surfaces, including flap entry and closure Ⓑ E1

D6102 Debridement and osseous contouring of a peri-implant defect or defects surrounding a single implant and includes surface cleaning of the exposed implant surfaces and flap entry and closure Ⓑ E1

D6103 Bone graft for repair of peri-implant defect - does not include flap entry and closure Ⓑ E1

Placement of a barrier membrane or biologic materials to aid in osseous regeneration, are reported separately.

D6104 Bone graft at time of implant placement Ⓑ E1

Placement of a barrier membrane, or biologic materials to aid in osseous regeneration are reported separately.

Implant Supported Prosthetics

D6110 Implant /abutment supported removable denture for edentulous arch - maxillary Ⓑ E1

D6111 Implant /abutment supported removable denture for edentulous arch - mandibular Ⓑ E1

D6112 Implant/abutment supported removable denture for partially edentulous arch - maxillary Ⓑ E1

D6113 Implant/abutment supported removable denture for partially edentulous arch - mandibular Ⓑ E1

D6114 Implant/abutment supported fixed denture for edentulous arch - maxillary Ⓑ E1

D6115 Implant/abutment supported fixed denture for edentulous arch - mandibular Ⓑ E1

D6116 Implant/abutment supported fixed denture for partially edentulous arch - maxillary Ⓑ E1

D6117 Implant/abutment supported fixed denture for partially edentulous arch - mandibular Ⓑ E1

D6118 Implant/abutment supported interim fixed denture for edentulous arch mandibular Ⓑ E1

Used when a period of healing is necessary prior to fabrication and placement of a permanent prosthetic.

D6119 Implant/abutment supported interim fixed denture for edentulous arch maxillary Ⓑ E1

Used when a period of healing is necessary prior to fabrication and placement of a permanent prosthetic.

D6120 Implant supported retainer - porcelain fused to titanium and titanium alloys E1

A metal-ceramic retainer for a fixed partial denture that gains retention, support, and stability from an implant.

D6121 Implant supported retainer for metal FPD - predominantly base alloys E1

A metal-ceramic retainer for a fixed partial denture that gains retention, support, and stability from an implant.

D6122 Implant supported retainer for metal FPD - noble alloys E1

A metal retainer for a fixed partial denture that gains retention, support, and stability from an implant.

D6123 Implant supported retainer for metal FPD - titanium and titanum alloys E1

A metal retainer for a fixed partial denture that gains retention, support, and stability from an implant.

D6190 Radiographic/surgical implant index, by report Ⓑ E1

An appliance, designed to relate osteotomy or fixture position to existing anatomic structures, to be utilized during radiographic exposure for treatment planning and/or during osteotomy creation for fixture installation.

▶ **D6191** Semi-precision abutment – placement

This procedure is the initial placement, or replacement, of a semi-precision abutment on the implant body.

▶ **D6192** Semi-precision attachment – placement

This procedure involves the luting of the initial, or replacement, semi-precision attachment to the removable prosthesis.

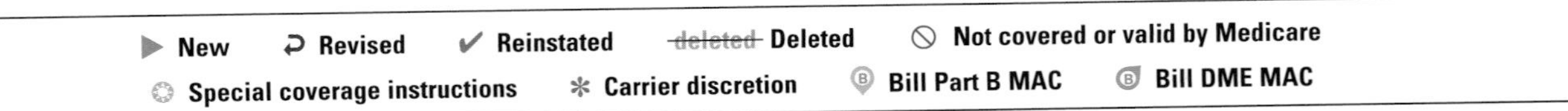

▶ New
Revised
Reinstated
~~deleted~~ Deleted
Not covered or valid by Medicare
Special coverage instructions
Carrier discretion
Bill Part B MAC
Bill DME MAC

D6194 Abutment supported retainer crown for FPD – titanium and titanium alloys E1

A retainer for a fixed partial denture that gains retention, support and stability from an abutment on an implant. May be cast or milled.

D6195 Abutment supported retainer - porcelain fused to titanium and titanium alloys E1

A metal retainer for a fixed partial denture that gains retention, support, and stability from an implant.

None

D6199 Unspecified implant procedure, by report E1

Use for procedure that is not adequately described by a code. Describe procedure.

Cross Reference 21299

Prosthodontics, fixed (D6205-D6999)

Fixed Partial Denture Pontics

D6205 Pontic - indirect resin based composite E1

Not to be used as a temporary or provisional prosthesis.

D6210 Pontic - cast high noble metal E1

D6211 Pontic - cast predominantly base metal E1

D6212 Pontic - cast noble metal E1

D6214 Pontic - titanium and titanium alloys E1

D6240 Pontic - porcelain fused to high noble metal E1

D6241 Pontic - porcelain fused to predominantly base metal E1

D6242 Pontic - porcelain fused to noble metal E1

IOM: 100-02, 15, 150

D6243 Pontic - porcelain fused to titanium and titanium alloys E1

D6245 Pontic - porcelain/ceramic E1

D6250 Pontic - resin with high noble metal E1

D6251 Pontic - resin with predominantly base metal E1

D6252 Pontic - resin with noble metal E1

D6253 Provisional pontic - further treatment or completion of diagnosis necessary prior to final impression E1

Not to be used as a temporary pontic for routine prosthetic fixed partial dentures.

Fixed Partial Denture Retainers – Inlays/Onlays

D6545 Retainer - cast metal for resin bonded fixed prosthesis E1

D6548 Retainer - porcelain/ceramic for resin bonded fixed prosthesis E1

D6549 Retainer - for resin bonded fixed prosthesis E1

D6600 Retainer inlay - porcelain/ceramic, two surfaces E1

D6601 Retainer inlay - porcelain/ceramic, three or more surfaces E1

D6602 Retainer inlay - cast high noble metal, two surfaces E1

D6603 Retainer inlay - cast high noble metal, three or more surfaces E1

D6604 Retainer inlay - cast predominantly base metal, two surfaces E1

D6605 Retainer inlay - cast predominantly base metal, three or more surfaces E1

D6606 Retainer inlay - cast noble metal, two surfaces E1

D6607 Retainer inlay - cast noble metal, three or more surfaces E1

D6608 Retainer onlay - porcelain/ceramic, two surfaces E1

D6609 Retainer onlay - porcelain/ceramic, three or more surfaces E1

D6610 Retainer onlay - cast high noble metal, two surfaces E1

D6611 Retainer onlay - cast high noble metal, three or more surfaces E1

D6612 Retainer onlay - cast predominantly base metal, two surfaces E1

D6613 Retainer onlay - cast predominantly base metal, three or more surfaces E1

D6614 Retainer onlay - cast noble metal, two surfaces E1

D6615 Retainer onlay - cast noble metal, three or more surfaces E1

D6624 Retainer inlay - titanium E1

D6634 Retainer onlay - titanium E1

Fixed Partial Denture Retainers – Crowns

D6710 Retainer crown - indirect resin based composite Ⓑ E1

Not to be used as a temporary or provisional prosthesis.

D6720 Retainer crown - resin with high noble metal Ⓑ E1

D6721 Retainer crown - resin with predominantly base metal Ⓑ E1

D6722 Retainer crown - resin with noble metal Ⓑ E1

D6740 Retainer crown - porcelain/ceramic Ⓑ E1

D6750 Retainer crown - porcelain fused to high noble metal Ⓑ E1

D6751 Retainer crown - porcelain fused to predominantly base metal Ⓑ E1

D6752 Retainer crown - porcelain fused to noble metal Ⓑ E1

D6753 Retainer crown - porcelain fused to titanium and titanium alloys E1

D6780 Retainer crown - 3/4 cast high noble metal Ⓑ E1

D6781 Retainer crown - 3/4 cast predominantly based metal Ⓑ E1

D6782 Retainer crown - 3/4 cast noble metal Ⓑ E1

D6783 Retainer crown - 3/4 porcelain/ceramic Ⓑ E1

D6784 Retainer crown 3/4 - titanium and titanium alloys E1

D6790 Retainer crown - full cast high noble metal Ⓑ E1

D6791 Retainer crown - full cast predominantly base metal Ⓑ E1

D6792 Retainer crown - full cast noble metal Ⓑ E1

D6793 Provisional retainer crown - further treatment or completion of diagnosis necessary prior to final impression Ⓑ E1

Not to be used as a temporary retainer crown for routine prosthetic fixed partial dentures.

D6794 Retainer crown - titanium and titanium alloys Ⓑ E1

Other Fixed Partial Denture Services

D6920 Connector bar Ⓑ S

A device attached to fixed partial denture retainer or coping which serves to stabilize and anchor a removable overdenture prosthesis.

D6930 Re-cement or re-bond fixed partial denture Ⓑ E1

D6940 Stress breaker Ⓑ E1

A non-rigid connector.

D6950 Precision attachment Ⓑ E1

A male and female pair constitutes one precision attachment, and is separate from the prosthesis.

D6980 Bridge repair necessitated by restorative material failure Ⓑ E1

D6985 Pediatric partial denture, fixed Ⓑ A E1

This prosthesis is used primarily for aesthetic purposes.

None

D6999 Unspecified fixed prosthodontic procedure, by report Ⓑ E1

Used for procedure that is not adequately described by a code. Describe procedure.

Oral and Maxillofacial Surgery (D7111-D7999)

Extractions (Includes Local Anesthesia, Suturing, If Needed, and Routine Postoperative Care)

D7111 Extraction, coronal remnants - primary tooth Ⓑ S

Removal of soft tissue-retained coronal remnants.

D7140 Extraction, erupted tooth or exposed root (elevation and/or forceps removal) Ⓑ S

Includes removal of tooth structure, minor smoothing of socket bone, and closure, as necessary.

D7210 Extraction, erupted tooth requiring removal of bone and/or sectioning of tooth, and including elevation of mucoperiosteal flap if indicated Ⓑ S

Includes related cutting of gingiva and bone, removal of tooth structure, minor smoothing of socket bone and closure.

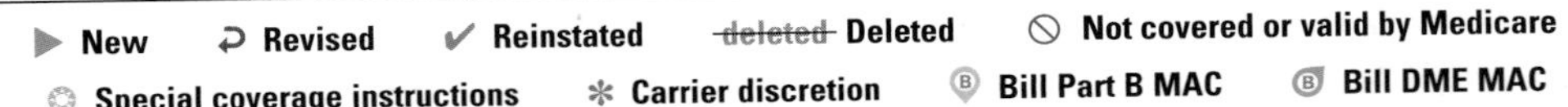
▶ New ⮌ Revised ✔ Reinstated ~~deleted~~ Deleted ⊘ Not covered or valid by Medicare
Special coverage instructions ✻ Carrier discretion Ⓑ Bill Part B MAC Ⓔ Bill DME MAC

D7220 Removal of impacted tooth - soft tissue ⓑ S

Occlusal surface of tooth covered by soft tissue; requires mucoperiosteal flap elevation.

D7230 Removal of impacted tooth - partially bony ⓑ S

Part of crown covered by bone; requires mucoperiosteal flap elevation and bone removal.

D7240 Removal of impacted tooth - completely bony ⓑ S

Most or all of crown covered by bone; requires mucoperiosteal flap elevation and bone removal.

D7241 Removal of impacted tooth - completely bony, with unusual surgical complications ⓑ S

Most or all of crown covered by bone; unusually difficult or complicated due to factors such as nerve dissection required, separate closure of maxillary sinus required or aberrant tooth position.

D7250 Removal of residual tooth roots (cutting procedure) ⓑ S

Includes cutting of soft tissue and bone, removal of tooth structure, and closure.

D7251 Coronectomy — intentional partial tooth removal ⓑ E1

Intentional partial tooth removal is performed when a neurovascular complication is likely if the entire impacted tooth is removed.

Other Surgical Procedures

⮐ **D7260** Oroantral fistula closure ⓑ S

Excision of fistulous tract between maxillary sinus and oral cavity and closure by advancement flap.

D7261 Primary closure of a sinus perforation ⓑ S

Subsequent to surgical removal of tooth, exposure of sinus requiring repair, or immediate closure of oroantral or oralnasal communication in absence of fistulous tract.

D7270 Tooth reimplantation and/or stabilization of accidentally evulsed or displaced tooth ⓑ E1

Includes splinting and/or stabilization.

D7272 Tooth transplantation (includes reimplantation from one site to another and splinting and/or stabilization) ⓑ E1

D7280 Exposure of an unerupted tooth ⓑ E1

An incision is made and the tissue is reflected and bone removed as necessary to expose the crown of an impacted tooth not intended to be extracted.

D7282 Mobilization of erupted or malpositioned tooth to aid eruption ⓑ E1

To move/luxate teeth to eliminate ankylosis; not in conjunction with an extraction.

D7283 Placement of device to facilitate eruption of impacted tooth ⓑ B

Placement of an orthodontic bracket, band or other device on an unerupted tooth, after its exposure, to aid in its eruption. Report the surgical exposure separately using D7280.

D7285 Incisional biopsy of oral tissue - hard (bone, tooth) ⓑ E1

For partial removal of specimen only. This procedure involves biopsy of osseous lesions and is not used for apicoectomy/periradicular surgery. This procedure does not entail an excision.

Cross Reference 20220, 20225, 20240, 20245

D7286 Incisional biopsy of oral tissue - soft ⓑ E1

For partial removal of an architecturally intact specimen only. This procedure is not used at the same time as codes for apicoectomy/ periradicular curettage. This procedure does not entail an excision.

Cross Reference 40808

D7287 Exfoliative cytological sample collection ⓑ E1

For collection of non-transepithelial cytology sample via mild scraping of the oral mucosa.

D7288 Brush biopsy - transepithelial sample collection ⓑ B

For collection of oral disaggregated transepithelial cells via rotational brushing of the oral mucosa.

D7290 Surgical repositioning of teeth ⓑ E1

Grafting procedure(s) is/are additional.

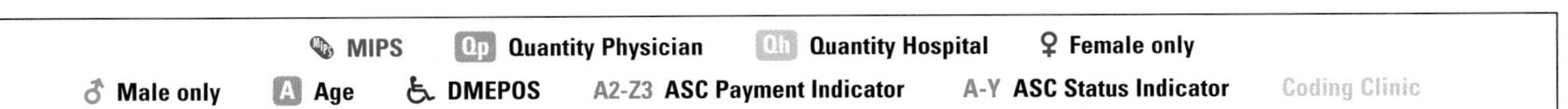
MIPS
Qp Quantity Physician
Qh Quantity Hospital
♀ Female only
♂ Male only
A Age
DMEPOS
A2-Z3 ASC Payment Indicator
A-Y ASC Status Indicator
Coding Clinic

D7291 Transseptal fiberotomy/supra-crestal fiberotomy, by report Ⓑ S

The supraosseous connective tissue attachment is surgically severed around the involved teeth. Where there are adjacent teeth, the transseptal fiberotomy of a single tooth will involve a minimum of three teeth. Since the incisions are within the gingival sulcus and tissue and the root surface is not instrumented, this procedure heals by the reunion of connective tissue with the root surface on which viable periodontal tissue is present (reattachment).

D7292 Placement of temporary anchorage device [screw retained plate] requiring flap; includes device removal Ⓑ E1

D7293 Placement of temporary anchorage device requiring flap; includes device removal Ⓑ E1

D7294 Placement of temporary anchorage device without flap; includes device removal Ⓑ E1

D7295 Harvest of bone for use in autogenous grafting procedure Ⓑ E1

Reported in addition to those autogenous graft placement procedures that do not include harvesting of bone.

D7296 Corticotomy one to three teeth or tooth spaces, per quadrant Ⓑ E1

This procedure involves creating multiple cuts, perforations, or removal of cortical, alveolar or basal bone of the jaw for the purpose of facilitating orthodontic repositioning of the dentition. This procedure includes flap entry and closure. Graft material and membrane, if used, should be reported separately.

D7297 Corticotomy four or more teeth or tooth spaces, per quadrant Ⓑ E1

This procedure involves creating multiple cuts, perforations, or removal of cortical, alveolar or basal bone of the jaw for the purpose of facilitating orthodontic repositioning of the dentition. This procedure includes flap entry and closure. Graft material and membrane, if used, should be reported separately.

Alveoloplasty – Preparation of Ridge

D7310 Alveoloplasty in conjunction with extractions - four or more teeth or tooth spaces, per quadrant Ⓑ E1

The alveoloplasty is distinct (separate procedure) from extractions. Usually in preparation for a prosthesis or other treatments such as radiation therapy and transplant surgery.

Cross Reference 41874

D7311 Alveoloplasty in conjunction with extractions - one to three teeth or tooth spaces, per quadrant Ⓑ E1

The alveoloplasty is distinct (separate procedure) from extractions. Usually in preparation for a prosthesis or other treatments such as radiation therapy and transplant surgery.

D7320 Alveoloplasty not in conjunction with extractions - four or more teeth or tooth spaces, per quadrant Ⓑ E1

No extractions performed in an edentulous area. See D7310 if teeth are being extracted concurrently with the alveoloplasty. Usually in preparation for a prosthesis or other treatments such as radiation therapy and transplant surgery.

Cross Reference 41870

D7321 Alveoloplasty not in conjunction with extractions - one to three teeth or tooth spaces, per quadrant Ⓑ B

No extractions performed in an edentulous area. See D7311 if teeth are being extracted concurrently with the alveoloplasty. Usually in preparation for a prosthesis or other treatments such as radiation therapy and transplant surgery.

Vestibuloplasty

D7340 Vestibuloplasty - ridge extension (second epithelialization) Ⓑ E1

Cross Reference 40840, 40842, 40843, 40844

D7350 Vestibuloplasty - ridge extension (including soft tissue grafts, muscle reattachments, revision of soft tissue attachment, and management of hypertrophied and hyperplastic tissue) Ⓑ E1

Cross Reference 40845

Excision of Soft Tissue Lesions

D7410 Excision of benign lesion up to 1.25 cm Ⓑ E1

D7411 Excision of benign lesion greater than 1.25 cm Ⓑ E1

D7412 Excision of benign lesion, complicated Ⓑ E1

Requires extensive undermining with advancement or rotational flap closure.

D7413 Excision of malignant lesion up to 1.25 cm Ⓑ E1

D7414 Excision of malignant lesion greater than 1.25 cm Ⓑ E1

D7415 Excision of malignant lesion, complicated Ⓑ E1

Requires extensive undermining with advancement or rotational flap closure.

Excision of Intra-Osseous Lesions

D7440 Excision of malignant tumor - lesion diameter up to 1.25 cm Ⓑ E1

D7441 Excision of malignant tumor - lesion diameter greater than 1.25 cm Ⓑ E1

D7450 Removal of benign odontogenic cyst or tumor - lesion diameter up to 1.25 cm Ⓑ E1

D7451 Removal of benign odontogenic cyst or tumor - lesion diameter greater than 1.25 cm Ⓑ E1

D7460 Removal of benign nonodontogenic cyst or tumor - lesion diameter up to 1.25 cm Ⓑ E1

D7461 Removal of benign nonodontogenic cyst or tumor - lesion diameter greater than 1.25 cm Ⓑ E1

Excision of Soft Tissue Lesions

D7465 Destruction of lesion(s) by physical or chemical methods, by report Ⓑ E1

Examples include using cryo, laser or electro surgery.

Cross Reference 41850

Excision of Bone Tissue

D7471 Removal of lateral exostosis (maxilla or mandible) Ⓑ E1

Cross Reference 21031, 21032

D7472 Removal of torus palatinus Ⓑ E1

D7473 Removal of torus mandibularis Ⓑ E1

D7485 Reduction of osseous tuberosity Ⓑ E1

D7490 Radical resection of maxilla or mandible Ⓑ E1

Partial resection of maxilla or mandible; removal of lesion and defect with margin of normal appearing bone. Reconstruction and bone grafts should be reported separately.

Cross Reference 21095

Surgical Incision

D7510 Incision and drainage of abscess - intraoral soft tissue Ⓑ E1

Involves incision through mucosa, including periodontal origins.

Cross Reference 41800

D7511 Incision and drainage of abscess - intraoral soft tissue - complicated (includes drainage of multiple fascial spaces) Ⓑ B

Incision is made intraorally and dissection is extended into adjacent fascial space(s) to provide adequate drainage of abscess/cellulitis.

D7520 Incision and drainage of abscess - extraoral soft tissue Ⓑ E1

Involves incision through skin.

Cross Reference 41800

D7521 Incision and drainage of abscess - extraoral soft tissue - complicated (includes drainage of multiple fascial spaces) Ⓑ B

Incision is made extraorally and dissection is extended into adjacent fascial space(s) to provide adequate drainage of abscess/cellulitis.

D7530 Removal of foreign body from mucosa, skin, or subcutaneous alveolar tissue Ⓑ E1

Cross Reference 41805, 41828

D7540 Removal of reaction-producing foreign bodies, musculoskeletal system Ⓑ E1

May include, but is not limited to, removal of splinters, pieces of wire, etc., from muscle and/or bone.

Cross Reference 20520, 41800, 41806

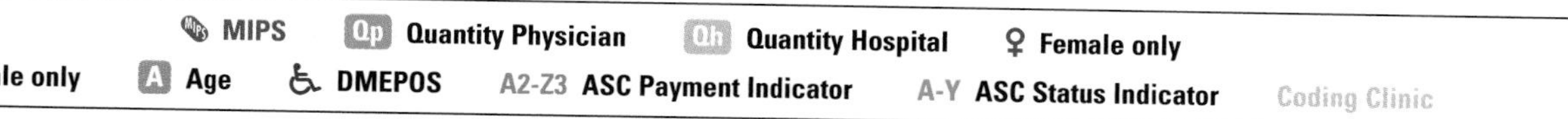
MIPS
Qp Quantity Physician
Qh Quantity Hospital
♀ Female only
♂ Male only
A Age
DMEPOS
A2-Z3 ASC Payment Indicator
A-Y ASC Status Indicator
Coding Clinic

D7550 Partial ostectomy/sequestrectomy for removal of non-vital bone Ⓑ E1

Removal of loose or sloughed-off dead bone caused by infection or reduced blood supply.

Cross Reference 20999

D7560 Maxillary sinusotomy for removal of tooth fragment or foreign body Ⓑ E1

Cross Reference 31020

Treatment of Closed Fractures

D7610 Maxilla - open reduction (teeth immobilized, if present) Ⓑ E1

Teeth may be wired, banded or splinted together to prevent movement. Incision required for interosseous fixation.

D7620 Maxilla - closed reduction (teeth immobilized if present) Ⓑ E1

No incision required to reduce fracture. See D7610 if interosseous fixation is applied.

D7630 Mandible - open reduction (teeth immobilized, if present) Ⓑ E1

Teeth may be wired, banded or splinted together to prevent movement. Incision required to reduce fracture.

D7640 Mandible - closed reduction (teeth immobilized if present) Ⓑ E1

No incision required to reduce fracture. See D7630 if interosseous fixation is applied.

D7650 Malar and/or zygomatic arch - open reduction Ⓑ E1

D7660 Malar and/or zygomatic arch - closed reduction Ⓑ E1

D7670 Alveolus - closed reduction, may include stabilization of teeth Ⓑ E1

Teeth may be wired, banded or splinted together to prevent movement.

D7671 Alveolus - open reduction, may include stabilization of teeth Ⓑ E1

Teeth may be wired, banded or splinted together to prevent movement.

D7680 Facial bones - complicated reduction with fixation and multiple surgical approaches Ⓑ E1

Facial bones include upper and lower jaw, cheek, and bones around eyes, nose, and ears.

Treatment of Open Fractures

D7710 Maxilla - open reduction Ⓑ E1

Incision required to reduce fracture.

Cross Reference 21346

D7720 Maxilla - closed reduction Ⓑ E1

Cross Reference 21345

D7730 Mandible - open reduction Ⓑ E1

Incision required to reduce fracture.

Cross Reference 21461, 21462

D7740 Mandible - closed reduction Ⓑ E1

Cross Reference 21455

D7750 Malar and/or zygomatic arch - open reduction Ⓑ E1

Incision required to reduce fracture.

Cross Reference 21360, 21365

D7760 Malar and/or zygomatic arch - closed reduction Ⓑ E1

Cross Reference 21355

D7770 Alveolus - open reduction stabilization of teeth Ⓑ E1

Fractured bone(s) are exposed to mouth or outside the face. Incision required to reduce fracture.

Cross Reference 21422

D7771 Alveolus, closed reduction stabilization of teeth Ⓑ E1

Fractured bone(s) are exposed to mouth or outside the face.

D7780 Facial bones - complicated reduction with fixation and multiple approaches Ⓑ E1

Incision required to reduce fracture. Facial bones include upper and lower jaw, cheek, and bones around eyes, nose, and ears.

Cross Reference 21433, 21435

Reduction of Dislocation and Management of Other Temporomandibular Joint Dysfunction

D7810 Open reduction of dislocation Ⓑ E1

Access to TMJ via surgical opening.

Cross Reference 21490

D7820 Closed reduction of dislocation Ⓑ E1

Joint manipulated into place; no surgical exposure.

Cross Reference 21480

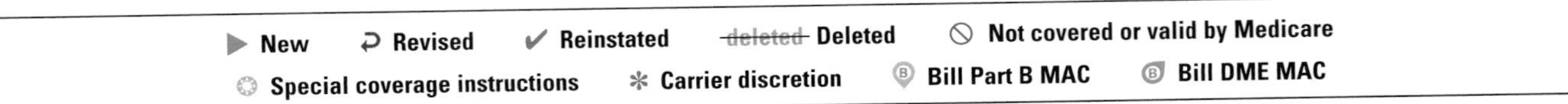
▶ New
Revised
✔ Reinstated
~~deleted~~ Deleted
Not covered or valid by Medicare
Special coverage instructions
✻ Carrier discretion
Ⓑ Bill Part B MAC
Bill DME MAC

D7830 Manipulation under anesthesia Ⓑ E1

Usually done under general anesthesia or intravenous sedation.

Cross Reference 00190

D7840 Condylectomy Ⓑ E1

Removal of all or portion of the mandibular condyle (separate procedure).

Cross Reference 21050

D7850 Surgical discectomy, with/without implant Ⓑ E1

Excision of the intra-articular disc of a joint.

Cross Reference 21060

D7852 Disc repair Ⓑ E1

Repositioning and/or sculpting of disc; repair of perforated posterior attachment.

Cross Reference 21299

D7854 Synovectomy Ⓑ E1

Excision of a portion or all of the synovial membrane of a joint.

Cross Reference 21299

D7856 Myotomy Ⓑ E1

Cutting of muscle for therapeutic purposes (separate procedure).

Cross Reference 21299

D7858 Joint reconstruction Ⓑ E1

Reconstruction of osseous components including or excluding soft tissues of the joint with autogenous, homologous, or alloplastic materials.

Cross Reference 21242, 21243

D7860 Arthrotomy Ⓑ E1

Cutting into joint (separate procedure).

D7865 Arthroplasty Ⓑ E1

Reduction of osseous components of the joint to create a pseudoarthrosis or eliminate an irregular remodeling pattern (osteophytes).

Cross Reference 21240

D7870 Arthrocentesis Ⓑ E1

Withdrawal of fluid from a joint space by aspiration.

Cross Reference 21060

D7871 Non-arthroscopic lysis and lavage Ⓑ E1

Inflow and outflow catheters are placed into the joint space. The joint is lavaged and manipulated as indicated in an effort to release minor adhesions and synovial vacuum phenomenon as well as to remove inflammation products from the joint space.

D7872 Arthroscopy - diagnosis, with or without biopsy Ⓑ E1

Cross Reference 29800

D7873 Arthroscopy: lavage and lysis of adhesions Ⓑ E1

Removal of adhesions using the arthroscope and lavage of the joint cavities.

Cross Reference 29804

D7874 Arthroscopy: disc repositioning and stabilization Ⓑ E1

Repositioning and stabilization of disc using arthroscopic techniques.

Cross Reference 29804

D7875 Arthroscopy: synovectomy Ⓑ E1

Removal of inflamed and hyperplastic synovium (partial/complete) via an arthroscopic technique.

Cross Reference 29804

D7876 Arthroscopy: discectomy Ⓑ E1

Removal of disc and remodeled posterior attachment via the arthroscope.

Cross Reference 29804

D7877 Arthroscopy: debridement Ⓑ E1

Removal of pathologic hard and/or soft tissue using the arthroscope.

Cross Reference 29804

D7880 Occlusal orthotic device, by report Ⓑ E1

Presently includes splints provided for treatment of temporomandibular joint dysfunction.

Cross Reference 21499

D7881 Occlusal orthotic device adjustment Ⓑ E1

D7899 Unspecified TMD therapy, by report Ⓑ E1

Used for procedure that is not adequately described by a code. Describe procedure.

Cross Reference 21499

Repair of Traumatic Wounds

D7910 Suture of recent small wounds up to 5 cm Ⓑ E1

Cross Reference 12011, 12013

Complicated Suturing (Reconstruction Requiring Delicate Handling of Tissue and Wide Undermining for Meticulous Closure)

D7911 Complicated suture - up to 5 cm Ⓑ E1

Cross Reference 12051, 12052

D7912 Complicated suture - greater than 5 cm Ⓑ E1

Cross Reference 13132

Other Repair Procedures

D7920 Skin graft (identify defect covered, location, and type of graft) Ⓑ E1

D7921 Collection and application of autologous blood concentrate product Ⓑ E1

D7922 Placement of intra-socket biological dressing to aid in hemostasis or clot stabilization, per site E1

This procedure can be performed at time and/or after extraction to aid in hemostasis. The socket is packed with a hemostatic agent to aid in hemostasis and or clot stabilization.

D7940 Osteoplasty - for orthognathic deformities Ⓑ S

Reconstruction of jaws for correction of congenital, developmental or acquired traumatic or surgical deformity.

D7941 Osteotomy - mandibular rami Ⓑ E1

Cross Reference 21193, 21195, 21196

D7943 Osteotomy - mandibular rami with bone graft; includes obtaining the graft Ⓑ E1

Cross Reference 21194

D7944 Osteotomy - segmented or subapical Ⓑ E1

Report by range of tooth numbers within segment.

Cross Reference 21198, 21206

D7945 Osteotomy - body of mandible Ⓑ E1

Sectioning of lower jaw. This includes exposure, bone cut, fixation, routine wound closure and normal post-operative follow-up care.

Cross Reference 21193, 21194, 21195, 21196

D7946 LeFort I (maxilla - total) Ⓑ E1

Sectioning of the upper jaw. This includes exposure, bone cuts, downfracture, repositioning, fixation, routine wound closure and normal post-operative follow-up care.

Cross Reference 21147

D7947 LeFort I (maxilla - segmented) Ⓑ E1

When reporting a surgically assisted palatal expansion without downfracture, this code would entail a reduced service and should be "by report."

Cross Reference 21145, 21146

D7948 LeFort II or LeFort III (osteoplasty of facial bones for midface hypoplasia or retrusion) - without bone graft Ⓑ E1

Sectioning of upper jaw. This includes exposure, bone cuts, downfracture, segmentation of maxilla, repositioning, fixation, routine wound closure and normal post-operative follow-up care.

Cross Reference 21150

D7949 LeFort II or LeFort III - with bone graft Ⓑ E1

Includes obtaining autografts.

D7950 Osseous, osteoperiosteal, or cartilage graft of the mandible or maxilla - autogenous or nonautogenous, by report Ⓑ E1

This procedure is for ridge augmentation or reconstruction to increase height, width and/or volume of residual alveolar ridge. It includes obtaining graft material. Placement of a barrier membrane, if used, should be reported separately.

Cross Reference 21247

D7951 Sinus augmentation with bone or bone substitutes Ⓑ E1

The augmentation of the sinus cavity to increase alveolar height for reconstruction of edentulous portions of the maxilla. This procedure is performed via a lateral open approach. This includes obtaining the bone or bone substitutes. Placement of a barrier membrane if used should be reported separately.

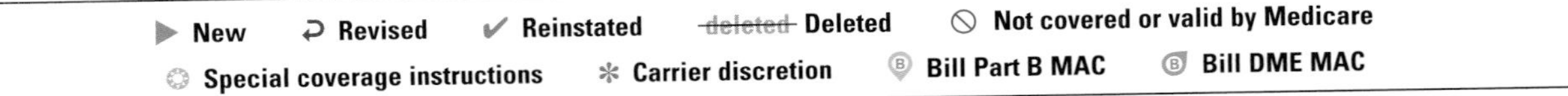

▶ New
⮌ Revised
✔ Reinstated
~~deleted~~ Deleted
⊘ Not covered or valid by Medicare
Special coverage instructions
✱ Carrier discretion
Ⓑ Bill Part B MAC
Ⓓ Bill DME MAC

D7952 Sinus augmentation via a vertical approach E1

The augmentation of the sinus to increase alveolar height by vertical access through the ridge crest by raising the floor of the sinus and grafting as necessary. This includes obtaining the bone or bone substitutes.

D7953 Bone replacement graft for ridge preservation - per site E1

Graft is placed in an extraction or implant removal site at the time of the extraction or removal to preserve ridge integrity (e.g., clinically indicated in preparation for implant reconstruction or where alveolar contour is critical to planned prosthetic reconstruction). Does not include obtaining graft material. Membrane, if used should be reported separately.

D7955 Repair of maxillofacial soft and/or hard tissue defect E1

Reconstruction of surgical, traumatic, or congenital defects of the facial bones, including the mandible, may utilize graft materials in conjunction with soft tissue procedures to repair and restore the facial bones to form and function. This does not include obtaining the graft and these procedures may require multiple surgical approaches. This procedure does not include edentulous maxilla and mandibular reconstruction for prosthetic considerations.

Cross Reference 21299

~~**D7960** Frenulectomy - also known as frenectomy or frenotomy - separate procedure not incidental to another procedure~~ ✖

~~Removal or release of mucosal and muscle elements of a buccal, labial or lingual frenum that is associated with a pathological condition, or interferes with proper oral development or treatment.~~

~~*Cross Reference 40819, 41010, 41115*~~

▶ **D7961** Buccal / labial frenectomy (frenulectomy)

▶ **D7962** Lingual frenectomy (frenulectomy)

D7963 Frenuloplasty E1

Excision of frenum with accompanying excision or repositioning of aberrant muscle and z-plasty or other local flap closure.

D7970 Excision of hyperplastic tissue - per arch E1

D7971 Excision of pericoronal gingival E1

Removal of inflammatory or hypertrophied tissues surrounding partially erupted/impacted teeth.

Cross Reference 41821

D7972 Surgical reduction of fibrous tuberosity E1

D7979 Non surgical sialolithotomy E1

A sialolith is removed from the gland or ductal portion of the gland without surgical incision into the gland or the duct of the gland; for example via manual manipulation, ductal dilation, or any other non-surgical method.

D7980 Surgical sialolithotomy E1

Procedure by which a stone within a salivary gland or its duct is removed, either intraorally or extraorally.

Cross Reference 42330, 42335, 42340

D7981 Excision of salivary gland, by report E1

Cross Reference 42408

D7982 Sialodochoplasty E1

Procedure for the repair of a defect and/or restoration of a portion of a salivary gland duct.

Cross Reference 42500

D7983 Closure of salivary fistula E1

Closure of an opening between a salivary duct and/or gland and the cutaneous surface, or an opening into the oral cavity through other than the normal anatomic pathway.

Cross Reference 42600

D7990 Emergency tracheotomy E1

Formation of a tracheal opening usually below the cricoid cartilage to allow for respiratory exchange.

Cross Reference 21070

D7991 Coronoidectomy E1

Removal of the coronoid process of the mandible.

Cross Reference 21070

▶ **D7993** Surgical placement of craniofacial implant – extra oral

Surgical placement of a craniofacial implant to aid in retention of an auricular, nasal, or orbital prosthesis.

MIPS | Qp Quantity Physician | Qh Quantity Hospital | ♀ Female only
♂ Male only | A Age | DMEPOS | A2-Z3 ASC Payment Indicator | A-Y ASC Status Indicator | Coding Clinic

▶ **D7994** Surgical placement: zygomatic implant

An implant placed in the zygomatic bone and exiting though the maxillary mucosal tissue providing support and attachment of a maxillary dental prosthesis.

D7995 Synthetic graft - mandible or facial bones, by report Ⓑ E1

Includes allogenic material.

Cross Reference 21299

D7996 Implant-mandible for augmentation purposes (excluding alveolar ridge), by report Ⓑ E1

Cross Reference 21299

D7997 Appliance removal (not by dentist who placed appliance), includes removal of archbar Ⓑ E1

D7998 Intraoral placement of a fixation device not in conjunction with a fracture Ⓑ E1

The placement of intermaxillary fixation appliance for documented medically accepted treatments not in association with fractures.

None

D7999 Unspecified oral surgery procedure, by report Ⓑ E1

Used for procedure that is not adequately described by a code. Describe procedure.

Cross Reference 21299

Orthodontics (D8010-D8999)

Limited Orthodontic Treatment

D8010 Limited orthodontic treatment of the primary dentition Ⓑ E1

D8020 Limited orthodontic treatment of the transitional dentition Ⓑ E1

D8030 Limited orthodontic treatment of the adolescent dentition Ⓑ A E1

D8040 Limited orthodontic treatment of the adult dentition Ⓑ A E1

Interceptive Orthodontic Treatment

D8050 Interceptive orthodontic treatment of the primary dentition Ⓑ E1

D8060 Interceptive orthodontic treatment of the transitional dentition Ⓑ E1

Comprehensive Orthodontic Treatment

D8070 Comprehensive orthodontic treatment of the transitional dentition Ⓑ E1

D8080 Comprehensive orthodontic treatment of the adolescent dentition Ⓑ A E1

D8090 Comprehensive orthodontic treatment of the adult dentition Ⓑ A E1

Minor Treatment to Control Harmful Habits

D8210 Removable appliance therapy Ⓑ E1

Removable indicates patient can remove; includes appliances for thumb sucking and tongue thrusting.

D8220 Fixed appliance therapy Ⓑ E1

Fixed indicates patient cannot remove appliance; includes appliances for thumb sucking and tongue thrusting.

Other Orthodontic Services

D8660 Pre-orthodontic treatment examination to monitor growth and development Ⓑ E1

Periodic observation of patient dentition, at intervals established by the dentist, to determine when orthodontic treatment should begin. Diagnostic procedures are documented separately.

D8670 Periodic orthodontic treatment visit Ⓑ E1

D8680 Orthodontic retention (removal of appliances, construction and placement of retainer(s)) Ⓑ E1

D8681 Removable orthodontic retainer adjustment Ⓑ E1

D8690 Orthodontic treatment (alternative billing to a contract fee) Ⓑ E1

Services provided by dentist other than original treating dentist. A method of payment between the provider and responsible party for services that reflect an open-ended fee arrangement.

D8695 Removal of fixed orthodontic appliances for reasons other than completion of treatment Ⓑ E1

D8696 Repair of orthodontic appliance - maxillary E1

Does not include bracket and standard fixed orthodontic appliances. It does include functional appliances and palatal expanders.

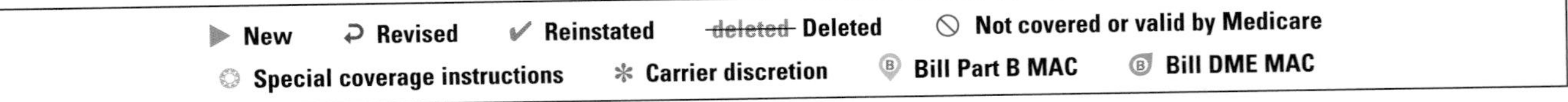
▶ New
Revised
Reinstated
~~deleted~~ Deleted
Not covered or valid by Medicare
Special coverage instructions
Carrier discretion
Bill Part B MAC
Bill DME MAC

D8697 Repair of orthodontic appliance - mandibular E1

Does not include bracket and standard fixed orthodontic appliances. It does include functional appliances and palatal expanders.

D8698 Re-cement or re-bond fixed retainer - maxillary E1

D8699 Re-cement or re-bond fixed retainer - mandibular E1

D8701 Repair of fixed retainer, includes reattachment - maxillary E1

D8702 Repair of fixed retainer, includes reattachment - mandibular E1

D8703 Replacement of lost or broken retainer - maxillary E1

D8704 Replacement of lost or broken retainer - mandibular E1

None

D8999 Unspecified orthodontic procedure, by report E1

Used for procedure that is not adequately described by a code. Describe procedure.

Adjunctive General Services (D9110-D9999)

Unclassified Treatment

D9110 Palliative (emergency) treatment of dental pain - minor procedures N

This is typically reported on a "per visit" basis for emergency treatment of dental pain.

D9120 Fixed partial denture sectioning E1

Separation of one or more connections between abutments and/or pontics when some portion of a fixed prosthesis is to remain intact and serviceable following sectioning and extraction or other treatment. Includes all recontouring and polishing of retained portions.

D9130 Temporomandibular joint dysfunction - non-invasive physical therapies E1

Anesthesia

D9210 Local anesthesia not in conjunction with operative or surgical procedures E1

Cross Reference 90784

D9211 Regional block anesthesia E1

Cross Reference 01995

D9212 Trigeminal division block anesthesia E1

Cross Reference 64400

D9215 Local anesthesia in conjunction with operative or surgical procedures E1

Cross Reference 90784

D9219 Evaluation for moderate sedation or general anesthesia A E1

D9222 Deep sedation/general anesthesia first 15 minutes E1

Anesthesia time begins when the doctor administering the anesthetic agent initiates the appropriate anesthesia and non-invasive monitoring protocol and remains in continuous attendance of the patient. Anesthesia services are considered completed when the patient may be safely left under the observation of trained personnel and the doctor may safely leave the room to attend to other patients or duties.

The level of anesthesia is determined by the anesthesia provider's documentation of the anesthetic effects upon the central nervous system and not dependent upon the route of administration.

D9223 Deep sedation/general anesthesia - each subsequent 15 minute increment E1

D9230 Inhalation of nitrous oxide/analgesia, anxiolysis N

D9239 Intravenous moderate (conscious) sedation/analgesia - first 15 minutes E1

Anesthesia time begins when the doctor administering the anesthetic agent initiates the appropriate anesthesia and non-invasive monitoring protocol and remains in continuous attendance of the patient. Anesthesia services are considered completed when the patient may be safely left under the observation of trained personnel and the doctor may safely leave the room to attend to other patients or duties.

The level of anesthesia is determined by the anesthesia provider's documentation of the anesthetic effects upon the central nervous system and not dependent upon the route of administration.

D9243 Intravenous moderate (conscious) sedation/analgesia - each subsequent 15 minute increment E1

D9248 Non-intravenous conscious sedation Ⓑ N

This includes non-IV minimal and moderate sedation. A medically controlled state of depressed consciousness while maintaining the patient's airway, protective reflexes and the ability to respond to stimulation or verbal commands. It includes non-intravenous administration of sedative and/or analgesic agent(s) and appropriate monitoring.

The level of anesthesia is determined by the anesthesia provider's documentation of the anesthetic's effects upon the central nervous system and not dependent upon the route of administration.

Professional Consultation

D9310 Consultation - diagnostic service provided by dentist or physician other than requesting dentist or physician Ⓑ E1

A patient encounter with a practitioner whose opinion or advice regarding evaluation and/or management of a specific problem; may be requested by another practitioner or appropriate source. The consultation includes an oral evaluation. The consulted practitioner may initiate diagnostic and/or therapeutic services.

D9311 Consultation with a medical health care professional Ⓑ E1

Treating dentist consults with a medical health care professional concerning medical issues that may affect patient's planned dental treatment.

Professional Visits

D9410 House/extended care facility call Ⓑ E1

Includes visits to nursing homes, long-term care facilities, hospice sites, institutions, etc. Report in addition to reporting appropriate code numbers for actual services performed.

D9420 Hospital or ambulatory surgical center call Ⓑ E1

Care provided outside the dentist's office to a patient who is in a hospital or ambulatory surgical center. Services delivered to the patient on the date of service are documented separately using the applicable procedure codes.

D9430 Office visit for observation (during regularly scheduled hours) - no other services performed Ⓑ E1

D9440 Office visit-after regularly scheduled hours Ⓑ E1

Cross Reference 99050

D9450 Case presentation, detailed and extensive treatment planning Ⓑ E1

Established patient. Not performed on same day as evaluation.

Drugs

D9610 Therapeutic parenteral drug, single administration Ⓑ E1

Includes single administration of antibiotics, steroids, anti-inflammatory drugs, or other therapeutic medications. This code should not be used to report administration of sedative, anesthetic or reversal agents.

D9612 Therapeutic parenteral drugs, two or more administrations, different medications Ⓑ E1

Includes multiple administrations of antibiotics, steroids, anti-inflammatory drugs or other therapeutic medications. This code should not be used to report administration of sedatives, anesthetic or reversal agents. This code should be reported when two or more different medications are necessary and should not be reported in addition to code D9610 on the same date.

D9613 Infiltration of sustained release therapeutic drug - single or multiple sites E1

D9630 Drugs or medicaments dispensed in the office for home use Ⓑ B

Includes, but is not limited to oral antibiotics, oral analgesics, and topical fluoride; does not include writing prescriptions.

Miscellaneous Services

D9910 Application of desensitizing medicament Ⓑ E1

Includes in-office treatment for root sensitivity. Typically reported on a "per visit" basis for application of topical fluoride. This code is not to be used for bases, liners or adhesives used under restorations.

▶ New ↺ Revised ✔ Reinstated ~~deleted~~ Deleted ⊘ Not covered or valid by Medicare
⊙ Special coverage instructions ✻ Carrier discretion Ⓑ Bill Part B MAC Ⓑ Bill DME MAC

D9911 Application of desensitizing resin for cervical and/or root surface, per tooth ⓑ E1

Typically reported on a "per tooth" basis for application of adhesive resins. This code is not to be used for bases, liners, or adhesives used under restorations.

D9920 Behavior management, by report ⓑ E1

May be reported in addition to treatment provided. Should be reported in 15-minute increments.

D9930 Treatment of complications (postsurgical) - unusual circumstances, by report ⓑ S

For example, treatment of a dry socket following extraction or removal of bony sequestrum.

D9932 Cleaning and inspection of removable complete denture, maxillary ⓑ E1

This procedure does not include any adjustments.

D9933 Cleaning and inspection of removable complete denture, mandibular ⓑ E1

This procedure does not include any adjustments.

D9934 Cleaning and inspection of removable partial denture, maxillary ⓑ E1

This procedure does not include any adjustments.

D9935 Cleaning and inspection of removable partial denture, mandibular ⓑ E1

This procedure does not include any adjustments.

D9941 Fabrication of athletic mouthguard ⓑ E1

Cross Reference 21089

D9942 Repair and/or reline of occlusal guard ⓑ E1

D9943 Occlusal guard adjustment ⓑ E1

D9944 Occlusal guard - hard appliance, full arch E1

D9945 Occlusal guard - soft appliance, full arch E1

D9946 Occlusal guard - hard appliance, partial arch ⓑ E1

D9950 Occlusion analysis - mounted case ⓑ S

Includes, but is not limited to, facebow, interocclusal records tracings, and diagnostic wax-up; for diagnostic casts, see D0470.

D9951 Occlusal adjustment - limited ⓑ S

May also be known as equilibration; reshaping the occlusal surfaces of teeth to create harmonious contact relationships between the maxillary and mandibular teeth. Presently includes discing/odontoplasty/enamoplasty. Typically reported on a "per visit" basis. This should not be reported when the procedure only involves bite adjustment in the routine post-delivery care for a direct/indirect restoration or fixed/removable prosthodontics.

D9952 Occlusal adjustment - complete ⓑ S

Occlusal adjustment may require several appointments of varying length, and sedation may be necessary to attain adequate relaxation of the musculature. Study casts mounted on an articulating instrument may be utilized for analysis of occlusal disharmony. It is designed to achieve functional relationships and masticatory efficiency in conjunction with restorative treatment, orthodontics, orthognathic surgery, or jaw trauma when indicated. Occlusal adjustment enhances the healing potential of tissues affected by the lesions of occlusal trauma.

D9961 Duplicate/copy of patient's records ⓑ E1

D9970 Enamel microabrasion ⓑ E1

The removal of discolored surface enamel defects resulting from altered mineralization or decalcification of the superficial enamel layer. Submit per treatment visit.

↩ **D9971** Odontoplasty - per tooth ⓑ E1

Removal/reshaping of enamel surfaces or projections

D9972 External bleaching - per arch - performed in office ⓑ E1

D9973 External bleaching - per tooth ⓑ E1

D9974 Internal bleaching - per tooth ⓑ E1

D9975 External bleaching for home application, per arch; includes materials and fabrication of custom trays ⓑ E1

Non-Clinical Procedures

D9985 Sales tax ⓑ E1

D9986 Missed appointment ⓑ E1

D9987 Cancelled appointment ⓑ E1

D9990 Certified translation or sign-language services - per visit ⓑ E1

D9991 Dental case management - addressing appointment compliance barriers Ⓑ E1

Individualized efforts to assist a patient to maintain scheduled appointments by solving transportation challenges or other barriers.

D9992 Dental case management - care coordination Ⓑ E1

Assisting in a patient's decisions regarding the coordination of oral health care services across multiple providers, provider types, specialty areas of treatment, health care settings, health care organizations and payment systems. This is the additional time and resources expended to provide experience or expertise beyond that possessed by the patient.

D9993 Dental case management - motivational interviewing Ⓑ E1

Patient-centered, personalized counseling using methods such as Motivational Interviewing (MI) to identify and modify behaviors interfering with positive oral health outcomes. This is a separate service from traditional nutritional or tobacco counseling.

D9994 Dental case management - patient education to improve oral health literacy Ⓑ E1

Individual, customized communication of information to assist the patient in making appropriate health decisions designed to improve oral health literacy, explained in a manner acknowledging economic circumstances and different cultural beliefs, values, attitudes, traditions and language preferences, and adopting information and services to these differences, which requires the expenditure of time and resources beyond that of an oral evaluation or case presentation.

D9995 Teledentistry synchronous; real-time encounter Ⓑ E1

Reported in addition to other procedures (e.g., diagnostic) delivered to the patient on the date of service.

D9996 Teledentistry asynchronous; information stored and forwarded to dentist for subsequent review Ⓑ E1

Reported in addition to other procedures (e.g., diagnostic) delivered to the patient on the date of service.

D9997 Dental case management - patients with special health care needs E1

Special treatment considerations for patients/individuals with physical, medical, developmental or cognitive conditions resulting in substantial functional limitations, which require that modifications be made to delivery of treatment to provide comprehensive oral health care services.

None

D9999 Unspecified adjunctive procedure, by report Ⓑ E1

Used for procedure that is not adequately described by a code. Describe procedure.

Cross Reference 21499

▶ New ⊋ Revised ✔ Reinstated ~~deleted~~ Deleted ⃠ Not covered or valid by Medicare
Special coverage instructions ✱ Carrier discretion Ⓑ Bill Part B MAC Ⓑ Bill DME MAC

DURABLE MEDICAL EQUIPMENT (E0100-E8002)

Canes

E0100 Cane, includes canes of all materials, adjustable or fixed, with tip Qp Qh Y

IOM: 100-02, 15, 110.1; 100-03, 4, 280.1; 100-03, 4, 280.2

E0105 Cane, quad or three prong, includes canes of all materials, adjustable or fixed, with tips Qp Qh Y

IOM: 100-02, 15, 110.1; 100-03, 4, 280.1; 100-03, 4, 280.2

Coding Clinic: 2016, Q3, P3

Crutches

E0110 Crutches, forearm, includes crutches of various materials, adjustable or fixed, pair, complete with tips and handgrips Qp Qh Y

Crutches are covered when prescribed for a patient who is normally ambulatory but suffers from a condition that impairs ambulation. Provides minimal to moderate weight support while ambulating.

IOM: 100-02, 15, 110.1; 100-03, 4, 280.1

E0111 Crutch forearm, includes crutches of various materials, adjustable or fixed, each, with tips and handgrips Qp Qh Y

IOM: 100-02, 15, 110.1; 100-03, 4, 280.1

E0112 Crutches, underarm, wood, adjustable or fixed, pair, with pads, tips, and handgrips Qp Qh Y

IOM: 100-02, 15, 110.1; 100-03, 4, 280.1

E0113 Crutch underarm, wood, adjustable or fixed, each, with pad, tip, and handgrip Qp Qh Y

IOM: 100-02, 15, 110.1; 100-03, 4, 280.1

E0114 Crutches, underarm, other than wood, adjustable or fixed, pair, with pads, tips and handgrips Qp Qh Y

IOM: 100-02, 15, 110.1; 100-03, 4, 280.1

E0116 Crutch, underarm, other than wood, adjustable or fixed, with pad, tip, handgrip, with or without shock absorber, each Qp Qh Y

IOM: 100-02, 15, 110.1; 100-03, 4, 280.1

E0117 Crutch, underarm, articulating, spring assisted, each Qp Qh Y

IOM: 100-02, 15, 110.1

* **E0118** Crutch substitute, lower leg platform, with or without wheels, each Qp Qh E1

Walkers

E0130 Walker, rigid (pickup), adjustable or fixed height Qp Qh Y

Standard walker criteria for payment: Individual has a mobility limitation that significantly impairs ability to participate in mobility-related activities of daily living that cannot be adequately or safely addressed by a cane. The patient is able to use the walker safely; the functional mobility deficit can be resolved with use of a standard walker.

IOM: 100-02, 15, 110.1; 100-03, 4, 280.1

E0135 Walker, folding (pickup), adjustable or fixed height Qp Qh Y

IOM: 100-02, 15, 110.1; 100-03, 4, 280.1

E0140 Walker, with trunk support, adjustable or fixed height, any type Qp Qh Y

IOM: 100-02, 15, 110.1; 100-03, 4, 280.1

E0141 Walker, rigid, wheeled, adjustable or fixed height Qp Qh Y

IOM: 100-02, 15, 110.1; 100-03, 4, 280.1

E0143 Walker, folding, wheeled, adjustable or fixed height Qp Qh Y

IOM: 100-02, 15, 110.1; 100-03, 4, 280.1

E0144 Walker, enclosed, four sided framed, rigid or folding, wheeled, with posterior seat Qp Qh Y

IOM: 100-02, 15, 110.1; 100-03, 4, 280.1

E0147 Walker, heavy duty, multiple braking system, variable wheel resistance Qp Qh Y

Heavy-duty walker is labeled as capable of supporting more than 300 pounds

IOM: 100-02, 15, 110.1; 100-03, 4, 280.1

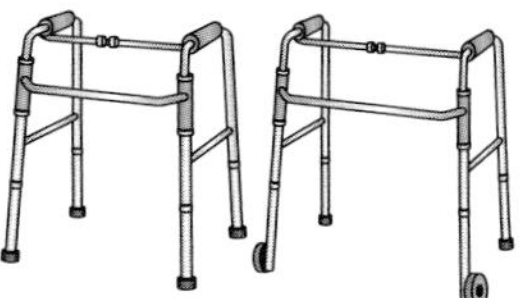

Figure 11 Walkers.

* **E0148** Walker, heavy duty, without wheels, rigid or folding, any type, each Ⓑ Qp Qh ♿ Y
  Heavy-duty walker is labeled as capable of supporting more than 300 pounds
* **E0149** Walker, heavy duty, wheeled, rigid or folding, any type Ⓑ Qp Qh ♿ Y
  Heavy-duty walker is labeled as capable of supporting more than 300 pounds
* **E0153** Platform attachment, forearm crutch, each Ⓑ Qp Qh ♿ Y
* **E0154** Platform attachment, walker, each Ⓑ Qp Qh ♿ Y
* **E0155** Wheel attachment, rigid pick-up walker, per pair Ⓑ Qp Qh ♿ Y

Attachments

* **E0156** Seat attachment, walker Ⓑ Qp Qh ♿ Y
* **E0157** Crutch attachment, walker, each Ⓑ Qp Qh ♿ Y
* **E0158** Leg extensions for walker, per set of four (4) Ⓑ Qp Qh ♿ Y
  Leg extensions are considered medically necessary DME for patients 6 feet tall or more.
* **E0159** Brake attachment for wheeled walker, replacement, each Ⓑ Qp Qh ♿ Y

Sitz Bath/Equipment

E0160 Sitz type bath or equipment, portable, used with or without commode Ⓑ Qp Qh ♿ Y
IOM: 100-03, 4, 280.1

E0161 Sitz type bath or equipment, portable, used with or without commode, with faucet attachment/s Ⓑ Qp Qh ♿ Y
IOM: 100-03, 4, 280.1

E0162 Sitz bath chair Ⓑ Qp Qh ♿ Y
IOM: 100-03, 4, 280.1

Commodes

E0163 Commode chair, mobile or stationary, with fixed arms Ⓑ Qp Qh ♿ Y
IOM: 100-02, 15, 110.1; 100-03, 4, 280.1

E0165 Commode chair, mobile or stationary, with detachable arms Ⓑ Qp Qh ♿ Y
IOM: 100-02, 15, 110.1; 100-03, 4, 280.1

E0167 Pail or pan for use with commode chair, replacement only Ⓑ Qp Qh ♿ Y
IOM: 100-03, 4, 280.1

* **E0168** Commode chair, extra wide and/or heavy duty, stationary or mobile, with or without arms, any type, each Ⓑ Qp Qh ♿ Y
  Extra-wide or heavy duty commode chair is labeled as capable of supporting more than 300 pounds
* **E0170** Commode chair with integrated seat lift mechanism, electric, any type Ⓑ Qp Qh ♿ Y
* **E0171** Commode chair with integrated seat lift mechanism, non-electric, any type Ⓑ Qp Qh ♿ Y

⊘ **E0172** Seat lift mechanism placed over or on top of toilet, any type Ⓑ Qp Qh E1
Medicare Statute 1861 SSA

* **E0175** Foot rest, for use with commode chair, each Ⓑ Qp Qh ♿ Y

Decubitus Care Equipment

E0181 Powered pressure reducing mattress overlay/pad, alternating, with pump, includes heavy duty Ⓑ Qp Qh ♿ Y
Requires the provider to determine medical necessity compliance. To demonstrate the requirements in the medical policy were met, attach KX.
IOM: 100-03, 4, 280.1; 100-08, 5, 5.2.3

E0182 Pump for alternating pressure pad, for replacement only Ⓑ Qp Qh ♿ Y
IOM: 100-03, 4, 280.1; 100-08, 5, 5.2.3

E0184 Dry pressure mattress Ⓑ Qp Qh ♿ Y
IOM: 100-03, 4, 280.1; 100-08, 5, 5.2.3

E0185 Gel or gel-like pressure pad for mattress, standard mattress length and width Ⓑ Qp Qh ♿ Y
IOM: 100-03, 4, 280.1; 100-08, 5, 5.2.3

E0186 Air pressure mattress Ⓑ Qp Qh ♿ Y
IOM: 100-03, 4, 280.1

E0187 Water pressure mattress Ⓑ Qp Qh ♿ Y
IOM: 100-03, 4, 280.1

E0188 Synthetic sheepskin pad Ⓑ Qp Qh ♿ Y
IOM: 100-03, 4, 280.1; 100-08, 5, 5.2.3

E0189 Lambswool sheepskin pad, any size Ⓑ Qp Qh ♿ Y
IOM: 100-03, 4, 280.1; 100-08, 5, 5.2.3

▶ New ⟲ Revised ✓ Reinstated ~~deleted~~ Deleted ⊘ Not covered or valid by Medicare
Special coverage instructions * Carrier discretion Ⓑ Bill Part B MAC Ⓑ Bill DME MAC

E0190 Positioning cushion/pillow/wedge, any shape or size, includes all components and accessories Qp Qh E1

IOM: 100-02, 15, 110.1

E0191 Heel or elbow protector, each Qp Qh Y

E0193 Powered air flotation bed (low air loss therapy) Qp Qh Y

E0194 Air fluidized bed Qp Qh Y

IOM: 100-03, 4, 280.1

E0196 Gel pressure mattress Qp Qh Y

IOM: 100-03, 4, 280.1

E0197 Air pressure pad for mattress, standard mattress length and width Qp Qh Y

IOM: 100-03, 4, 280.1

E0198 Water pressure pad for mattress, standard mattress length and width Qp Qh Y

IOM: 100-03, 4, 280.1

E0199 Dry pressure pad for mattress, standard mattress length and width Qp Qh Y

IOM: 100-03, 4, 280.1

Heat/Cold Application

E0200 Heat lamp, without stand (table model), includes bulb, or infrared element Qp Qh Y

Covered when medical review determines patient's medical condition is one for which application of heat by heat lamp is therapeutically effective

IOM: 100-02, 15, 110.1; 100-03, 4, 280.1

E0202 Phototherapy (bilirubin) light with photometer Qp Qh Y

E0203 Therapeutic lightbox, minimum 10,000 lux, table top model Qp Qh E1

IOM: 100-03, 4, 280.1

E0205 Heat lamp, with stand, includes bulb, or infrared element Qp Qh Y

IOM: 100-02, 15, 110.1; 100-03, 4, 280.1

E0210 Electric heat pad, standard Qp Qh Y

Flexible device containing electric resistive elements producing heat; has fabric cover to prevent burns; with or without timing devices for automatic shut-off

IOM: 100-03, 4, 280.1

E0215 Electric heat pad, moist Qp Qh Y

Flexible device containing electric resistive elements producing heat. Must have component that will absorb and retain liquid (water).

IOM: 100-03, 4, 280.1

E0217 Water circulating heat pad with pump Qp Qh Y

Consists of flexible pad containing series of channels through which water is circulated by means of electrical pumping mechanism and heated in external reservoir

IOM: 100-03, 4, 280.1

E0218 Fluid circulating cold pad with pump, any type Qp Qh Y

IOM: 100-03, 4, 280.1

E0221 Infrared heating pad system Qp Qh Y

E0225 Hydrocollator unit, includes pads Qp Qh Y

IOM: 100-02, 15, 230; 100-03, 4, 280.1

E0231 Non-contact wound warming device (temperature control unit, AC adapter and power cord) for use with warming card and wound cover Qp Qh E1

IOM: 100-02, 16, 20

E0232 Warming card for use with the non-contact wound warming device and non-contact wound warming wound cover Qp Qh E1

IOM: 100-02, 16, 20

E0235 Paraffin bath unit, portable, (see medical supply code A4265 for paraffin) Qp Qh Y

Ordered by physician and patient's condition expected to be relieved by long-term use of modality

IOM: 100-02, 15, 230; 100-03, 4, 280.1

E0236 Pump for water circulating pad Qp Qh Y

IOM: 100-03, 4, 280.1

E0239 Hydrocollator unit, portable Qp Qh Y

IOM: 100-02, 15, 230; 100-03, 4, 280.1

Bath and Toilet Aids

E0240 Bath/shower chair, with or without wheels, any size Qp Qh E1

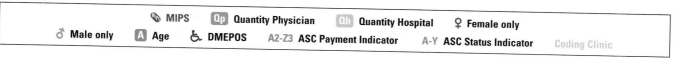

IOM: 100-03, 4, 280.1

⊘ **E0241** Bath tub wall rail, each Ⓑ Qp Qh E1
IOM: 100-02, 15, 110.1; 100-03, 4, 280.1

⊘ **E0242** Bath tub rail, floor base Ⓑ Qp Qh E1
IOM: 100-02, 15, 110.1; 100-03, 4, 280.1

⊘ **E0243** Toilet rail, each Ⓑ Qp Qh E1
IOM: 100-02, 15, 110.1; 100-03, 4, 280.1

⊘ **E0244** Raised toilet seat Ⓑ Qp Qh E1
IOM: 100-03, 4, 280.1

⊘ **E0245** Tub stool or bench Ⓑ Qp Qh E1
IOM: 100-03, 4, 280.1

* **E0246** Transfer tub rail attachment Ⓑ Qp Qh E1

E0247 Transfer bench for tub or toilet with or without commode opening Ⓑ Qp Qh E1
IOM: 100-03, 4, 280.1

E0248 Transfer bench, heavy duty, for tub or toilet with or without commode opening Ⓑ Qp Qh E1
Heavy duty transfer bench is labeled as capable of supporting more than 300 pounds
IOM: 100-03, 4, 280.1

Pad for Heating Unit

E0249 Pad for water circulating heat unit, for replacement only Ⓑ Qp Qh ♿ Y
Describes durable replacement pad used with water circulating heat pump system
IOM: 100-03, 4, 280.1

Hospital Beds and Accessories

E0250 Hospital bed, fixed height, with any type side rails, with mattress Ⓑ Qp Qh ♿ Y
IOM: 100-02, 15, 110.1; 100-03, 4, 280.7

E0251 Hospital bed, fixed height, with any type side rails, without mattress Ⓑ Qp Qh ♿ Y
IOM: 100-02, 15, 110.1; 100-03, 4, 280.7

E0255 Hospital bed, variable height, hi-lo, with any type side rails, with mattress Ⓑ Qp Qh ♿ Y
IOM: 100-02, 15, 110.1; 100-03, 4, 280.7

E0256 Hospital bed, variable height, hi-lo, with any type side rails, without mattress Ⓑ Qp Qh ♿ Y
IOM: 100-02, 15, 110.1; 100-03, 4, 280.7

E0260 Hospital bed, semi-electric (head and foot adjustment), with any type side rails, with mattress Ⓑ Qp Qh ♿ Y
IOM: 100-02, 15, 110.1; 100-03, 4, 280.7

E0261 Hospital bed, semi-electric (head and foot adjustment), with any type side rails, without mattress Ⓑ Qp Qh ♿ Y
IOM: 100-02, 15, 110.1; 100-03, 4, 280.7

E0265 Hospital bed, total electric (head, foot and height adjustments), with any type side rails, with mattress Ⓑ Qp Qh ♿ Y
IOM: 100-02, 15, 110.1; 100-03, 4, 280.7

E0266 Hospital bed, total electric (head, foot and height adjustments), with any type side rails, without mattress Ⓑ Qp Qh ♿ Y
IOM: 100-02, 15, 110.1; 100-03, 4, 280.7

⊘ **E0270** Hospital bed, institutional type includes: oscillating, circulating and Stryker frame, with mattress Ⓑ Qp Qh E1
IOM: 100-03, 4, 280.1

E0271 Mattress, innerspring Ⓑ Qp Qh ♿ Y
IOM: 100-03, 4, 280.1; 100-03, 4, 280.7

E0272 Mattress, foam rubber Ⓑ Qp Qh ♿ Y
IOM: 100-03, 4, 280.1; 100-03, 4, 280.7

⊘ **E0273** Bed board Ⓑ Qp Qh E1
IOM: 100-03, 4, 280.1

⊘ **E0274** Over-bed table Ⓑ Qp Qh E1
IOM: 100-03, 4, 280.1

E0275 Bed pan, standard, metal or plastic Ⓑ Qp Qh ♿ Y
IOM: 100-03, 4, 280.1

E0276 Bed pan, fracture, metal or plastic Ⓑ Qp Qh ♿ Y
IOM: 100-03, 4, 280.1

E0277 Powered pressure-reducing air mattress Ⓑ Qp Qh ♿ Y
IOM: 100-03, 4, 280.1

* **E0280** Bed cradle, any type Ⓑ Qp Qh ♿ Y

E0290 Hospital bed, fixed height, without side rails, with mattress Ⓑ Qp Qh ♿ Y
IOM: 100-02, 15, 110.1; 100-03, 4, 280.7

▶ New ↩ Revised ✔ Reinstated ~~deleted~~ Deleted ⊘ Not covered or valid by Medicare
Special coverage instructions * Carrier discretion Bill Part B MAC Ⓑ Bill DME MAC

E0291 Hospital bed, fixed height, without side rails, without mattress Qp Qh Y

IOM: 100-02, 15, 110.1; 100-03, 4, 280.7

E0292 Hospital bed, variable height, hi-lo, without side rails, with mattress Qp Qh Y

IOM: 100-02, 15, 110.1; 100-03, 4, 280.7

E0293 Hospital bed, variable height, hi-lo, without side rails, without mattress Qp Qh Y

IOM: 100-02, 15, 110.1; 100-03, 4, 280.7

E0294 Hospital bed, semi-electric (head and foot adjustment), without side rails, with mattress Qp Qh Y

IOM: 100-02, 15, 110.1; 100-03, 4, 280.7

E0295 Hospital bed, semi-electric (head and foot adjustment), without side rails, without mattress Qp Qh Y

IOM: 100-02, 15, 110.1; 100-03, 4, 280.7

E0296 Hospital bed, total electric (head, foot and height adjustments), without side rails, with mattress Qp Qh Y

IOM: 100-02, 15, 110.1; 100-03, 4, 280.7

E0297 Hospital bed, total electric (head, foot and height adjustments), without side rails, without mattress Qp Qh Y

IOM: 100-02, 15, 110.1; 100-03, 4, 280.7

* **E0300** Pediatric crib, hospital grade, fully enclosed, with or without top enclosure Qp Qh A Y

E0301 Hospital bed, heavy duty, extra wide, with weight capacity greater than 350 pounds, but less than or equal to 600 pounds, with any type side rails, without mattress Qp Qh Y

IOM: 100-03, 4, 280.7

E0302 Hospital bed, extra heavy duty, extra wide, with weight capacity greater than 600 pounds, with any type side rails, without mattress Qp Qh Y

IOM: 100-03, 4, 280.7

E0303 Hospital bed, heavy duty, extra wide, with weight capacity greater than 350 pounds, but less than or equal to 600 pounds, with any type side rails, with mattress Qp Qh Y

IOM: 100-03, 4, 280.7

E0304 Hospital bed, extra heavy duty, extra wide, with weight capacity greater than 600 pounds, with any type side rails, with mattress Qp Qh Y

IOM: 100-03, 4, 280.7

E0305 Bed side rails, half length Qp Qh Y

IOM: 100-03, 4, 280.7

E0310 Bed side rails, full length Qp Qh Y

IOM: 100-03, 4, 280.7

E0315 Bed accessory: board, table, or support device, any type Qp Qh E1

IOM: 100-03, 4, 280.1

* **E0316** Safety enclosure frame/canopy for use with hospital bed, any type Qp Qh Y

E0325 Urinal; male, jug-type, any material Qp Qh ♂ Y

IOM: 100-03, 4, 280.1

E0326 Urinal; female, jug-type, any material Qp Qh ♀ Y

IOM: 100-03, 4, 280.1

* **E0328** Hospital bed, pediatric, manual, 360 degree side enclosures, top of headboard, footboard and side rails up to 24 inches above the spring, includes mattress Qp Qh A Y

* **E0329** Hospital bed, pediatric, electric or semi-electric, 360 degree side enclosures, top of headboard, footboard and side rails up to 24 inches above the spring, includes mattress Qp Qh A Y

* **E0350** Control unit for electronic bowel irrigation/evacuation system Qp Qh E1

Pulsed Irrigation Enhanced Evacuation (PIEE) is pulsed irrigation of severely impacted fecal material and may be necessary for patients who have not responded to traditional bowel program.

* **E0352** Disposable pack (water reservoir bag, speculum, valving mechanism and collection bag/box) for use with the electronic bowel irrigation/evacuation system Qp Qh E1

Therapy kit includes 1 B-Valve circuit, 2 containment bags, 1 lubricating jelly, 1 bed pad, 1 tray liner-waste disposable bag, and 2 hose clamps

* **E0370** Air pressure elevator for heel Qp Qh E1

MIPS | Qp Quantity Physician | Qh Quantity Hospital | ♀ Female only
♂ Male only | A Age | DMEPOS | A2-Z3 ASC Payment Indicator | A-Y ASC Status Indicator | Coding Clinic

✻ **E0371** Non powered advanced pressure reducing overlay for mattress, standard mattress length and width Ⓑ Qp Qh ♿ Y

Patient has at least one large Stage III or Stage IV pressure sore (greater than 2 × 2 cm.) on trunk, with only two turning surfaces on which to lie

✻ **E0372** Powered air overlay for mattress, standard mattress length and width Ⓑ Qp Qh ♿ Y

✻ **E0373** Non powered advanced pressure reducing mattress Ⓑ Qp Qh ♿ Y

Oxygen and Related Respiratory Equipment

◌ **E0424** Stationary compressed gaseous oxygen system, rental; includes container, contents, regulator, flowmeter, humidifier, nebulizer, cannula or mask, and tubing Ⓑ Qp Qh ♿ Y

IOM: 100-03, 4, 280.1; 100-04, 20, 30.6

◌ **E0425** Stationary compressed gas system, purchase; includes regulator, flowmeter, humidifier, nebulizer, cannula or mask, and tubing Ⓑ Qp Qh E1

IOM: 100-03, 4, 280.1; 100-04, 20, 30.6

◌ **E0430** Portable gaseous oxygen system, purchase; includes regulator, flowmeter, humidifier, cannula or mask, and tubing Ⓑ Qp Qh E1

IOM: 100-03, 4, 280.1; 100-04, 20, 30.6

◌ **E0431** Portable gaseous oxygen system, rental; includes portable container, regulator, flowmeter, humidifier, cannula or mask, and tubing Ⓑ Qp Qh ♿ Y

IOM: 100-03, 4, 280.1; 100-04, 20, 30.6

✻ **E0433** Portable liquid oxygen system, rental; home liquefier used to fill portable liquid oxygen containers, includes portable containers, regulator, flowmeter, humidifier, cannula or mask and tubing, with or without supply reservoir and contents gauge Ⓑ Qh ♿ Y

◌ **E0434** Portable liquid oxygen system, rental; includes portable container, supply reservoir, humidifier, flowmeter, refill adaptor, contents gauge, cannula or mask, and tubing Ⓑ Qp Qh ♿ Y

Fee schedule payments for stationary oxygen system rentals are all-inclusive and represent monthly allowance for beneficiary. Non-Medicare payers may rent device to beneficiaries, or arrange for purchase of device.

IOM: 100-03, 4, 280.1; 100-04, 20, 30.6

◌ **E0435** Portable liquid oxygen system, purchase; includes portable container, supply reservoir, flowmeter, humidifier, contents gauge, cannula or mask, tubing and refill adaptor Ⓑ Qp Qh E1

IOM: 100-03, 4, 280.1; 100-04, 20, 30.6

◌ **E0439** Stationary liquid oxygen system, rental; includes container, contents, regulator, flowmeter, humidifier, nebulizer, cannula or mask, and tubing Ⓑ Qp Qh ♿ Y

This allowance includes payment for equipment, contents, and accessories furnished during rental month

IOM: 100-03, 4, 280.1; 100-04, 20, 30.6

◌ **E0440** Stationary liquid oxygen system, purchase; includes use of reservoir, contents indicator, regulator, flowmeter, humidifier, nebulizer, cannula or mask, and tubing Ⓑ Qp Qh E1

IOM: 100-03, 4, 280.1; 100-04, 20, 30.6

◌ **E0441** Stationary oxygen contents, gaseous, 1 month's supply = 1 unit Ⓑ Qp Qh ♿ Y

IOM: 100-03, 4, 280.1; 100-04, 20, 30.6

◌ **E0442** Stationary oxygen contents, liquid, 1 month's supply = 1 unit Ⓑ Qp Qh ♿ Y

IOM: 100-03, 4, 280.1; 100-04, 20, 30.6

◌ **E0443** Portable oxygen contents, gaseous, 1 month's supply = 1 unit Ⓑ Qp Qh ♿ Y

IOM: 100-03, 4, 280.1; 100-04, 20, 30.6

◌ **E0444** Portable oxygen contents, liquid, 1 month's supply = 1 unit Ⓑ Qp Qh ♿ Y

IOM: 100-03, 4, 280.1; 100-04, 20, 30.6

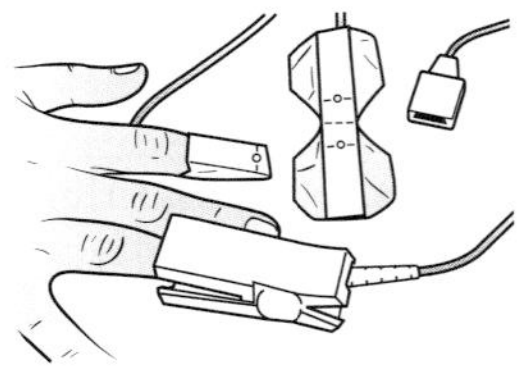

Figure 12 Oximeter device.

▶ New ↩ Revised ✔ Reinstated ~~deleted~~ Deleted ⊘ Not covered or valid by Medicare
◌ Special coverage instructions ✻ Carrier discretion Ⓑ Bill Part B MAC Ⓑ Bill DME MAC

* **E0445** Oximeter device for measuring blood oxygen levels non-invasively Qp Qh N

* **E0446** Topical oxygen delivery system, not otherwise specified, includes all supplies and accessories Qp Qh A

E0447 Portable oxygen contents, liquid, 1 month's supply = 1 unit, prescribed amount at rest or nighttime exceeds 4 liters per minute (lpm) Y

E0455 Oxygen tent, excluding croup or pediatric tents Qp Qh Y

IOM: 100-03, 4, 280.1; 100-04, 20, 30.6

E0457 Chest shell (cuirass) Qp Qh E1

E0459 Chest wrap Qp Qh E1

* **E0462** Rocking bed with or without side rails Qp Qh Y

E0465 Home ventilator, any type, used with invasive interface (e.g., tracheostomy tube) Qp Qh Y

IOM: 100-03, 4, 280.1

E0466 Home ventilator, any type, used with non-invasive interface (e.g., mask, chest shell) Qp Qh Y

IOM: 100-03, 4, 280.1

E0467 Home ventilator, multi-function respiratory device, also performs any or all of the additional functions of oxygen concentration, drug nebulization, aspiration, and cough stimulation, includes all accessories, components and supplies for all functions Y

E0470 Respiratory assist device, bi-level pressure capability, without backup rate feature, used with noninvasive interface, e.g., nasal or facial mask (intermittent assist device with continuous positive airway pressure device) Qp Qh Y

IOM: 100-03, 4, 240.2

E0471 Respiratory assist device, bi-level pressure capability, with back-up rate feature, used with noninvasive interface, e.g., nasal or facial mask (intermittent assist device with continuous positive airway pressure device) Qp Qh Y

IOM: 100-03, 4, 240.2

E0472 Respiratory assist device, bi-level pressure capability, with backup rate feature, used with invasive interface, e.g., tracheostomy tube (intermittent assist device with continuous positive airway pressure device) Qp Qh Y

IOM: 100-03, 4, 240.2

E0480 Percussor, electric or pneumatic, home model Qp Qh Y

IOM: 100-03, 4, 240.2

E0481 Intrapulmonary percussive ventilation system and related accessories Qp Qh E1

IOM: 100-03, 4, 240.2

* **E0482** Cough stimulating device, alternating positive and negative airway pressure Qp Qh Y

* **E0483** High frequency chest wall oscillation system, includes all accessories and supplies, each Qp Qh Y

* **E0484** Oscillatory positive expiratory pressure device, non-electric, any type, each Qp Qh Y

* **E0485** Oral device/appliance used to reduce upper airway collapsibility, adjustable or non-adjustable, prefabricated, includes fitting and adjustment Qp Qh Y

* **E0486** Oral device/appliance used to reduce upper airway collapsibility, adjustable or non-adjustable, custom fabricated, includes fitting and adjustment Qp Qh Y

E0487 Spirometer, electronic, includes all accessories Qp Qh N

IPPB Machines

E0500 IPPB machine, all types, with built-in nebulization; manual or automatic valves; internal or external power source Qp Qh Y

IOM: 100-03, 4, 240.2

Humidifiers/Nebulizers/Compressors for Use with Oxygen IPPB Equipment

E0550 Humidifier, durable for extensive supplemental humidification during IPPB treatments or oxygen delivery Qp Qh Y

IOM: 100-03, 4, 240.2

E0555 Humidifier, durable, glass or autoclavable plastic bottle type, for use with regulator or flowmeter Qp Qh Y

IOM: 100-03, 4, 280.1; 100-04, 20, 30.6

E0560 Humidifier, durable for supplemental humidification during IPPB treatment or oxygen delivery Qp Qh Y

IOM: 100-03, 4, 280.1

MIPS | Qp Quantity Physician | Qh Quantity Hospital | ♀ Female only | ♂ Male only | A Age | DMEPOS | A2-Z3 ASC Payment Indicator | A-Y ASC Status Indicator | Coding Clinic

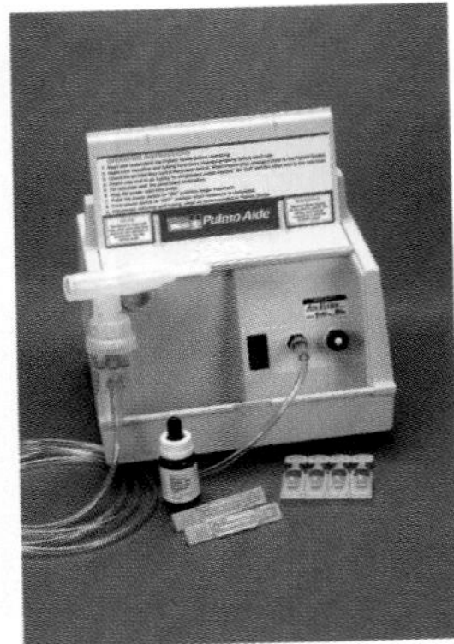

Figure 13 Nebulizer

* **E0561** Humidifier, non-heated, used with positive airway pressure device Ⓑ Qp Qh ♿ Y

* **E0562** Humidifier, heated, used with positive airway pressure device Ⓑ Qp Qh ♿ Y

* **E0565** Compressor, air power source for equipment which is not self-contained or cylinder driven Ⓑ Qp Qh ♿ Y

○ **E0570** Nebulizer, with compressor Ⓑ Qp Qh ♿ Y

IOM: 100-03, 4, 240.2; 100-03, 4, 280.1

* **E0572** Aerosol compressor, adjustable pressure, light duty for intermittent use Ⓑ Qp Qh ♿ Y

* **E0574** Ultrasonic/electronic aerosol generator with small volume nebulizer Ⓑ Qp Qh ♿ Y

○ **E0575** Nebulizer, ultrasonic, large volume Ⓑ Qp Qh ♿ Y

IOM: 100-03, 4, 240.2

○ **E0580** Nebulizer, durable, glass or autoclavable plastic, bottle type, for use with regulator or flowmeter Ⓑ Qp Qh ♿ Y

IOM: 100-03, 4, 240.2; 100-03, 4, 280.1

○ **E0585** Nebulizer, with compressor and heater Ⓑ Qp Qh ♿ Y

IOM: 100-03, 4, 240.2; 100-03, 4, 280.1

Suction Pump/CPAP

○ **E0600** Respiratory suction pump, home model, portable or stationary, electric Ⓑ Qp Qh ♿ Y

IOM: 100-03, 4, 240.2

○ **E0601** Continuous positive airway pressure (CPAP) device Ⓑ Qp Qh ♿ Y

IOM: 100-03, 4, 240.4

Breast Pump

* **E0602** Breast pump, manual, any type Ⓑ Qp Qh ♀ ♿ Y

Bill either manual breast pump or breast pump kit

* **E0603** Breast pump, electric (AC and/or DC), any type Ⓑ Qp Qh ♀ N

* **E0604** Breast pump, hospital grade, electric (AC and/or DC), any type Ⓑ Qp Qh ♀ A

Other Breathing Aids

○ **E0605** Vaporizer, room type Ⓑ Qp Qh ♿ Y

IOM: 100-03, 4, 240.2

○ **E0606** Postural drainage board Ⓑ Qp Qh ♿ Y

IOM: 100-03, 4, 240.2

Monitoring Equipment

○ **E0607** Home blood glucose monitor Ⓑ Qp Qh ♿ Y

Document recipient or caregiver is competent to monitor equipment and that device is designed for home rather than clinical use

IOM: 100-03, 4, 280.1; 100-03, 1, 40.2

○ **E0610** Pacemaker monitor, self-contained, (checks battery depletion, includes audible and visible check systems) Ⓑ Qp Qh ♿ Y

IOM: 100-03, 1, 20.8

○ **E0615** Pacemaker monitor, self-contained, checks battery depletion and other pacemaker components, includes digital/visible check systems Ⓑ Qp Qh ♿ Y

IOM: 100-03, 1, 20.8

* **E0616** Implantable cardiac event recorder with memory, activator and programmer Ⓑ Qp Qh N

Assign when two 30-day pre-symptom external loop recordings fail to establish a definitive diagnosis

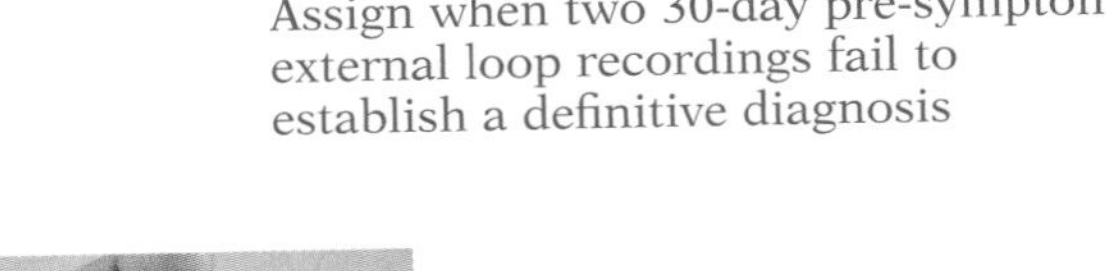

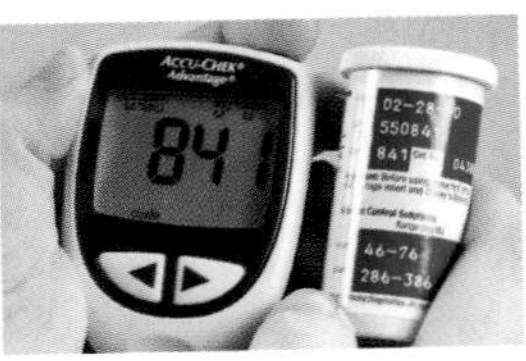
ACCU-CHEK
Advantage
84

Figure 14 Glucose monitor.

▶ New ⮌ Revised ✔ Reinstated ~~deleted~~ Deleted ⊘ Not covered or valid by Medicare
○ Special coverage instructions * Carrier discretion Ⓑ Bill Part B MAC Ⓑ Bill DME MAC

* **E0617** External defibrillator with integrated electrocardiogram analysis Ⓑ Qp Qh ♿ Y
* **E0618** Apnea monitor, without recording feature Ⓑ Qp Qh ♿ Y
* **E0619** Apnea monitor, with recording feature Ⓑ Qp Qh ♿ Y
* **E0620** Skin piercing device for collection of capillary blood, laser, each Ⓑ Qp Qh ♿ Y

Patient Lifts

E0621 Sling or seat, patient lift, canvas or nylon Ⓑ Qp Qh ♿ Y

IOM: 100-03, 4, 240.2, 280.4

⊘ **E0625** Patient lift, bathroom or toilet, not otherwise classified Ⓑ Qp Qh E1

IOM: 100-03, 4, 240.2

E0627 Seat lift mechanism, electric, any type Ⓑ Qp Qh ♿ Y

IOM: 100-03, 4, 280.4; 100-04, 4, 20

E0629 Seat lift mechanism, non-electric, any type Ⓑ Qp Qh ♿ Y

IOM: 100-04, 4, 20

E0630 Patient lift, hydraulic or mechanical, includes any seat, sling, strap(s) or pad(s) Ⓑ Qp Qh ♿ Y

IOM: 100-03, 4, 240.2

E0635 Patient lift, electric, with seat or sling Ⓑ Qp Qh ♿ Y

IOM: 100-03, 4, 240.2

* **E0636** Multipositional patient support system, with integrated lift, patient accessible controls Ⓑ Qp Qh ♿ Y

⊘ **E0637** Combination sit to stand frame/table system, any size including pediatric, with seat lift feature, with or without wheels Ⓑ Qp Qh E1

IOM: 100-03, 4, 240.2

⊘ **E0638** Standing frame/table system, one position (e.g., upright, supine or prone stander), any size including pediatric, with or without wheels Ⓑ Qp Qh E1

IOM: 100-03, 4, 240.2

* **E0639** Patient lift, moveable from room to room with disassembly and reassembly, includes all components/ accessories Ⓑ Qp Qh ♿ E1
* **E0640** Patient lift, fixed system, includes all components/ accessories Ⓑ Qp Qh ♿ E1

⊘ **E0641** Standing frame/table system, multi-position (e.g., three-way stander), any size including pediatric, with or without wheels Ⓑ Qp Qh E1

IOM: 100-03, 4, 240.2

⊘ **E0642** Standing frame/table system, mobile (dynamic stander), any size including pediatric Ⓑ Qp Qh E1

IOM: 100-03, 4, 240.2

Pneumatic Compressor and Appliances

E0650 Pneumatic compressor, non-segmental home model Ⓑ Qp Qh ♿ Y

Lymphedema pumps are classified as segmented or nonsegmented, depending on whether distinct segments of devices can be inflated sequentially.

IOM: 100-03, 4, 280.6

E0651 Pneumatic compressor, segmental home model without calibrated gradient pressure Ⓑ Qp Qh ♿ Y

IOM: 100-03, 4, 280.6

E0652 Pneumatic compressor, segmental home model with calibrated gradient pressure Ⓑ Qp Qh ♿ Y

IOM: 100-03, 4, 280.6

E0655 Non-segmental pneumatic appliance for use with pneumatic compressor, half arm Ⓑ Qp Qh ♿ Y

IOM: 100-03, 4, 280.6

E0656 Segmental pneumatic appliance for use with pneumatic compressor, trunk Ⓑ Qp Qh ♿ Y

E0657 Segmental pneumatic appliance for use with pneumatic compressor, chest Ⓑ Qp Qh ♿ Y

E0660 Non-segmental pneumatic appliance for use with pneumatic compressor, full leg Ⓑ Qp Qh ♿ Y

IOM: 100-03, 4, 280.6

E0665 Non-segmental pneumatic appliance for use with pneumatic compressor, full arm Ⓑ Qp Qh ♿ Y

IOM: 100-03, 4, 280.6

E0666 Non-segmental pneumatic appliance for use with pneumatic compressor, half leg Ⓑ Qp Qh ♿ Y

IOM: 100-03, 4, 280.6

E0667 Segmental pneumatic appliance for use with pneumatic compressor, full leg Y

IOM: 100-03, 4, 280.6

E0668 Segmental pneumatic appliance for use with pneumatic compressor, full arm Y

IOM: 100-03, 4, 280.6

E0669 Segmental pneumatic appliance for use with pneumatic compressor, half leg Y

IOM: 100-03, 4, 280.6

E0670 Segmental pneumatic appliance for use with pneumatic compressor, integrated, 2 full legs and trunk Y

IOM: 100-03, 4, 280.6

E0671 Segmental gradient pressure pneumatic appliance, full leg Y

IOM: 100-03, 4, 280.6

E0672 Segmental gradient pressure pneumatic appliance, full arm Y

IOM: 100-03, 4, 280.6

E0673 Segmental gradient pressure pneumatic appliance, half leg Y

IOM: 100-03, 4, 280.6

* **E0675** Pneumatic compression device, high pressure, rapid inflation/deflation cycle, for arterial insufficiency (unilateral or bilateral system) Y

* **E0676** Intermittent limb compression device (includes all accessories), not otherwise specified Y

Ultraviolet Light Therapy Systems

* **E0691** Ultraviolet light therapy system, includes bulbs/lamps, timer and eye protection; treatment area 2 square feet or less Y

* **E0692** Ultraviolet light therapy system panel, includes bulbs/lamps, timer and eye protection, 4 foot panel Y

* **E0693** Ultraviolet light therapy system panel, includes bulbs/lamps, timer and eye protection, 6 foot panel Y

* **E0694** Ultraviolet multidirectional light therapy system in 6 foot cabinet, includes bulbs/lamps, timer and eye protection Y

Safety Equipment

* **E0700** Safety equipment, device or accessory, any type E1

E0705 Transfer device, any type, each B

Restraints

* **E0710** Restraints, any type (body, chest, wrist or ankle) E1

Transcutaneous and/or Neuromuscular Electrical Nerve Stimulators (TENS)

E0720 Transcutaneous electrical nerve stimulation (TENS) device, two lead, localized stimulation Y

A Certificate of Medical Necessity (CMN) is not needed for a TENS rental, but is needed for purchase.

IOM: 100-03, 2, 160.2; 100-03, 4, 280.1

E0730 Transcutaneous electrical nerve stimulation (TENS) device, four or more leads, for multiple nerve stimulation Y

IOM: 100-03, 2, 160.2; 100-03, 4, 280.1

E0731 Form-fitting conductive garment for delivery of TENS or NMES (with conductive fibers separated from the patient's skin by layers of fabric) Y

IOM: 100-03, 2, 160.13

E0740 Non-implanted pelvic floor electrical stimulator, complete system Y

IOM: 100-03, 4, 230.8

* **E0744** Neuromuscular stimulator for scoliosis Y

E0745 Neuromuscular stimulator, electronic shock unit Y

IOM: 100-03, 2, 160.12

E0746 Electromyography (EMG), biofeedback device N

IOM: 100-03, 1, 30.1

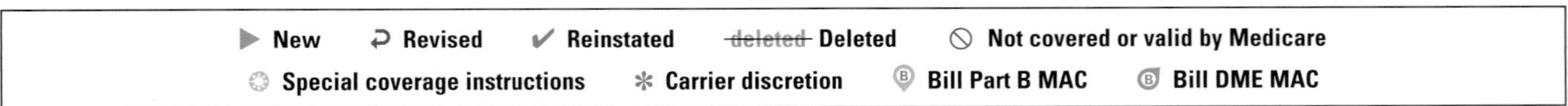

New
Revised
Reinstated
deleted Deleted
Not covered or valid by Medicare
Special coverage instructions
Carrier discretion
Bill Part B MAC
Bill DME MAC

E0747 Osteogenesis stimulator, electrical, non-invasive, other than spinal applications Qp Qh Y

Devices are composed of two basic parts: Coils that wrap around cast and pulse generator that produces electric current

E0748 Osteogenesis stimulator, electrical, non-invasive, spinal applications Qp Qh Y

Device should be applied within 30 days as adjunct to spinal fusion surgery

E0749 Osteogenesis stimulator, electrical, surgically implanted Qp Qh N

* **E0755** Electronic salivary reflex stimulator (intra-oral/non-invasive) Qp Qh E1

* **E0760** Osteogenesis stimulator, low intensity ultrasound, non-invasive Qp Qh Y

Ultrasonic osteogenesis stimulator may not be used concurrently with other noninvasive stimulators

E0761 Non-thermal pulsed high frequency radiowaves, high peak power electromagnetic energy treatment device Qp Qh E1

* **E0762** Transcutaneous electrical joint stimulation device system, includes all accessories Qp Qh B

E0764 Functional neuromuscular stimulator, transcutaneous stimulation of sequential muscle groups of ambulation with computer control, used for walking by spinal cord injured, entire system, after completion of training program Qp Qh Y

IOM: 100-03, 2, 160.12

* **E0765** FDA approved nerve stimulator, with replaceable batteries, for treatment of nausea and vomiting Qp Qh Y

* **E0766** Electrical stimulation device used for cancer treatment, includes all accessories, any type Qp Qh Y

E0769 Electrical stimulation or electromagnetic wound treatment device, not otherwise classified Qp Qh B

IOM: 100-04, 32, 11.1

E0770 Functional electrical stimulator, transcutaneous stimulation of nerve and/or muscle groups, any type, complete system, not otherwise specified Qp Qh Y

Infusion Supplies

* **E0776** IV pole Qp Qh Y

PEN: On Fee Schedule

* **E0779** Ambulatory infusion pump, mechanical, reusable, for infusion 8 hours or greater Qp Qh Y

Requires prior authorization and copy of invoice

This is a capped rental infusion pump modifier. The correct monthly modifier (KH, KI, KJ) is used to indicate which month the rental is for (i.e., KH, month 1; KI, months 2 and 3; KJ, months 4 through 13).

* **E0780** Ambulatory infusion pump, mechanical, reusable, for infusion less than 8 hours Qp Qh Y

Requires prior authorization and copy of invoice

E0781 Ambulatory infusion pump, single or multiple channels, electric or battery operated with administrative equipment, worn by patient Qp Qh Y

IOM: 100-03, 1, 50.3

E0782 Infusion pump, implantable, non-programmable (includes all components, e.g., pump, cathether, connectors, etc.) Qp Qh N

IOM: 100-03, 1, 50.3

E0783 Infusion pump system, implantable, programmable (includes all components, e.g., pump, catheter, connectors, etc.) Qp Qh N

IOM: 100-03, 1, 50.3

E0784 External ambulatory infusion pump, insulin Qp Qh Y

IOM: 100-03, 4, 280.14

E0785 Implantable intraspinal (epidural/intrathecal) catheter used with implantable infusion pump, replacement Qp Qh N

IOM: 100-03, 1, 50.3

E0786 Implantable programmable infusion pump, replacement (excludes implantable intraspinal catheter) Qp Qh N

IOM: 100-03, 1, 50.3

* **E0787** External ambulatory infusion pump, insulin, dosage rate adjustment using therapeutic continuous glucose sensing Y

MIPS | Qp Quantity Physician | Qh Quantity Hospital | ♀ Female only | ♂ Male only | A Age | DMEPOS | A2-Z3 ASC Payment Indicator | A-Y ASC Status Indicator | Coding Clinic

E0791 Parenteral infusion pump, stationary, single or multi-channel Y

IOM: 100-02, 15, 120; 100-03, 3, 180.2; 100-04, 20, 100.2.2

Traction Equipment and Orthopedic Devices

E0830 Ambulatory traction device, all types, each N

IOM: 100-03, 4, 280.1

E0840 Traction frame, attached to headboard, cervical traction Y

IOM: 100-03, 4, 280.1

* **E0849** Traction equipment, cervical, free-standing stand/frame, pneumatic, applying traction force to other than mandible Y

E0850 Traction stand, free standing, cervical traction Y

IOM: 100-03, 4, 280.1

* **E0855** Cervical traction equipment not requiring additional stand or frame Y

* **E0856** Cervical traction device, with inflatable air bladder(s) Y

E0860 Traction equipment, overdoor, cervical Y

IOM: 100-03, 4, 280.1

E0870 Traction frame, attached to footboard, extremity traction, (e.g., Buck's) Y

IOM: 100-03, 4, 280.1

E0880 Traction stand, free standing, extremity traction Y

IOM: 100-03, 4, 280.1

E0890 Traction frame, attached to footboard, pelvic traction Y

IOM: 100-03, 4, 280.1

E0900 Traction stand, free standing, pelvic traction (e.g., Buck's) Y

IOM: 100-03, 4, 280.1

E0910 Trapeze bars, A/K/A patient helper, attached to bed, with grab bar Y

IOM: 100-03, 4, 280.1

E0911 Trapeze bar, heavy duty, for patient weight capacity greater than 250 pounds, attached to bed, with grab bar Y

IOM: 100-03, 4, 280.1

E0912 Trapeze bar, heavy duty, for patient weight capacity greater than 250 pounds, free standing, complete with grab bar Y

IOM: 100-03, 4, 280.1

E0920 Fracture frame, attached to bed, includes weights Y

IOM: 100-03, 4, 280.1

E0930 Fracture frame, free standing, includes weights Y

IOM: 100-03, 4, 280.1

E0935 Continuous passive motion exercise device for use on knee only Y

To qualify for coverage, use of device must commence within two days following surgery

IOM: 100-03, 4, 280.1

E0936 Continuous passive motion exercise device for use other than knee E1

E0940 Trapeze bar, free standing, complete with grab bar Y

IOM: 100-03, 4, 280.1

E0941 Gravity assisted traction device, any type Y

IOM: 100-03, 4, 280.1

* **E0942** Cervical head harness/halter Y

* **E0944** Pelvic belt/harness/boot Y

* **E0945** Extremity belt/harness Y

E0946 Fracture, frame, dual with cross bars, attached to bed (e.g., Balken, 4 poster) Y

IOM: 100-03, 4, 280.1

E0947 Fracture frame, attachments for complex pelvic traction Y

IOM: 100-03, 4, 280.1

E0948 Fracture frame, attachments for complex cervical traction Y

IOM: 100-03, 4, 280.1

Wheelchair Accessories

E0950 Wheelchair accessory, tray, each Y

IOM: 100-03, 4, 280.1

▶ New ↩ Revised ✓ Reinstated ~~deleted~~ Deleted ⊘ Not covered or valid by Medicare
Special coverage instructions * Carrier discretion Bill Part B MAC Bill DME MAC

* **E0951** Heel loop/holder, any type, with or without ankle strap, each Ⓑ Qp Qh ♿ Y

E0952 Toe loop/holder, any type, each Ⓑ Qp Qh ♿ Y

IOM: 100-03, 4, 280.1

* **E0953** Wheelchair accessory, lateral thigh or knee support, any type, including fixed mounting hardware, each Y

* **E0954** Wheelchair accessory, foot box, any type, includes attachment and mounting hardware, each foot Y

* **E0955** Wheelchair accessory, headrest, cushioned, any type, including fixed mounting hardware, each Ⓑ Qp Qh ♿ Y

* **E0956** Wheelchair accessory, lateral trunk or hip support, any type, including fixed mounting hardware, each Ⓑ Qp Qh ♿ Y

* **E0957** Wheelchair accessory, medial thigh support, any type, including fixed mounting hardware, each Ⓑ Qp Qh ♿ Y

E0958 Manual wheelchair accessory, one-arm drive attachment, each Ⓑ Qp Qh ♿ Y

IOM: 100-03, 4, 280.1

* **E0959** Manual wheelchair accessory, adapter for amputee, each Ⓑ Qp Qh ♿ B

IOM: 100-03, 4, 280.1

* **E0960** Wheelchair accessory, shoulder harness/straps or chest strap, including any type mounting hardware Ⓑ Qp Qh ♿ Y

* **E0961** Manual wheelchair accessory, wheel lock brake extension (handle), each Ⓑ Qp Qh ♿ B

IOM: 100-03, 4, 280.1

* **E0966** Manual wheelchair accessory, headrest extension, each Ⓑ Qp Qh ♿ B

IOM: 100-03, 4, 280.1

E0967 Manual wheelchair accessory, hand rim with projections, any type, replacement only, each Ⓑ Qp Qh ♿ Y

IOM: 100-03, 4, 280.1

E0968 Commode seat, wheelchair Ⓑ Qp Qh ♿ Y

IOM: 100-03, 4, 280.1

E0969 Narrowing device, wheelchair Ⓑ ♿ Y

IOM: 100-03, 4, 280.1

⊘ **E0970** No. 2 footplates, except for elevating leg rest Ⓑ Qp Qh E1

IOM: 100-03, 4, 280.1

Cross Reference K0037, K0042

* **E0971** Manual wheelchair accessory, anti-tipping device, each Ⓑ Qp Qh ♿ B

IOM: 100-03, 4, 280.1

Cross Reference K0021

E0973 Wheelchair accessory, adjustable height, detachable armrest, complete assembly, each Ⓑ Qp Qh ♿ B

IOM: 100-03, 4, 280.1

E0974 Manual wheelchair accessory, anti-rollback device, each Ⓑ Qp Qh ♿ B

IOM: 100-03, 4, 280.1

* **E0978** Wheelchair accessory, positioning belt/safety belt/pelvic strap, each Ⓑ Qp Qh ♿ B

* **E0980** Safety vest, wheelchair Ⓑ ♿ Y

* **E0981** Wheelchair accessory, seat upholstery, replacement only, each Ⓑ Qp Qh ♿ Y

* **E0982** Wheelchair accessory, back upholstery, replacement only, each Ⓑ Qp Qh ♿ Y

* **E0983** Manual wheelchair accessory, power add-on to convert manual wheelchair to motorized wheelchair, joystick control Ⓑ Qp Qh ♿ Y

* **E0984** Manual wheelchair accessory, power add-on to convert manual wheelchair to motorized wheelchair, tiller control Ⓑ Qp Qh ♿ Y

* **E0985** Wheelchair accessory, seat lift mechanism Ⓑ Qp Qh ♿ Y

* **E0986** Manual wheelchair accessory, push-rim activated power assist system Ⓑ Qp Qh ♿ Y

* **E0988** Manual wheelchair accessory, lever-activated, wheel drive, pair Ⓑ Qp Qh ♿ Y

* **E0990** Wheelchair accessory, elevating leg rest, complete assembly, each Ⓑ Qp Qh ♿ B

IOM: 100-03, 4, 280.1

* **E0992** Manual wheelchair accessory, solid seat insert Ⓑ Qp Qh ♿ B

E0994 Arm rest, each Ⓑ Qp Qh ♿ Y

IOM: 100-03, 4, 280.1

* **E0995** Wheelchair accessory, calf rest/pad, replacement only, each Ⓑ Qp Qh ♿ B

IOM: 100-03, 4, 280.1

✻ **E1002** Wheelchair accessory, power seating system, tilt only Ⓑ Qp Qh ♿ Y

✻ **E1003** Wheelchair accessory, power seating system, recline only, without shear reduction Ⓑ Qp Qh ♿ Y

✻ **E1004** Wheelchair accessory, power seating system, recline only, with mechanical shear reduction Ⓑ Qp Qh ♿ Y

✻ **E1005** Wheelchair accessory, power seating system, recline only, with power shear reduction Ⓑ Qp Qh ♿ Y

✻ **E1006** Wheelchair accessory, power seating system, combination tilt and recline, without shear reduction Ⓑ Qp Qh ♿ Y

✻ **E1007** Wheelchair accessory, power seating system, combination tilt and recline, with mechanical shear reduction Ⓑ Qp Qh ♿ Y

✻ **E1008** Wheelchair accessory, power seating system, combination tilt and recline, with power shear reduction Ⓑ Qp Qh ♿ Y

✻ **E1009** Wheelchair accessory, addition to power seating system, mechanically linked leg elevation system, including pushrod and leg rest, each Ⓑ Qp Qh ♿ Y

✻ **E1010** Wheelchair accessory, addition to power seating system, power leg elevation system, including leg rest, pair Ⓑ Qp Qh ♿ Y

⊛ **E1011** Modification to pediatric size wheelchair, width adjustment package (not to be dispensed with initial chair) Ⓑ Qp Qh A ♿ Y

IOM: 100-03, 4, 280.1

✻ **E1012** Wheelchair accessory, addition to power seating system, center mount power elevating leg rest/platform, complete system, any type, each Qp Qh ♿ Y

⊛ **E1014** Reclining back, addition to pediatric size wheelchair Ⓑ Qp Qh A ♿ Y

IOM: 100-03, 4, 280.1

⊛ **E1015** Shock absorber for manual wheelchair, each Ⓑ Qp Qh ♿ Y

IOM: 100-03, 4, 280.1

⊛ **E1016** Shock absorber for power wheelchair, each Ⓑ Qp Qh ♿ Y

IOM: 100-03, 4, 280.1

⊛ **E1017** Heavy duty shock absorber for heavy duty or extra heavy duty manual wheelchair, each Ⓑ Qp Qh ♿ Y

IOM: 100-03, 4, 280.1

⊛ **E1018** Heavy duty shock absorber for heavy duty or extra heavy duty power wheelchair, each Ⓑ Qp Qh ♿ Y

IOM: 100-03, 4, 280.1

⊛ **E1020** Residual limb support system for wheelchair, any type Ⓑ Qp Qh ♿ Y

IOM: 100-03, 3, 280.3

✻ **E1028** Wheelchair accessory, manual swing-away, retractable or removable mounting hardware for joystick, other control interface or positioning accessory Ⓑ Qp Qh ♿ Y

✻ **E1029** Wheelchair accessory, ventilator tray, fixed Ⓑ Qp Qh ♿ Y

✻ **E1030** Wheelchair accessory, ventilator tray, gimbaled Ⓑ Qp Qh ♿ Y

Rollabout Chair, Transfer System, Transport Chair

⊛ **E1031** Rollabout chair, any and all types with casters 5" or greater Ⓑ Qp Qh ♿ Y

IOM: 100- 03, 4, 280.1

⊛ **E1035** Multi-positional patient transfer system, with integrated seat, operated by care giver, patient weight capacity up to and including 300 lbs Ⓑ Qp Qh ♿ Y

IOM: 100-02, 15, 110

✻ **E1036** Multi-positional patient transfer system, extra-wide, with integrated seat, operated by caregiver, patient weight capacity greater than 300 lbs Ⓑ Qh ♿ Y

⊛ **E1037** Transport chair, pediatric size Ⓑ Qp Qh A ♿ Y

IOM: 100-03, 4, 280.1

⊛ **E1038** Transport chair, adult size, patient weight capacity up to and including 300 pounds Ⓑ Qp Qh A ♿ Y

IOM: 100-03, 4, 280.1

✻ **E1039** Transport chair, adult size, heavy duty, patient weight capacity greater than 300 pounds Ⓑ Qp Qh A ♿ Y

Wheelchair: Fully Reclining

⊛ **E1050** Fully-reclining wheelchair, fixed full length arms, swing away detachable elevating leg rests Ⓑ Qp Qh ♿ Y

IOM: 100-03, 4, 280.1

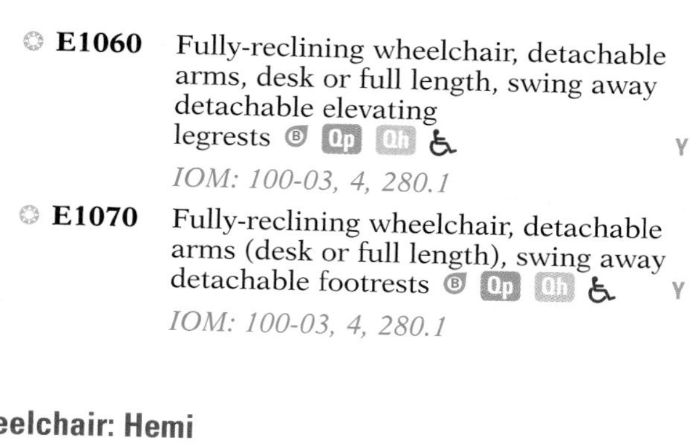

E1060 Fully-reclining wheelchair, detachable arms, desk or full length, swing away detachable elevating legrests Y

IOM: 100-03, 4, 280.1

E1070 Fully-reclining wheelchair, detachable arms (desk or full length), swing away detachable footrests Y

IOM: 100-03, 4, 280.1

Wheelchair: Hemi

E1083 Hemi-wheelchair, fixed full length arms, swing away detachable elevating leg rest Y

IOM: 100-03, 4, 280.1

E1084 Hemi-wheelchair, detachable arms desk or full length arms, swing away detachable elevating leg rests Y

IOM: 100-03, 4, 280.1

E1085 Hemi-wheelchair, fixed full length arms, swing away detachable foot rests E1

IOM: 100-03, 4, 280.1

Cross Reference K0002

E1086 Hemi-wheelchair, detachable arms desk or full length, swing away detachable footrests E1

IOM: 100-03, 4, 280.1

Cross Reference K0002

Wheelchair: High-strength Lightweight

E1087 High strength lightweight wheelchair, fixed full length arms, swing away detachable elevating leg rests Y

IOM: 100-03, 4, 280.1

E1088 High strength lightweight wheelchair, detachable arms desk or full length, swing away detachable elevating leg rests Y

IOM: 100-03, 4, 280.1

E1089 High strength lightweight wheelchair, fixed length arms, swing away detachable footrest E1

IOM: 100-03, 4, 280.1

Cross Reference K0004

E1090 High strength lightweight wheelchair, detachable arms desk or full length, swing away detachable foot rests E1

IOM: 100-03, 4, 280.1

Cross Reference K0004

Wheelchair: Wide Heavy Duty

E1092 Wide heavy duty wheelchair, detachable arms (desk or full length), swing away detachable elevating leg rests Y

IOM: 100-03, 4, 280.1

E1093 Wide heavy duty wheelchair, detachable arms (desk or full length arms), swing away detachable foot rests Y

IOM: 100-03, 4, 280.1

Wheelchair: Semi-reclining

E1100 Semi-reclining wheelchair, fixed full length arms, swing away detachable elevating leg rests Y

IOM: 100-03, 4, 280.1

E1110 Semi-reclining wheelchair, detachable arms (desk or full length), elevating leg rest Y

IOM: 100-03, 4, 280.1

Wheelchair: Standard

E1130 Standard wheelchair, fixed full length arms, fixed or swing away detachable footrests E1

IOM: 100-03, 4, 280.1

Cross Reference K0001

E1140 Wheelchair, detachable arms, desk or full length, swing away detachable footrests E1

IOM: 100-03, 4, 280.1

Cross Reference K0001

E1150 Wheelchair, detachable arms, desk or full length, swing away detachable elevating legrests Y

IOM: 100-03, 4, 280.1

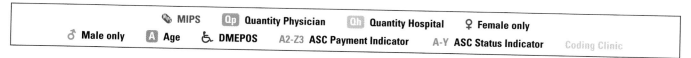
MIPS
Qp Quantity Physician
Qh Quantity Hospital
Female only
Male only
A Age
DMEPOS
A2-Z3 ASC Payment Indicator
A-Y ASC Status Indicator
Coding Clinic

E1160 Wheelchair, fixed full length arms, swing away detachable elevating legrests Y

IOM: 100-03, 4, 280.1

* **E1161** Manual adult size wheelchair, includes tilt in space Y

Wheelchair: Amputee

E1170 Amputee wheelchair, fixed full length arms, swing away detachable elevating legrests Y

IOM: 100-03, 4, 280.1

E1171 Amputee wheelchair, fixed full length arms, without footrests or legrest Y

IOM: 100-03, 4, 280.1

E1172 Amputee wheelchair, detachable arms (desk or full length) without footrests or legrest Y

IOM: 100-03, 4, 280.1

E1180 Amputee wheelchair, detachable arms (desk or full length) swing away detachable footrests Y

IOM: 100-03, 4, 280.1

E1190 Amputee wheelchair, detachable arms (desk or full length), swing away detachable elevating legrests Y

IOM: 100-03, 4, 280.1

E1195 Heavy duty wheelchair, fixed full length arms, swing away detachable elevating legrests Y

IOM: 100-03, 4, 280.1

E1200 Amputee wheelchair, fixed full length arms, swing away detachable footrest Y

IOM: 100-03, 4, 280.1

Wheelchair: Other and Accessories

E1220 Wheelchair; specially sized or constructed (indicate brand name, model number, if any) and justification Y

IOM: 100-03, 4, 280.3

E1221 Wheelchair with fixed arm, footrests Y

IOM: 100-03, 4, 280.3

E1222 Wheelchair with fixed arm, elevating legrests Y

IOM: 100-03, 4, 280.3

E1223 Wheelchair with detachable arms, footrests Y

IOM: 100-03, 4, 280.3

E1224 Wheelchair with detachable arms, elevating legrests Y

IOM: 100-03, 4, 280.3

E1225 Wheelchair accessory, manual semi-reclining back, (recline greater than 15 degrees, but less than 80 degrees), each Y

IOM: 100-03, 4, 280.3

E1226 Wheelchair accessory, manual fully reclining back, (recline greater than 80 degrees), each B

IOM: 100-03, 4, 280.1

E1227 Special height arms for wheelchair Y

IOM: 100-03, 4, 280.3

E1228 Special back height for wheelchair Y

IOM: 100-03, 4, 280.3

Wheelchair: Pediatric

* **E1229** Wheelchair, pediatric size, not otherwise specified Y

E1230 Power operated vehicle (three or four wheel non-highway), specify brand name and model number Y

Patient is unable to operate manual wheelchair; patient capable of safely operating controls for scooter; patient can transfer safely in and out of scooter

IOM: 100-08, 5, 5.2.3

E1231 Wheelchair, pediatric size, tilt-in-space, rigid, adjustable, with seating system Y

IOM: 100-03, 4, 280.1

E1232 Wheelchair, pediatric size, tilt-in-space, folding, adjustable, with seating system Y

IOM: 100-03, 4, 280.1

E1233 Wheelchair, pediatric size, tilt-in-space, rigid, adjustable, without seating system Y

IOM: 100-03, 4, 280.1

E1234 Wheelchair, pediatric size, tilt-in-space, folding, adjustable, without seating system Qp Qh A Y
IOM: 100-03, 4, 280.1

E1235 Wheelchair, pediatric size, rigid, adjustable, with seating system Qp Qh A Y
IOM: 100-03, 4, 280.1

E1236 Wheelchair, pediatric size, folding, adjustable, with seating system Qp Qh A Y
IOM: 100-03, 4, 280.1

E1237 Wheelchair, pediatric size, rigid, adjustable, without seating system Qp Qh A Y
IOM: 100-03, 4, 280.1

E1238 Wheelchair, pediatric size, folding, adjustable, without seating system Qp Qh A Y
IOM: 100-03, 4, 280.1

* E1239 Power wheelchair, pediatric size, not otherwise specified Qh A Y

Wheelchair: Lightweight

E1240 Lightweight wheelchair, detachable arms (desk or full length), swing-away detachable elevating leg rests Qp Qh Y
IOM: 100-03, 4, 280.1

E1250 Lightweight wheelchair, fixed full length arms, swing away detachable footrest Qp Qh E1
IOM: 100-03, 4, 280.1
Cross Reference K0003

E1260 Lightweight wheelchair, detachable arms (desk or full length), swing-away detachable footrest Qp Qh E1
IOM: 100-03, 4, 280.1
Cross Reference K0003

E1270 Lightweight wheelchair, fixed full length arms, swing away detachable elevating legrests Qp Qh Y
IOM: 100-03, 4, 280.1

Wheelchair: Heavy Duty

E1280 Heavy duty wheelchair, detachable arms (desk or full length), elevating legrests Qp Qh Y
IOM: 100-03, 4, 280.1

E1285 Heavy duty wheelchair, fixed full length arms, swing away detachable footrest Qp Qh E1
IOM: 100-03, 4, 280.1
Cross Reference K0006

E1290 Heavy duty wheelchair, detachable arms (desk or full length), swing-away detachable footrest Qp Qh E1
IOM: 100-03, 4, 280.1
Cross Reference K0006

E1295 Heavy duty wheelchair, fixed full length arms, elevating legrest Qp Qh Y
IOM: 100-03, 4, 280.1

E1296 Special wheelchair seat height from floor Y
IOM: 100-03, 4, 280.3

E1297 Special wheelchair seat depth, by upholstery Y
IOM: 100-03, 4, 280.3

E1298 Special wheelchair seat depth and/or width, by construction Y
IOM: 100-03, 4, 280.3

Whirlpool Equipment

E1300 Whirlpool, portable (overtub type) Qp Qh E1
IOM: 100-03, 4, 280.1

E1310 Whirlpool, non-portable (built-in type) Qp Qh Y
IOM: 100-03, 4, 280.1

Additional Oxygen Related Equipment

* E1352 Oxygen accessory, flow regulator capable of positive inspiratory pressure Qp Qh Y

E1353 Regulator Qp Qh Y
IOM: 100-03, 4, 240.2

* E1354 Oxygen accessory, wheeled cart for portable cylinder or portable concentrator, any type, replacement only, each Qp Qh Y

E1355 Stand/rack Qp Qh Y
IOM: 100-03, 4, 240.2

* E1356 Oxygen accessory, battery pack/cartridge for portable concentrator, any type, replacement only, each Qp Qh Y

MIPS Qp Quantity Physician Qh Quantity Hospital ♀ Female only
♂ Male only A Age DMEPOS A2-Z3 ASC Payment Indicator A-Y ASC Status Indicator Coding Clinic

* **E1357** Oxygen accessory, battery charger for portable concentrator, any type, replacement only, each Ⓔ Qp Qh Y
* **E1358** Oxygen accessory, DC power adapter for portable concentrator, any type, replacement only, each Ⓔ Qp Qh Y
* **E1372** Immersion external heater for nebulizer Ⓔ Qp Qh ♿ Y

  IOM: 100-03, 4, 240.2
* **E1390** Oxygen concentrator, single delivery port, capable of delivering 85 percent or greater oxygen concentration at the prescribed flow rate Ⓔ Qp Qh ♿ Y

  IOM: 100-03, 4, 240.2
* **E1391** Oxygen concentrator, dual delivery port, capable of delivering 85 percent or greater oxygen concentration at the prescribed flow rate, each Ⓔ Qp Qh ♿ Y

  IOM: 100-03, 4, 240.2
* **E1392** Portable oxygen concentrator, rental Ⓔ Qp Qh ♿ Y

  IOM: 100-03, 4, 240.2
* **E1399** Durable medical equipment, miscellaneous Ⓑ Ⓔ Y

  Example: Therapeutic exercise putty; rubber exercise tubing; anti-vibration gloves

  On DMEPOS fee schedule as a payable replacement for miscellaneous implanted or non-implanted items
* **E1405** Oxygen and water vapor enriching system with heated delivery Ⓔ Qp Qh ♿ Y

  IOM: 100-03, 4, 240.2
* **E1406** Oxygen and water vapor enriching system without heated delivery Ⓔ Qp Qh ♿ Y

  IOM: 100-03, 4, 240.2

Artificial Kidney Machines and Accessories

* **E1500** Centrifuge, for dialysis Ⓔ Qp Qh A
* **E1510** Kidney, dialysate delivery system, kidney machine, pump recirculating, air removal system, flowrate meter, power off, heater and temperature control with alarm, I.V. poles, pressure gauge, concentrate container Ⓔ Qp Qh A
* **E1520** Heparin infusion pump for hemodialysis Ⓔ Qp Qh A
* **E1530** Air bubble detector for hemodialysis, each, replacement Ⓔ Qp Qh A
* **E1540** Pressure alarm for hemodialysis, each, replacement Ⓔ Qp Qh A
* **E1550** Bath conductivity meter for hemodialysis, each Ⓔ Qp Qh A
* **E1560** Blood leak detector for hemodialysis, each, replacement Ⓔ Qp Qh A
* **E1570** Adjustable chair, for ESRD patients Ⓔ Qp Qh A
* **E1575** Transducer protectors/fluid barriers for hemodialysis, any size, per 10 Ⓔ Qp Qh A
* **E1580** Unipuncture control system for hemodialysis Ⓔ Qp Qh A
* **E1590** Hemodialysis machine Ⓔ Qp Qh A
* **E1592** Automatic intermittent peritoneal dialysis system Ⓔ Qp Qh A
* **E1594** Cycler dialysis machine for peritoneal dialysis Ⓔ Qp Qh A
* **E1600** Delivery and/or installation charges for hemodialysis equipment Ⓔ Qp Qh A
* **E1610** Reverse osmosis water purification system, for hemodialysis Ⓔ Qp Qh A

  IOM: 100-03, 4, 230.7
* **E1615** Deionizer water purification system, for hemodialysis Ⓔ Qp Qh A

  IOM: 100-03, 4, 230.7
* **E1620** Blood pump for hemodialysis replacement Ⓔ Qp Qh A
* **E1625** Water softening system, for hemodialysis Ⓔ Qp Qh A

  IOM: 100-03, 4, 230.7
* **E1630** Reciprocating peritoneal dialysis system Ⓔ Qp Qh A
* **E1632** Wearable artificial kidney, each Ⓔ Qp Qh A
* **E1634** Peritoneal dialysis clamps, each Ⓔ Qp Qh B

  IOM: 100-04, 8, 60.4.2; 100-04, 8, 90.1; 100-04, 18, 80; 100-04, 18, 90
* **E1635** Compact (portable) travel hemodialyzer system Ⓔ Qp Qh A
* **E1636** Sorbent cartridges, for hemodialysis, per 10 Ⓔ Qp Qh A
* **E1637** Hemostats, each Ⓔ Qp Qh A
* **E1639** Scale, each Ⓔ Qp Qh A
* **E1699** Dialysis equipment, not otherwise specified Ⓔ A

Jaw Motion Rehabilitation System

* **E1700** Jaw motion rehabilitation system Qp Qh DMEPOS Y
  Must be prescribed by physician
* **E1701** Replacement cushions for jaw motion rehabilitation system, pkg. of 6 Qp Qh DMEPOS Y
* **E1702** Replacement measuring scales for jaw motion rehabilitation system, pkg. of 200 Qp Qh DMEPOS Y

Other Orthopedic Devices

* **E1800** Dynamic adjustable elbow extension/flexion device, includes soft interface material Qp Qh DMEPOS Y
* **E1801** Static progressive stretch elbow device, extension and/or flexion, with or without range of motion adjustment, includes all components and accessories Qp Qh DMEPOS Y
* **E1802** Dynamic adjustable forearm pronation/supination device, includes soft interface material Qp Qh DMEPOS Y
* **E1805** Dynamic adjustable wrist extension/flexion device, includes soft interface material Qp Qh DMEPOS Y
* **E1806** Static progressive stretch wrist device, flexion and/or extension, with or without range of motion adjustment, includes all components and accessories Qp Qh DMEPOS Y
* **E1810** Dynamic adjustable knee extension/flexion device, includes soft interface material Qp Qh DMEPOS Y
* **E1811** Static progressive stretch knee device, extension and/or flexion, with or without range of motion adjustment, includes all components and accessories Qp Qh DMEPOS Y
* **E1812** Dynamic knee, extension/flexion device with active resistance control Qp Qh DMEPOS Y
* **E1815** Dynamic adjustable ankle extension/flexion device, includes soft interface material Qp Qh DMEPOS Y
* **E1816** Static progressive stretch ankle device, flexion and/or extension, with or without range of motion adjustment, includes all components and accessories Qp Qh DMEPOS Y
* **E1818** Static progressive stretch forearm pronation/supination device with or without range of motion adjustment, includes all components and accessories Qp Qh DMEPOS Y
* **E1820** Replacement soft interface material, dynamic adjustable extension/flexion device Qp Qh DMEPOS Y
* **E1821** Replacement soft interface material/cuffs for bi-directional static progressive stretch device Qp Qh DMEPOS Y
* **E1825** Dynamic adjustable finger extension/flexion device, includes soft interface material Qp Qh DMEPOS Y
* **E1830** Dynamic adjustable toe extension/flexion device, includes soft interface material Qp Qh DMEPOS Y
* **E1831** Static progressive stretch toe device, extension and/or flexion, with or without range of motion adjustment, includes all components and accessories Qp Qh DMEPOS Y
* **E1840** Dynamic adjustable shoulder flexion/abduction/rotation device, includes soft interface material Qp Qh DMEPOS Y
* **E1841** Static progressive stretch shoulder device, with or without range of motion adjustment, includes all components and accessories Qp Qh DMEPOS Y

Miscellaneous

* **E1902** Communication board, non-electronic augmentative or alternative communication device Qp Qh Y
* **E2000** Gastric suction pump, home model, portable or stationary, electric Qp Qh DMEPOS Y
* **E2100** Blood glucose monitor with integrated voice synthesizer Qp Qh DMEPOS Y
  IOM: 100-03, 4, 230.16
* **E2101** Blood glucose monitor with integrated lancing/blood sample Qp Qh DMEPOS Y
  IOM: 100-03, 4, 230.16
* **E2120** Pulse generator system for tympanic treatment of inner ear endolymphatic fluid Qp Qh DMEPOS Y

MIPS | Qp Quantity Physician | Qh Quantity Hospital | ♀ Female only
♂ Male only | A Age | DMEPOS | A2-Z3 ASC Payment Indicator | A-Y ASC Status Indicator | Coding Clinic

Wheelchair Assessories: Manual and Power

* ✻ **E2201** Manual wheelchair accessory, nonstandard seat frame, width greater than or equal to 20 inches and less than 24 inches Ⓑ Qp Qh ♿ Y
* ✻ **E2202** Manual wheelchair accessory, nonstandard seat frame width, 24-27 inches Ⓑ Qp Qh ♿ Y
* ✻ **E2203** Manual wheelchair accessory, nonstandard seat frame depth, 20 to less than 22 inches Ⓑ Qp Qh ♿ Y
* ✻ **E2204** Manual wheelchair accessory, nonstandard seat frame depth, 22 to 25 inches Ⓑ Qp Qh ♿ Y
* ✻ **E2205** Manual wheelchair accessory, handrim without projections (includes ergonomic or contoured), any type, replacement only, each Ⓑ Qp Qh ♿ Y
* ✻ **E2206** Manual wheelchair accessory, wheel lock assembly, complete, replacement only, each Ⓑ Qp Qh ♿ Y
* ✻ **E2207** Wheelchair accessory, crutch and cane holder, each Ⓑ Qp Qh ♿ Y
* ✻ **E2208** Wheelchair accessory, cylinder tank carrier, each Ⓑ Qp Qh ♿ Y
* ✻ **E2209** Accessory arm trough, with or without hand support, each Ⓑ Qp Qh ♿ Y
* ✻ **E2210** Wheelchair accessory, bearings, any type, replacement only, each Ⓑ Qp Qh ♿ Y
* ✻ **E2211** Manual wheelchair accessory, pneumatic propulsion tire, any size, each Ⓑ Qp Qh ♿ Y
* ✻ **E2212** Manual wheelchair accessory, tube for pneumatic propulsion tire, any size, each Ⓑ Qp Qh ♿ Y
* ✻ **E2213** Manual wheelchair accessory, insert for pneumatic propulsion tire (removable), any type, any size, each Ⓑ Qp Qh ♿ Y
* ✻ **E2214** Manual wheelchair accessory, pneumatic caster tire, any size, each Ⓑ Qp Qh ♿ Y
* ✻ **E2215** Manual wheelchair accessory, tube for pneumatic caster tire, any size, each Ⓑ Qp Qh ♿ Y
* ✻ **E2216** Manual wheelchair accessory, foam filled propulsion tire, any size, each Ⓑ Qp Qh ♿ Y
* ✻ **E2217** Manual wheelchair accessory, foam filled caster tire, any size, each Ⓑ Qp Qh ♿ Y
* ✻ **E2218** Manual wheelchair accessory, foam propulsion tire, any size, each Ⓑ Qp Qh ♿ Y
* ✻ **E2219** Manual wheelchair accessory, foam caster tire, any size, each Ⓑ Qp Qh ♿ Y
* ✻ **E2220** Manual wheelchair accessory, solid (rubber/plastic) propulsion tire, any size, replacement only, each Ⓑ Qp Qh ♿ Y
* ✻ **E2221** Manual wheelchair accessory, solid (rubber/plastic) caster tire (removable), any size, replacement only, each Ⓑ Qp Qh ♿ Y
* ✻ **E2222** Manual wheelchair accessory, solid (rubber/plastic) caster tire with integrated wheel, any size, replacement only, each Ⓑ Qp Qh ♿ Y
* ✻ **E2224** Manual wheelchair accessory, propulsion wheel excludes tire, any size, replacement only, each Ⓑ Qp Qh ♿ Y
* ✻ **E2225** Manual wheelchair accessory, caster wheel excludes tire, any size, replacement only, each Ⓑ Qp Qh ♿ Y
* ✻ **E2226** Manual wheelchair accessory, caster fork, any size, replacement only, each Ⓑ Qp Qh ♿ Y
* ✻ **E2227** Manual wheelchair accessory, gear reduction drive wheel, each Ⓑ Qp Qh ♿ Y
* ✻ **E2228** Manual wheelchair accessory, wheel braking system and lock, complete, each Ⓑ Qp Qh ♿ Y
* ✻ **E2230** Manual wheelchair accessory, manual standing system Ⓑ Qp Qh Y
* ✻ **E2231** Manual wheelchair accessory, solid seat support base (replaces sling seat), includes any type mounting hardware Ⓑ Qp Qh ♿ Y
* ✻ **E2291** Back, planar, for pediatric size wheelchair including fixed attaching hardware Ⓑ Qp Qh A Y
* ✻ **E2292** Seat, planar, for pediatric size wheelchair including fixed attaching hardware Ⓑ Qp Qh A Y
* ✻ **E2293** Back, contoured, for pediatric size wheelchair including fixed attaching hardware Ⓑ Qp Qh A Y
* ✻ **E2294** Seat, contoured, for pediatric size wheelchair including fixed attaching hardware Ⓑ Qp Qh A Y
* ✻ **E2295** Manual wheelchair accessory, for pediatric size wheelchair, dynamic seating frame, allows coordinated movement of multiple positioning features Ⓑ Qp Qh A Y
* ✻ **E2300** Wheelchair accessory, power seat elevation system, any type Ⓑ Qp Qh Y

▶ New ↻ Revised ✔ Reinstated ~~deleted~~ Deleted ⊘ Not covered or valid by Medicare
Special coverage instructions ✻ Carrier discretion Ⓑ Bill Part B MAC Ⓑ Bill DME MAC

* **E2301** Wheelchair accessory, power standing system, any type Qp Qh Y

* **E2310** Power wheelchair accessory, electronic connection between wheelchair controller and one power seating system motor, including all related electronics, indicator feature, mechanical function selection switch, and fixed mounting hardware Qp Qh Y

* **E2311** Power wheelchair accessory, electronic connection between wheelchair controller and two or more power seating system motors, including all related electronics, indicator feature, mechanical function selection switch, and fixed mounting hardware Qp Qh Y

* **E2312** Power wheelchair accessory, hand or chin control interface, mini-proportional remote joystick, proportional, including fixed mounting hardware Qp Qh Y

* **E2313** Power wheelchair accessory, harness for upgrade to expandable controller, including all fasteners, connectors and mounting hardware, each Qp Qh Y

* **E2321** Power wheelchair accessory, hand control interface, remote joystick, nonproportional, including all related electronics, mechanical stop switch, and fixed mounting hardware Qp Qh Y

* **E2322** Power wheelchair accessory, hand control interface, multiple mechanical switches, nonproportional, including all related electronics, mechanical stop switch, and fixed mounting hardware Qp Qh Y

* **E2323** Power wheelchair accessory, specialty joystick handle for hand control interface, prefabricated Qp Qh Y

* **E2324** Power wheelchair accessory, chin cup for chin control interface Qp Qh Y

* **E2325** Power wheelchair accessory, sip and puff interface, nonproportional, including all related electronics, mechanical stop switch, and manual swingaway mounting hardware Qp Qh Y

* **E2326** Power wheelchair accessory, breath tube kit for sip and puff interface Qp Qh Y

* **E2327** Power wheelchair accessory, head control interface, mechanical, proportional, including all related electronics, mechanical direction change switch, and fixed mounting hardware Qp Qh Y

* **E2328** Power wheelchair accessory, head control or extremity control interface, electronic, proportional, including all related electronics and fixed mounting hardware Qp Qh Y

* **E2329** Power wheelchair accessory, head control interface, contact switch mechanism, nonproportional, including all related electronics, mechanical stop switch, mechanical direction change switch, head array, and fixed mounting hardware Qp Qh Y

* **E2330** Power wheelchair accessory, head control interface, proximity switch mechanism, nonproportional, including all related electronics, mechanical stop switch, mechanical direction change switch, head array, and fixed mounting hardware Qp Qh Y

* **E2331** Power wheelchair accessory, attendant control, proportional, including all related electronics and fixed mounting hardware Qp Qh Y

* **E2340** Power wheelchair accessory, nonstandard seat frame width, 20-23 inches Qp Qh Y

* **E2341** Power wheelchair accessory, nonstandard seat frame width, 24-27 inches Qp Qh Y

* **E2342** Power wheelchair accessory, nonstandard seat frame depth, 20 or 21 inches Qp Qh Y

* **E2343** Power wheelchair accessory, nonstandard seat frame depth, 22-25 inches Qp Qh Y

* **E2351** Power wheelchair accessory, electronic interface to operate speech generating device using power wheelchair control interface Qp Qh Y

* **E2358** Power wheelchair accessory, Group 34 non-sealed lead acid battery, each Qp Qh Y

* **E2359** Power wheelchair accessory, Group 34 sealed lead acid battery, each (e.g., gel cell, absorbed glassmat) Qp Qh Y

* **E2360** Power wheelchair accessory, 22 NF non-sealed lead acid battery, each Y

MIPS Qp Quantity Physician Qh Quantity Hospital ♀ Female only
♂ Male only A Age DMEPOS A2-Z3 ASC Payment Indicator A-Y ASC Status Indicator Coding Clinic

* **E2361** Power wheelchair accessory, 22NF sealed lead acid battery, each (e.g., gel cell, absorbed glassmat) Qp Qh Y
* **E2362** Power wheelchair accessory, group 24 non-sealed lead acid battery, each Y
* **E2363** Power wheelchair accessory, group 24 sealed lead acid battery, each (e.g., gel cell, absorbed glassmat) Qp Qh Y
* **E2364** Power wheelchair accessory, U-1 non-sealed lead acid battery, each Y
* **E2365** Power wheelchair accessory, U-1 sealed lead acid battery, each (e.g., gel cell, absorbed glassmat) Qp Qh Y
* **E2366** Power wheelchair accessory, battery charger, single mode, for use with only one battery type, sealed or non-sealed, each Qp Qh Y
* **E2367** Power wheelchair accessory, battery charger, dual mode, for use with either battery type, sealed or non-sealed, each Qp Qh Y
* **E2368** Power wheelchair component, drive wheel motor, replacement only Qp Qh Y
* **E2369** Power wheelchair component, drive wheel gear box, replacement only Qp Qh Y
* **E2370** Power wheelchair component, integrated drive wheel motor and gear box combination, replacement only Qp Qh Y
* **E2371** Power wheelchair accessory, group 27 sealed lead acid battery, (e.g., gel cell, absorbed glass mat), each Qp Qh Y
* **E2372** Power wheelchair accessory, group 27 non-sealed lead acid battery, each Y
* **E2373** Power wheelchair accessory, hand or chin control interface, compact remote joystick, proportional, including fixed mounting hardware Qp Qh Y

E2374 Power wheelchair accessory, hand or chin control interface, standard remote joystick (not including controller), proportional, including all related electronics and fixed mounting hardware, replacement only Qp Qh Y

E2375 Power wheelchair accessory, non-expandable controller, including all related electronics and mounting hardware, replacement only Qp Qh Y

E2376 Power wheelchair accessory, expandable controller, including all related electronics and mounting hardware, replacement only Qp Qh Y

E2377 Power wheelchair accessory, expandable controller, including all related electronics and mounting hardware, upgrade provided at initial issue Qp Qh Y

* **E2378** Power wheelchair component, actuator, replacement only Qp Qh Y

E2381 Power wheelchair accessory, pneumatic drive wheel tire, any size, replacement only, each Qp Qh Y

E2382 Power wheelchair accessory, tube for pneumatic drive wheel tire, any size, replacement only, each Qp Qh Y

E2383 Power wheelchair accessory, insert for pneumatic drive wheel tire (removable), any type, any size, replacement only, each Qp Qh Y

E2384 Power wheelchair accessory, pneumatic caster tire, any size, replacement only, each Qp Qh Y

E2385 Power wheelchair accessory, tube for pneumatic caster tire, any size, replacement only, each Qp Qh Y

E2386 Power wheelchair accessory, foam filled drive wheel tire, any size, replacement only, each Qp Qh Y

E2387 Power wheelchair accessory, foam filled caster tire, any size, replacement only, each Qp Qh Y

E2388 Power wheelchair accessory, foam drive wheel tire, any size, replacement only, each Qp Qh Y

E2389 Power wheelchair accessory, foam caster tire, any size, replacement only, each Qp Qh Y

E2390 Power wheelchair accessory, solid (rubber/plastic) drive wheel tire, any size, replacement only, each Qp Qh Y

E2391 Power wheelchair accessory, solid (rubber/plastic) caster tire (removable), any size, replacement only, each Qp Qh Y

E2392 Power wheelchair accessory, solid (rubber/plastic) caster tire with integrated wheel, any size, replacement only, each Qp Qh Y

▶ New ↩ Revised ✔ Reinstated ~~deleted~~ Deleted ⊘ Not covered or valid by Medicare
Special coverage instructions * Carrier discretion Bill Part B MAC Bill DME MAC

◌ **E2394** Power wheelchair accessory, drive wheel excludes tire, any size, replacement only, each Ⓑ Qp Qh ♿ Y

◌ **E2395** Power wheelchair accessory, caster wheel excludes tire, any size, replacement only, each Ⓑ Qp Qh ♿ Y

◌ **E2396** Power wheelchair accessory, caster fork, any size, replacement only, each Ⓑ Qp Qh ♿ Y

* **E2397** Power wheelchair accessory, lithium-based battery, each Ⓑ Qp Qh ♿ Y

* **E2398** Wheelchair accessory, dynamic positioning hardware for back Y

Negative Pressure

* **E2402** Negative pressure wound therapy electrical pump, stationary or portable Ⓑ Qp Qh ♿ Y

Document at least every 30 calendar days the quantitative wound characteristics, including wound surface area (length, width and depth).

Medicare coverage up to a maximum of 15 dressing kits (A6550) per wound per month unless documentation states that the wound size requires more than one dressing kit for each dressing change.

Speech Device

◌ **E2500** Speech generating device, digitized speech, using pre-recorded messages, less than or equal to 8 minutes recording time Ⓑ Qp Qh ♿ Y

IOM: 100-03, 1, 50.1

◌ **E2502** Speech generating device, digitized speech, using pre-recorded messages, greater than 8 minutes but less than or equal to 20 minutes recording time Ⓑ Qp Qh ♿ Y

IOM: 100-03, 1, 50.1

◌ **E2504** Speech generating device, digitized speech, using pre-recorded messages, greater than 20 minutes but less than or equal to 40 minutes recording time Ⓑ Qp Qh ♿ Y

IOM: 100-03, 1, 50.1

◌ **E2506** Speech generating device, digitized speech, using pre-recorded messages, greater than 40 minutes recording time Ⓑ Qp Qh ♿ Y

IOM: 100-03, 1, 50.1

◌ **E2508** Speech generating device, synthesized speech, requiring message formulation by spelling and access by physical contact with the device Ⓑ Qp Qh ♿ Y

IOM: 100-03, 1, 50.1

◌ **E2510** Speech generating device, synthesized speech, permitting multiple methods of message formulation and multiple methods of device access Ⓑ Qp Qh ♿ Y

IOM: 100-03, 1, 50.1

◌ **E2511** Speech generating software program, for personal computer or personal digital assistant Ⓑ Qp Qh ♿ Y

IOM: 100-03, 1, 50.1

◌ **E2512** Accessory for speech generating device, mounting system Ⓑ Qp Qh ♿ Y

IOM: 100-03, 1, 50.1

◌ **E2599** Accessory for speech generating device, not otherwise classified Ⓑ Y

IOM: 100-03, 1, 50.1

Wheelchair: Cushion

* **E2601** General use wheelchair seat cushion, width less than 22 inches, any depth Ⓑ Qp Qh ♿ Y

* **E2602** General use wheelchair seat cushion, width 22 inches or greater, any depth Ⓑ Qp Qh ♿ Y

* **E2603** Skin protection wheelchair seat cushion, width less than 22 inches, any depth Ⓑ Qp Qh ♿ Y

* **E2604** Skin protection wheelchair seat cushion, width 22 inches or greater, any depth Ⓑ Qp Qh ♿ Y

* **E2605** Positioning wheelchair seat cushion, width less than 22 inches, any depth Ⓑ Qp Qh ♿ Y

* **E2606** Positioning wheelchair seat cushion, width 22 inches or greater, any depth Ⓑ Qp Qh ♿ Y

* **E2607** Skin protection and positioning wheelchair seat cushion, width less than 22 inches, any depth Ⓑ Qp Qh ♿ Y

* **E2608** Skin protection and positioning wheelchair seat cushion, width 22 inches or greater, any depth Ⓑ Qp Qh ♿ Y

* **E2609** Custom fabricated wheelchair seat cushion, any size Ⓑ Qp Qh Y

* **E2610** Wheelchair seat cushion, powered Ⓑ B

* **E2611** General use wheelchair back cushion, width less than 22 inches, any height, including any type mounting hardware Ⓔ Qp Qh ♿ Y
* **E2612** General use wheelchair back cushion, width 22 inches or greater, any height, including any type mounting hardware Ⓔ Qp Qh ♿ Y
* **E2613** Positioning wheelchair back cushion, posterior, width less than 22 inches, any height, including any type mounting hardware Ⓔ Qp Qh ♿ Y
* **E2614** Positioning wheelchair back cushion, posterior, width 22 inches or greater, any height, including any type mounting hardware Ⓔ Qp Qh ♿ Y
* **E2615** Positioning wheelchair back cushion, posterior-lateral, width less than 22 inches, any height, including any type mounting hardware Ⓔ Qp Qh ♿ Y
* **E2616** Positioning wheelchair back cushion, posterior-lateral, width 22 inches or greater, any height, including any type mounting hardware Ⓔ Qp Qh ♿ Y
* **E2617** Custom fabricated wheelchair back cushion, any size, including any type mounting hardware Ⓔ Qp Qh Y
* **E2619** Replacement cover for wheelchair seat cushion or back cushion, each Ⓔ Qp Qh ♿ Y
* **E2620** Positioning wheelchair back cushion, planar back with lateral supports, width less than 22 inches, any height, including any type mounting hardware Ⓔ Qp Qh ♿ Y
* **E2621** Positioning wheelchair back cushion, planar back with lateral supports, width 22 inches or greater, any height, including any type mounting hardware Ⓔ Qp Qh ♿ Y

Wheelchair: Skin Protection

* **E2622** Skin protection wheelchair seat cushion, adjustable, width less than 22 inches, any depth Ⓔ Qp Qh ♿ Y
* **E2623** Skin protection wheelchair seat cushion, adjustable, width 22 inches or greater, any depth Ⓔ Qp Qh ♿ Y
* **E2624** Skin protection and positioning wheelchair seat cushion, adjustable, width less than 22 inches, any depth Ⓔ Qp Qh ♿ Y
* **E2625** Skin protection and positioning wheelchair seat cushion, adjustable, width 22 inches or greater, any depth Ⓔ Qp Qh ♿ Y

Wheelchair: Arm Support

* **E2626** Wheelchair accessory, shoulder elbow, mobile arm support attached to wheelchair, balanced, adjustable Ⓔ Qp Qh ♿ Y
* **E2627** Wheelchair accessory, shoulder elbow, mobile arm support attached to wheelchair, balanced, adjustable rancho type Ⓔ Qp Qh ♿ Y
* **E2628** Wheelchair accessory, shoulder elbow, mobile arm support attached to wheelchair, balanced, reclining Ⓔ Qp Qh ♿ Y
* **E2629** Wheelchair accessory, shoulder elbow, mobile arm support attached to wheelchair, balanced, friction arm support (friction dampening to proximal and distal joints) Ⓔ Qp Qh ♿ Y
* **E2630** Wheelchair accessory, shoulder elbow, mobile arm support, monosuspension arm and hand support, overhead elbow forearm hand sling support, yoke type suspension support Ⓔ Qp Qh ♿ Y
* **E2631** Wheelchair accessory, addition to mobile arm support, elevating proximal arm Ⓔ Qp Qh ♿ Y
* **E2632** Wheelchair accessory, addition to mobile arm support, offset or lateral rocker arm with elastic balance control Ⓔ Qp Qh ♿ Y
* **E2633** Wheelchair accessory, addition to mobile arm support, supinator Ⓔ Qp Qh ♿ Y

Pediatric Gait Trainer

⃠ **E8000** Gait trainer, pediatric size, posterior support, includes all accessories and components Ⓔ A E1

⃠ **E8001** Gait trainer, pediatric size, upright support, includes all accessories and components Ⓔ A E1

⃠ **E8002** Gait trainer, pediatric size, anterior support, includes all accessories and components Ⓔ A E1

TEMPORARY PROCEDURES/ PROFESSIONAL SERVICES (G0000-G9999)

NOTE: Series "G", "K", and "Q" in the Level II coding are reserved for CMS assignment. "G", "K", and "Q" codes are temporary national codes for items or services requiring uniform national coding between one year's update and the next. Sometimes "temporary" codes remain for more than one update. If "G", "K", and "Q" codes are not converted to permanent codes in Level I or Level II series in the following update, they will remain active until converted in following years or until CMS notifies contractors to delete them. All active "G", "K", and "Q" codes at the time of update will be included on the update file for contractors. In addition, deleted codes are retained on the file for informational purposes, with a deleted indicator, for four years.

Vaccine Administration

* **G0008** Administration of influenza virus vaccine Qp Qh — S

  Coinsurance and deductible do not apply. If provided, report significant, separately identifiable E/M for medically necessary services (Z23).

  Coding Clinic: 2016, Q4, P3

* **G0009** Administration of pneumococcal vaccine Qp Qh — S

  Reported once in a lifetime based on risk; Medicare covers cost of vaccine and administration (Z23)

  Copayment, coinsurance, and deductible waived. (https://www.cms.gov/MLNProducts/downloads/MPS_QuickReferenceChart_1.pdf)

  Coding Clinic: 2016, Q4, P3

* **G0010** Administration of hepatitis B vaccine Qp Qh — S

  Report for other than OPPs. Coinsurance and deductible apply; Medicare covers both cost of vaccine and administration (Z23)

  Copayment/coinsurance and deductible are waived. (https://www.cms.gov/MLNProducts/downloads/MPS_QuickReferenceChart_1.pdf)

  Coding Clinic: 2016, Q4, P3

Semen Analysis

* **G0027** Semen analysis; presence and/or motility of sperm excluding Huhner Qp Qh ♂ — Q4

  Laboratory Certification: Hematology

Administration, Payment and Care Management Services

* **G0068** Professional services for the administration of anti-infective, pain management, chelation, pulmonary hypertension, or other intravenous infusion drug or biological (excluding chemotherapy or other highly complex drug or biological) inotropic for each infusion drug administration calendar day in the individual's home, each 15 minutes — A

* **G0069** Professional services for the administration of subcutaneous immunotherapy or other subcutaneous infusion drug or biological for each infusion drug administration calendar day in the individual's home, each 15 minutes — A

* **G0070** Professional services for the administration of intravenous chemotherapy or other intravenous highly complex drug or biological infusion for each infusion drug administration calendar day in the individual's home, each 15 minutes — A

* **G0071** Payment for communication technology-based services for 5 minutes or more of a virtual (non-face-to-face) communication between an rural health clinic (RHC) or federally qualified health center (FQHC) practitioner and RHC or FQHC patient, or 5 minutes or more of remote evaluation of recorded video and/or images by an RHC or FQHC practitioner, occurring in lieu of an office visit; RHC or FQHC only — A

* **G0076** Brief (20 minutes) care management home visit for a new patient. For use only in a Medicare-approved CMMI model. (Services must be furnished within a beneficiary's home, domiciliary, rest home, assisted living and/or nursing facility.) — B

* **G0077** Limited (30 minutes) care management home visit for a new patient. For use only in a Medicare-approved CMMI model. (Services must be furnished within a beneficiary's home, domiciliary, rest home, assisted living and/or nursing facility.) — B

MIPS | Qp Quantity Physician | Qh Quantity Hospital | ♀ Female only
♂ Male only | A Age | DMEPOS | A2-Z3 ASC Payment Indicator | A-Y ASC Status Indicator | Coding Clinic

✻ **G0078** Moderate (45 minutes) care management home visit for a new patient. For use only in a Medicare-approved CMMI model. (Services must be furnished within a beneficiary's home, domiciliary, rest home, assisted living and/or nursing facility.) Ⓑ B

✻ **G0079** Comprehensive (60 minutes) care management home visit for a new patient. For use only in a Medicare-approved CMMI model. (Services must be furnished within a beneficiary's home, domiciliary, rest home, assisted living and/or nursing facility.) Ⓑ B

✻ **G0080** Extensive (75 minutes) care management home visit for a new patient. For use only in a Medicare-approved CMMI model. (Services must be furnished within a beneficiary's home, domiciliary, rest home, assisted living and/or nursing facility.) Ⓑ B

✻ **G0081** Brief (20 minutes) care management home visit for an existing patient. For use only in a Medicare-approved CMMI model. (Services must be furnished within a beneficiary's home, domiciliary, rest home, assisted living and/or nursing facility.) Ⓑ B

✻ **G0082** Limited (30 minutes) care management home visit for an existing patient. For use only in a Medicare-approved CMMI model. (Services must be furnished within a beneficiary's home, domiciliary, rest home, assisted living and/or nursing facility.) Ⓑ B

✻ **G0083** Moderate (45 minutes) care management home visit for an existing patient. For use only in a Medicare-approved CMMI model. (Services must be furnished within a beneficiary's home, domiciliary, rest home, assisted living and/or nursing facility.) Ⓑ B

✻ **G0084** Comprehensive (60 minutes) care management home visit for an existing patient. For use only in a Medicare-approved CMMI model. (Services must be furnished within a beneficiary's home, domiciliary, rest home, assisted living and/or nursing facility.) Ⓑ B

✻ **G0085** Extensive (75 minutes) care management home visit for an existing patient. For use only in a Medicare-approved CMMI model. (Services must be furnished within a beneficiary's home, domiciliary, rest home, assisted living and/or nursing facility.) Ⓑ B

✻ **G0086** Limited (30 minutes) care management home care plan oversight. For use only in a Medicare-approved CMMI model. (Services must be furnished within a beneficiary's home, domiciliary, rest home, assisted living and/or nursing facility.) Ⓑ B

✻ **G0087** Comprehensive (60 minutes) care management home care plan oversight. For use only in a Medicare-approved CMMI model. (Services must be furnished within a beneficiary's home, domiciliary, rest home, assisted living and/or nursing facility.) Ⓑ B

▶ ✻ **G0088** Professional services, initial visit, for the administration of anti-infective, pain management, chelation, pulmonary hypertension, inotropic, or other intravenous infusion drug or biological (excluding chemotherapy or other highly complex drug or biological) for each infusion drug administration calendar day in the individual's home, each 15 minutes A

▶ ✻ **G0089** Professional services, initial visit, for the administration of subcutaneous immunotherapy or other subcutaneous infusion drug or biological for each infusion drug administration calendar day in the individual's home, each 15 minutes A

▶ ✻ **G0090** Professional services, initial visit, for the administration of intravenous chemotherapy or other highly complex infusion drug or biological for each infusion drug administration calendar day in the individual's home, each 15 minutes A

Screening Services

MIPS ◌ **G0101** Cervical or vaginal cancer screening; pelvic and clinical breast examination Ⓑ Qp Qh S

Covered once every two years and annually if high risk for cervical/vaginal cancer, or if childbearing age patient has had an abnormal Pap smear in preceding three years. High risk diagnosis, Z77.9

Coding Clinic: 2002, Q4, P8

MIPS ◌ **G0102** Prostate cancer screening; digital rectal examination Ⓑ Qp Qh N

Covered annually by Medicare (Z12.5). Not separately payable with an E/M code (99201-99499).

IOM: 100-02, 6, 10; 100-04, 4, 240; 100-04, 18, 50.1

▶ New ⟲ Revised ✓ Reinstated ~~deleted~~ Deleted ⊘ Not covered or valid by Medicare
◌ Special coverage instructions ✻ Carrier discretion Ⓑ Bill Part B MAC Ⓑ Bill DME MAC

G0103 Prostate cancer screening; prostate specific antigen test (PSA) Ⓑ Qp Qh A

Covered annually by Medicare (Z12.5)

IOM: 100-02, 6, 10; 100-04, 4, 240; 100-04, 18, 50

Laboratory Certification: Routine chemistry

MIPS **G0104** Colorectal cancer screening; flexible sigmoidoscopy Ⓑ Qp Qh T

Covered once every 48 months for beneficiaries age 50+

Co-insurance waived under Section 4104.

Coding Clinic: 2011, Q2, P4

MIPS **G0105** Colorectal cancer screening; colonoscopy on individual at high risk Ⓑ Qp Qh T

Screening colonoscopy covered once every 24 months for high risk for developing colorectal cancer. May use modifier 53 if appropriate (physician fee schedule).

Co-insurance waived under Section 4104.

Coding Clinic: 2018, Q2, P4; 2011, Q2, P4

MIPS **G0106** Colorectal cancer screening; alternative to G0104, screening sigmoidoscopy, barium enema Ⓑ Qp Qh S

Barium enema (not high risk) (alternative to G0104). Covered once every 4 years for beneficiaries age 50+. Use modifier 26 for professional component only.

Coding Clinic: 2011, Q2, P4

Diabetes Management Training Services

MIPS * **G0108** Diabetes outpatient self-management training services, individual, per 30 minutes Ⓑ Qp Qh A

Report for beneficiaries diagnosed with diabetes.

Effective January 2011, DSMT will be included in the list of reimbursable Medicare telehealth services.

* **G0109** Diabetes outpatient self-management training services, group session (2 or more) per 30 minutes Ⓑ Qp Qh A

Report for beneficiaries diagnosed with diabetes.

Effective January 2011, DSMT will be included in the list of reimbursable Medicare telehealth services.

Screening Services

MIPS * **G0117** Glaucoma screening for high risk patients furnished by an optometrist or ophthalmologist Ⓑ Qp Qh S

Covered once per year (full 11 months between screenings). Bundled with all other ophthalmic services provided on same day. Diagnosis code Z13.5.

MIPS * **G0118** Glaucoma screening for high risk patient furnished under the direct supervision of an optometrist or ophthalmologist Ⓑ Qp Qh S

Covered once per year (full 11 months between screenings). Diagnosis code Z13.5.

MIPS **G0120** Colorectal cancer screening; alternative to G0105, screening colonoscopy, barium enema. Ⓑ Qp Qh S

Barium enema for patients with a high risk of developing colorectal. Covered once every 2 years. Used as an alternative to G0105. Use modifier 26 for professional component only.

MIPS **G0121** Colorectal cancer screening; colonoscopy on individual not meeting criteria for high risk Ⓑ Qp Qh T

Screening colonoscopy for patients that are not high risk. Covered once every 10 years, but not within 48 months of a G0104. For non-Medicare patients report 45378.

Co-insurance waived under Section 4104.

Coding Clinic: 2018, Q2, P4

MIPS ⊘ **G0122** Colorectal cancer screening; barium enema Ⓑ E1

Medicare: this service is denied as noncovered, because it fails to meet the requirements of the benefit. The beneficiary is liable for payment.

G0123 Screening cytopathology, cervical or vaginal (any reporting system), collected in preservative fluid, automated thin layer preparation, screening by cytotechnologist under physician supervision Ⓑ Qp Qh ♀ A

Use G0123 or G0143 or G0144 or G0145 or G0147 or G0148 or P3000 for Pap smears NOT requiring physician interpretation (technical component).

IOM: 100-03, 3, 190.2; 100-04, 18, 30

Laboratory Certification: Cytology

G0124 Screening cytopathology, cervical or vaginal (any reporting system), collected in preservative fluid, automated thin layer preparation, requiring interpretation by physician Qp Qh ♀ B

Report professional component for Pap smears requiring physician interpretation.

IOM: 100-03, 3, 190.2; 100-04, 18, 30

Laboratory Certification: Cytology

Miscellaneous Services, Diagnostic and Therapeutic

G0127 Trimming of dystrophic nails, any number Qp Qh Q1

Must be used with a modifier (Q7, Q8, or Q9) to show that the foot care service is needed because the beneficiary has a systemic disease. Limit 1 unit of service.

IOM: 100-02, 15, 290

G0128 Direct (face-to-face with patient) skilled nursing services of a registered nurse provided in a comprehensive outpatient rehabilitation facility, each 10 minutes beyond the first 5 minutes Qp Qh B

A separate nursing service that is clearly identifiable in the Plan of Treatment and not part of other services. Documentation must support this service. Examples include: Insertion of a urinary catheter, intramuscular injections, bowel disimpaction, nursing assessment, and education. Restricted coverage by Medicare.

Medicare Statute 1833(a)

* **G0129** Occupational therapy services requiring the skills of a qualified occupational therapist, furnished as a component of a partial hospitalization treatment program, per session (45 minutes or more) Qh P

G0130 Single energy x-ray absorptiometry (SEXA) bone density study, one or more sites; appendicular skeleton (peripheral) (e.g., radius, wrist, heel) Qp Qh Z3 S

Covered every 24 months (more frequently if medically necessary). Use modifier 26 for professional component only.

Preventive service; no deductible

IOM: 100-03, 2, 150.3; 100-04, 13, 140.1

* **G0141** Screening cytopathology smears, cervical or vaginal, performed by automated system, with manual rescreening, requiring interpretation by physician Qp Qh ♀ B

Co-insurance, copay, and deductible waived

Report professional component for Pap smears requiring physician interpretation. Refer to diagnosis of Z92.89, Z12.4, Z12.72, or Z12.89 to report appropriate risk level.

Laboratory Certification: Cytology

* **G0143** Screening cytopathology, cervical or vaginal (any reporting system), collected in preservative fluid, automated thin layer preparation, with manual screening and rescreening by cytotechnologist under physician supervision Qp Qh ♀ A

Co-insurance, copay, and deductible waived

Laboratory Certification: Cytology

* **G0144** Screening cytopathology, cervical or vaginal (any reporting system), collected in preservative fluid, automated thin layer preparation, with screening by automated system, under physician supervision Qp Qh ♀ A

Co-insurance, copay, and deductible waived

Laboratory Certification: Cytology

* **G0145** Screening cytopathology, cervical or vaginal (any reporting system), collected in preservative fluid, automated thin layer preparation, with screening by automated system and manual rescreening under physician supervision Qp Qh ♀ A

Co-insurance, copay, and deductible waived

Laboratory Certification: Cytology

* **G0147** Screening cytopathology smears, cervical or vaginal; performed by automated system under physician supervision Qp Qh ♀ A

Co-insurance, copay, and deductible waived

Laboratory Certification: Cytology

* **G0148** Screening cytopathology smears, cervical or vaginal; performed by automated system with manual rescreening Qp Qh ♀ A

Co-insurance, copay, and deductible waived

Laboratory Certification: Cytology

▶ New ↩ Revised ✔ Reinstated ~~deleted~~ Deleted ⃠ Not covered or valid by Medicare
Special coverage instructions * Carrier discretion Bill Part B MAC Bill DME MAC

* **G0151** Services performed by a qualified physical therapist in the home health or hospice setting, each 15 minutes B
* **G0152** Services performed by a qualified occupational therapist in the home health or hospice setting, each 15 minutes B
* **G0153** Services performed by a qualified speech-language pathologist in the home health or hospice setting, each 15 minutes B
* **G0155** Services of clinical social worker in home health or hospice settings, each 15 minutes B
* **G0156** Services of home health/health aide in home health or hospice settings, each 15 minutes B
* **G0157** Services performed by a qualified physical therapist assistant in the home health or hospice setting, each 15 minutes B
* **G0158** Services performed by a qualified occupational therapist assistant in the home health or hospice setting, each 15 minutes B
* **G0159** Services performed by a qualified physical therapist, in the home health setting, in the establishment or delivery of a safe and effective physical therapy maintenance program, each 15 minutes B
* **G0160** Services performed by a qualified occupational therapist, in the home health setting, in the establishment or delivery of a safe and effective occupational therapy maintenance program, each 15 minutes B
* **G0161** Services performed by a qualified speech-language pathologist, in the home health setting, in the establishment or delivery of a safe and effective speech-language pathology maintenance program, each 15 minutes B
* **G0162** Skilled services by a registered nurse (RN) for management and evaluation of the plan of care; each 15 minutes (the patient's underlying condition or complication requires an RN to ensure that essential non-skilled care achieves its purpose in the home health or hospice setting) B

  Transmittal No. 824 (CR7182)

G0166 External counterpulsation, per treatment session Qp Qh Q1

IOM: 100-03, 1, 20.20

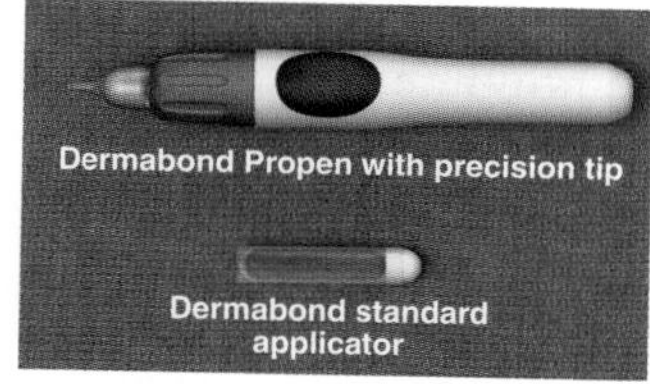
Dermabond Propen with precision tip
Dermabond standard applicator

Figure 15 Tissue adhesive.

* **G0168** Wound closure utilizing tissue adhesive(s) only Qp Qh B

  Report for wound closure with only tissue adhesive. If a practitioner utilizes tissue adhesive in addition to staples or sutures to close a wound, HCPCS code G0168 is not separately reportable, but is included in the tissue repair.

  The only closure material used for a simple repair, coverage based on payer.

  Coding Clinic: 2005, Q1, P5; 2001, Q4, P12; Q3, P13

* **G0175** Scheduled interdisciplinary team conference (minimum of three exclusive of patient care nursing staff) with patient present Qp Qh V

G0176 Activity therapy, such as music, dance, art or play therapies not for recreation, related to the care and treatment of patient's disabling mental health problems, per session (45 minutes or more) Qh P

Paid in partial hospitalization

G0177 Training and educational services related to the care and treatment of patient's disabling mental health problems per session (45 minutes or more) Qp Qh N

Paid in partial hospitalization

* **G0179** Physician recertification for Medicare-covered home health services under a home health plan of care (patient not present), including contacts with home health agency and review of reports of patient status required by physicians to affirm the initial implementation of the plan of care that meets patient's needs, per recertification period Qp Qh M

  The recertification code is used after a patient has received services for at least 60 days (or one certification period) when the physician signs the certification after the initial certification period.

MIPS | Qp Quantity Physician | Qh Quantity Hospital | ♀ Female only | ♂ Male only | A Age | DMEPOS | A2-Z3 ASC Payment Indicator | A-Y ASC Status Indicator | Coding Clinic

* **G0180** Physician certification for Medicare-covered home health services under a home health plan of care (patient not present), including contacts with home health agency and review of reports of patient status required by physicians to affirm the initial implementation of the plan of care that meets patient's needs, per certification period Ⓑ Qp Qh M

This code can be billed only when the patient has not received Medicare covered home health services for at least 60 days.

* **G0181** Physician supervision of a patient receiving Medicare-covered services provided by a participating home health agency (patient not present) requiring complex and multidisciplinary care modalities involving regular physician development and/or revision of care plans, review of subsequent reports of patient status, review of laboratory and other studies, communication (including telephone calls) with other health care professionals involved in the patient's care, integration of new information into the medical treatment plan and/or adjustment of medical therapy, within a calendar month, 30 minutes or more Ⓑ Qp Qh M

Coding Clinic: 2015, Q2, P10

* **G0182** Physician supervision of a patient under a Medicare-approved hospice (patient not present) requiring complex and multidisciplinary care modalities involving regular physician development and/or revision of care plans, review of subsequent reports of patient status, review of laboratory and other studies, communication (including telephone calls) with other health care professionals involved in the patient's care, integration of new information into the medical treatment plan and/or adjustment of medical therapy, within a calendar month, 30 minutes or more Ⓑ Qp Qh M

Coding Clinic: 2015, Q2, P10

* **G0186** Destruction of localized lesion of choroid (for example, choroidal neovascularization); photocoagulation, feeder vessel technique (one or more sessions) Ⓑ Qp Qh T

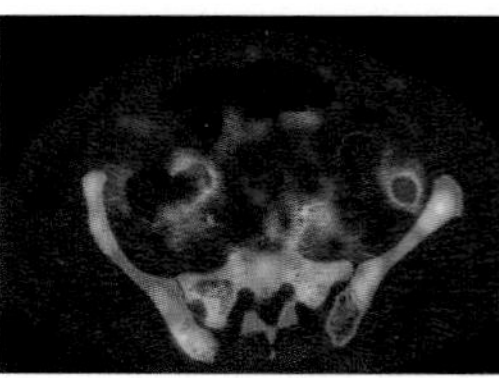

Figure 16 PET scan.

⊘ **G0219** PET imaging whole body; melanoma for non-covered indications Ⓑ E1

Example: Assessing regional lymph nodes in melanoma.

IOM: 100-03, 4, 220.6

Coding Clinic: 2007, Q1, P6

⊘ **G0235** PET imaging, any site, not otherwise specified Ⓑ Qp Qh E1

Example: Prostate cancer diagnosis and initial staging.

IOM: 100-03, 4, 220.6

Coding Clinic: 2007, Q1, P6

* **G0237** Therapeutic procedures to increase strength or endurance of respiratory muscles, face to face, one on one, each 15 minutes (includes monitoring) Ⓑ Qp Qh S

* **G0238** Therapeutic procedures to improve respiratory function, other than described by G0237, one on one, face to face, per 15 minutes (includes monitoring) Ⓑ Qp Qh S

* **G0239** Therapeutic procedures to improve respiratory function or increase strength or endurance of respiratory muscles, two or more individuals (includes monitoring) Ⓑ Qp Qh S

G0245 Initial physician evaluation and management of a diabetic patient with diabetic sensory neuropathy resulting in a loss of protective sensation (LOPS) which must include (1) the diagnosis of LOPS, (2) a patient history, (3) a physical examination that consist of at least the following elements: (A) visual inspection of the forefoot, hindfoot and toe web spaces, (B) evaluation of a protective sensation, (C) evaluation of foot structure and biomechanics, (D) evaluation of vascular status and skin integrity, and (E) evaluation and recommendation of footwear, and (4) patient education Ⓑ Qp Qh V

IOM: 100-03, 1, 70.2.1

▶ New ↻ Revised ✓ Reinstated ~~deleted~~ Deleted ⊘ Not covered or valid by Medicare
Special coverage instructions * Carrier discretion Ⓑ Bill Part B MAC Ⓓ Bill DME MAC

G0246 Follow-up physician evaluation and management of a diabetic patient with diabetic sensory neuropathy resulting in a loss of protective sensation (LOPS) to include at least the following: (1) a patient history, (2) a physical examination that includes: (A) visual inspection of the forefoot, hindfoot and toe web spaces, (B) evaluation of protective sensation, (C) evaluation of foot structure and biomechanics, (D) evaluation of vascular status and skin integrity, and (E) evaluation and recommendation of footwear, and (3) patient education Qp Qh V

IOM: 100-03, 1, 70.2.1; 100-02, 15, 290

G0247 Routine foot care by a physician of a diabetic patient with diabetic sensory neuropathy resulting in a loss of protective sensation (LOPS) to include, the local care of superficial wounds (i.e., superficial to muscle and fascia) and at least the following if present: (1) local care of superficial wounds, (2) debridement of corns and calluses, and (3) trimming and debridement of nails Qp Qh Q1

IOM: 100-03, 1, 70.2.1

G0248 Demonstration, prior to initiation, of home INR monitoring for patient with either mechanical heart valve(s), chronic atrial fibrillation, or venous thromboembolism who meets Medicare coverage criteria, under the direction of a physician; includes: face-to-face demonstration of use and care of the INR monitor, obtaining at least one blood sample, provision of instructions for reporting home INR test results, and documentation of patient's ability to perform testing and report results Qp Qh V

G0249 Provision of test materials and equipment for home INR monitoring of patient with either mechanical heart valve(s), chronic atrial fibrillation, or venous thromboembolism who meets Medicare coverage criteria; includes provision of materials for use in the home and reporting of test results to physician; testing not occurring more frequently than once a week; testing materials, billing units of service include 4 tests Qp Qh V

G0250 Physician review, interpretation, and patient management of home INR testing for patient with either mechanical heart valve(s), chronic atrial fibrillation, or venous thromboembolism who meets Medicare coverage criteria; testing not occurring more frequently than once a week; billing units of service include 4 tests Qp Qh M

G0252 PET imaging, full and partial-ring PET scanners only, for initial diagnosis of breast cancer and/or surgical planning for breast cancer (e.g., initial staging of axillary lymph nodes) E1

IOM: 100-03, 4, 220.6

Coding Clinic: 2007, Q1, P6

G0255 Current perception threshold/sensory nerve conduction test (SNCT), per limb, any nerve E1

IOM: 100-03, 2, 160.23

G0257 Unscheduled or emergency dialysis treatment for an ESRD patient in a hospital outpatient department that is not certified as an ESRD facility Qp Qh S

Coding Clinic: 2003, Q1, P9

G0259 Injection procedure for sacroiliac joint; arthrography Qp Qh N

Replaces 27096 for reporting injections for Medicare beneficiaries

Used by Part A only (facility), not priced by Part B Medicare.

G0260 Injection procedure for sacroiliac joint; provision of anesthetic, steroid and/or other therapeutic agent, with or without arthrography Qp Qh T

ASCs report when a therapeutic sacroiliac joint injection is administered in ASC

* **G0268** Removal of impacted cerumen (one or both ears) by physician on same date of service as audiologic function testing Qp Qh N

Report only when a physician, not an audiologist, performs the procedure.

Use with DX H61.2- when performed by physician.

Coding Clinic: 2016, Q2, P2-3; 2003, Q1, P12

MIPS | Qp Quantity Physician | Qh Quantity Hospital | ♀ Female only
♂ Male only | A Age | DMEPOS | A2-Z3 ASC Payment Indicator | A-Y ASC Status Indicator | Coding Clinic

G0269 Placement of occlusive device into either a venous or arterial access site, post surgical or interventional procedure (e.g., angioseal plug, vascular plug) Ⓑ Qh N

Report for replacement of vasoseal. Hospitals may report the closure device as a supply with C1760. Bundled status on Physician Fee Schedule.

Coding Clinic: 2011, Q3, P4; 2010, Q4, P6

* **G0270** Medical nutrition therapy; reassessment and subsequent intervention(s) following second referral in same year for change in diagnosis, medical condition or treatment regimen (including additional hours needed for renal disease), individual, face to face with the patient, each 15 minutes Ⓑ Qp Qh A

Requires physician referral for beneficiaries with diabetes or renal disease. Services must be provided by dietitian/nutritionist. Co-insurance and deductible waived.

* **G0271** Medical nutrition therapy, reassessment and subsequent intervention(s) following second referral in same year for change in diagnosis, medical condition, or treatment regimen (including additional hours needed for renal disease), group (2 or more individuals), each 30 minutes Ⓑ Qp Qh A

Requires physician referral for beneficiaries with diabetes or renal disease. Services must be provided by dietitian/nutritionist. Co-insurance and deductible waived.

G0276 Blinded procedure for lumbar stenosis, percutaneous image-guided lumbar decompression (PILD) or placebo-control, performed in an approved coverage with evidence development (CED) clinical trial Ⓑ Qp Qh J1

G0277 Hyperbaric oxygen under pressure, full body chamber, per 30 minute interval Ⓑ Qp Qh S

IOM: 100-03, 1, 20.29

Coding Clinic: 2015, Q3, P7

* **G0278** Iliac and/or femoral artery angiography, non-selective, bilateral or ipsilateral to catheter insertion, performed at the same time as cardiac catheterization and/or coronary angiography, includes positioning or placement of the catheter in the distal aorta or ipsilateral femoral or iliac artery, injection of dye, production of permanent images, and radiologic supervision and interpretation (list separately in addition to primary procedure) Ⓑ Qp Qh N

Medicare specific code not reported for iliac injection used as a guiding shot for a closure device

Coding Clinic: 2011, Q3, P4; 2006, Q4, P7

* **G0279** Diagnostic digital breast tomosynthesis, unilateral or bilateral (list separately in addition to G0204 or G0206) Ⓑ A

* **G0281** Electrical stimulation, (unattended), to one or more areas, for chronic stage III and stage IV pressure ulcers, arterial ulcers, diabetic ulcers, and venous stasis ulcers not demonstrating measurable signs of healing after 30 days of conventional care, as part of a therapy plan of care Ⓑ Qp Qh A

Reported by encounter/areas and not by site. Therapists report G0281 and G0283 rather than 97014.

⊘ **G0282** Electrical stimulation, (unattended), to one or more areas, for wound care other than described in G0281 Ⓑ E1

IOM: 100-03, 4, 270.1

* **G0283** Electrical stimulation (unattended), to one or more areas for indication(s) other than wound care, as part of a therapy plan of care Ⓑ Qp Qh A

Reported by encounter/areas and not by site. Therapists report G0281 and G0283 rather than 97014.

* **G0288** Reconstruction, computed tomographic angiography of aorta for surgical planning for vascular surgery Ⓑ Qp Qh N

▶ New ⮌ Revised ✔ Reinstated ~~deleted~~ Deleted ⊘ Not covered or valid by Medicare
Special coverage instructions * Carrier discretion Ⓑ Bill Part B MAC Ⓑ Bill DME MAC

✻ **G0289** Arthroscopy, knee, surgical, for removal of loose body, foreign body, debridement/shaving of articular cartilage (chondroplasty) at the time of other surgical knee arthroscopy in a different compartment of the same knee Ⓑ Qp Qh N

Add-on code reported with knee arthroscopy code for major procedure performed-reported once per extra compartment

"The code may be reported twice (or with a unit of two) if the physician performs these procedures in two compartments, in addition to the compartment where the main procedure was performed." (http://www.ama-assn.org/resources/doc/cpt/orthopaedics.pdf)

G0293 Noncovered surgical procedure(s) using conscious sedation, regional, general or spinal anesthesia in a Medicare qualifying clinical trial, per day Ⓑ Qp Qh Q1

G0294 Noncovered procedure(s) using either no anesthesia or local anesthesia only, in a Medicare qualifying clinical trial, per day Ⓑ Qp Qh Q1

⊘ **G0295** Electromagnetic therapy, to one or more areas, for wound care other than described in G0329 or for other uses Ⓑ E1

IOM: 100-03, 4, 270.1

✻ **G0296** Counseling visit to discuss need for lung cancer screening (LDCT) using low dose CT scan (service is for eligibility determination and shared decision making) Ⓑ Qp Qh S

~~G0297 Low dose CT scan (LDCT) for lung cancer screening~~ ✖

✻ **G0299** Direct skilled nursing services of a registered nurse (RN) in the home health or hospice setting, each 15 minutes Ⓑ B

✻ **G0300** Direct skilled nursing services of a licensed practical nurse (LPN) in the home health or hospice setting, each 15 minutes Ⓑ B

✻ **G0302** Pre-operative pulmonary surgery services for preparation for LVRS, complete course of services, to include a minimum of 16 days of services Ⓑ Qp Qh S

✻ **G0303** Pre-operative pulmonary surgery services for preparation for LVRS, 10 to 15 days of services Ⓑ Qp Qh S

✻ **G0304** Pre-operative pulmonary surgery services for preparation for LVRS, 1 to 9 days of services Ⓑ Qp Qh S

✻ **G0305** Post-discharge pulmonary surgery services after LVRS, minimum of 6 days of services Ⓑ Qp Qh S

✻ **G0306** Complete CBC, automated (HgB, HCT, RBC, WBC, without platelet count) and automated WBC differential count Ⓑ Qp Qh Q4

Laboratory Certification: Hematology

✻ **G0307** Complete CBC, automated (HgB, HCT, RBC, WBC; without platelet count) Ⓑ Qp Qh Q4

Laboratory Certification: Hematology

G0328 Colorectal cancer screening; fecal occult blood test, immunoassay, 1-3 simultaneous Ⓑ Qp Qh A

Co-insurance and deductible waived

Reported for Medicare patients 501; one FOBT per year, with either G0107 (guaiac-based) or G0328 (immunoassay-based)

Laboratory Certification: Routine chemistry, Hematology

Coding Clinic: 2012, Q2, P9

✻ **G0329** Electromagnetic therapy, to one or more areas for chronic stage III and stage IV pressure ulcers, arterial ulcers, and diabetic ulcers and venous stasis ulcers not demonstrating measurable signs of healing after 30 days of conventional care as part of a therapy plan of care Ⓑ Qp Qh A

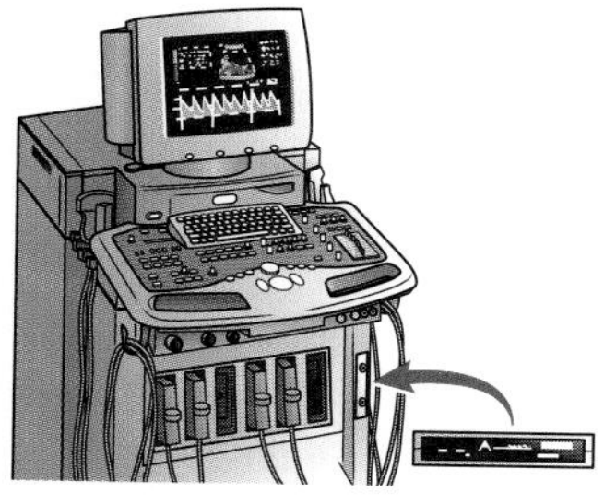

US machine

Electromagnetic device

Figure 17 Electromagnetic device.

MIPS | Qp Quantity Physician | Qh Quantity Hospital | ♀ Female only
♂ Male only | A Age | DMEPOS | A2-Z3 ASC Payment Indicator | A-Y ASC Status Indicator | Coding Clinic

G0333 Pharmacy dispensing fee for inhalation drug(s); initial 30-day supply as a beneficiary Qp Qh M

Medicare will reimburse an initial dispensing fee to a pharmacy for initial 30-day period of inhalation drugs furnished through DME.

* **G0337** Hospice evaluation and counseling services, pre-election Qp Qh B

* **G0339** Image-guided robotic linear accelerator-based stereotactic radiosurgery, complete course of therapy in one session or first session of fractionated treatment Qp Qh B

* **G0340** Image-guided robotic linear accelerator-based stereotactic radiosurgery, delivery including collimator changes and custom plugging, fractionated treatment, all lesions, per session, second through fifth sessions, maximum five sessions per course of treatment Qp Qh B

G0341 Percutaneous islet cell transplant, includes portal vein catheterization and infusion Qp Qh C

IOM: 100-03, 4, 260.3; 100-04, 32, 70

G0342 Laparoscopy for islet cell transplant, includes portal vein catheterization and infusion Qp Qh C

IOM: 100-03, 4, 260.3

G0343 Laparotomy for islet cell transplant, includes portal vein catheterization and infusion Qp Qh C

IOM: 100-03, 4, 260.3

G0372 Physician service required to establish and document the need for a power mobility device Qp Qh M

Providers should bill the E/M code and G0372 on the same claim.

Hospital Services: Observation and Emergency Department

G0378 Hospital observation service, per hour Qh N

Report all related services in addition to G0378. Report units of hours spent in observation (rounded to the nearest hour). Hospitals report the ED or clinic visit with a CPT code or, if applicable, G0379 (direct admit to observation) and G0378 (hospital observation services, per hour).

Coding Clinic: 2007, Q1, P10; 2006, Q3, P7-8

G0379 Direct admission of patient for hospital observation care Qp Qh J2

Report all related services in addition to G0379. Report units of hours spent in observation (rounded to the nearest hour). Hospitals report the ED or clinic visit with a CPT code or, if applicable, G0379 (direct admit to observation) and G0378 (hospital observation services, per hour).

Coding Clinic: 2007, Q1, P7

* **G0380** Level 1 hospital emergency department visit provided in a type B emergency department; (the ED must meet at least one of the following requirements: (1) it is licensed by the state in which it is located under applicable state law as an emergency room or emergency department; (2) it is held out to the public (by name, posted signs, advertising, or other means) as a place that provides care for emergency medical conditions on an urgent basis without requiring a previously scheduled appointment; or (3) during the calendar year immediately preceding the calendar year in which a determination under 42 CFR 489.24 is being made, based on a representative sample of patient visits that occurred during that calendar year, it provides at least one-third of all of its outpatient visits for the treatment of emergency medical conditions on an urgent basis without requiring a previously scheduled appointment) Qh J2

Coding Clinic: 2009, Q1, P4; 2007, Q2, P1

* **G0381** Level 2 hospital emergency department visit provided in a type B emergency department; (the ED must meet at least one of the following requirements: (1) it is licensed by the state in which it is located under applicable state law as an emergency room or emergency department; (2) it is held out to the public (by name, posted signs, advertising, or other means) as a place that provides care for emergency medical conditions on an urgent basis without requiring a previously scheduled appointment; or (3) during the calendar year immediately preceding the calendar year in which a determination under 42 CFR 489.24 is being made, based on a representative sample of patient visits that occurred during that calendar year, it provides at least one-third of all of its outpatient visits for the treatment of emergency medical conditions on an urgent basis without requiring a previously scheduled appointment) Ⓑ Qh J2

Coding Clinic: 2009, Q1, P4; 2007, Q2, P1

* **G0382** Level 3 hospital emergency department visit provided in a type B emergency department; (the ED must meet at least one of the following requirements: (1) it is licensed by the state in which it is located under applicable state law as an emergency room or emergency department; (2) it is held out to the public (by name, posted signs, advertising, or other means) as a place that provides care for emergency medical conditions on an urgent basis without requiring a previously scheduled appointment; or (3) during the calendar year immediately preceding the calendar year in which a determination under 42 CFR 489.24 is being made, based on a representative sample of patient visits that occurred during that calendar year, it provides at least one-third of all of its outpatient visits for the treatment of emergency medical conditions on an urgent basis without requiring a previously scheduled appointment) Ⓑ Qh J2

Coding Clinic: 2009, Q1, P4; 2007, Q2, P1

* **G0383** Level 4 hospital emergency department visit provided in a type B emergency department; (the ED must meet at least one of the following requirements: (1) it is licensed by the state in which it is located under applicable state law as an emergency room or emergency department; (2) it is held out to the public (by name, posted signs, advertising, or other means) as a place that provides care for emergency medical conditions on an urgent basis without requiring a previously scheduled appointment; or (3) during the calendar year immediately preceding the calendar year in which a determination under 42 CFR 489.24 is being made, based on a representative sample of patient visits that occurred during that calendar year, it provides at least one-third of all of its outpatient visits for the treatment of emergency medical conditions on an urgent basis without requiring a previously scheduled appointment) Ⓑ Qh J2

Coding Clinic: 2009, Q1, P4; 2007, Q2, P1

* **G0384** Level 5 hospital emergency department visit provided in a type B emergency department; (the ED must meet at least one of the following requirements: (1) it is licensed by the state in which it is located under applicable state law as an emergency room or emergency department; (2) it is held out to the public (by name, posted signs, advertising, or other means) as a place that provides care for emergency medical conditions on an urgent basis without requiring a previously scheduled appointment; or (3) during the calendar year immediately preceding the calendar year in which a determination under 42 CFR 489.24 is being made, based on a representative sample of patient visits that occurred during that calendar year, it provides at least one-third of all of its outpatient visits for the treatment of emergency medical conditions on an urgent basis without requiring a previously scheduled appointment) Ⓑ Qh J2

Coding Clinic: 2009, Q1, P4; 2007, Q2, P1

Trauma Response Team

G0390 Trauma response team associated with hospital critical care service Ⓑ Qh S

Coding Clinic: 2007, Q2, P5

Alcohol Substance Abuse Assessment and Intervention

G0396 Alcohol and/or substance (other than tobacco) misuse structured assessment (e.g., audit) and brief intervention 15 to 30 minutes Op Qh S

Bill instead of 99408 and 99409

G0397 Alcohol and/or substance (other than tobacco) misuse structured assessment (e.g., audit) and intervention, greater than 30 minutes Op Qh S

Bill instead of 99408 and 99409

Home Sleep Study Test

* **G0398** Home sleep study test (HST) with type II portable monitor, unattended; minimum of 7 channels: EEG, EOG, EMG, ECG/heart rate, airflow, respiratory effort and oxygen saturation Op Qh S

* **G0399** Home sleep test (HST) with type III portable monitor, unattended; minimum of 4 channels: 2 respiratory movement/airflow, 1 ECG/heart rate and 1 oxygen saturation Op Qh S

* **G0400** Home sleep test (HST) with type IV portable monitor, unattended; minimum of 3 channels Op Qh S

Initial Examination for Medicare Enrollment

* **G0402** Initial preventive physical examination; face-to-face visit, services limited to new beneficiary during the first 12 months of Medicare enrollment Op Qh V

Depending on circumstances, 99201-99215 may be assigned with modifier 25 to report an E/M service as a significant, separately identifiable service in addition to the Initial Preventive Physical Examination (IPPE), G0402.

Copayment and coinsurance waived, deductible waived.

Coding Clinic: 2009, Q4, P8

Electrocardiogram

* **G0403** Electrocardiogram, routine ECG with 12 leads; performed as a screening for the initial preventive physical examination with interpretation and report Op Qh M

Optional service may be ordered or performed at discretion of physician. Once in a lifetime screening, stemming from a referral from Initial Preventive Physical Examination (IPPE). Both deductible and co-payment apply.

* **G0404** Electrocardiogram, routine ECG with 12 leads; tracing only, without interpretation and report, performed as a screening for the initial preventive physical examination Op Qh S

* **G0405** Electrocardiogram, routine ECG with 12 leads; interpretation and report only, performed as a screening for the initial preventive physical examination Op Qh B

Follow-up Telehealth Consultation

* **G0406** Follow-up inpatient consultation, limited, physicians typically spend 15 minutes communicating with the patient via telehealth Op Qh B

These telehealth modifers are required when billing for telehealth services with codes G0406-G0408 and G0425-G0427:

- GT, via interactive audio and video telecommunications system
- GQ, via asynchronous telecommunications system

* **G0407** Follow-up inpatient consultation, intermediate, physicians typically spend 25 minutes communicating with the patient via telehealth Op Qh B

* **G0408** Follow-up inpatient consultation, complex, physicians typically spend 35 minutes communicating with the patient via telehealth Op Qh B

New | Revised | Reinstated | ~~deleted~~ Deleted | Not covered or valid by Medicare | Special coverage instructions | * Carrier discretion | Bill Part B MAC | Bill DME MAC

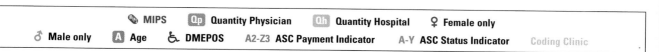

Psychological Services

MIPS ✻ **G0409** Social work and psychological services, directly relating to and/or furthering the patient's rehabilitation goals, each 15 minutes, face-to-face; individual (services provided by a CORF-qualified social worker or psychologist in a CORF) Ⓑ B

MIPS ✻ **G0410** Group psychotherapy other than of a multiple-family group, in a partial hospitalization setting, approximately 45 to 50 minutes Ⓑ Qp Qh P

Coding Clinic: 2009, Q4, P9, 10

MIPS ✻ **G0411** Interactive group psychotherapy, in a partial hospitalization setting, approximately 45 to 50 minutes Ⓑ Qp Qh P

Coding Clinic: 2009, Q4, P9, 10

Fracture Treatment

✻ **G0412** Open treatment of iliac spine(s), tuberosity avulsion, or iliac wing fracture(s), unilateral or bilateral for pelvic bone fracture patterns which do not disrupt the pelvic ring, includes internal fixation, when performed Ⓑ Qp Qh C

✻ **G0413** Percutaneous skeletal fixation of posterior pelvic bone fracture and/or dislocation, for fracture patterns which disrupt the pelvic ring, unilateral or bilateral, (includes ilium, sacroiliac joint and/or sacrum) Ⓑ Qp Qh J1

✻ **G0414** Open treatment of anterior pelvic bone fracture and/or dislocation for fracture patterns which disrupt the pelvic ring, unilateral or bilateral, includes internal fixation when performed (includes pubic symphysis and/or superior/inferior rami) Ⓑ Qp Qh C

✻ **G0415** Open treatment of posterior pelvic bone fracture and/or dislocation, for fracture patterns which disrupt the pelvic ring, unilateral or bilateral, includes internal fixation, when performed (includes ilium, sacroiliac joint and/or sacrum) Ⓑ Qp Qh C

Surgical Pathology: Prostate Biopsy

✻ **G0416** Surgical pathology, gross and microscopic examinations for prostate needle biopsy, any method Ⓑ Qp Qh ♂ Q2

This testing requires a facility to have either a CLIA certificate of registration (certificate type code 9), a CLIA certificate of compliance (certificate type code 1), or a CLIA certificate of accreditation (certificate type code 3). A facility without a valid, current, CLIA certificate, with a current CLIA certificate of waiver (certificate type code 2) or with a current CLIA certificate for provider-performed microscopy procedures (certificate type code 4), must not be permitted to be paid for these tests. This code has a TC, 26 (physician), or global component.

Laboratory Certification: Histopathology

Coding Clinic: 2013, Q2, P6

Educational Services

✻ **G0420** Face-to-face educational services related to the care of chronic kidney disease; individual, per session, per one hour Ⓑ Qp Qh A

CKD is kidney damage of 3 months or longer, regardless of the cause of kidney damage. Sessions billed in increments of one hour (if session is less than one hour, it must last at least 31 minutes to be billable. Sessions less than one hour and longer than 31 minutes are billable as one session. No more than 6 sessions of KDE services in a beneficiary's lifetime.

✻ **G0421** Face-to-face educational services related to the care of chronic kidney disease; group, per session, per one hour Ⓑ Qp Qh A

Group setting: 2 to 20, report codes G0420 and G0421 with diagnosis code N18.4.

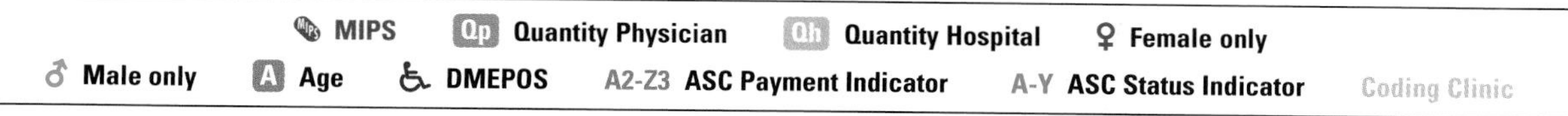
MIPS
Qp Quantity Physician
Qh Quantity Hospital
♀ Female only
♂ Male only
A Age
DMEPOS
A2-Z3 ASC Payment Indicator
A-Y ASC Status Indicator
Coding Clinic

Cardiac and Pulmonary Rehabilitation

✻ **G0422** Intensive cardiac rehabilitation; with or without continuous ECG monitoring with exercise, per session Ⓑ Qp Qh S

Includes the same service as 93798 but at a greater frequency; may be reported with as many as six hourly sessions on a single date of service. Includes medical nutrition services to reduce cardiac disease risk factors.

✻ **G0423** Intensive cardiac rehabilitation; with or without continuous ECG monitoring; without exercise, per session Ⓑ Qp Qh S

Includes the same service as 93797 but at a greater frequency; may be reported with as many as six hourly sessions on a single date of service. Includes medical nutrition services to reduce cardiac disease risk factors.

✻ **G0424** Pulmonary rehabilitation, including exercise (includes monitoring), one hour, per session, up to two sessions per day Ⓑ Qp Qh S

Includes therapeutic services and all related monitoring services to improve respiratory function. Do not report with G0237, G0238, or G0239.

Initial Telehealth Consultation

✻ **G0425** Telehealth consultation, emergency department or initial inpatient, typically 30 minutes communicating with the patient via telehealth Ⓑ Qp Qh B

Problem Focused: Problem focused history and examination, with straightforward medical decision-making complexity. Typically 30 minutes communicating with patient via telehealth.

✻ **G0426** Initial inpatient telehealth consultation, emergency department or initial inpatient, typically 50 minutes communicating with the patient via telehealth Ⓑ Qp Qh B

Detailed: Detailed history and examination, with moderate medical decision-making complexity. Typically 50 minutes communicating with patient via telehealth.

✻ **G0427** Initial inpatient telehealth consultation, emergency department or initial inpatient, typically 70 minutes or more communicating with the patient via telehealth Ⓑ Qp Qh B

Comprehensive: Comprehensive history and examination, with high medical decision-making complexity. Typically 70 minutes or more communicating with patient via telehealth.

Fillers

⃠ **G0428** Collagen meniscus implant procedure for filling meniscal defects (e.g., cmi, collagen scaffold, menaflex) Ⓑ E1

✻ **G0429** Dermal filler injection(s) for the treatment of facial lipodystrophy syndrome (LDS) (e.g., as a result of highly active antiretroviral therapy) Ⓑ Qp Qh T

Designated for dermal fillers Sculptra and Radiesse (Medicare). (https://www.cms.gov/ContractorLearningResources/downloads/JA6953.pdf)

Coding Clinic: 2010, Q3, P8

Laboratory Screening

✻ **G0432** Infectious agent antibody detection by enzyme immunoassay (EIA) technique, HIV-1 and/or HIV-2, screening Ⓑ Qp Qh A

Laboratory Certification: Virology, General immunology

Coding Clinic: 2010, Q2, P10

✻ **G0433** Infectious agent antibody detection by enzyme-linked immunosorbent assay (ELISA) technique, HIV-1 and/or HIV-2, screening Ⓑ Qp Qh A

Laboratory Certification: Virology, General immunology

Coding Clinic: 2010, Q2, P10

✻ **G0435** Infectious agent antibody detection by rapid antibody test, HIV-1 and/or HIV-2, screening Ⓑ Qp Qh A

Coding Clinic: 2010, Q2, P10

Counselling, Wellness, and Screening Services

MIPS ✻ **G0438** Annual wellness visit; includes a personalized prevention plan of service (pps), initial visit Ⓑ Qp Qh A

MIPS ✻ **G0439** Annual wellness visit, includes a personalized prevention plan of service (pps), subsequent visit Ⓑ Qp Qh A

MIPS ✻ **G0442** Annual alcohol misuse screening, 15 minutes Ⓑ Qp Qh S

Coding Clinic: 2012, Q1, P7

MIPS ✻ **G0443** Brief face-to-face behavioral counseling for alcohol misuse, 15 minutes Ⓑ Qp Qh S

Coding Clinic: 2012, Q1, P7

MIPS ✻ **G0444** Annual depression screening, 15 minutes Ⓑ Qp Qh S

MIPS ✻ **G0445** High intensity behavioral counseling to prevent sexually transmitted infection; face-to-face, individual, includes: education, skills training and guidance on how to change sexual behavior; performed semi-annually, 30 minutes Ⓑ Qp Qh S

MIPS ✻ **G0446** Annual, face-to-face intensive behavioral therapy for cardiovascular disease, individual, 15 minutes Ⓑ Qp Qh S

Coding Clinic: 2012, Q2, P8

MIPS ✻ **G0447** Face-to-face behavioral counseling for obesity, 15 minutes Ⓑ Qp Qh S

Coding Clinic: 2012, Q1, P8

✻ **G0448** Insertion or replacement of a permanent pacing cardioverter-defibrillator system with transvenous lead(s), single or dual chamber with insertion of pacing electrode, cardiac venous system, for left ventricular pacing Ⓑ Qp Qh B

✻ **G0451** Development testing, with interpretation and report, per standardized instrument form Ⓑ Qp Qh Q3

Miscellaneous Services

✻ **G0452** Molecular pathology procedure; physician interpretation and report Ⓑ Qp Qh B

✻ **G0453** Continuous intraoperative neurophysiology monitoring, from outside the operating room (remote or nearby), per patient (attention directed exclusively to one patient), each 15 minutes (list in addition to primary procedure) Ⓑ Qp Qh N

✻ **G0454** Physician documentation of face-to-face visit for durable medical equipment determination performed by nurse practitioner, physician assistant or clinical nurse specialist Ⓑ Qp Qh B

✻ **G0455** Preparation with instillation of fecal microbiota by any method, including assessment of donor specimen Ⓑ Qp Qh Q1

Coding Clinic: 2013, Q3, P8

✻ **G0458** Low dose rate (LDR) prostate brachytherapy services, composite rate Ⓑ Qp Qh B

✻ **G0459** Inpatient telehealth pharmacologic management, including prescription, use, and review of medication with no more than minimal medical psychotherapy Ⓑ Qp Qh B

✻ **G0460** Autologous platelet rich plasma for chronic wounds/ulcers, including phlebotomy, centrifugation, and all other preparatory procedures, administration and dressings, per treatment Ⓑ Qp Qh T

MIPS ✻ **G0463** Hospital outpatient clinic visit for assessment and management of a patient Ⓑ Qp Qh J2

✻ **G0464** Colorectal cancer screening; stool-based DNA and fecal occult hemoglobin (e.g., KRAS, NDRG4 and BMP3) Ⓑ

Cross Reference 81528

Laboratory Certification: General immunology, Routine chemistry,Clinical cytogenetics

Federally Qualified Health Center Visits

✻ **G0466** Federally qualified health center (FQHC) visit, new patient; a medically-necessary, face-to-face encounter (one-on-one) between a new patient and a FQHC practitioner during which time one or more FQHC services are rendered and includes a typical bundle of Medicare-covered services that would be furnished per diem to a patient receiving a FQHC visit Ⓑ Qp Qh A

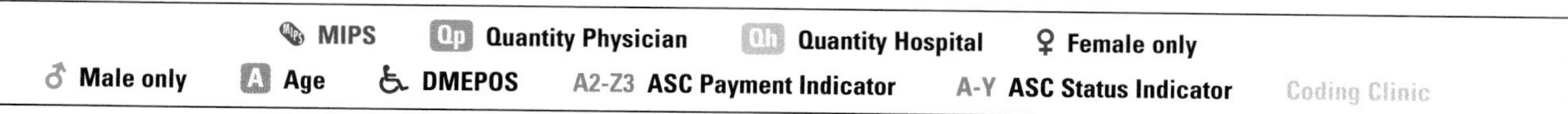
MIPS
Qp Quantity Physician
Qh Quantity Hospital
♀ Female only
♂ Male only
A Age
DMEPOS
A2-Z3 ASC Payment Indicator
A-Y ASC Status Indicator
Coding Clinic

✻ **G0467** Federally qualified health center (FQHC) visit, established patient; a medically-necessary, face-to-face encounter (one-on-one) between an established patient and a FQHC practitioner during which time one or more FQHC services are rendered and includes a typical bundle of Medicare-covered services that would be furnished per diem to a patient receiving a FQHC visit Ⓑ Qp Qh A

✻ **G0468** Federally qualified health center (FQHC) visit, IPPE or AWV; a FQHC visit that includes an initial preventive physical examination (IPPE) or annual wellness visit (AWV) and includes a typical bundle of Medicare-covered services that would be furnished per diem to a patient receiving an IPPE or AWV Ⓑ Qp Qh A

✻ **G0469** Federally qualified health center (FQHC) visit, mental health, new patient; a medically-necessary, face-to-face mental health encounter (one-on-one) between a new patient and a FQHC practitioner during which time one or more FQHC services are rendered and includes a typical bundle of Medicare-covered services that would be furnished per diem to a patient receiving a mental health visit Ⓑ Qp Qh A

✻ **G0470** Federally qualified health center (FQHC) visit, mental health, established patient; a medically-necessary, face-to-face mental health encounter (one-on-one) between an established patient and a FQHC practitioner during which time one or more FQHC services are rendered and includes a typical bundle of Medicare-covered services that would be furnished per diem to a patient receiving a mental health visit Ⓑ Qp Qh A

Other Miscellaneous Services

✻ **G0471** Collection of venous blood by venipuncture or urine sample by catheterization from an individual in a skilled nursing facility (SNF) or by a laboratory on behalf of a home health agency (HHA) Ⓑ Qp Qh A

◌ **G0472** Hepatitis C antibody screening, for individual at high risk and other covered indication(s) Ⓑ Qp Qh A

Medicare Statute 1861SSA

Laboratory Certification: General immunology

✻ **G0473** Face-to-face behavioral counseling for obesity, group (2-10), 30 minutes Ⓑ Qp Qh S

✻ **G0475** HIV antigen/antibody, combination assay, screening Ⓑ Qp Qh A

Laboratory Certification: Virology, General immunology

✻ **G0476** Infectious agent detection by nucleic acid (DNA or RNA); human papillomavirus (HPV), high-risk types (e.g., 16, 18, 31, 33, 35, 39, 45, 51, 52, 56, 58, 59, 68) for cervical cancer screening, must be performed in addition to pap test Ⓑ Qp Qh A

Laboratory Certification: Virology

Drug Tests

✻ **G0480** Drug test(s), definitive, utilizing drug identification methods able to identify individual drugs and distinguish between structural isomers (but not necessarily stereoisomers), including, but not limited to GC/MS (any type, single or tandem) and LC/MS (any type, single or tandem and excluding immunoassays (e.g., IA, EIA, ELISA, EMIT, FPIA) and enzymatic methods (e.g., alcohol dehydrogenase)); qualitative or quantitative, all sources(s), includes specimen validity testing, per day, 1-7 drug class(es), including metabolite(s) if performed Ⓑ Qp Qh Q4

Coding Clinic: 2018, Q1, P5

✻ **G0481** Drug test(s), definitive, utilizing drug identification methods able to identify individual drugs and distinguish between structural isomers (but not necessarily stereoisomers), including, but not limited to GC/MS (any type, single or tandem) and LC/MS (any type, single or tandem and excluding immunoassays (e.g., IA, EIA, ELISA, EMIT, FPIA) and enzymatic methods (e.g., alcohol dehydrogenase)); qualitative or quantitative, all sources(s), includes specimen validity testing, per day, 8-14 drug class(es), including metabolite(s) if performed Ⓑ Qp Qh Q4

Coding Clinic: 2018, Q1, P5

* **G0482** Drug test(s), definitive, utilizing drug identification methods able to identify individual drugs and distinguish between structural isomers (but not necessarily stereoisomers), including, but not limited to GC/MS (any type, single or tandem) and LC/MS (any type, single or tandem and excluding immunoassays (e.g., IA, EIA, ELISA, EMIT, FPIA) and enzymatic methods (e.g., alcohol dehydrogenase); qualitative or quantitative, all sources(s), includes specimen validity testing, per day, 15-21 drug class(es), including metabolite(s) if performed Qp Qh Q4

  Coding Clinic: 2018, Q1, P5

* **G0483** Drug test(s), definitive, utilizing drug identification methods able to identify individual drugs and distinguish between structural isomers (but not necessarily stereoisomers), including, but not limited to GC/MS (any type, single or tandem) and LC/MS (any type, single or tandem and excluding immunoassays (e.g., IA, EIA, ELISA, EMIT, FPIA) and enzymatic methods (e.g., alcohol dehydrogenase); qualitative or quantitative, all sources(s), includes specimen validity testing, per day, 22 or more drug class(es), including metabolite(s) if performed Qp Qh Q4

  Coding Clinic: 2018, Q1, P5

Home Health Nursing Visit: Area of Shortage

* **G0490** Face-to-face home health nursing visit by a rural health clinic (RHC) or federally qualified health center (FQHC) in an area with a shortage of home health agencies (services limited to RN or LPN only) A

Dialysis Procedure

* **G0491** Dialysis procedure at a Medicare certified ESRD facility for acute kidney injury without ESRD Qp Qh B
* **G0492** Dialysis procedure with single evaluation by a physician or other qualified health care professional for acute kidney injury without ESRD Qp Qh B

Home Health or Hospice: Skilled Services

* **G0493** Skilled services of a registered nurse (RN) for the observation and assessment of the patient's condition, each 15 minutes (the change in the patient's condition requires skilled nursing personnel to identify and evaluate the patient's need for possible modification of treatment in the home health or hospice setting) B
* **G0494** Skilled services of a licensed practical nurse (LPN) for the observation and assessment of the patient's condition, each 15 minutes (the change in the patient's condition requires skilled nursing personnel to identify and evaluate the patient's need for possible modification of treatment in the home health or hospice setting) B
* **G0495** Skilled services of a registered nurse (RN), in the training and/or education of a patient or family member, in the home health or hospice setting, each 15 minutes B
* **G0496** Skilled services of a licensed practical nurse (LPN), in the training and/or education of a patient or family member, in the home health or hospice setting, each 15 minutes B

Chemotherapy Administration

* **G0498** Chemotherapy administration, intravenous infusion technique; initiation of infusion in the office/clinic setting using office/clinic pump/supplies, with continuation of the infusion in the community setting (e.g., home, domiciliary, rest home or assisted living) using a portable pump provided by the office/clinic, includes follow up office/clinic visit at the conclusion of the infusion Qp Qh S

Hepatitis B Screening

* **G0499** Hepatitis B screening in non-pregnant, high risk individual includes hepatitis B surface antigen (HBsAG), antibodies to HBsAG (anti-HBs) and antibodies to hepatitis B core antigen (anti-hbc), and is followed by a neutralizing confirmatory test, when performed, only for an initially reactive HBsAG result Qp Qh A

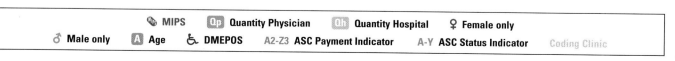

  Laboratory Certification: Virology

Moderate Sedation Services

* **G0500** Moderate sedation services provided by the same physician or other qualified health care professional performing a gastrointestinal endoscopic service that sedation supports, requiring the presence of an independent trained observer to assist in the monitoring of the patient's level of consciousness and physiological status; initial 15 minutes of intra-service time; patient age 5 years or older (additional time may be reported with 99153, as appropriate) Ⓑ Qp Qh N

Resource-Intensive Service

* **G0501** Resource-intensive services for patients for whom the use of specialized mobility-assistive technology (such as adjustable height chairs or tables, patient lift, and adjustable padded leg supports) is medically necessary and used during the provision of an office/outpatient, evaluation and management visit (list separately in addition to primary service) Ⓑ N

Psychiatric Care Management

* **G0506** Comprehensive assessment of and care planning for patients requiring chronic care management services (list separately in addition to primary monthly care management service) Ⓑ Qp Qh N

Critical Care Telehealth Consultation

* **G0508** Telehealth consultation, critical care, initial, physicians typically spend 60 minutes communicating with the patient and providers via telehealth Ⓑ Qp Qh B

* **G0509** Telehealth consultation, critical care, subsequent, physicians typically spend 50 minutes communicating with the patient and providers via telehealth Ⓑ Qp Qh B

Rural Health Clinic: Management and Care

G0511 Rural health clinic or federally qualified health center (RHC or FQHC) only, general care management, 20 minutes or more of clinical staff time for chronic care management services or behavioral health integration services directed by an RHC or FQHC practitioner (physician, NP, PA, or CNM), per calendar month A

G0512 Rural health clinic or federally qualified health center (RHC/FQHC) only, psychiatric collaborative care model (psychiatric CoCM), 60 minutes or more of clinical staff time for psychiatric CoCM services directed by an RHC or FQHC practitioner (physician, NP, PA, or CNM) and including services furnished by a behavioral health care manager and consultation with a psychiatric consultant, per calendar month A

Prolonged Preventive Services

* **G0513** Prolonged preventive service(s) (beyond the typical service time of the primary procedure), in the office or other outpatient setting requiring direct patient contact beyond the usual service; first 30 minutes (list separately in addition to code for preventive service) N

* **G0514** Prolonged preventive service(s) (beyond the typical service time of the primary procedure), in the office or other outpatient setting requiring direct patient contact beyond the usual service; each additional 30 minutes (list separately in addition to code G0513 for additional 30 minutes of preventive service) N

▶ New ↩ Revised ✔ Reinstated ~~deleted~~ Deleted ⊘ Not covered or valid by Medicare
Special coverage instructions * Carrier discretion Ⓑ Bill Part B MAC Ⓑ Bill DME MAC

Non-biodegradable Drug Delivery Implants: Removal and Insertion

* G0516 Insertion of non-biodegradable drug delivery implants, 4 or more (services for subdermal rod implant) Q1

* G0517 Removal of non-biodegradable drug delivery implants, 4 or more (services for subdermal implants) Q1

* G0518 Removal with reinsertion, non-biodegradable drug delivery implants, 4 or more (services for subdermal implants) Q1

Drug Test

* G0659 Drug test(s), definitive, utilizing drug identification methods able to identify individual drugs and distinguish between structural isomers (but not necessarily stereoisomers), including but not limited to GC/MS (any type, single or tandem) and LC/MS (any type, single or tandem), excluding immunoassays (e.g., IA, EIA, ELISA, EMIT, FPIA) and enzymatic methods (e.g., alcohol dehydrogenase), performed without method or drug-specific calibration, without matrix-matched quality control material, or without use of stable isotope or other universally recognized internal standard(s) for each drug, drug metabolite or drug class per specimen; qualitative or quantitative, all sources, includes specimen validity testing, per day, any number of drug classes Q4

Quality Care Measures: Cataract Surgery

* G0913 Improvement in visual function achieved within 90 days following cataract surgery M

* G0914 Patient care survey was not completed by patient M

* G0915 Improvement in visual function not achieved within 90 days following cataract surgery M

* G0916 Satisfaction with care achieved within 90 days following cataract surgery M

* G0917 Patient satisfaction survey was not completed by patient M

* G0918 Satisfaction with care not achieved within 90 days following cataract surgery M

Clinical Decision Support Mechanism

~~G1000 Clinical decision support mechanism applied pathways, as defined by the Medicare Appropriate Use Criteria Program~~ ✖

* G1001 Clinical decision support mechanism eviCore, as defined by the Medicare Appropriate Use Criteria Program E1

* G1002 Clinical decision support mechanism MedCurrent, as defined by the Medicare Appropriate Use Criteria Program E1

* G1003 Clinical decision support mechanism Medicalis, as defined by the Medicare Appropriate Use Criteria Program E1

* G1004 Clinical decision support mechanism National Decision Support Company, as defined by the Medicare Appropriate Use Criteria Program E1

~~G1005 Clinical decision support mechanism National Imaging Associates, as defined by the Medicare Appropriate Use Criteria Program~~ ✖

~~G1006 Clinical decision support mechanism Test Appropriate, as defined by the Medicare Appropriate Use Criteria Program~~ ✖

* G1007 Clinical decision support mechanism AIM Specialty Health, as defined by the Medicare Appropriate Use Criteria Program E1

* G1008 Clinical decision support mechanism Cranberry Peak, as defined by the Medicare Appropriate Use Criteria Program E1

* G1009 Clinical decision support mechanism Sage Health Management Solutions, as defined by the Medicare Appropriate Use Criteria Program E1

* G1010 Clinical decision support mechanism Stanson, as defined by the Medicare Appropriate Use Criteria Program E1

* G1011 Clinical decision support mechanism, qualified tool not otherwise specified, as defined by the Medicare Appropriate Use Criteria Program E1

▶ * G1012 Clinical decision support mechanism AgileMD, as defined by the Medicare appropriate use criteria program E1

▶ * G1013 Clinical decision support mechanism EvidenceCare imaging advisor, as defined by the Medicare appropriate use criteria program E1

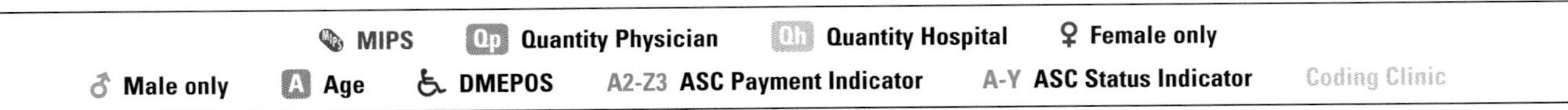
MIPS
Qp Quantity Physician
Qh Quantity Hospital
♀ Female only
♂ Male only
A Age
DMEPOS
A2-Z3 ASC Payment Indicator
A-Y ASC Status Indicator
Coding Clinic

▶ * **G1014** Clinical decision support mechanism InveniQA semantic answers in medicine, as defined by the Medicare appropriate use criteria program E1

▶ * **G1015** Clinical decision support mechanism Reliant Medical Group, as defined by the Medicare appropriate use criteria program E1

▶ * **G1016** Clinical decision support mechanism Speed of Care, as defined by the Medicare appropriate use criteria program E1

▶ * **G1017** Clinical decision support mechanism HealthHelp, as defined by the Medicare appropriate use criteria program E1

▶ * **G1018** Clinical decision support mechanism Infinx, as defined by the Medicare appropriate use criteria program E1

▶ * **G1019** Clinical decision support mechanism LogicNets, as defined by the Medicare appropriate use criteria program E1

▶ * **G1020** Clinical decision support mechanism Curbside Clinical Augmented Workflow, as defined by the Medicare appropriate use criteria program E1

▶ * **G1021** Clinical decision support mechanism E*HealthLine clinical decision support mechanism, as defined by the Medicare appropriate use criteria program E1

▶ * **G1022** Clinical decision support mechanism Intermountain clinical decision support mechanism, as defined by the Medicare appropriate use criteria program E1

▶ * **G1023** Clinical decision support mechanism Persivia clinical decision support, as defined by the Medicare appropriate use criteria program E1

Therapy, Evaluation and Assessment

* **G2000** Blinded administration of convulsive therapy procedure, either electroconvulsive therapy (ECT, current covered gold standard) or magnetic seizure therapy (MST, non-covered experimental therapy), performed in an approved IDE-based clinical trial, per treatment session S

* **G2010** Remote evaluation of recorded video and/or images submitted by an established patient (e.g., store and forward), including interpretation with follow-up with the patient within 24 business hours, not originating from a related E/M service provided within the previous 7 days nor leading to an E/M service or procedure within the next 24 hours or soonest available appointment M

↩ * **G2011** Alcohol and/or substance (other than tobacco) misuse structured assessment (e.g., audit, dast), and brief intervention, 5-14 minutes S

* **G2012** Brief communication technology-based service, e.g., virtual check-in, by a physician or other qualified health care professional who can report evaluation and management services, provided to an established patient, not originating from a related E/M service provided within the previous 7 days nor leading to an E/M service or procedure within the next 24 hours or soonest available appointment; 5-10 minutes of medical discussion M

* **G2021** Health care practitioners rendering treatment in place (TIP) E1

* **G2022** A model participant (ambulance supplier/provider), the beneficiary refuses services covered under the model (transport to an alternate destination/treatment in place) E1

▶ * **G2023** Specimen collection for severe acute respiratory syndrome coronavirus 2 (SARS-CoV-2) (coronavirus disease [COVID-19]), any specimen source B

▶ * **G2024** Specimen collection for severe acute respiratory syndrome coronavirus 2 (SARS-CoV-2) (coronavirus disease [COVID-19]) from an individual in a SNF or by a laboratory on behalf of a HHA, any specimen source B

▶ * **G2025** Payment for a telehealth distant site service furnished by a rural health clinic (RHC) or federally qualified health center (FQHC) only A

~~G2058 Chronic care management services, each additional 20 minutes of clinical staff time directed by a physician or other qualified health care professional, per calendar month (list separately in addition to code for primary procedure). (Do not report G2058 for care management services of less than 20 minutes additional to the first 20 minutes of chronic care management services during a calendar month.) (Use G2058 in conjunction with 99490.) (Do not report 99490, G2058 in the same calendar month as 99487, 99489, 99491.)~~ ✖

⮐ * **G2061** Qualified nonphysician healthcare professional online assessment and management service, for an established patient, for up to seven days, cumulative time during the 7 days; 5-10 minutes M

⮐ * **G2062** Qualified nonphysician healthcare professional online assessment and management service, for an established patient, for up to seven days, cumulative time during the 7 days; 11-20 minutes M

⮐ * **G2063** Qualified nonphysician qualified healthcare professional assessment and management service, for an established patient, for up to seven days, cumulative time during the 7 days; 21 or more minutes M

* **G2064** Comprehensive care management services for a single high-risk disease, e.g., principal care management, at least 30 minutes of physician or other qualified health care professional time per calendar month with the following elements: one complex chronic condition lasting at least 3 months, which is the focus of the care plan; the condition is of sufficient severity to place patient at risk of hospitalization or have been the cause of a recent hospitalization; the condition requires development or revision of disease-specific care plan; the condition requires frequent adjustments in the medication regimen; and/or the management of the condition is unusually complex due to comorbidities M

* **G2065** Comprehensive care management for a single high-risk disease services, e.g., principal care management, at least 30 minutes of clinical staff time directed by a physician or other qualified health care professional, per calendar month with the following elements: one complex chronic condition lasting at least 3 months, which is the focus of the care plan; the condition is of sufficient severity to place patient at risk of hospitalization or have been cause of a recent hospitalization; the condition requires development or revision of disease-specific care plan; the condition requires frequent adjustments in the medication regimen; and/or the management of the condition is unusually complex due to comorbidities S

* **G2066** Interrogation device evaluation(s), (remote) up to 30 days; implantable cardiovascular physiologic monitor system, implantable loop recorder system, or subcutaneous cardiac rhythm monitor system, remote data acquisition(s), receipt of transmissions and technician review, technical support and distribution of results Q1

* **G2067** Medication assisted treatment, methadone; weekly bundle including dispensing and/or administration, substance use counseling, individual and group therapy, and toxicology testing, if performed (provision of the services by a Medicare-enrolled opioid treatment program) E1

* **G2068** Medication assisted treatment, buprenorphine (oral); weekly bundle including dispensing and/or administration, substance use counseling, individual and group therapy, and toxicology testing if performed (provision of the services by a Medicare-enrolled opioid treatment program) E1

* **G2069** Medication assisted treatment, buprenorphine (injectable); weekly bundle including dispensing and/or administration, substance use counseling, individual and group therapy, and toxicology testing if performed (provision of the services by a Medicare-enrolled opioid treatment program) E1

* **G2070** Medication assisted treatment, buprenorphine (implant insertion); weekly bundle including dispensing and/or administration, substance use counseling, individual and group therapy, and toxicology testing if performed (provision of the services by a Medicare-enrolled opioid treatment program) E1

* **G2071** Medication assisted treatment, buprenorphine (implant removal); weekly bundle including dispensing and/or administration, substance use counseling, individual and group therapy, and toxicology testing if performed (provision of the services by a Medicare-enrolled opioid treatment program) E1

* **G2072** Medication assisted treatment, buprenorphine (implant insertion and removal); weekly bundle including dispensing and/or administration, substance use counseling, individual and group therapy, and toxicology testing if performed (provision of the services by a Medicare-enrolled opioid treatment program) E1

* **G2073** Medication assisted treatment, naltrexone; weekly bundle including dispensing and/or administration, substance use counseling, individual and group therapy, and toxicology testing if performed (provision of the services by a Medicare-enrolled opioid treatment program) E1

* **G2074** Medication assisted treatment, weekly bundle not including the drug, including substance use counseling, individual and group therapy, and toxicology testing if performed (provision of the services by a Medicare-enrolled opioid treatment program) E1

* **G2075** Medication assisted treatment, medication not otherwise specified; weekly bundle including dispensing and/or administration, substance use counseling, individual and group therapy, and toxicology testing, if performed (provision of the services by a Medicare-enrolled opioid treatment program) E1

* **G2076** Intake activities, including initial medical examination that is a complete, fully documented physical evaluation and initial assessment by a program physician or a primary care physician, or an authorized healthcare professional under the supervision of a program physician qualified personnel that includes preparation of a treatment plan that includes the patient's short-term goals and the tasks the patient must perform to complete the short-term goals; the patient's requirements for education, vocational rehabilitation, and employment; and the medical, psycho-social, economic, legal, or other supportive services that a patient needs, conducted by qualified personnel (provision of the services by a Medicare-enrolled opioid treatment program); list separately in addition to code for primary procedure E1

* **G2077** Periodic assessment; assessing periodically by qualified personnel to determine the most appropriate combination of services and treatment (provision of the services by a Medicare-enrolled opioid treatment program); list separately in addition to code for primary procedure E1

* **G2078** Take-home supply of methadone; up to 7 additional day supply (provision of the services by a Medicare-enrolled opioid treatment program); list separately in addition to code for primary procedure E1

* **G2079** Take-home supply of buprenorphine (oral); up to 7 additional day supply (provision of the services by a Medicare-enrolled opioid treatment program); list separately in addition to code for primary procedure E1

* **G2080** Each additional 30 minutes of counseling in a week of medication assisted treatment, (provision of the services by a Medicare-enrolled opioid treatment program); list separately in addition to code for primary procedure E1

* **G2081** Patients age 66 and older in institutional special needs plans (SNP) or residing in long-term care with a POS code 32, 33, 34, 54 or 56 for more than 90 days during the measurement period M

✻ **G2082** Office or other outpatient visit for the evaluation and management of an established patient that requires the supervision of a physician or other qualified health care professional and provision of up to 56 mg of esketamine nasal self-administration, includes 2 hours post-administration observation S

✻ **G2083** Office or other outpatient visit for the evaluation and management of an established patient that requires the supervision of a physician or other qualified health care professional and provision of greater than 56 mg esketamine nasal self-administration, includes 2 hours post-administration observation S

✻ **G2086** Office-based treatment for opioid use disorder, including development of the treatment plan, care coordination, individual therapy and group therapy and counseling; at least 70 minutes in the first calendar month S

✻ **G2087** Office-based treatment for opioid use disorder, including care coordination, individual therapy and group therapy and counseling; at least 60 minutes in a subsequent calendar month S

✻ **G2088** Office-based treatment for opioid use disorder, including care coordination, individual therapy and group therapy and counseling; each additional 30 minutes beyond the first 120 minutes (list separately in addition to code for primary procedure) N

~~G2089 Most recent hemoglobin A1c (HbA1c) level 7.0 to 9.0%~~ ✖

✻ **G2090** Patients 66 years of age and older with at least one claim/encounter for frailty during the measurement period and a dispensed medication for dementia during the measurement period or the year prior to the measurement period N1 M

✻ **G2091** Patients 66 years of age and older with at least one claim/encounter for frailty during the measurement period and either one acute inpatient encounter with a diagnosis of advanced illness or two outpatient, observation, ED or nonacute inpatient encounters on different dates of service with an advanced illness diagnosis during the measurement period or the year prior to the measurement period N1 M

✻ **G2092** Angiotensin converting enzyme (ACE) inhibitor or angiotensin receptor blocker (ARB) or angiotensin receptor-neprilysin inhibitor (AMI) therapy prescribed or currently being taken N1 M

✻ **G2093** Documentation of medical reason(s) for not prescribing ACE inhibitor or ARB or AMI therapy (e.g., hypotensive patients who are at immediate risk of cardiogenic shock, hospitalized patients who have experienced marked azotemia, allergy, intolerance, other medical reasons) N1 M

✻ **G2094** Documentation of patient reason(s) for not prescribing ACE inhibitor or ARB or AMI therapy (e.g., patient declined, other patient reasons) N1 M

✻ **G2095** Documentation of system reason(s) for not prescribing ACE inhibitor or ARB or AMI therapy (e.g., other system reasons) N1 M

✻ **G2096** Angiotensin converting enzyme (ACE) inhibitor or angiotensin receptor blocker (ARB) or angiotensin receptor-neprilysin inhibitor (AMI) therapy was not prescribed, reason not given N1 M

⤺ ✻ **G2097** Episodes where the patient had a competing diagnosis within three days after the episode date (e.g., intestinal infection, pertussis, bacterial infection, Lyme disease, otitis media, acute sinusitis, acute pharyngitis, acute tonsillitis, chronic sinusitis, infection of the pharynx/larynx/tonsils/adenoids, prostatitis, cellulitis, mastoiditis, or bone infections, acute lymphadenitis, impetigo, skin staph infections, pneumonia/gonococcal infections, venereal disease (syphilis, chlamydia, inflammatory diseases [female reproductive organs]), infections of the kidney, cystitis or UTI N1 M

✻ **G2098** Patients 66 years of age and older with at least one claim/encounter for frailty during the measurement period and a dispensed medication for dementia during the measurement period or the year prior to the measurement period N1 M

MIPS
Qp Quantity Physician
Qh Quantity Hospital
♀ Female only
♂ Male only
A Age
DMEPOS
A2-Z3 ASC Payment Indicator
A-Y ASC Status Indicator
Coding Clinic

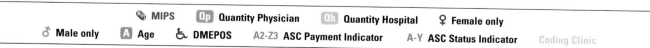

✻ **G2099** Patients 66 years of age and older with at least one claim/encounter for frailty during the measurement period and either one acute inpatient encounter with a diagnosis of advanced illness or two outpatient, observation, ED or nonacute inpatient encounters on different dates of service with an advanced illness diagnosis during the measurement period or the year prior to the measurement period N1 M

✻ **G2100** Patients 66 years of age and older with at least one claim/encounter for frailty during the measurement period and a dispensed medication for dementia during the measurement period or the year prior to the measurement period N1 M

✻ **G2101** Patients 66 years of age and older with at least one claim/encounter for frailty during the measurement period and either one acute inpatient encounter with a diagnosis of advanced illness or two outpatient, observation, ED or nonacute inpatient encounters on different dates of service with an advanced illness diagnosis during the measurement period or the year prior to the measurement period N1 M

~~G2102 Dilated retinal eye exam with interpretation by an ophthalmologist or optometrist documented and reviewed~~ ✖

~~G2103 Seven standard field stereoscopic photos with interpretation by an ophthalmologist or optometrist documented and reviewed~~ ✖

~~G2104 Eye imaging validated to match diagnosis from seven standard field stereoscopic photos results documented and reviewed~~ ✖

↩ ✻ **G2105** Patients age 66 or older in institutional special needs plans (SNP) or residing in long-term care with POS code 32, 33, 34, 54 or 56 for more than 90 days consecutive during the measurement period N1 M

✻ **G2106** Patients 66 years of age and older with at least one claim/encounter for frailty during the measurement period and a dispensed medication for dementia during the measurement period or the year prior to the measurement period N1 M

✻ **G2107** Patients 66 years of age and older with at least one claim/encounter for frailty during the measurement period and either one acute inpatient encounter with a diagnosis of advanced illness or two outpatient, observation, ED or nonacute inpatient encounters on different dates of service with an advanced illness diagnosis during the measurement period or the year prior to the measurement period N1 M

↩ ✻ **G2108** Patients age 66 or older in institutional special needs plans (SNP) or residing in long-term care with POS code 32, 33, 34, 54 or 56 for more than 90 days consecutive during the measurement period N1 M

✻ **G2109** Patients 66 years of age and older with at least one claim/encounter for frailty during the measurement period and a dispensed medication for dementia during the measurement period or the year prior to the measurement period N1 M

✻ **G2110** Patients 66 years of age and older with at least one claim/encounter for frailty during the measurement period and either one acute inpatient encounter with a diagnosis of advanced illness or two outpatient, observation, ED or nonacute inpatient encounters on different dates of service with an advanced illness diagnosis during the measurement period or the year prior to the measurement period N1 M

✻ **G2112** Patient receiving <=5 mg daily prednisone (or equivalent), or RA activity is worsening, or glucocorticoid use is for less than 6 months N1 M

✻ **G2113** Patient receiving >5 mg daily prednisone (or equivalent) for longer than 6 months, and improvement or no change in disease activity N1 M

~~G2114 Patients 66-80 years of age with at least one claim/encounter for frailty during the measurement period and a dispensed medication for dementia during the measurement period or the year prior to the measurement period~~ ✖

↩ ✻ **G2115** Patients 66-80 years of age with at least one claim/encounter for frailty during the measurement period and a dispensed medication for dementia during the measurement period or the year prior to the measurement period N1 M

▶ New ↩ Revised ✔ Reinstated ~~deleted~~ Deleted ⊘ Not covered or valid by Medicare
Special coverage instructions ✻ Carrier discretion Ⓑ Bill Part B MAC Ⓔ Bill DME MAC

G2116 Patients 66-80 years of age with at least one claim/encounter for frailty during the measurement period and either one acute inpatient encounter with a diagnosis of advanced illness or two outpatient, observation, ED or nonacute inpatient encounters on different dates of service with an advanced illness diagnosis during the measurement period or the year prior to the measurement period N1 M

~~G2117 Patients 66-80 years of age with at least one claim/encounter for frailty during the measurement period and either one acute inpatient encounter with a diagnosis of advanced illness or two outpatient, observation, ED or nonacute inpatient encounters on different dates of service with an advanced illness diagnosis during the measurement period or the year prior to the measurement period~~

G2118 Patients 81 years of age and older with at least one claim/encounter for frailty during the measurement period N1 M

~~G2119 Within the past 2 years, calcium and/or vitamin D optimization has been ordered or performed~~

~~G2120 Within the past 2 years, calcium and/or vitamin D optimization has not been ordered or performed~~

G2121 Psychosis, depression, anxiety, apathy, and impulse control disorder assessed N1 M

G2122 Psychosis, depression, anxiety, apathy, and impulse control disorder not assessed N1 M

~~G2123 Patients 66-80 years of age and had at least one claim/encounter for frailty during the measurement period and either one acute inpatient encounter with a diagnosis of advanced illness or two outpatient, observation, ED or nonacute inpatient encounters on different dates of service with an advanced illness diagnosis during the measurement period or the year prior to the measurement period~~

~~G2124 Patients 66-80 years of age and had at least one claim/encounter for frailty during the measurement period and a dispensed dementia medication~~

G2125 Patients 81 years of age and older with at least one claim/encounter for frailty during the six months prior to the measurement period through December 31 of the measurement period N1 M

G2126 Patients 66-80 years of age with at least one claim/encounter for frailty during the measurement period and either one acute inpatient encounter with a diagnosis of advanced illness or two outpatient, observation, ED or nonacute inpatient encounters on different dates of service with an advanced illness diagnosis during the measurement period or the year prior to the measurement period N1 M

G2127 Patients 66-80 years of age with at least one claim/encounter for frailty during the measurement period and a dispensed dementia medication N1 M

G2128 Documentation of medical reason(s) for not on a daily aspirin or other antiplatelet (e.g. history of gastrointestinal bleed, intra-cranial bleed, blood disorders, idiopathic thrombocytopenic purpura [ITP], gastric bypass or documentation of active anticoagulant use during the measurement period) N1 M

G2129 Procedure-related BP's not taken during an outpatient visit. Examples include same day surgery, ambulatory service center, G.I. lab, dialysis, infusion center, chemotherapy N1 M

~~G2130 Patients age 66 or older in institutional special needs plans (SNP) or residing in long-term care with POS code 32, 33, 34, 54 or 56 for more than 90 days during the measurement period~~

~~G2131 Patients 81 years and older with a diagnosis of frailty~~

~~G2132 Patients 66-80 years of age with at least one claim/encounter for frailty during the measurement period and a dispensed medication for dementia during the measurement period or the year prior to the measurement period~~

~~G2133 Patients 66-80 years of age with at least one claim/encounter for frailty during the measurement period and either one acute inpatient encounter with a diagnosis of advanced illness or two outpatient, observation, ED or nonacute inpatient encounters on different dates of service with an advanced illness diagnosis during the measurement period or the year prior to the measurement period~~

~~G2134 Patients 66 years of age or older with at least one claim/encounter for frailty during the measurement period and a dispensed medication for dementia during the measurement period or the year prior to the measurement period~~

~~G2135 Patients 66 years of age or older with at least one claim/encounter for frailty during the measurement period and either one acute inpatient encounter with a diagnosis of advanced illness or two outpatient, observation, ED or nonacute inpatient encounters on different dates of service with an advanced illness diagnosis during the measurement period or the year prior to the measurement period~~ ✖

✻ **G2136** Back pain measured by the Visual Analog Scale (VAS) at three months (6 - 20 weeks) postoperatively was less than or equal to 3.0 or back pain measured by the Visual Analog Scale (VAS) within three months preoperatively and at three months (6 - 20 weeks) postoperatively demonstrated an improvement of 5.0 points or greater N1 M

✻ **G2137** Back pain measured by the Visual Analog Scale (VAS) at three months (6 - 20 weeks) postoperatively was greater than 3.0 and back pain measured by the Visual Analog Scale (VAS) within three months preoperatively and at three months (6 - 20 weeks) postoperatively demonstrated a change of less than an improvement of 5.0 points N1 M

✻ **G2138** Back pain as measured by the Visual Analog Scale (VAS) at one year (9 to 15 months) postoperatively was less than or equal to 3.0 or back pain measured by the Visual Analog Scale (VAS) within three months preoperatively and at one year (9 to 15 months) postoperatively demonstrated a change of 5.0 points or greater N1 M

✻ **G2139** Back pain measured by the Visual Analog Scale (VAS) pain at one year (9 to 15 months) postoperatively was greater than 3.0 and back pain measured by the Visual Analog Scale (VAS) within three months preoperatively and at one year (9 to 15 months) postoperatively demonstrated a change of less than 5.0 N1 M

✻ **G2140** Leg pain measured by the Visual Analog Scale (VAS) at three months (6 - 20 weeks) postoperatively was less than or equal to 3.0 or leg pain measured by the Visual Analog Scale (VAS) within three months preoperatively and at three months (6 - 20 weeks) postoperatively demonstrated an improvement of 5.0 points or greater N1 M

✻ **G2141** Leg pain measured by the Visual Analog Scale (VAS) at three months (6 - 20 weeks) postoperatively was greater than 3.0 and leg pain measured by the Visual Analog Scale (VAS) within three months preoperatively and at three months (6 - 20 weeks) postoperatively demonstrated less than an improvement of 5.0 points N1 M

✻ **G2142** Functional status measured by the Oswestry Disability Index (ODI version 2.1a) at one year (9 to 15 months) postoperatively was less than or equal to 22 or functional status measured by the ODI version 2.1a within three months preoperatively and at one year (9 to 15 months) postoperatively demonstrated a change of 30 points or greater N1 M

✻ **G2143** Functional status measured by the Oswestry Disability Index (ODI version 2.1a) at one year (9 to 15 months) postoperatively was greater than 22 and functional status measured by the ODI version 2.1a within three months preoperatively and at one year (9 to 15 months) postoperatively demonstrated a change of less than 30 points N1 M

✻ **G2144** Functional status measured by the Oswestry Disability Index (ODI version 2.1a) at three months (6 - 20 weeks) postoperatively was less than or equal to 22 or functional status measured by the ODI version 2.1a within three months preoperatively and at three months (6 - 20 weeks) postoperatively demonstrated a change of 30 points or greater

✻ **G2145** Functional status measured by the Oswestry Disability Index (ODI version 2.1a) at three months (6 - 20 weeks) postoperatively was greater than 22 and functional status measured by the ODI version 2.1a within three months preoperatively and at three months (6 - 20 weeks) postoperatively demonstrated a change of less than 30 points N1 M

✻ **G2146** Leg pain as measured by the Visual Analog Scale (VAS) at one year (9 to 15 months) postoperatively was less than or equal to 3.0 or leg pain measured by the Visual Analog Scale (VAS) within three months preoperatively and at one year (9 to 15 months) postoperatively demonstrated an improvement of 5.0 points or greater N1 M

* **G2147** Leg pain measured by the Visual Analog Scale (VAS) at one year (9 to 15 months) postoperatively was greater than 3.0 and leg pain measured by the Visual Analog Scale (VAS) within three months preoperatively and at one year (9 to 15 months) postoperatively demonstrated less than an improvement of 5.0 points N1 M

* **G2148** Performance met: multimodal pain management was used N1 M

* **G2149** Documentation of medical reason(s) for not using multimodal pain management (e.g., allergy to multiple classes of analgesics, intubated patient, hepatic failure, patient reports no pain during PACU stay, other medical reason(s)) N1 M

* **G2150** Performance not met: multimodal pain management was not used N1 M

↩ * **G2151** Documentation stating patient has a diagnosis of a degenerative neurological condition such as ALS, MS, Parkinson's diagnosed at any time before or during the episode of care N1 M

↩ * **G2152** Risk-adjusted functional status change residual score for the neck impairment successfully calculated and the score was equal to zero (0) or greater than zero (> 0) N1 M

~~G2153 In hospice or using hospice services during the measurement period~~ ✖

~~G2154 Patient received at least one Td vaccine or one Tdap vaccine between nine years prior to the start of the measurement period and the end of the measurement period~~ ✖

~~G2155 Patient had history of at least one of the following contraindications any time during or before the measurement period: anaphylaxis due to Tdap vaccine, anaphylaxis due to Td vaccine or its components; encephalopathy due to Tdap or Td vaccination (post tetanus vaccination encephalitis, post diphtheria vaccination encephalitis or post pertussis vaccination encephalitis)~~ ✖

~~G2156 Patient did not receive at least one Td vaccine or one Tdap vaccine between nine years prior to the start of the measurement period and the end of the measurement period; or have history of at least one of the following contraindications any time during or before the measurement period: anaphylaxis due to Tdap vaccine, anaphylaxis due to Td vaccine or its components; encephalopathy due to Tdap or Td vaccination (post tetanus vaccination encephalitis, post diphtheria vaccination encephalitis or post pertussis vaccination encephalitis)~~ ✖

~~G2157 Patients received both the 13-valent pneumococcal conjugate vaccine and the 23-valent pneumococcal polysaccharide vaccine at least 12 months apart, with the first occurrence after the age of 60 before or during the measurement period~~ ✖

~~G2158 Patient had prior pneumococcal vaccine adverse reaction any time during or before the measurement period~~ ✖

~~G2159 Patient did not receive both the 13-valent pneumococcal conjugate vaccine and the 23-valent pneumococcal polysaccharide vaccine at least 12 months apart, with the first occurrence after the age of 60 before or during measurement period; or have prior pneumococcal vaccine adverse reaction any time during or before the measurement period~~ ✖

~~G2160 Patient received at least one dose of the herpes zoster live vaccine or two doses of the herpes zoster recombinant vaccine (at least 28 days apart) anytime on or after the patient's 50th birthday before or during the measurement period~~ ✖

~~G2161 Patient had prior adverse reaction caused by zoster vaccine or its components any time during or before the measurement period~~ ✖

~~G2162 Patient did not receive at least one dose of the herpes zoster live vaccine or two doses of the herpes zoster recombinant vaccine (at least 28 days apart) anytime on or after the patient's 50th birthday before or during the measurement period; or have prior adverse reaction caused by zoster vaccine or its components any time during or before the measurement period~~ ✖

~~G2163 Patient received an influenza vaccine on or between July 1 of the year prior to the measurement period and June 30 of the measurement period~~ ✖

~~G2164 Patient had a prior influenza virus vaccine adverse reaction any time before or during the measurement period~~ ✖

~~G2165 Patient did not receive an influenza vaccine on or between July 1 of the year prior to the measurement period and June 30 of the measurement period; or did not have a prior influenza virus vaccine adverse reaction any time before or during the measurement period~~ ✖

MIPS | Qp Quantity Physician | Qh Quantity Hospital | ♀ Female only
♂ Male only | A Age | DMEPOS | A2-Z3 ASC Payment Indicator | A-Y ASC Status Indicator | Coding Clinic

~~G2166 Patient refused to participate at admission and/or discharge; patient unable to complete the neck FS prom at admission or discharge due to cognitive deficit, visual deficit, motor deficit, language barrier, or low reading level, and a suitable proxy/recorder is not available; patient self-discharged early; medical reason~~ ✖

↻ ✻ **G2167** Risk-adjusted functional status change residual score for the neck impairment successfully calculated and the score was less than zero (< 0) N1 M

▶ ✻ **G2168** Services performed by a physical therapist assistant in the home health setting in the delivery of a safe and effective physical therapy maintenance program, each 15 minutes B

▶ ✻ **G2169** Services performed by an occupational therapist assistant in the home health setting in the delivery of a safe and effective occupational therapy maintenance program, each 15 minutes B

▶ ✻ **G2170** Percutaneous arteriovenous fistula creation (AVF), direct, any site, by tissue approximation using thermal resistance energy, and secondary procedures to redirect blood flow (e.g., transluminal balloon angioplasty, coil embolization) when performed, and includes all imaging and radiologic guidance, supervision and interpretation, when performed J1

▶ ✻ **G2171** Percutaneous arteriovenous fistula creation (AVF), direct, any site, using magnetic-guided arterial and venous catheters and radiofrequency energy, including flow-directing procedures (e.g., vascular coil embolization with radiologic supervision and interpretation, wen performed) and fistulogram(s), angiography, enography, and/or ultrasound, with radiologic supervision and interpretation, when performed J1

▶ ✻ **G2173** URI episodes where the patient had a competing comorbid condition during the 12 months prior to or on the episode date (e.g., tuberculosis, neutropenia, cystic fibrosis, chronic bronchitis, pulmonary edema, respiratory failure, rheumatoid lung disease) M

▶ ✻ **G2174** URI episodes when the patient had a new or refill prescription of antibiotics (table 1) in the 30 days prior to or on the episode date M

▶ ✻ **G2175** Episodes where the patient had a competing comorbid condition during the 12 months prior to or on the episode date (e.g., tuberculosis, neutropenia, cystic fibrosis, chronic bronchitis, pulmonary edema, respiratory failure, rheumatoid lung disease) M

▶ ✻ **G2176** Outpatient, ED, or observation visits that result in an inpatient admission M

▶ ✻ **G2177** Acute bronchitis/bronchiolitis episodes when the patient had a new or refill prescription of antibiotics (table 1) in the 30 days prior to or on the episode date

▶ ✻ **G2178** Clinician documented that patient was not an eligible candidate for lower extremity neurological exam measure, for example patient bilateral amputee; patient has condition that would not allow them to accurately respond to a neurological exam (dementia, Alzheimer's, etc.); patient has previously documented diabetic peripheral neuropathy with loss of protective sensation M

▶ ✻ **G2179** Clinician documented that patient had medical reason for not performing lower extremity neurological exam M

▶ ✻ **G2180** Clinician documented that patient was not an eligible candidate for evaluation of footwear as patient is bilateral lower extremity amputee M

▶ ✻ **G2181** BMI not documented due to medical reason or patient refusal of height or weight measurement M

▶ ✻ **G2182** Patient receiving first-time biologic disease modifying anti-rheumatic drug therapy M

▶ ✻ **G2183** Documentation patient unable to communicate and informant not available M

▶ ✻ **G2184** Patient does not have a caregiver M

▶ ✻ **G2185** Documentation caregiver is trained and certified in dementia care M

▶ ✻ **G2186** Patient /caregiver dyad has been referred to appropriate resources and connection to those resources is confirmed M

▶ ✻ **G2187** Patients with clinical indications for imaging of the head: Head trauma M

▶ ✻ **G2188** Patients with clinical indications for imaging of the head: New or change in headache above 50 years of age M

▶ New ↻ Revised ✔ Reinstated ~~deleted~~ Deleted ⊘ Not covered or valid by Medicare
Special coverage instructions ✻ Carrier discretion Ⓑ Bill Part B MAC Ⓓ Bill DME MAC

▶ * **G2189** Patients with clinical indications for imaging of the head: Abnormal neurologic exam M

▶ * **G2190** Patients with clinical indications for imaging of the head: Headache radiating to the neck M

▶ * **G2191** Patients with clinical indications for imaging of the head: Positional headaches M

▶ * **G2192** Patients with clinical indications for imaging of the head: Temporal headaches in patients over 55 years of age M

▶ * **G2193** Patients with clinical indications for imaging of the head: New onset headache in pre-school children or younger (<6 years of age) M

▶ * **G2194** Patients with clinical indications for imaging of the head: New onset headache in pediatric patients with disabilities for which headache is a concern as inferred from behavior M

▶ * **G2195** Patients with clinical indications for imaging of the head: Occipital headache in children M

▶ * **G2196** Patient identified as an unhealthy alcohol user when screened for unhealthy alcohol use using a systematic screening method M

▶ * **G2197** Patient screened for unhealthy alcohol use using a systematic screening method and not identified as an unhealthy alcohol user M

▶ * **G2198** Documentation of medical reason(s) for not screening for unhealthy alcohol use using a systematic screening method (e.g., limited life expectancy, other medical reasons) M

▶ * **G2199** Patient not screened for unhealthy alcohol use using a systematic screening method, reason not given M

▶ * **G2200** Patient identified as an unhealthy alcohol user received brief counseling M

▶ * **G2201** Patient identified as an unhealthy alcohol user received brief counseling M

▶ * **G2202** Patient did not receive brief counseling if identified as an unhealthy alcohol user, reason not given M

▶ * **G2203** Documentation of medical reason(s) for not providing brief counseling if identified as an unhealthy alcohol user (e.g., limited life expectancy, other medical reasons) M

▶ * **G2204** Patients between 50 and 85 years of age who received a screening colonoscopy during the performance period M

▶ * **G2205** Patients with pregnancy during adjuvant treatment course M

▶ * **G2206** Patient received adjuvant treatment course including both chemotherapy and her 2-targeted therapy M

▶ * **G2207** Reason for not administering adjuvant treatment course including both chemotherapy and her 2-targeted therapy (e.g., poor performance status (ECOG 3-4; Karnofsky = 50), cardiac contraindications, insufficient renal function, insufficient hepatic function, other active or secondary cancer diagnoses, other medical contraindications, patients who died during initial treatment course or transferred during or after initial treatment course) M

▶ * **G2208** Patient did not receive adjuvant treatment course including both chemotherapy and her 2-targeted therapy M

▶ * **G2209** Patient refused to participate M

▶ * **G2210** Risk-adjusted functional status change residual score for the neck impairment not measured because the patient did not complete the neck fs prom at initial evaluation and/or near discharge, reason not given M

▶ * **G2211** Visit complexity inherent to evaluation and management associated with medical care services that serve as the continuing focal point for all needed health care services and/or with medical care services that are part of ongoing care related to a patient's single, serious condition or a complex condition. (Add-on code, list separately in addition to office/outpatient evaluation and management visit, new or established) N

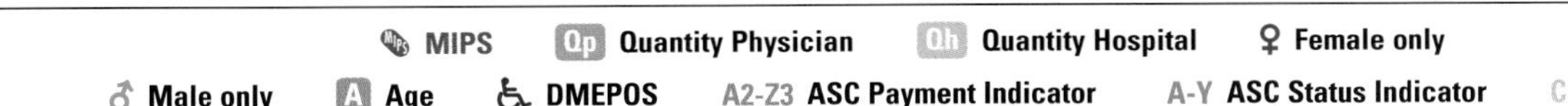

▶ ✻ **G2212** Prolonged office or other outpatient evaluation and management service(s) beyond the maximum required time of the primary procedure which has been selected using total time on the date of the primary service; each additional 15 minutes by the physician or qualified healthcare professional, with or without direct patient contact (list separately in addition to CPT codes 99205, 99215 for office or other outpatient evaluation and management services) (do not report G2212 on the same date of service as 99354, 99355, 99358, 99359, 99415, 99416). (Do not report G2212 for any time unit less than 15 minutes) N

▶ ✻ **G2213** Initiation of medication for the treatment of opioid use disorder in the emergency department setting, including assessment, referral to ongoing care, and arranging access to supportive services (list separately in addition to code for primary procedure) N

▶ ✻ **G2214** Initial or subsequent psychiatric collaborative care management, first 30 minutes in a month of behavioral health care manager activities, in consultation with a psychiatric consultant, and directed by the treating physician or other qualified health care professional S

▶ ✻ **G2215** Take-home supply of nasal naloxone (provision of the services by a Medicare-enrolled opioid treatment program); list separately in addition to code for primary procedure A

▶ ✻ **G2216** Take-home supply of injectable naloxone (provision of the services by a Medicare-enrolled opioid treatment program); list separately in addition to code for primary procedure A

▶ ✻ **G2250** Remote assessment of recorded video and/or images submitted by an established patient (e.g., store and forward), including interpretation with follow-up with the patient within 24 business hours, not originating from a related service provided within the previous 7 days nor leading to a service or procedure within the next 24 hours or soonest available appointment A

▶ ✻ **G2251** Brief communication technology-based service, e.g., virtual check-in, by a qualified health care professional who cannot report Evaluation and Management services, provided to an established patient, not originating from a related service provided within the previous 7 days nor leading to a service or procedure within the next 24 hours or soonest available appointment; 5-10 minutes of clinical discussion A

▶ ✻ **G2252** Brief communication technology-based service, e.g., virtual check-in, by a physician or other qualified health care professional who can report Evaluation and Management services, provided to an established patient, not originating from a related e/m service provided within the previous 7 days nor leading to an e/m service or procedure within the next 24 hours or soonest available appointment; 11-20 minutes of medical discussion A

Guidance

⚙ **G6001** Ultrasonic guidance for placement of radiation therapy fields Ⓑ Qp Qh B

✻ **G6002** Stereoscopic x-ray guidance for localization of target volume for the delivery of radiation therapy Ⓑ Qp Qh B

Radiation Treatment

✻ **G6003** Radiation treatment delivery, single treatment area, single port or parallel opposed ports, simple blocks or no blocks: up to 5 mev Ⓑ Qp Qh B

✻ **G6004** Radiation treatment delivery, single treatment area, single port or parallel opposed ports, simple blocks or no blocks: 6-10 mev Ⓑ Qp Qh B

✻ **G6005** Radiation treatment delivery, single treatment area, single port or parallel opposed ports, simple blocks or no blocks: 11-19 mev Ⓑ Qp Qh B

✻ **G6006** Radiation treatment delivery, single treatment area, single port or parallel opposed ports, simple blocks or no blocks: 20 mev or greater Ⓑ Qp Qh B

✻ **G6007** Radiation treatment delivery, 2 separate treatment areas, 3 or more ports on a single treatment area, use of multiple blocks: up to 5 mev Ⓑ Qp Qh B

✻ **G6008** Radiation treatment delivery, 2 separate treatment areas, 3 or more ports on a single treatment area, use of multiple blocks: 6-10 mev Ⓑ Qp Qh B

✻ **G6009** Radiation treatment delivery, 2 separate treatment areas, 3 or more ports on a single treatment area, use of multiple blocks: 11-19 mev Ⓑ Qp Qh B

✻ **G6010** Radiation treatment delivery, 2 separate treatment areas, 3 or more ports on a single treatment area, use of multiple blocks: 20 mev or greater Ⓑ Qp Qh B

✻ **G6011** Radiation treatment delivery, 3 or more separate treatment areas, custom blocking, tangential ports, wedges, rotational beam, compensators, electron beam; up to 5 mev Ⓑ Qp Qh B

✻ **G6012** Radiation treatment delivery, 3 or more separate treatment areas, custom blocking, tangential ports, wedges, rotational beam, compensators, electron beam; 6-10 mev Ⓑ Qp Qh B

✻ **G6013** Radiation treatment delivery, 3 or more separate treatment areas, custom blocking, tangential ports, wedges, rotational beam, compensators, electron beam; 11-19 mev Ⓑ Qp Qh B

✻ **G6014** Radiation treatment delivery, 3 or more separate treatment areas, custom blocking, tangential ports, wedges, rotational beam, compensators, electron beam; 20 mev or greater Ⓑ Qp Qh B

✻ **G6015** Intensity modulated treatment delivery, single or multiple fields/arcs, via narrow spatially and temporally modulated beams, binary, dynamic MLC, per treatment session Ⓑ Qp Qh B

✻ **G6016** Compensator-based beam modulation treatment delivery of inverse planned treatment using 3 or more high resolution (milled or cast) compensator, convergent beam modulated fields, per treatment session Ⓑ Qp Qh B

✻ **G6017** Intra-fraction localization and tracking of target or patient motion during delivery of radiation therapy (e.g., 3D positional tracking, gating, 3D surface tracking), each fraction of treatment Ⓑ Qp Qh B

Quality Measures

✻ **G8395** Left ventricular ejection fraction (LVEF) >=40% or documentation as normal or mildly depressed left ventricular systolic function Ⓑ M

✻ **G8396** Left ventricular ejection fraction (LVEF) not performed or documented Ⓑ M

MIPS ✻ **G8397** Dilated macular or fundus exam performed, including documentation of the presence or absence of macular edema and level of severity of retinopathy Ⓑ M

~~G8398 Dilated macular or fundus exam not performed~~ ✖

MIPS ✻ **G8399** Patient with documented results of a central dual-energy x-ray absorptiometry (DXA) ever being performed Ⓑ M

MIPS ✻ **G8400** Patient with central dual-energy x-ray absorptiometry (DXA) results not documented Ⓑ M

MIPS ✻ **G8404** Lower extremity neurological exam performed and documented Ⓑ M

MIPS ✻ **G8405** Lower extremity neurological exam not performed Ⓑ M

MIPS ✻ **G8410** Footwear evaluation performed and documented Ⓑ M

MIPS ✻ **G8415** Footwear evaluation was not performed Ⓑ M

MIPS ✻ **G8416** Clinician documented that patient was not an eligible candidate for footwear evaluation measure Ⓑ M

MIPS ✻ **G8417** BMI is documented above normal parameters and a follow-up plan is documented Ⓑ M

MIPS ✻ **G8418** BMI is documented below normal parameters and a follow-up plan is documented Ⓑ M

MIPS ✻ **G8419** BMI is documented outside normal parameters, no follow-up plan documented, no reason given Ⓑ M

MIPS ✻ **G8420** BMI is documented within normal parameters and no follow-up plan is required Ⓑ M

MIPS ✻ **G8421** BMI not documented and no reason is given Ⓑ M

MIPS ✻ **G8422** BMI not documented, documentation the patient is not eligible for BMI calculation Ⓑ M

* G8427 Eligible clinician attests to documenting in the medical record they obtained, updated, or reviewed the patient's current medications Ⓑ M
* G8428 Current list of medications not documented as obtained, updated, or reviewed by the eligible clinician, reason not given Ⓑ M
* G8430 Documentation of a medical reason(s) for not documenting, updating, or reviewing the patient's current medications list (e.g., patient is in an urgent or emergent medical situation) Ⓑ M
* G8431 Screening for depression is documented as being positive and a follow-up plan is documented Ⓑ M
* G8432 Depression screening not documented, reason not given Ⓑ M
* G8433 Screening for depression not completed, documented reason Ⓑ M

~~G8442 Pain assessment not documented as being performed, documentation the patient is not eligible for a pain assessment using a standardized tool at the time of the encounter~~ ✖

* G8450 Beta-blocker therapy prescribed Ⓑ M
* G8451 beta therapy for LVEF <40% not prescribed for reasons documented by the clinician (e.g., low blood pressure, fluid overload, asthma, patients recently treated with an intravenous positive inotropic agent, allergy, intolerance, other medical reasons, patient declined, other patient reasons or other reasons attributable to the healthcare system) Ⓑ M
* G8452 Beta-blocker therapy not prescribed Ⓑ M
* G8465 High or very high risk of recurrence of prostate cancer Ⓑ ♂ M
* G8473 Angiotensin converting enzyme (ACE) inhibitor or angiotensin receptor blocker (ARB) therapy prescribed Ⓑ M
* G8474 Angiotensin converting enzyme (ACE) inhibitor or angiotensin receptor blocker (ARB) therapy not prescribed for reasons documented by the clinician (e.g., allergy, intolerance, pregnancy, renal failure due to ACE inhibitor, diseases of the aortic or mitral valve, other medical reasons) or (e.g., patient declined, other patient reasons) or (e.g., lack of drug availability, other reasons attributable to the health care system) Ⓑ M
* G8475 Angiotensin converting enzyme (ACE) inhibitor or angiotensin receptor blocker (ARB) therapy not prescribed, reason not given Ⓑ M
* G8476 Most recent blood pressure has a systolic measurement of <140 mmHg and a diastolic measurement of <90 mmHg Ⓑ M
* G8477 Most recent blood pressure has a systolic measurement of >=140 mmHg and/or a diastolic measurement of >=90 mmHg Ⓑ M
* G8478 Blood pressure measurement not performed or documented, reason not given Ⓑ M
* G8482 Influenza immunization administered or previously received Ⓑ M
* G8483 Influenza immunization was not administered for reasons documented by clinician (e.g., patient allergy or other medical reasons, patient declined or other patient reasons, vaccine not available or other system reasons) Ⓑ M
* G8484 Influenza immunization was not administered, reason not given Ⓑ M
* G8506 Patient receiving angiotensin converting enzyme (ACE) inhibitor or angiotensin receptor blocker (ARB) therapy Ⓑ M

~~G8509 Pain assessment documented as positive using a standardized tool, follow-up plan not documented, reason not given~~ ✖

* G8510 Screening for depression is documented as negative, a follow-up plan is not required Ⓑ M
* G8511 Screening for depression documented as positive, follow up plan not documented, reason not given Ⓑ M
* G8535 Elder maltreatment screen not documented; documentation that patient is not eligible for the elder maltreatment screen at the time of the encounter Ⓑ A M
* G8536 No documentation of an elder maltreatment screen, reason not given Ⓑ A M
* G8539 Functional outcome assessment documented as positive using a standardized tool and a care plan based on identified deficiencies on the date of functional outcome assessment is documented Ⓑ M

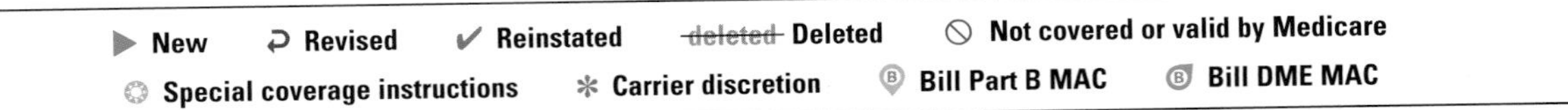
▶ New
Revised
✔ Reinstated
deleted Deleted
⊘ Not covered or valid by Medicare
Special coverage instructions
✻ Carrier discretion
Ⓑ Bill Part B MAC
Ⓑ Bill DME MAC

* **G8540** Functional outcome assessment not documented as being performed, documentation the patient is not eligible for a functional outcome assessment using a standardized tool at the time of the encounter M
* **G8541** Functional outcome assessment using a standardized tool not documented, reason not given M
* **G8542** Functional outcome assessment using a standardized tool is documented; no functional deficiencies identified, care plan not required M
* **G8543** Documentation of a positive functional outcome assessment using a standardized tool; care plan not documented, reason not given M
* **G8559** Patient referred to a physician (preferably a physician with training in disorders of the ear) for an otologic evaluation M
* **G8560** Patient has a history of active drainage from the ear within the previous 90 days M
* **G8561** Patient is not eligible for the referral for otologic evaluation for patients with a history of active drainage measure M
* **G8562** Patient does not have a history of active drainage from the ear within the previous 90 days M
* **G8563** Patient not referred to a physician (preferably a physician with training in disorders of the ear) for an otologic evaluation, reason not given M
* **G8564** Patient was referred to a physician (preferably a physician with training in disorders of the ear) for an otologic evaluation, reason not specified M
* **G8565** Verification and documentation of sudden or rapidly progressive hearing loss M
* **G8566** Patient is not eligible for the "referral for otologic evaluation for sudden or rapidly progressive hearing loss" measure M
* **G8567** Patient does not have verification and documentation of sudden or rapidly progressive hearing loss M
* **G8568** Patient was not referred to a physician (preferably a physician with training in disorders of the ear) for an otologic evaluation, reason not given M
* **G8569** Prolonged postoperative intubation (>24 hrs) required M
* **G8570** Prolonged postoperative intubation (>24 hrs) not required M

~~G8571 Development of deep sternal wound infection/mediastinitis within 30 days postoperatively~~

~~G8572 No deep sternal wound infection/mediastinitis~~

~~G8573 Stroke following isolated CABG surgery~~

~~G8574 No stroke following isolated CABG surgery~~

* **G8575** Developed postoperative renal failure or required dialysis M
* **G8576** No postoperative renal failure/dialysis not required M
* **G8577** Re-exploration required due to mediastinal bleeding with or without tamponade, graft occlusion, valve disfunction, or other cardiac reason M
* **G8578** Re-exploration not required due to mediastinal bleeding with or without tamponade, graft occlusion, valve dysfunction, or other cardiac reason M
* **G8598** Aspirin or another antiplatelet therapy used M
* **G8599** Aspirin or another antiplatelet therapy not used, reason not given M
* **G8600** IV T-PA initiated within three hours (<=180 minutes) of time last known well M
* **G8601** IV alteplase not initiated within three hours (<=180 minutes) of time last known well for reasons documented by clinician (e.g. patient enrolled in clinical trial for stroke, patient admitted for elective carotid intervention, patient received tenecteplase [tnk]) M
* **G8602** IV T-PA not initiated within three hours (<=180 minutes) of time last known well, reason not given M

~~G8627 Surgical procedure performed within 30 days following cataract surgery for major complications (e.g., retained nuclear fragments, endophthalmitis, dislocated or wrong power IOL, retinal detachment, or wound dehiscence)~~

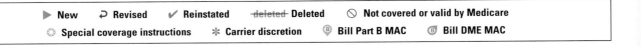

~~G8628~~ ~~Surgical procedure not performed within 30 days following cataract surgery for major complications (e.g., retained nuclear fragments, endophthalmitis, dislocated or wrong power IOL, retinal detachment, or wound dehiscence)~~ ✖

* G8633 Pharmacologic therapy (other than minerals/vitamins) for osteoporosis prescribed Ⓑ M

* G8635 Pharmacologic therapy for osteoporosis was not prescribed, reason not given Ⓑ M

* G8647 Risk-adjusted functional status change residual score for the knee impairment successfully calculated and the score was equal to zero (0) or greater than zero (>0) Ⓑ M

* G8648 Risk-adjusted functional status change residual score for the knee impairment successfully calculated and the score was less than zero (<0) Ⓑ M

⊃ * G8650 Risk-adjusted functional status change residual scores for the knee impairment not measured because the patient did not complete the LEPT prom at initial evaluation and/or near discharge, reason not given Ⓑ M

* G8651 Risk-adjusted functional status change residual score for the hip impairment successfully calculated and the score was equal to zero (0) or greater than zero (>0) Ⓑ M

* G8652 Risk-adjusted functional status change residual score for the hip impairment successfully calculated and the score was less than zero (<0) Ⓑ M

⊃ * G8654 Risk-adjusted functional status change residual scores for the hip impairment not measured because the patient did not complete LEPT prom at initial evaluation and/or follow up status survey near discharge, reason not given Ⓑ M

* G8655 Risk-adjusted functional status change residual score for the foot or ankle impairment successfully calculated and the score was equal to zero (0) or greater than zero (>0) Ⓑ M

* G8656 Risk-adjusted functional status change residual score for the foot or ankle impairment successfully calculated and the score was less than zero (<0) Ⓑ M

⊃ * G8658 Risk-adjusted functional status change residual scores for the lower leg, foot or ankle impairment not measured because the patient did not complete LEPT prom at initial evaluation and/or follow up status survey near discharge, reason not given Ⓑ M

* G8659 Risk-adjusted functional status change residual score for the low back impairment successfully calculated and the score was equal to zero (0) or greater than zero (>0) Ⓑ M

* G8660 Risk-adjusted functional status change residual score for the low back impairment successfully calculated and the score was less than zero (<0) Ⓑ M

* G8661 Risk-adjusted functional status change residual scores for the low back impairment not measured because the patient did not complete FOTO'S status survey near discharge, patient not appropriate Ⓑ M

* G8662 Risk-adjusted functional status change residual scores for the low back impairment not measured because the patient did not complete the low back FS prom at initial evaluation and/or near discharge, reason not given Ⓑ M

* G8663 Risk-adjusted functional status change residual score for the shoulder impairment successfully calculated and the score was equal to zero (0) or greater than zero (>0) Ⓑ M

* G8664 Risk-adjusted functional status change residual score for the shoulder impairment successfully calculated and the score was less than zero (<0) Ⓑ M

* G8666 Risk-adjusted functional status change residual scores for the shoulder impairment not measured because the patient did not complete the shoulder FS prom at initial evaluation and/or near discharge, reason not given Ⓑ M

* G8667 Risk-adjusted functional status change residual score for the elbow, wrist or hand impairment successfully calculated and the score was equal to zero (0) or greater than zero (>0) Ⓑ M

* G8668 Risk-adjusted functional status change residual score for the elbow, wrist or hand impairment successfully calculated and the score was less than zero (<0) Ⓑ M

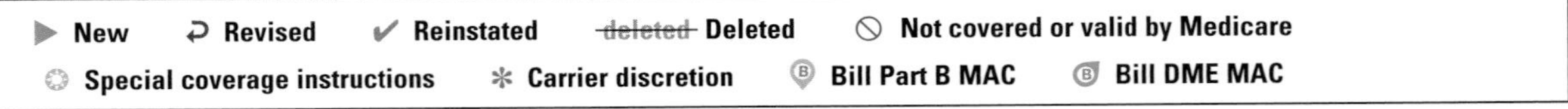
▶ New
⊃ Revised
✔ Reinstated
~~deleted~~ Deleted
⊘ Not covered or valid by Medicare
Special coverage instructions
* Carrier discretion
Ⓑ Bill Part B MAC
Ⓔ Bill DME MAC

* G8670 Risk-adjusted functional status change residual scores for the elbow, wrist or hand impairment not measured because the patient did not complete the the elbow/wrist/hand FS prom at initial evaluation near discharge, reason not given M

~~G8671 Risk-adjusted functional status change residual score for the neck, cranium, mandible, thoracic spine, ribs, or other general orthopaedic impairment successfully calculated and the score was equal to zero (0) or greater than zero (>0)~~

~~G8672 Risk-adjusted functional status change residual score for the neck, cranium, mandible, thoracic spine, ribs, or other general orthopaedic impairment successfully calculated and the score was less than zero (<0)~~

~~G8674 Risk-adjusted functional status change residual scores for the neck, cranium, mandible, thoracic spine, ribs, or other general orthopaedic impairment not measured because the patient did not complete the general orthopedic FS prom at initial evaluation near discharge, reason not given~~

* G8694 Left ventriucular ejection fraction (LVEF) <40% or documentation of moderate or severe LVSD M

* G8708 Patient not prescribed or dispensed antibiotic M

* G8709 URI episodes when the patient had competing diagnoses on or three days after the episode date (e.g., intestinal infection, pertussis, bacterial infection, Lyme disease, otitis media, acute sinusitis, acute pharyngitis, acute tonsillitis, chronic sinusitis, infection of the pharynx/larynx/tonsils/adenoids, prostatitis, cellulitis, mastoiditis, or bone infections, acute lymphadenitis, impetigo, skin staph infections, pneumonia/gonococcal infections, venereal disease [syphilis, chlamydia, inflammatory diseases (female reproductive organs)], infections of the kidney, cystitis or UTI, and acne) M

* G8710 Patient prescribed or dispensed antibiotic M

* G8711 Prescribed or dispensed antibiotic M

* G8712 Antibiotic not prescribed or dispensed M

* G8721 PT category (primary tumor), PN category (regional lymph nodes), and histologic grade were documented in pathology report M

* G8722 Documentation of medical reason(s) for not including the PT category, the PN category or the histologic grade in the pathology report (e.g., re-excision without residual tumor; non-carcinomasanal canal) M

* G8723 Specimen site is other than anatomic location of primary tumor M

* G8724 PT category, PN category and histologic grade were not documented in the pathology report, reason not given M

~~G8730 Pain assessment documented as positive using a standardized tool and a follow-up plan is documented~~

~~G8731 Pain assessment using a standardized tool is documented as negative, no follow-up plan required~~

~~G8732 No documentation of pain assessment, reason not given~~

* G8733 Elder maltreatment screen documented as positive and a follow-up plan is documented A M

* G8734 Elder maltreatment screen documented as negative, no follow-up required A M

* G8735 Elder maltreatment screen documented as positive, follow-up plan not documented, reason not given A M

* G8749 Absence of signs of melanoma (tenderness, jaundice, localized neurologic signs such as weakness, or any other sign suggesting systemic spread) or absence of symptoms of melanoma (cough, dyspnea, pain, paresthesia, or any other symptom suggesting the possibility of systemic spread of melanoma) M

* G8752 Most recent systolic blood pressure <140 mmhg M

* G8753 Most recent systolic blood pressure >=140 mmhg M

* G8754 Most recent diastolic blood pressure <90 mmhg M

* G8755 Most recent diastolic blood pressure >=90 mmhg M

* G8756 No documentation of blood pressure measurement, reason not given M

* G8783 Normal blood pressure reading documented, follow-up not required M

* G8785 Blood pressure reading not documented, reason not given M

* G8797 Specimen site other than anatomic location of esophagus M

MIPS | Qp Quantity Physician | Qh Quantity Hospital | ♀ Female only | ♂ Male only | A Age | DMEPOS | A2-Z3 ASC Payment Indicator | A-Y ASC Status Indicator | Coding Clinic

* G8798 Specimen site other than anatomic location of prostate Ⓑ M

* G8806 Performance of trans-abdominal or trans-vaginal ultrasound and pregnancy location documented Ⓑ M

* G8807 Trans-abdominal or trans-vaginal ultrasound not performed for reasons documented by clinician (e.g., patient has visited the ED multiple times within 72 hours, patient has a documented intrauterine pregnancy [IUP]) Ⓑ M

* G8808 Trans-abdominal or trans-vaginal ultrasound not performed, reason not given Ⓑ M

~~G8809 Rh-immunoglobulin (RhoGAM) ordered~~ ✖

~~G8810 Rh-immunoglobulin (RhoGAM) not ordered for reasons documented by clinician (e.g., patient had prior documented report of RhoGAM within 12 weeks, patient refusal)~~ ✖

~~G8811 Documentation RH-immunoglobulin (RhoGAM) was not ordered, reason not given~~ ✖

* G8815 Documented reason in the medical records for why the statin therapy was not prescribed (i.e., lower extremity bypass was for a patient with non-artherosclerotic disease) Ⓑ M

* G8816 Statin medication prescribed at discharge Ⓑ M

* G8817 Statin therapy not prescribed at discharge, reason not given Ⓑ M

* G8818 Patient discharge to home no later than post-operative day #7 Ⓑ M

* G8825 Patient not discharged to home by post-operative day #7 Ⓑ M

* G8826 Patient discharge to home no later than post-operative day #2 following EVAR Ⓑ M

* G8833 Patient not discharged to home by post-operative day #2 following EVAR Ⓑ M

* G8834 Patient discharged to home no later than post-operative day #2 following CEA Ⓑ M

* G8838 Patient not discharged to home by post-operative day #2 following CEA Ⓑ M

* G8839 Sleep apnea symptoms assessed, including presence or absence of snoring and daytime sleepiness Ⓑ M

* G8840 Documentation of reason(s) for not documenting an assessment of sleep symptoms (e.g., patient didn't have initial daytime sleepiness, patient visited between initial testing and initiation of therapy) Ⓑ M

* G8841 Sleep apnea symptoms not assessed, reason not given Ⓑ M

* G8842 Apnea Hypopnea Index (AHI) or Respiratory Disturbance Index (RDI) measured at the time of initial diagnosis Ⓑ M

* G8843 Documentation of reason(s) for not measuring an Apnea Hypopnea Index (AHI) or a Respiratory Disturbance Index (RDI) at the time of initial diagnosis (e.g., psychiatric disease, dementia, patient declined, financial, insurance coverage, test ordered but not yet completed) Ⓑ M

* G8844 Apnea Hypopnea Index (AHI) or Respiratory Disturbance Index (RDI) not measured at the time of initial diagnosis, reason not given Ⓑ M

* G8845 Positive airway pressure therapy prescribed Ⓑ M

* G8846 Moderate or severe obstructive sleep apnea (Apnea Hypopnea Index (AHI) or Respiratory Disturbance Index (RDI) of 15 or greater) Ⓑ M

* G8849 Documentation of reason(s) for not prescribing positive airway pressure therapy (e.g., patient unable to tolerate, alternative therapies use, patient declined, financial, insurance coverage) Ⓑ M

* G8850 Positive airway pressure therapy not prescribed, reason not given Ⓑ M

* G8851 Objective measurement of adherence to positive airway pressure therapy, documented Ⓑ M

* G8852 Positive airway pressure therapy prescribed Ⓑ M

* G8854 Documentation of reason(s) for not objectively measuring adherence to positive airway pressure therapy (e.g., patient didn't bring data from continuous positive airway pressure [CPAP], therapy was not yet initiated, not available on machine) Ⓑ M

* G8855 Objective measurement of adherence to positive airway pressure therapy not performed, reason not given Ⓑ M

* G8856 Referral to a physician for an otologic evaluation performed Ⓑ M

* ✻ **G8857** Patient is not eligible for the referral for otologic evaluation measure (e.g., patients who are already under the care of a physician for acute or chronic dizziness) M
* ✻ **G8858** Referral to a physician for an otologic evaluation not performed, reason not given M
* ✻ **G8863** Patients not assessed for risk of bone loss, reason not given M
* ✻ **G8864** Pneumococcal vaccine administered or previously received M
* ✻ **G8865** Documentation of medical reason(s) for not administering or previously receiving pneumococcal vaccine (e.g., patient allergic reaction, potential adverse drug reaction) M
* ✻ **G8866** Documentation of patient reason(s) for not administering or previously receiving pneumococcal vaccine (e.g., patient refusal) M
* ✻ **G8867** Pneumococcal vaccine not administered or previously received, reason not given M
* ✻ **G8869** Patient has documented immunity to hepatitis B and initiating anti-TNF therapy M
* ~~G8872 Excised tissue evaluated by imaging intraoperatively to confirm successful inclusion of targeted lesion~~ ✖
* ~~G8873 Patients with needle localization specimens which are not amenable to intraoperative imaging such as MRI needle wire localization, or targets which are tentatively identified on mammogram or ultrasound which do not contain a biopsy marker but which can be verified on intraoperative inspection or pathology (e.g., needle biopsy site where the biopsy marker is remote from the actual biopsy site)~~ ✖
* ~~G8874 Excised tissue not evaluated by imaging intraoperatively to confirm successful inclusion of targeted lesion~~ ✖
* ✻ **G8875** Clinician diagnosed breast cancer preoperatively by a minimally invasive biopsy method M
* ✻ **G8876** Documentation of reason(s) for not performing minimally invasive biopsy to diagnose breast cancer preoperatively (e.g., lesion too close to skin, implant, chest wall, etc., lesion could not be adequately visualized for needle biopsy, patient condition prevents needle biopsy [weight, breast thickness, etc.], duct excision without imaging abnormality, prophylactic mastectomy, reduction mammoplasty, excisional biopsy performed by another physician) M
* ✻ **G8877** Clinician did not attempt to achieve the diagnosis of breast cancer preoperatively by a minimally invasive biopsy method, reason not given M
* ✻ **G8878** Sentinel lymph node biopsy procedure performed M
* ✻ **G8880** Documentation of reason(s) sentinel lymph node biopsy not performed (e.g., reasons could include but not limited to: non-invasive cancer, incidental discovery of breast cancer on prophylactic mastectomy, incidental discovery of breast cancer on reduction mammoplasty, pre-operative biopsy proven lymph node (LN) metastases, inflammatory carcinoma, stage 3 locally advanced cancer, recurrent invasive breast cancer, clinically node positive after neoadjuvant systemic therapy, patient refusal after informed consent; patient with significant age, comorbidities, or limited life expectancy and favorable tumor; adjuvant systemic therapy unlikely to change) M
* ✻ **G8881** Stage of breast cancer is greater than T1N0M0 or T2N0M0 M
* ✻ **G8882** Sentinel lymph node biopsy procedure not performed, reason not given M
* ✻ **G8883** Biopsy results reviewed, communicated, tracked and documented M
* ✻ **G8884** Clinician documented reason that patient's biopsy results were not reviewed M
* ✻ **G8885** Biopsy results not reviewed, communicated, tracked or documented M
* ✻ **G8907** Patient documented not to have experienced any of the following events: a burn prior to discharge; a fall within the facility; wrong site/side/patient/procedure/implant event; or a hospital transfer or hospital admission upon discharge from the facility M
* ✻ **G8908** Patient documented to have received a burn prior to discharge M
* ✻ **G8909** Patient documented not to have received a burn prior to discharge M
* ✻ **G8910** Patient documented to have experienced a fall within ASC M
* ✻ **G8911** Patient documented not to have experienced a fall within ambulatory surgical center M

MIPS | Qp Quantity Physician | Qh Quantity Hospital | ♀ Female only
♂ Male only | A Age | DMEPOS | A2-Z3 ASC Payment Indicator | A-Y ASC Status Indicator | Coding Clinic

✻ **G8912** Patient documented to have experienced a wrong site, wrong side, wrong patient, wrong procedure or wrong implant event Ⓑ M

✻ **G8913** Patient documented not to have experienced a wrong site, wrong side, wrong patient, wrong procedure or wrong implant event Ⓑ M

✻ **G8914** Patient documented to have experienced a hospital transfer or hospital admission upon discharge from ASC Ⓑ M

✻ **G8915** Patient documented not to have experienced a hospital transfer or hospital admission upon discharge from ASC Ⓑ M

✻ **G8916** Patient with preoperative order for IV antibiotic surgical site infection (SSI) prophylaxis, antibiotic initiated on time Ⓑ M

✻ **G8917** Patient with preoperative order for IV antibiotic surgical site infection (SSI) prophylaxis, antibiotic not initiated on time Ⓑ M

✻ **G8918** Patient without preoperative order for IV antibiotic surgical site infection(SSI) prophylaxis Ⓑ M

MIPS ✻ **G8923** Left ventricular ejection fraction (LVEF) <40% or documentation of moderately or severely depressed left ventricular systolic function Ⓑ M

MIPS ↻ ✻ **G8924** Spirometry test results demonstrate FEV1/FVC <70%, FEV 1 <60% predicted and patient has COPD symptoms (e.g., dyspnea, cough/sputum, wheezing) Ⓑ M

MIPS ✻ **G8925** Spirometry test results demonstrate FEV1 >=60% FEV1/FVC >=70%, predicted or patient does not have COPD symptoms Ⓑ M

MIPS ✻ **G8926** Spirometry test not performed or documented, reason not given Ⓑ M

MIPS ✻ **G8934** Left ventricular ejection fraction (LVEF) <40% or documentation of moderately or severely depressed left ventricular systolic function Ⓑ M

MIPS ✻ **G8935** Clinician prescribed angiotensin converting enzyme (ACE) inhibitor or angiotensin receptor blocker (ARB) therapy Ⓑ M

~~G8936 Clinician documented that patient was not an eligible candidate for angiotensin converting enzyme (ACE) inhibitor or angiotensin receptor blocker (ARB) therapy (e.g., allergy, intolerance, pregnancy, renal failure due to ace inhibitor, diseases of the aortic or mitral valve, other medical reasons) or (e.g., patient declined, other patient reasons) or (e.g., lack of drug availability, other reasons attributable to the health care system)~~ ✖

MIPS ✻ **G8937** Clinician did not prescribe angiotensin converting enzyme (ACE) inhibitor or angiotensin receptor blocker (ARB) therapy, reason not given Ⓑ M

MIPS ↻ ✻ **G8938** BMI is documented as being outside of normal parameters, follow-up plan is not documented, documentation the patient is not eligible Ⓑ M

MIPS ✻ **G8939** Pain assessment documented as positive, follow-up plan not documented, documentation the patient is not eligible at the time of the encounter at the time of the encounter Ⓑ M

MIPS ✻ **G8941** Elder maltreatment screen documented as positive, follow-up plan not documented, documentation the patient is not eligible for follow-up plan at the time of the encounter Ⓑ A M

MIPS ✻ **G8942** Functional outcomes assessment using a standardized tool is documented within the previous 30 days and care plan, based on identified deficiencies on the date of the functional outcome assessment, is documented Ⓑ M

MIPS ✻ **G8944** AJCC melanoma cancer stage 0 through IIC melanoma Ⓑ M

MIPS ✻ **G8946** Minimally invasive biopsy method attempted but not diagnostic of breast cancer (e.g., high risk lesion of breast such as atypical ductal hyperplasia, lobular neoplasia, atypical lobular hyperplasia, lobular carcinoma in situ, atypical columnar hyperplasia, flat epithelial atypia, radial scar, complex sclerosing lesion, papillary lesion, or any lesion with spindle cells) Ⓑ M

MIPS ✻ **G8950** Pre-hypertensive or hypertensive blood pressure reading documented, and the indicated follow-up documented Ⓑ M

MIPS ✻ **G8952** Pre-hypertensive or hypertensive blood pressure reading documented, indicated follow-up not documented, reason not given Ⓑ M

MIPS ✻ **G8955** Most recent assessment of adequacy of volume management documented Ⓑ M

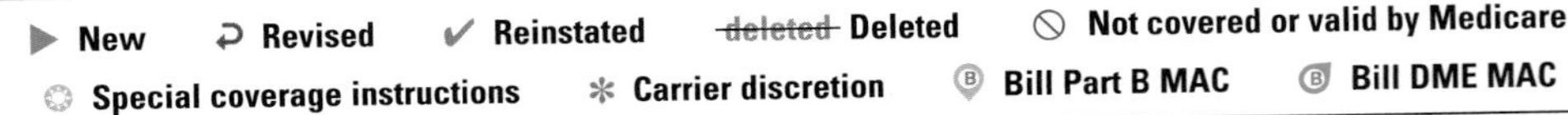
▶ New ↻ Revised ✔ Reinstated ~~deleted~~ Deleted ⃠ Not covered or valid by Medicare
Special coverage instructions ✻ Carrier discretion Ⓑ Bill Part B MAC Ⓓ Bill DME MAC

G8956 Patient receiving maintenance hemodialysis in an outpatient dialysis facility M

G8958 Assessment of adequacy of volume management not documented, reason not given M

~~G8959 Clinician treating major depressive disorder communicates to clinician treating comorbid condition~~

~~G8960 Clinician treating major depressive disorder did not communicate to clinician treating comorbid condition, reason not given~~

G8961 Cardiac stress imaging test primarily performed on low-risk surgery patient for preoperative evaluation within 30 days preceding this surgery M

G8962 Cardiac stress imaging test performed on patient for any reason including those who did not have low risk surgery or test that was performed more than 30 days preceding low risk surgery M

G8963 Cardiac stress imaging performed primarily for monitoring of asymptomatic patient who had PCI within 2 years M

G8964 Cardiac stress imaging test performed primarily for any other reason than monitoring of asymptomatic patient who had PCI within 2 years (e.g., symptomatic patient, patient greater than 2 years since PCI, initial evaluation, etc.) M

G8965 Cardiac stress imaging test primarily performed on low CHD risk patient for initial detection and risk assessment M

G8966 Cardiac stress imaging test performed on symptomatic or higher than low CHD risk patient or for any reason other than initial detection and risk assessment M

G8967 Warfarin or another FDA-approved oral anticoagulant is prescribed M

G8968 Documentation of medical reason(s) for not prescribing warfarin or another FDA-approved anticoagulant (e.g., atrial appendage device in place) M

G8969 Documentation of patient reason(s) for not prescribing warfarin or another oral anticoagulant that is FDA approved for the prevention of thromboembolism (e.g., patient choice of having atrial appendage device placed) M

G8970 No risk factors or one moderate risk factor for thromboembolism M

~~G8973 Most recent hemoglobin (Hgb) level <10 g/dl~~

~~G8974 Hemoglobin level measurement not documented, reason not given~~

~~G8975 Documentation of medical reason(s) for patient having a hemoglobin level <10 g/dl (e.g., patients who have non-renal etiologies of anemia [e.g., sickle cell anemia or other hemoglobinopathies, hypersplenism, primary bone marrow disease, anemia related to chemotherapy for diagnosis of malignancy, postoperative bleeding, active bloodstream or peritoneal infection], other medical reasons)~~

~~G8976 Most recent hemoglobin (Hgb) level >=10 g/dl~~

Coordinated Care

G9001 Coordinated care fee, initial rate B

G9002 Coordinated care fee, maintenance rate B

G9003 Coordinated care fee, risk adjusted high, initial B

G9004 Coordinated care fee, risk adjusted low, initial B

G9005 Coordinated care fee, risk adjusted maintenance B

G9006 Coordinated care fee, home monitoring B

G9007 Coordinated care fee, scheduled team conference B

G9008 Coordinated care fee, physician coordinated care oversight services B

G9009 Coordinated care fee, risk adjusted maintenance, level 3 B

G9010 Coordinated care fee, risk adjusted maintenance, level 4 B

G9011 Coordinated care fee, risk adjusted maintenance, level 5 B

G9012 Other specified case management services not elsewhere classified B

Demonstration Project

G9013 ESRD demo basic bundle Level I E1

G9014 ESRD demo expanded bundle including venous access and related services E1

G9016 Smoking cessation counseling, individual, in the absence of or in addition to any other evaluation and management service, per session (6-10 minutes) [demo project code only] E1

MIPS | Qp Quantity Physician | Qh Quantity Hospital | ♀ Female only | ♂ Male only | A Age | DMEPOS | A2-Z3 ASC Payment Indicator | A-Y ASC Status Indicator | Coding Clinic

⊘ **G9050** Oncology; primary focus of visit; work-up, evaluation, or staging at the time of cancer diagnosis or recurrence (for use in a Medicare-approved demonstration project) Ⓑ E1

⊘ **G9051** Oncology; primary focus of visit; treatment decision-making after disease is staged or restaged, discussion of treatment options, supervising/ coordinating active cancer directed therapy or managing consequences of cancer directed therapy (for use in a Medicare-approved demonstration project) Ⓑ E1

⊘ **G9052** Oncology; primary focus of visit; surveillance for disease recurrence for patient who has completed definitive cancer-directed therapy and currently lacks evidence of recurrent disease; cancer directed therapy might be considered in the future (for use in a Medicare-approved demonstration project) Ⓑ E1

⊘ **G9053** Oncology; primary focus of visit; expectant management of patient with evidence of cancer for whom no cancer directed therapy is being administered or arranged at present; cancer directed therapy might be considered in the future (for use in a Medicare-approved demonstration project) Ⓑ E1

⊘ **G9054** Oncology; primary focus of visit; supervising, coordinating or managing care of patient with terminal cancer or for whom other medical illness prevents further cancer treatment; includes symptom management, end-of-life care planning, management of palliative therapies (for use in a Medicare-approved demonstration project) Ⓑ E1

⊘ **G9055** Oncology; primary focus of visit; other, unspecified service not otherwise listed (for use in a Medicare-approved demonstration project) Ⓑ E1

⊘ **G9056** Oncology; practice guidelines; management adheres to guidelines (for use in a Medicare-approved demonstration project) Ⓑ E1

⊘ **G9057** Oncology; practice guidelines; management differs from guidelines as a result of patient enrollment in an institutional review board approved clinical trial (for use in a Medicare-approved demonstration project) Ⓑ E1

⊘ **G9058** Oncology; practice guidelines; management differs from guidelines because the treating physician disagrees with guideline recommendations (for use in a Medicare-approved demonstration project) Ⓑ E1

⊘ **G9059** Oncology; practice guidelines; management differs from guidelines because the patient, after being offered treatment consistent with guidelines, has opted for alternative treatment or management, including no treatment (for use in a Medicare-approved demonstration project) Ⓑ E1

⊘ **G9060** Oncology; practice guidelines; management differs from guidelines for reason(s) associated with patient comorbid illness or performance status not factored into guidelines (for use in a Medicare-approved demonstration project) Ⓑ E1

⊘ **G9061** Oncology; practice guidelines; patient's condition not addressed by available guidelines (for use in a Medicare-approved demonstration project) Ⓑ E1

⊘ **G9062** Oncology; practice guidelines; management differs from guidelines for other reason(s) not listed (for use in a Medicare-approved demonstration project) Ⓑ E1

✻ **G9063** Oncology; disease status; limited to non-small cell lung cancer; extent of disease initially established as stage I (prior to neo-adjuvant therapy, if any) with no evidence of disease progression, recurrence, or metastases (for use in a Medicare-approved demonstration project) Ⓑ M

✻ **G9064** Oncology; disease status; limited to non-small cell lung cancer; extent of disease initially established as stage II (prior to neo-adjuvant therapy, if any) with no evidence of disease progression, recurrence, or metastases (for use in a Medicare-approved demonstration project) Ⓑ M

✻ **G9065** Oncology; disease status; limited to non-small cell lung cancer; extent of disease initially established as stage IIIA (prior to neo-adjuvant therapy, if any) with no evidence of disease progression, recurrence, or metastases (for use in a Medicare-approved demonstration project) Ⓑ M

▶ New ⤾ Revised ✔ Reinstated ~~deleted~~ Deleted ⊘ Not covered or valid by Medicare
Special coverage instructions ✻ Carrier discretion Ⓑ Bill Part B MAC Ⓑ Bill DME MAC

✻ **G9066** Oncology; disease status; limited to non-small cell lung cancer; stage IIIB-IV at diagnosis, metastatic, locally recurrent, or progressive (for use in a Medicare-approved demonstration project) Ⓑ M

✻ **G9067** Oncology; disease status; limited to non-small cell lung cancer; extent of disease unknown, staging in progress, or not listed (for use in a Medicare-approved demonstration project) Ⓑ M

✻ **G9068** Oncology; disease status; limited to small cell and combined small cell/non-small cell; extent of disease initially established as limited with no evidence of disease progression, recurrence, or metastases (for use in a Medicare-approved demonstration project) Ⓑ M

✻ **G9069** Oncology; disease status; small cell lung cancer, limited to small cell and combined small cell/non-small cell; extensive stage at diagnosis, metastatic, locally recurrent, or progressive (for use in a Medicare-approved demonstration project) Ⓑ M

✻ **G9070** Oncology; disease status; small cell lung cancer, limited to small cell and combined small cell/non-small cell; extent of disease unknown, staging in progress, or not listed (for use in a Medicare-approved demonstration project) Ⓑ M

✻ **G9071** Oncology; disease status; invasive female breast cancer (does not include ductal carcinoma in situ); adenocarcinoma as predominant cell type; stage I or stage IIA-IIB; or T3, N1, M0; and ER and/or PR positive; with no evidence of disease progression, recurrence, or metastases (for use in a Medicare-approved demonstration project) Ⓑ ♀ M

✻ **G9072** Oncology; disease status; invasive female breast cancer (does not include ductal carcinoma in situ); adenocarcinoma as predominant cell type; stage I, or stage IIA-IIB; or T3, N1, M0; and ER and PR negative; with no evidence of disease progression, recurrence, or metastases (for use in a Medicare-approved demonstration project) Ⓑ ♀ M

✻ **G9073** Oncology; disease status; invasive female breast cancer (does not include ductal carcinoma in situ); adenocarcinoma as predominant cell type; stage IIIA-IIIB; and not T3, N1, M0; and ER and/or PR positive; with no evidence of disease progression, recurrence, or metastases (for use in a Medicare-approved demonstration project) Ⓑ ♀ M

✻ **G9074** Oncology; disease status; invasive female breast cancer (does not include ductal carcinoma in situ); adenocarcinoma as predominant cell type; stage IIIA-IIIB; and not T3, N1, M0; and ER and PR negative; with no evidence of disease progression, recurrence, or metastases (for use in a Medicare-approved demonstration project) Ⓑ ♀ M

✻ **G9075** Oncology; disease status; invasive female breast cancer (does not include ductal carcinoma in situ); adenocarcinoma as predominant cell type; M1 at diagnosis, metastatic, locally recurrent, or progressive (for use in a Medicare-approved demonstration project) Ⓑ ♀ M

✻ **G9077** Oncology; disease status; prostate cancer, limited to adenocarcinoma as predominant cell type; T1-T2c and Gleason 2-7 and PSA < or equal to 20 at diagnosis with no evidence of disease progression, recurrence, or metastases (for use in a Medicare-approved demonstration project) Ⓑ ♂ M

✻ **G9078** Oncology; disease status; prostate cancer, limited to adenocarcinoma as predominant cell type; T2 or T3a Gleason 8-10 or PSA >20 at diagnosis with no evidence of disease progression, recurrence, or metastases (for use in a Medicare-approved demonstration project) Ⓑ ♂ M

✻ **G9079** Oncology; disease status; prostate cancer, limited to adenocarcinoma as predominant cell type; T3b-T4, any N; any T, N1 at diagnosis with no evidence of disease progression, recurrence, or metastases (for use in a Medicare-approved demonstration project) Ⓑ ♂ M

✻ **G9080** Oncology; disease status; prostate cancer, limited to adenocarcinoma; after initial treatment with rising PSA or failure of PSA decline (for use in a Medicare-approved demonstration project) Ⓑ ♂ M

* **G9083** Oncology; disease status; prostate cancer, limited to adenocarcinoma; extent of disease unknown, staging in progress, or not listed (for use in a Medicare-approved demonstration project) Ⓑ ♂ M

* **G9084** Oncology; disease status; colon cancer, limited to invasive cancer, adenocarcinoma as predominant cell type; extent of disease initially established as T1-3, N0, M0 with no evidence of disease progression, recurrence, or metastases (for use in a Medicare-approved demonstration project) Ⓑ M

* **G9085** Oncology; disease status; colon cancer, limited to invasive cancer, adenocarcinoma as predominant cell type; extent of disease initially established as T4, N0, M0 with no evidence of disease progression, recurrence, or metastases (for use in a Medicare-approved demonstration project) Ⓑ M

* **G9086** Oncology; disease status; colon cancer, limited to invasive cancer, adenocarcinoma as predominant cell type; extent of disease initially established as T1-4, N1-2, M0 with no evidence of disease progression, recurrence, or metastases (for use in a Medicare-approved demonstration project) Ⓑ M

* **G9087** Oncology; disease status; colon cancer, limited to invasive cancer, adenocarcinoma as predominant cell type; M1 at diagnosis, metastatic, locally recurrent, or progressive with current clinical, radiologic, or biochemical evidence of disease (for use in a Medicare-approved demonstration project) Ⓑ M

* **G9088** Oncology; disease status; colon cancer, limited to invasive cancer, adenocarcinoma as predominant cell type; M1 at diagnosis, metastatic, locally recurrent, or progressive without current clinical, radiologic, or biochemical evidence of disease (for use in a Medicare-approved demonstration project) Ⓑ M

* **G9089** Oncology; disease status; colon cancer, limited to invasive cancer, adenocarcinoma as predominant cell type; extent of disease unknown, staging in progress, or not listed (for use in a Medicare-approved demonstration project) Ⓑ M

* **G9090** Oncology; disease status; rectal cancer, limited to invasive cancer, adenocarcinoma as predominant cell type; extent of disease initially established as T1-2, N0, M0 (prior to neo-adjuvant therapy, if any) with no evidence of disease progression, recurrence, or metastases (for use in a Medicare-approved demonstration project) Ⓑ M

* **G9091** Oncology; disease status; rectal cancer, limited to invasive cancer, adenocarcinoma as predominant cell type; extent of disease initially established as T3, N0, M0 (prior to neo-adjuvant therapy, if any) with no evidence of disease progression, recurrence, or metastases (for use in a Medicare-approved demonstration project) Ⓑ M

* **G9092** Oncology; disease status; rectal cancer, limited to invasive cancer, adenocarcinoma as predominant cell type; extent of disease initially established as T1-3, N1-2, M0 (prior to neo-adjuvant therapy, if any) with no evidence of disease progression, recurrence or metastases (for use in a Medicare-approved demonstration project) Ⓑ M

* **G9093** Oncology; disease status; rectal cancer, limited to invasive cancer, adenocarcinoma as predominant cell type; extent of disease initially established as T4, any N, M0 (prior to neo-adjuvant therapy, if any) with no evidence of disease progression, recurrence, or metastases (for use in a Medicare-approved demonstration project) Ⓑ M

* **G9094** Oncology; disease status; rectal cancer, limited to invasive cancer, adenocarcinoma as predominant cell type; M1 at diagnosis, metastatic, locally recurrent, or progressive (for use in a Medicare-approved demonstration project) Ⓑ M

* **G9095** Oncology; disease status; rectal cancer, limited to invasive cancer, adenocarcinoma as predominant cell type; extent of disease unknown, staging in progress, or not listed (for use in a Medicare-approved demonstration project) Ⓑ M

* **G9096** Oncology; disease status; esophageal cancer, limited to adenocarcinoma or squamous cell carcinoma as predominant cell type; extent of disease initially established as T1-T3, N0-N1 or NX (prior to neo-adjuvant therapy, if any) with no evidence of disease progression, recurrence, or metastases (for use in a Medicare-approved demonstration project) M

* **G9097** Oncology; disease status; esophageal cancer, limited to adenocarcinoma or squamous cell carcinoma as predominant cell type; extent of disease initially established as T4, any N, M0 (prior to neo-adjuvant therapy, if any) with no evidence of disease progression, recurrence, or metastases (for use in a Medicare-approved demonstration project) M

* **G9098** Oncology; disease status; esophageal cancer, limited to adenocarcinoma or squamous cell carcinoma as predominant cell type; M1 at diagnosis, metastatic, locally recurrent, or progressive (for use in a Medicare-approved demonstration project) M

* **G9099** Oncology; disease status; esophageal cancer, limited to adenocarcinoma or squamous cell carcinoma as predominant cell type; extent of disease unknown, staging in progress, or not listed (for use in a Medicare-approved demonstration project) M

* **G9100** Oncology; disease status; gastric cancer, limited to adenocarcinoma as predominant cell type; post R0 resection (with or without neoadjuvant therapy) with no evidence of disease recurrence, progression, or metastases (for use in a Medicare-approved demonstration project) M

* **G9101** Oncology; disease status; gastric cancer, limited to adenocarcinoma as predominant cell type; post R1 or R2 resection (with or without neoadjuvant therapy) with no evidence of disease progression, or metastases (for use in a Medicare-approved demonstration project) M

* **G9102** Oncology; disease status; gastric cancer, limited to adenocarcinoma as predominant cell type; clinical or pathologic M0, unresectable with no evidence of disease progression, or metastases (for use in a Medicare-approved demonstration project) M

* **G9103** Oncology; disease status; gastric cancer, limited to adenocarcinoma as predominant cell type; clinical or pathologic M1 at diagnosis, metastatic, locally recurrent, or progressive (for use in a Medicare-approved demonstration project) M

* **G9104** Oncology; disease status; gastric cancer, limited to adenocarcinoma as predominant cell type; extent of disease unknown, staging in progress, or not listed (for use in a Medicare-approved demonstration project) M

* **G9105** Oncology; disease status; pancreatic cancer, limited to adenocarcinoma as predominant cell type; post R0 resection without evidence of disease progression, recurrence, or metastases (for use in a Medicare-approved demonstration project) M

* **G9106** Oncology; disease status; pancreatic cancer, limited to adenocarcinoma; post R1 or R2 resection with no evidence of disease progression or metastases (for use in a Medicare-approved demonstration project) M

* **G9107** Oncology; disease status; pancreatic cancer, limited to adenocarcinoma; unresectable at diagnosis, M1 at diagnosis, metastatic, locally recurrent, or progressive (for use in a Medicare-approved demonstration project) M

* **G9108** Oncology; disease status; pancreatic cancer, limited to adenocarcinoma; extent of disease unknown, staging in progress, or not listed (for use in a Medicare-approved demonstration project) M

* **G9109** Oncology; disease status; head and neck cancer, limited to cancers of oral cavity, pharynx and larynx with squamous cell as predominant cell type; extent of disease initially established as T1-T2 and N0, M0 (prior to neo-adjuvant therapy, if any) with no evidence of disease progression, recurrence, or metastases (for use in a Medicare-approved demonstration project) M

* **G9110** Oncology; disease status; head and neck cancer, limited to cancers of oral cavity, pharynx, and larynx with squamous cell as predominant cell type; extent of disease initially established as T3-4 and/ or N1-3, M0 (prior to neo-adjuvant therapy, if any) with no evidence of disease progression, recurrence, or metastases (for use in a Medicare-approved demonstration project) M

* **G9111** Oncology; disease status; head and neck cancer, limited to cancers of oral cavity, pharynx and larynx with squamous cell as predominant cell type; M1 at diagnosis, metastatic, locally recurrent, or progressive (for use in a Medicare-approved demonstration project) Ⓑ M

* **G9112** Oncology; disease status; head and neck cancer, limited to cancers of oral cavity, pharynx and larynx with squamous cell as predominant cell type; extent of disease unknown, staging in progress, or not listed (for use in a Medicare-approved demonstration project) Ⓑ M

* **G9113** Oncology; disease status; ovarian cancer, limited to epithelial cancer; pathologic stage IA-B (grade 1) without evidence of disease progression, recurrence, or metastases (for use in a Medicare-approved demonstration project) Ⓑ ♀ M

* **G9114** Oncology; disease status; ovarian cancer, limited to epithelial cancer; pathologic stage IA-B (grade 2-3); or stage IC (all grades); or stage II; without evidence of disease progression, recurrence, or metastases (for use in a Medicare-approved demonstration project) Ⓑ ♀ M

* **G9115** Oncology; disease status; ovarian cancer, limited to epithelial cancer; pathologic stage III-IV; without evidence of progression, recurrence, or metastases (for use in a Medicare-approved demonstration project) Ⓑ ♀ M

* **G9116** Oncology; disease status; ovarian cancer, limited to epithelial cancer; evidence of disease progression, or recurrence and/or platinum resistance (for use in a Medicare-approved demonstration project) Ⓑ ♀ M

* **G9117** Oncology; disease status; ovarian cancer, limited to epithelial cancer; extent of disease unknown, staging in progress, or not listed (for use in a Medicare-approved demonstration project) Ⓑ ♀ M

* **G9123** Oncology; disease status; chronic myelogenous leukemia, limited to Philadelphia chromosome positive and/or BCR-ABL positive; chronic phase not in hematologic, cytogenetic, or molecular remission (for use in a Medicare-approved demonstration project) Ⓑ M

* **G9124** Oncology; disease status; chronic myelogenous leukemia, limited to Philadelphia chromosome positive and/or BCR-ABL positive; accelerated phase not in hematologic cytogenetic, or molecular remission (for use in a Medicare-approved demonstration project) Ⓑ M

* **G9125** Oncology; disease status; chronic myelogenous leukemia, limited to Philadelphia chromosome positive and/or BCR-ABL positive; blast phase not in hematologic, cytogenetic, or molecular remission (for use in a Medicare-approved demonstration project) Ⓑ M

* **G9126** Oncology; disease status; chronic myelogenous leukemia, limited to Philadelphia chromosome positive and/or BCR-ABL positive; in hematologic, cytogenetic, or molecular remission (for use in a Medicare-approved demonstration project) Ⓑ M

* **G9128** Oncology: disease status; limited to multiple myeloma, systemic disease; smouldering, stage I (for use in a Medicare-approved demonstration project) Ⓑ M

* **G9129** Oncology; disease status; limited to multiple myeloma, systemic disease; stage II or higher (for use in a Medicare-approved demonstration project) Ⓑ M

* **G9130** Oncology; disease status; limited to multiple myeloma, systemic disease; extent of disease unknown, staging in progress, or not listed (for use in a Medicare-approved demonstration project) Ⓑ M

* **G9131** Oncology; disease status; invasive female breast cancer (does not include ductal carcinoma in situ); adenocarcinoma as predominant cell type; extent of disease unknown, staging in progress, or not listed (for use in a Medicare-approved demonstration project) Ⓑ ♀ M

* **G9132** Oncology; disease status; prostate cancer, limited to adenocarcinoma; hormone-refractory/androgen-independent (e.g., rising PSA on anti-androgen therapy or post-orchiectomy); clinical metastases (for use in a Medicare-approved demonstration project) Ⓑ ♂ M

✻ **G9133** Oncology; disease status; prostate cancer, limited to adenocarcinoma; hormone-responsive; clinical metastases or M1 at diagnosis (for use in a Medicare-approved demonstration project) ♂ M

✻ **G9134** Oncology; disease status; non-Hodgkin's lymphoma, any cellular classification; stage I, II at diagnosis, not relapsed, not refractory (for use in a Medicare-approved demonstration project) M

✻ **G9135** Oncology; disease status; non-Hodgkin's lymphoma, any cellular classification; stage III, IV, not relapsed, not refractory (for use in a Medicare-approved demonstration project) M

✻ **G9136** Oncology; disease status; non-Hodgkin's lymphoma, transformed from original cellular diagnosis to a second cellular classification (for use in a Medicare-approved demonstration project) M

✻ **G9137** Oncology; disease status; non-Hodgkin's lymphoma, any cellular classification; relapsed/refractory (for use in a Medicare-approved demonstration project) M

✻ **G9138** Oncology; disease status; non-Hodgkin's lymphoma, any cellular classification; diagnostic evaluation, stage not determined, evaluation of possible relapse or non-response to therapy, or not listed (for use in a Medicare-approved demonstration project) M

✻ **G9139** Oncology; disease status; chronic myelogenous leukemia, limited to Philadelphia chromosome positive and/or BCR-ABL positive; extent of disease unknown, staging in progress, not listed (for use in a Medicare-approved demonstration project) M

✻ **G9140** Frontier extended stay clinic demonstration; for a patient stay in a clinic approved for the CMS demonstration project; the following measures should be present: the stay must be equal to or greater than 4 hours; weather or other conditions must prevent transfer or the case falls into a category of monitoring and observation cases that are permitted by the rules of the demonstration; there is a maximum frontier extended stay clinic (FESC) visit of 48 hours, except in the case when weather or other conditions prevent transfer; payment is made on each period up to 4 hours, after the first 4 hours A

Warfarin Responsiveness Testing

✻ **G9143** Warfarin responsiveness testing by genetic technique using any method, any number of specimen(s) Qp Qh N

This would be a once-in-a-lifetime test unless there is a reason to believe that the patient's personal genetic characteristics would change over time. (https://www.cms.gov/ContractorLearningResources/downloads/JA6715.pdf)

Laboratory Certification: General immunology, Hematology

Coding Clinic: 2010, Q2, P10

Outpatient IV Insulin Treatment

⊘ **G9147** Outpatient intravenous insulin treatment (OIVIT) either pulsatile or continuous, by any means, guided by the results of measurements for: respiratory quotient; and/or urine urea nitrogen (UUN); and/or arterial, venous or capillary glucose; and/or potassium concentration E1

On December 23, 2009, CMS issued a national non-coverage decision on the use of OIVIT. CR 6775.

Not covered on Physician Fee Schedule

Coding Clinic: 2010, Q2, P10

Quality Assurance

✻ **G9148** National Committee for Quality Assurance - level 1 medical home M

✻ **G9149** National Committee for Quality Assurance - level 2 medical home M

✻ **G9150** National Committee for Quality Assurance - level 3 medical home M

✻ **G9151** MAPCP demonstration - state provided services M

✻ **G9152** MAPCP demonstration - community health teams M

✻ **G9153** MAPCP demonstration - physician incentive pool M

Wheelchair Evaluation

* **G9156** Evaluation for wheelchair requiring face to face visit with physician Ⓑ Qp Qh M

Cardiac Monitoring

* **G9157** Transesophageal doppler measurement of cardiac output (including probe placement, image acquisition, and interpretation per course of treatment) for monitoring purposes Ⓑ Qp Qh B

Bundled Payment Care Improvement

* **G9187** Bundled payments for care improvement initiative home visit for patient assessment performed by a qualified health care professional for individuals not considered homebound including, but not limited to, assessment of safety, falls, clinical status, fluid status, medication reconciliation/management, patient compliance with orders/plan of care, performance of activities of daily living, appropriateness of care setting; (for use only in the Medicare-approved bundled payments for care improvement initiative); may not be billed for a 30-day period covered by a transitional care management code Ⓑ Qp Qh E1

Quality Measures: Miscellaneous

* **G9188** Beta-blocker therapy not prescribed, reason not given Ⓑ M
* **G9189** Beta-blocker therapy prescribed or currently being taken Ⓑ M
* **G9190** Documentation of medical reason(s) for not prescribing beta-blocker therapy (e.g., allergy, intolerance, other medical reasons) Ⓑ M
* **G9191** Documentation of patient reason(s) for not prescribing beta-blocker therapy (e.g., patient declined, other patient reasons) Ⓑ M
* **G9192** Documentation of system reason(s) for not prescribing beta-blocker therapy (e.g., other reasons attributable to the health care system) Ⓑ M
* **G9196** Documentation of medical reason(s) for not ordering a first or second generation cephalosporin for antimicrobial prophylaxis (e.g., patients enrolled in clinical trials, patients with documented infection prior to surgical procedure of interest, patients who were receiving antibiotics more than 24 hours prior to surgery [except colon surgery patients taking oral prophylactic antibiotics], patients who were receiving antibiotics within 24 hours prior to arrival [except colon surgery patients taking oral prophylactic antibiotics], other medical reason(s)) Ⓑ M
* **G9197** Documentation of order for first or second generation cephalosporin for antimicrobial prophylaxis Ⓑ M
* **G9198** Order for first or second generation cephalosporin for antimicrobial prophylaxis was not documented, reason not given Ⓑ M
* **G9212** DSM-IV-TM criteria for major depressive disorder documented at the initial evaluation Ⓑ M
* **G9213** DSM-IV-TR criteria for major depressive disorder not documented at the initial evaluation, reason not otherwise specified Ⓑ M
* **G9223** Pneumocystis jiroveci pneumonia prophylaxis prescribed within 3 months of low CD4+ cell count below 500 cells/mm3 or a CD4 percentage below 15% Ⓑ M
* **G9225** Foot exam was not performed, reason not given Ⓑ M
* **G9226** Foot examination performed (includes examination through visual inspection, sensory exam with 10-g monofilament plus testing any one of the following: vibration using 128-hz tuning fork, pinprick sensation, ankle reflexes, or vibration perception threshold, and pulse exam; report when all of the 3 components are completed) Ⓑ M
* **G9227** Functional outcome assessment documented, care plan not documented, documentation the patient is not eligible for a care plan at the time of the encounter Ⓑ M
* **G9228** Chlamydia, gonorrhea and syphilis screening results documented (report when results are present for all of the 3 screenings) Ⓑ M

▶ New ↻ Revised ✓ Reinstated ~~deleted~~ Deleted ⊘ Not covered or valid by Medicare
Special coverage instructions * Carrier discretion Ⓑ Bill Part B MAC Ⓑ Bill DME MAC

* ✻ **G9229** Chlamydia, gonorrhea, and syphilis screening results not documented (patient refusal is the only allowed exception) M
* ✻ **G9230** Chlamydia, gonorrhea, and syphilis not screened, reason not given M
* ✻ **G9231** Documentation of end stage renal disease (ESRD), dialysis, renal transplant before or during the measurement period or pregnancy during the measurement period M
* ~~G9232 Clinician treating major depressive disorder did not communicate to clinician treating comorbid condition for specified patient reason (e.g., patient is unable to communicate the diagnosis of a comorbid condition; the patient is unwilling to communicate the diagnosis of a comorbid condition; or the patient is unaware of the comorbid condition, or any other specified patient reason)~~ ✖
* ~~G9239 Documentation of reasons for patient initiating maintenance hemodialysis with a catheter as the mode of vascular access (e.g., patient has a maturing arteriovenous fistula (AVF)/arteriovenous graft (AVG), time-limited trial of hemodialysis, other medical reasons, patient declined AVF/AVG, other patient reasons, patient followed by reporting nephrologist for fewer than 90 days, other system reasons)~~ ✖
* ~~G9240 Patient whose mode of vascular access is a catheter at the time maintenance hemodialysis is initiated~~ ✖
* ~~G9241 Patient whose mode of vascular access is not a catheter at the time maintenance hemodialysis is initiated~~ ✖
* ✻ **G9242** Documentation of viral load equal to or greater than 200 copies/ml or viral load not performed M
* ✻ **G9243** Documentation of viral load less than 200 copies/ml M
* ✻ **G9246** Patient did not have at least one medical visit in each 6 month period of the 24 month measurement period, with a minimum of 60 days between medical visits M
* ✻ **G9247** Patient had at least one medical visit in each 6 month period of the 24 month measurement period, with a minimum of 60 days between medical visits M
* ✻ **G9250** Documentation of patient pain brought to a comfortable level within 48 hours from initial assessment M
* ✻ **G9251** Documentation of patient with pain not brought to a comfortable level within 48 hours from initial assessment M
* ✻ **G9254** Documentation of patient discharged to home later than post-operative day 2 following CAS M
* ✻ **G9255** Documentation of patient discharged to home no later than post operative day 2 following CAS M
* ~~G9256 Documentation of patient death following CAS~~ ✖
* ~~G9257 Documentation of patient stroke following CAS~~ ✖
* ~~G9258 Documentation of patient stroke following CEA~~ ✖
* ~~G9259 Documentation of patient survival and absence of stroke following CAS~~ ✖
* ~~G9260 Documentation of patient death following CEA~~ ✖
* ~~G9261 Documentation of patient survival and absence of stroke following CEA~~ ✖
* ~~G9262 Documentation of patient death in the hospital following endovascular AAA repair~~ ✖
* ~~G9263 Documentation of patient discharged alive following endovascular AAA repair~~ ✖
* ~~G9264 Documentation of patient receiving maintenance hemodialysis for greater than or equal to 90 days with a catheter for documented reasons (e.g., other medical reasons, patient declined arteriovenous fistula (AVF)/arteriovenous graft (AVG), other patient reasons)~~ ✖
* ~~G9265 Patient receiving maintenance hemodialysis for greater than or equal to 90 days with a catheter as the mode of vascular access~~ ✖
* ~~G9266 Patient receiving maintenance hemodialysis for greater than or equal to 90 days without a catheter as the mode of vascular access~~ ✖
* ✻ **G9267** Documentation of patient with one or more complications or mortality within 30 days M
* ✻ **G9268** Documentation of patient with one or more complications within 90 days M
* ✻ **G9269** Documentation of patient without one or more complications and without mortality within 30 days M
* ✻ **G9270** Documentation of patient without one or more complications within 90 days M
* ✻ **G9273** Blood pressure has a systolic value of <140 and a diastolic value of <90 M

MIPS | Qp Quantity Physician | Qh Quantity Hospital | ♀ Female only
♂ Male only | A Age | DMEPOS | A2-Z3 ASC Payment Indicator | A-Y ASC Status Indicator | Coding Clinic

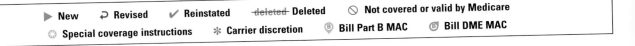

* **G9274** Blood pressure has a systolic value of = 140 and a diastolic value of = 90 or systolic value <140 and diastolic value = 90 or systolic value = 140 and diastolic value <90 Ⓑ M

* **G9275** Documentation that patient is a current non-tobacco user Ⓑ M

* **G9276** Documentation that patient is a current tobacco user Ⓑ M

* **G9277** Documentation that the patient is on daily aspirin or anti-platelet or has documentation of a valid contraindication or exception to aspirin/anti-platelet; contraindications/exceptions include anti-coagulant use, allergy to aspirin or anti-platelets, history of gastrointestinal bleed and bleeding disorder; additionally, the following exceptions documented by the physician as a reason for not taking daily aspirin or anti-platelet are acceptable (use of non-steroidal anti-inflammatory agents, documented risk for drug interaction, uncontrolled hypertension defined as >180 systolic or >110 diastolic or gastroesophageal reflux) Ⓑ M

* **G9278** Documentation that the patient is not on daily aspirin or anti-platelet regimen Ⓑ M

* **G9279** Pneumococcal screening performed and documentation of vaccination received prior to discharge Ⓑ M

* **G9280** Pneumococcal vaccination not administered prior to discharge, reason not specified Ⓑ M

* **G9281** Screening performed and documentation that vaccination not indicated/patient refusal Ⓑ M

* **G9282** Documentation of medical reason(s) for not reporting the histological type or NSCLC-NOS classification with an explanation (e.g., biopsy taken for other purposes in a patient with a history of non-small cell lung cancer or other documented medical reasons) Ⓑ M

* **G9283** Non-small-cell lung cancer biopsy and cytology specimen report documents classification into specific histologic type or classified as NSCLC-NOS with an explanation Ⓑ M

* **G9284** Non-small-cell lung cancer biopsy and cytology specimen report does not document classification into specific histologic type or classified as NSCLC-NOS with an explanation Ⓑ M

* **G9285** Specimen site other than anatomic location of lung or is not classified as non-small-cell lung cancer Ⓑ M

* **G9286** Antibiotic regimen prescribed within 10 days after onset of symptoms Ⓑ M

* **G9287** Antibiotic regimen not prescribed within 10 days after onset of symptoms Ⓑ M

* **G9288** Documentation of medical reason(s) for not reporting the histological type or NSCLC-NOS classification with an explanation (e.g., a solitary fibrous tumor in a person with a history of non-small cell carcinoma or other documented medical reasons) Ⓑ M

* **G9289** Non-small cell lung cancer biopsy and cytology specimen report documents classification into specific histologic type or classified as NSCLC-NOS with an explanation Ⓑ M

* **G9290** Non-small cell lung cancer biopsy and cytology specimen report does not document classification into specific histologic type or classified as NSCLC-NOS with an explanation Ⓑ M

* **G9291** Specimen site other than anatomic location of lung, is not classified as non-small-cell lung cancer or classified as NSCLC-NOS Ⓑ M

* **G9292** Documentation of medical reason(s) for not reporting PT category and a statement on thickness and ulceration and for PT1, mitotic rate (e.g., negative skin biopsies in a patient with a history of melanoma or other documented medical reasons) Ⓑ M

* **G9293** Pathology report does not include the PT category and a statement on thickness and ulceration and for PT1, mitotic rate Ⓑ M

* **G9294** Pathology report includes the PT category and a statement on thickness and ulceration and for PT1, mitotic rate Ⓑ M

* **G9295** Specimen site other than anatomic cutaneous location Ⓑ M

* **G9296** Patients with documented shared decision-making including discussion of conservative (non-surgical) therapy (e.g., NSAIDs, analgesics, weight loss, exercise, injections) prior to the procedure Ⓑ M

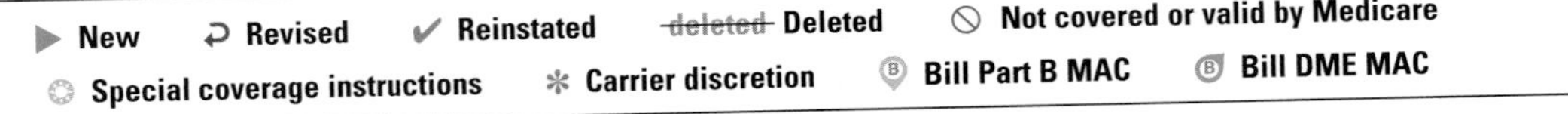
▶ New
Revised
✓ Reinstated
~~deleted~~ Deleted
Not covered or valid by Medicare
Special coverage instructions
* Carrier discretion
Ⓑ Bill Part B MAC
Ⓑ Bill DME MAC

MIPS * **G9297** Shared decision-making including discussion of conservative (non-surgical) therapy (e.g., NSAIDs, analgesics, weight loss, exercise, injections) prior to the procedure not documented, reason not given B M

MIPS * **G9298** Patients who are evaluated for venous thromboembolic and cardiovascular risk factors within 30 days prior to the procedure (e.g., history of DVT, PE, MI, arrhythmia and stroke) B M

MIPS * **G9299** Patients who are not evaluated for venous thromboembolic and cardiovascular risk factors within 30 days prior to the procedure (e.g., history of DVT, PE, MI, arrhythmia and stroke, reason not given) B M

~~G9300 Documentation of medical reason(s) for not completely infusing the prophylactic antibiotic prior to the inflation of the proximal tourniquet (e.g., a tourniquet was not used)~~ ✖

~~G9301 Patients who had the prophylactic antibiotic completely infused prior to the inflation of the proximal tourniquet~~ ✖

~~G9302 Prophylactic antibiotic not completely infused prior to the inflation of the proximal tourniquet, reason not given~~ ✖

~~G9303 Operative report does not identify the prosthetic implant specifications including the prosthetic implant manufacturer, the brand name of the prosthetic implant and the size of each prosthetic implant, reason not given~~ ✖

~~G9304 Operative report identifies the prosthetic implant specifications including the prosthetic implant manufacturer, the brand name of the prosthetic implant and the size of each prosthetic implant~~ ✖

MIPS * **G9305** Intervention for presence of leak of endoluminal contents through an anastomosis not required B M

MIPS * **G9306** Intervention for presence of leak of endoluminal contents through an anastomosis required B M

MIPS * **G9307** No return to the operating room for a surgical procedure, for complications of the principal operative procedure, within 30 days of the principal operative procedure B M

MIPS * **G9308** Unplanned return to the operating room for a surgical procedure, for complications of the principal operative procedure, within 30 days of the principal operative procedure B M

MIPS * **G9309** No unplanned hospital readmission within 30 days of principal procedure B M

MIPS * **G9310** Unplanned hospital readmission within 30 days of principal procedure B M

MIPS * **G9311** No surgical site infection B M

MIPS * **G9312** Surgical site infection B M

MIPS * **G9313** Amoxicillin, with or without clavulanate, not prescribed as first line antibiotic at the time of diagnosis for documented reason B M

MIPS * **G9314** Amoxicillin, with or without clavulanate, not prescribed as first line antibiotic at the time of diagnosis, reason not given B M

MIPS * **G9315** Documentation amoxicillin, with or without clavulanate, prescribed as a first line antibiotic at the time of diagnosis B M

MIPS * **G9316** Documentation of patient-specific risk assessment with a risk calculator based on multi-institutional clinical data, the specific risk calculator used, and communication of risk assessment from risk calculator with the patient or family B M

MIPS * **G9317** Documentation of patient-specific risk assessment with a risk calculator based on multi-institutional clinical data, the specific risk calculator used, and communication of risk assessment from risk calculator with the patient or family not completed B M

MIPS * **G9318** Imaging study named according to standardized nomenclature B M

MIPS * **G9319** Imaging study not named according to standardized nomenclature, reason not given B M

* **G9321** Count of previous CT (any type of CT) and cardiac nuclear medicine (myocardial perfusion) studies documented in the 12-month period prior to the current study B M

* **G9322** Count of previous CT and cardiac nuclear medicine (myocardial perfusion) studies not documented in the 12-month period prior to the current study, reason not given B M

~~G9326 CT studies performed not reported to a radiation dose index registry that is capable of collecting at a minimum all necessary data elements, reason not given~~ ✖

~~G9327 CT studies performed reported to a radiation dose index registry that is capable of collecting at a minimum all necessary data elements~~ ✖

~~G9329 DICOM format image data available to non-affiliated external healthcare facilities or entities on a secure, media free, reciprocally searchable basis with patient authorization for at least a 12-month period after the study not documented in final report, reason not given~~ ✖

~~G9340 Final report documented that DICOM format image data available to non-affiliated external healthcare facilities or entities on a secure, media-free, reciprocally searchable basis with patient authorization for at least a 12-month period after the study~~ ✖

✱ **G9341** Search conducted for prior patient CT studies completed at non-affiliated external healthcare facilities or entities within the past 12-months and are available through a secure, authorized, media-free, shared archive prior to an imaging study being performed Ⓑ M

✱ **G9342** Search not conducted prior to an imaging study being performed for prior patient CT studies completed at non-affiliated external healthcare facilities or entities within the past 12-months and are available through a secure, authorized, media-free, shared archive, reason not given Ⓑ M

✱ **G9344** Due to system reasons search not conducted for DICOM format images for prior patient CT imaging studies completed at non-affiliated external healthcare facilities or entities within the past 12 months that are available through a secure, authorized, media-free, shared archive (e.g., non-affiliated external healthcare facilities or entities does not have archival abilities through a shared archival system) Ⓑ M

✱ **G9345** Follow-up recommendations documented according to recommended guidelines for incidentally detected pulmonary nodules (e.g., follow-up CT imaging studies needed or that no follow-up is needed) based at a minimum on nodule size and patient risk factors Ⓑ M

✱ **G9347** Follow-up recommendations not documented according to recommended guidelines for incidentally detected pulmonary nodules, reason not given Ⓑ M

✱ **G9348** CT scan of the paranasal sinuses ordered at the time of diagnosis for documented reasons Ⓑ M

✱ **G9349** CT scan of the paranasal sinuses ordered at the time of diagnosis or received within 28 days after date of diagnosis Ⓑ M

✱ **G9350** CT scan of the paranasal sinuses not ordered at the time of diagnosis or received within 28 days after date of diagnosis Ⓑ M

✱ **G9351** More than one CT scan of the paranasal sinuses ordered or received within 90 days after diagnosis Ⓑ M

✱ **G9352** More than one CT scan of the paranasal sinuses ordered or received within 90 days after the date of diagnosis, reason not given Ⓑ M

✱ **G9353** More than one CT scan of the paranasal sinuses ordered or received within 90 days after the date of diagnosis for documented reasons (e.g., patients with complications, second CT obtained prior to surgery, other medical reasons) Ⓑ M

✱ **G9354** One CT scan or no CT scan of the paranasal sinuses ordered within 90 days after the date of diagnosis Ⓑ M

↩ ✱ **G9355** Early elective delivery by c-section, or early induction not performed (less than 39 weeks gestation) Ⓑ M

↩ ✱ **G9356** Early elective delivery by c-section, or early induction performed (less than 39 weeks gestation) Ⓑ M

✱ **G9357** Post-partum screenings, evaluations and education performed Ⓑ M

✱ **G9358** Post-partum screenings, evaluations and education not performed Ⓑ M

✱ **G9359** Documentation of negative or managed positive TB screen with further evidence that TB is not active prior to the treatment with a biologic immune response modifier Ⓑ M

✱ **G9360** No documentation of negative or managed positive TB screen Ⓑ M

✱ **G9361** Medical indication for induction [documentation of reason(s) for elective delivery (c-section) or early induction (e.g., hemorrhage and placental complications, hypertension, preeclampsia and eclampsia, rupture of membranes-premature or prolonged, maternal conditions complicating pregnancy/delivery, fetal conditions complicating pregnancy/delivery, late pregnancy, prior uterine surgery, or participation in clinical trial)] Ⓑ M

✱ **G9364** Sinusitis caused by, or presumed to be caused by, bacterial infection Ⓑ M

▶ New ↩ Revised ✔ Reinstated ~~deleted~~ Deleted ⊘ Not covered or valid by Medicare
Special coverage instructions ✱ Carrier discretion Ⓑ Bill Part B MAC Ⓔ Bill DME MAC

~~G9365 One high-risk medication ordered~~ ✖

~~G9366 One high-risk medication not ordered~~ ✖

MIPS * **G9367** At least two different high-risk medications ordered Ⓑ M

MIPS * **G9368** At least two different high-risk medications not ordered Ⓑ M

MIPS * **G9380** Patient offered assistance with end of life issues during the measurement period Ⓑ M

MIPS * **G9382** Patient not offered assistance with end of life issues during the measurement period Ⓑ M

MIPS * **G9383** Patient received screening for HCV infection within the 12 month reporting period Ⓑ M

MIPS * **G9384** Documentation of medical reason(s) for not receiving annual screening for HCV infection (e.g., decompensated cirrhosis indicating advanced disease [i.e., ascites, esophageal variceal bleeding, hepatic encephalopathy], hepatocellular carcinoma, waitlist for organ transplant, limited life expectancy, other medical reasons) Ⓑ M

MIPS * **G9385** Documentation of patient reason(s) for not receiving annual screening for HCV infection (e.g., patient declined, other patient reasons) Ⓑ M

MIPS * **G9386** Screening for HCV infection not received within the 12 month reporting period, reason not given Ⓑ M

MIPS ~~G9389 Unplanned rupture of the posterior capsule requiring vitrectomy during cataract surgery~~ ✖

~~G9390 No unplanned rupture of the posterior capsule requiring vitrectomy during cataract surgery~~ ✖

* **G9393** Patient with an initial PHQ-9 score greater than nine who achieves remission at 12 months as demonstrated by a 12 month (+/- 30 days) PHQ-9 score of less than five Ⓑ M

* **G9394** Patient who had a diagnosis of bipolar disorder or personality disorder, death, permanent nursing home resident or receiving hospice or palliative care any time during the measurement or assessment period Ⓑ M

* **G9395** Patient with an initial PHQ-9 score greater than nine who did not achieve remission at 12 months as demonstrated by a 12 month (+/- 30 days) PHQ-9 score greater than or equal to five Ⓑ M

* **G9396** Patient with an initial PHQ-9 score greater than nine who was not assessed for remission at 12 months (+/- 30 days) Ⓑ M

MIPS * **G9399** Documentation in the patient record of a discussion between the physician/clinician and the patient that includes all of the following: treatment choices appropriate to genotype, risks and benefits, evidence of effectiveness, and patient preferences toward the outcome of the treatment Ⓑ M

MIPS * **G9400** Documentation of medical or patient reason(s) for not discussing treatment options; medical reasons: patient is not a candidate for treatment due to advanced physical or mental health comorbidity (including active substance use); currently receiving antiviral treatment; successful antiviral treatment (with sustained virologic response) prior to reporting period; other documented medical reasons; patient reasons: patient unable or unwilling to participate in the discussion or other patient reasons Ⓑ M

MIPS ⊋ * **G9401** No documentation in the patient record of a discussion between the physician or other qualified health care professional and the patient that includes all of the following: treatment choices appropriate to genotype, risks and benefits, evidence of effectiveness, and patient preferences toward treatment Ⓑ M

MIPS ⊋ * **G9402** Patient received follow-up within 30 days after discharge Ⓑ M

MIPS * **G9403** Clinician documented reason patient was not able to complete 30 day follow-up from acute inpatient setting discharge (e.g., patient death prior to follow-up visit, patient non-compliant for visit follow-up) Ⓑ M

MIPS * **G9404** Patient did not receive follow-up on the date of discharge or within 30 days after discharge Ⓑ M

MIPS * **G9405** Patient received follow-up within 7 days after discharge Ⓑ M

MIPS * **G9406** Clinician documented reason patient was not able to complete 7 day follow-up from acute inpatient setting discharge (i.e patient death prior to follow-up visit, patient non-compliance for visit follow-up) Ⓑ M

MIPS * **G9407** Patient did not receive follow-up on or within 7 days after discharge Ⓑ M

* **G9408** Patients with cardiac tamponade and/or pericardiocentesis occurring within 30 days Ⓑ M

* **G9409** Patients without cardiac tamponade and/or pericardiocentesis occurring within 30 days Ⓑ M

* **G9410** Patient admitted within 180 days, status post CIED implantation, replacement, or revision with an infection requiring device removal or surgical revision Ⓑ M

* **G9411** Patient not admitted within 180 days, status post CIED implantation, replacement, or revision with an infection requiring device removal or surgical revision Ⓑ M

* **G9412** Patient admitted within 180 days, status post CIED implantation, replacement, or revision with an infection requiring device removal or surgical revision Ⓑ M

* **G9413** Patient not admitted within 180 days, status post CIED implantation, replacement, or revision with an infection requiring device removal or surgical revision Ⓑ M

* **G9414** Patient had one dose of meningococcal vaccine (serogroups a, c, w, y) on or between the patient's 11th and 13th birthdays Ⓑ M

⊋ * **G9415** Patient did not have one dose of meningococcal (serogroups a, c, w, y) vaccine on or between the patient's 11th and 13th birthdays Ⓑ M

* **G9416** Patient had one tetanus, diphtheria toxoids and acellular pertussis vaccine (Tdap) or one tetanus, diphtheria toxoids vaccine (Td) on or between the patient's 10th and 13th birthdays Ⓑ M

* **G9417** Patient did not have one tetanus, diphtheria toxoids and acellular pertussis vaccine (Tdap) on or between the patient's 10th and 13th birthdays Ⓑ M

* **G9418** Primary non-small cell lung cancer biopsy and cytology specimen report documents classification into specific histologic type or classified as NSCLC-NOS with an explanation Ⓑ M

* **G9419** Documentation of medical reason(s) for not including the histological type or NSCLC-NOS classification with an explanation (e.g., biopsy taken for other purposes in a patient with a history of primary non-small cell lung cancer or other documented medical reasons) Ⓑ M

* **G9420** Specimen site other than anatomic location of lung or is not classified as primary non-small cell lung cancer Ⓑ M

* **G9421** Primary non-small cell lung cancer biopsy and cytology specimen report does not document classification into specific histologic type or classified as NSCLC-NOS with an explanation Ⓑ M

* **G9422** Primary lung carcinoma resection report documents pT category, pN category and for non-small cell lung cancer, histologic type (squamous cell carcinoma, adenocarcinoma and not nsclc-nos) Ⓑ M

* **G9423** Documentation of medical reason for not including pT category, pN category and histologic type [for patient with appropriate exclusion criteria (e.g., metastatic disease, benign tumors, malignant tumors other than carcinomas, inadequate surgical specimens)] Ⓑ M

* **G9424** Specimen site other than anatomic location of lung, or classified as NSCLC-NOS Ⓑ M

* **G9425** Primary lung carcinoma resection report does not document pT category, pN category and for non-small cell lung cancer, histologic type (squamous cell carcinoma,adenocarcinoma) Ⓑ M

* **G9426** Improvement in median time from ED arrival to initial ED oral or parenteral pain medication administration performed for ED admitted patients Ⓑ M

* **G9427** Improvement in median time from ED arrival to initial ED oral or parenteral pain medication administration not performed for ED admitted patients Ⓑ M

* **G9428** Pathology report includes the pT category and a statement on thickness, ulceration and mitotic rate Ⓑ M

* **G9429** Documentation of medical reason(s) for not including pT category and a statement on thickness, ulceration and mitotic rate (e.g., negative skin biopsies in a patient with a history of melanoma or other documented medical reasons) Ⓑ M

* **G9430** Specimen site other than anatomic cutaneous location Ⓑ M

* **G9431** Pathology report does not include the pT category and a statement on thickness, ulceration and mitotic rate Ⓑ M

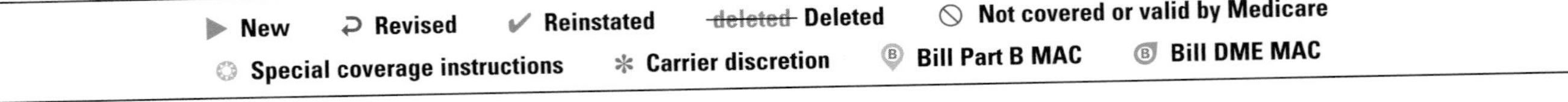

▶ New
⊋ Revised
✓ Reinstated
~~deleted~~ Deleted
⊘ Not covered or valid by Medicare
Special coverage instructions
* Carrier discretion
Ⓑ Bill Part B MAC
Ⓔ Bill DME MAC

* **G9432** Asthma well-controlled based on the ACT, C-ACT, ACQ, or ATAQ score and results documented M

* **G9434** Asthma not well-controlled based on the ACT, C-ACT, ACQ, or ATAQ score, or specified asthma control tool not used, reason not given M

* **G9448** Patients who were born in the years 1945 to 1965 M

* **G9449** History of receiving blood transfusions prior to 1992 M

* **G9450** History of injection drug use M

* **G9451** Patient received one-time screening for HCV infection M

* **G9452** Documentation of medical reason(s) for not receiving one-time screening for HCV infection (e.g., decompensated cirrhosis indicating advanced disease [i.e., ascites, esophageal variceal bleeding, hepatic encephalopathy], hepatocellular carcinoma, waitlist for organ transplant, limited life expectancy, other medical reasons) M

* **G9453** Documentation of patient reason(s) for not receiving one-time screening for HCV infection (e.g., patient declined, other patient reasons) M

* **G9454** One-time screening for HCV infection not received within 12 month reporting period and no documentation of prior screening for HCV infection, reason not given M

* **G9455** Patient underwent abdominal imaging with ultrasound, contrast enhanced CT or contrast MRI for HCC M

* **G9456** Documentation of medical or patient reason(s) for not ordering or performing screening for HCC. medical reason: comorbid medical conditions with expected survival <5 years, hepatic decompensation and not a candidate for liver transplantation, or other medical reasons; patient reasons: patient declined or other patient reasons (e.g., cost of tests, time related to accessing testing equipment) M

* **G9457** Patient did not undergo abdominal imaging and did not have a documented reason for not undergoing abdominal imaging in the submission period M

* **G9458** Patient documented as tobacco user and received tobacco cessation intervention (must include at least one of the following: advice given to quit smoking or tobacco use, counseling on the benefits of quitting smoking or tobacco use, assistance with or referral to external smoking or tobacco cessation support programs, or current enrollment in smoking or tobacco use cessation program) if identified as a tobacco user M

* **G9459** Currently a tobacco non-user M

* **G9460** Tobacco assessment or tobacco cessation intervention not performed, reason not given M

* **G9468** Patient not receiving corticosteroids greater than or equal to 10 mg/day of prednisone equivalents for 60 or greater consecutive days or a single prescription equating to 600 mg prednisone or greater for all fills M

~~G9469 Patients who have received or are receiving corticosteroids greater than or equal to 10 mg/day of prednisone equivalents for 90 or greater consecutive days or a single prescription equating to 900 mg prednisone or greater for all fills~~ ✖

* **G9470** Patients not receiving corticosteroids greater than or equal to 10 mg/day of prednisone equivalents for 60 or greater consecutive days or a single prescription equating to 600 mg prednisone or greater for all fills M

* **G9471** Within the past 2 years, central dual-energy x-ray absorptiometry (DXA) not ordered or documented M

* **G9473** Services performed by chaplain in the hospice setting, each 15 minutes B

* **G9474** Services performed by dietary counselor in the hospice setting, each 15 minutes B

* **G9475** Services performed by other counselor in the hospice setting, each 15 minutes B

* **G9476** Services performed by volunteer in the hospice setting, each 15 minutes B

* **G9477** Services performed by care coordinator in the hospice setting, each 15 minutes B

* **G9478** Services performed by other qualified therapist in the hospice setting, each 15 minutes B

* **G9479** Services performed by qualified pharmacist in the hospice setting, each 15 minutes B

MIPS | Qp Quantity Physician | Qh Quantity Hospital | ♀ Female only
♂ Male only | A Age | DMEPOS | A2-Z3 ASC Payment Indicator | A-Y ASC Status Indicator | Coding Clinic

* **G9480** Admission to Medicare Care Choice Model program (MCCM) Ⓑ Qp Qh B

* **G9481** Remote in-home visit for the evaluation and management of a new patient for use only in the Medicare-approved comprehensive care for joint replacement model, which requires these 3 key components: a problem focused history; a problem focused examination; and straightforward medical decision making, furnished in real time using interactive audio and video technology. Counseling and coordination of care with other physicians, other qualified health care professionals or agencies are provided consistent with the nature of the problem(s) and the needs of the patient or the family or both. Usually, the presenting problem(s) are self limited or minor. Typically, 10 minutes are spent with the patient or family or both via real time, audio and video intercommunications technology Ⓑ B

* **G9482** Remote in-home visit for the evaluation and management of a new patient for use only in the Medicare-approved comprehensive care for joint replacement model, which requires these 3 key components: an expanded problem focused history; an expanded problem focused examination; straightforward medical decision making, furnished in real time using interactive audio and video technology. Counseling and coordination of care with other physicians, other qualified health care professionals or agencies are provided consistent with the nature of the problem(s) and the needs of the patient or the family or both. Usually, the presenting problem(s) are of low to moderate severity. Typically, 20 minutes are spent with the patient or family or both via real time, audio and video intercommunications technology Ⓑ B

* **G9483** Remote in-home visit for the evaluation and management of a new patient for use only in the Medicare-approved comprehensive care for joint replacement model, which requires these 3 key components: a detailed history; a detailed examination; medical decision making of low complexity, furnished in real time using interactive audio and video technology. Counseling and coordination of care with other physicians, other qualified health care professionals or agencies are provided consistent with the nature of the problem(s) and the needs of the patient or the family or both. Usually, the presenting problem(s) are of moderate severity. Typically, 30 minutes are spent with the patient or family or both via real time, audio and video intercommunications technology Ⓑ B

* **G9484** Remote in-home visit for the evaluation and management of a new patient for use only in the Medicare-approved comprehensive care for joint replacement model, which requires these 3 key components: a comprehensive history; a comprehensive examination; medical decision making of moderate complexity, furnished in real time using interactive audio and video technology. Counseling and coordination of care with other physicians, other qualified health care professionals or agencies are provided consistent with the nature of the problem(s) and the needs of the patient or the family or both. Usually, the presenting problem(s) are of moderate to high severity. Typically, 45 minutes are spent with the patient or family or both via real time, audio and video intercommunications technology Ⓑ B

✻ **G9485** Remote in-home visit for the evaluation and management of a new patient for use only in the Medicare-approved comprehensive care for joint replacement model, which requires these 3 key components: a comprehensive history; a comprehensive examination; medical decision making of high complexity, furnished in real time using interactive audio and video technology. Counseling and coordination of care with other physicians, other qualified health care professionals or agencies are provided consistent with the nature of the problem(s) and the needs of the patient or the family or both. Usually, the presenting problem(s) are of moderate to high severity. Typically, 60 minutes are spent with the patient or family or both via real time, audio and video intercommunications technology Ⓑ B

✻ **G9486** Remote in-home visit for the evaluation and management of an established patient for use only in the Medicare-approved comprehensive care for joint replacement model, which requires at least 2 of the following 3 key components: a problem focused history; a problem focused examination; straightforward medical decision making, furnished in real time using interactive audio and video technology. Counseling and coordination of care with other physicians, other qualified health care professionals or agencies are provided consistent with the nature of the problem(s) and the needs of the patient or the family or both. Usually, the presenting problem(s) are self limited or minor. Typically, 10 minutes are spent with the patient or family or both via real time, audio and video intercommunications technology Ⓑ B

✻ **G9487** Remote in-home visit for the evaluation and management of an established patient for use only in the Medicare-approved comprehensive care for joint replacement model, which requires at least 2 of the following 3 key components: an expanded problem focused history; an expanded problem focused examination; medical decision making of low complexity, furnished in real time using interactive audio and video technology. Counseling and coordination of care with other physicians, other qualified health care professionals or agencies are provided consistent with the nature of the problem(s) and the needs of the patient or the family or both. Usually, the presenting problem(s) are of low to moderate severity. Typically, 15 minutes are spent with the patient or family or both via real time, audio and video intercommunications technology Ⓑ B

✻ **G9488** Remote in-home visit for the evaluation and management of an established patient for use only in the Medicare-approved comprehensive care for joint replacement model, which requires at least 2 of the following 3 key components: a detailed history; a detailed examination; medical decision making of moderate complexity, furnished in real time using interactive audio and video technology. Counseling and coordination of care with other physicians, other qualified health care professionals or agencies are provided consistent with the nature of the problem(s) and the needs of the patient or the family or both. Usually, the presenting problem(s) are of moderate to high severity. Typically, 25 minutes are spent with the patient or family or both via real time, audio and video intercommunications technology Ⓑ B

* **G9489** Remote in-home visit for the evaluation and management of an established patient for use only in the Medicare-approved comprehensive care for joint replacement model, which requires at least 2 of the following 3 key components: a comprehensive history; a comprehensive examination; medical decision making of high complexity, furnished in real time using interactive audio and video technology. Counseling and coordination of care with other physicians, other qualified health care professionals or agencies are provided consistent with the nature of the problem(s) and the needs of the patient or the family or both. Usually, the presenting problem(s) are of moderate to high severity. Typically, 40 minutes are spent with the patient or family or both via real time, audio and video intercommunications technology Ⓑ B

* **G9490** Comprehensive care for joint replacement model, home visit for patient assessment performed by clinical staff for an individual not considered homebound, including, but not necessarily limited to patient assessment of clinical status, safety/fall prevention, functional status/ambulation, medication reconciliation/management, compliance with orders/plan of care, performance of activities of daily living, and ensuring beneficiary connections to community and other services. (for use only in the Medicare-approved CJR model); may not be billed for a 30 day period covered by a transitional care management code Ⓑ B

* **G9497** Received instruction from the anesthesiologist or proxy prior to the day of surgery to abstain from smoking on the day of surgery Ⓑ M

* **G9498** Antibiotic regimen prescribed Ⓑ M

* **G9500** Radiation exposure indices, or exposure time and number of fluorographic images in final report for procedures using fluoroscopy, documented Ⓑ M

* **G9501** Radiation exposure indices, or exposure time and number of fluorographic images not documented in final report for procedure using fluoroscopy, reason not given Ⓑ M

* **G9502** Documentation of medical reason for not performing foot exam (i.e., patients who have had either a bilateral amputation above or below the knee, or both a left and right amputation above or below the knee before or during the measurement period) Ⓑ M

~~G9503 Patient taking tamsulosin hydrochloride~~ ✖

* **G9504** Documented reason for not assessing Hepatitis B virus (HBV) status (e.g. patient not initiating anti-TNF therapy, patient declined) prior to initiating anti-TNF therapy Ⓑ M

* **G9505** Antibiotic regimen prescribed within 10 days after onset of symptoms for documented medical reason Ⓑ M

* **G9506** Biologic immune response modifier prescribed Ⓑ M

* **G9507** Documentation that the patient is on a statin medication or has documentation of a valid contraindication or exception to statin medications; contraindications/exceptions that can be defined by diagnosis codes include pregnancy during the measurement period, active liver disease, rhabdomyolysis, end stage renal disease on dialysis and heart failure; provider documented contraindications/exceptions include breastfeeding during the measurement period, woman of child-bearing age not actively taking birth control, allergy to statin, drug interaction (HIV protease inhibitors, nefazodone, cyclosporine, gemfibrozil, and danazol) and intolerance (with supporting documentation of trying a statin at least once within the last 5 years or diagnosis codes for myostitis or toxic myopathy related to drugs) Ⓑ M

* **G9508** Documentation that the patient is not on a statin medication Ⓑ M

* **G9509** Adult patients 18 years of age or older with major depression or dysthymia who reached remission at 12 months as demonstrated by a 12 month (+/-60 days) PHQ-9 or PHQ-9m score of less than 5 Ⓑ M

* **G9510** Adult patients 18 years of age or older with major depression or dysthymia who did not reach remission at twelve months as demonstrated by a twelve month (+/-60 days) PHQ-9 or PHQ-9m score of less than 5. Either PHQ-9 or PHQ-9m score was not assessed or is greater than or equal to 5 Ⓑ M

* **G9511** Index event date PHQ-9 score greater than 9 documented during the 12 month denominator identification period Ⓑ M

* **G9512** Individual had a PDC of 0.8 or greater Ⓑ M

* **G9513** Individual did not have a PDC of 0.8 or greater Ⓑ M

▶ New ↻ Revised ✔ Reinstated ~~deleted~~ Deleted ⊘ Not covered or valid by Medicare
◌ Special coverage instructions * Carrier discretion Ⓑ Bill Part B MAC Ⓑ Bill DME MAC

* ✻ **G9514** Patient required a return to the operating room within 90 days of surgery Ⓑ M
* ✻ **G9515** Patient did not require a return to the operating room within 90 days of surgery Ⓑ M
* ✻ **G9516** Patient achieved an improvement in visual acuity, from their preoperative level, within 90 days of surgery Ⓑ M
* ✻ **G9517** Patient did not achieve an improvement in visual acuity, from their preoperative level, within 90 days of surgery, reason not given Ⓑ M
* ✻ **G9518** Documentation of active injection drug use Ⓑ M
* ✻ **G9519** Patient achieves final refraction (spherical equivalent) +/-1.0 diopters of their planned refraction within 90 days of surgery Ⓑ M
* ✻ **G9520** Patient does not achieve final refraction (spherical equivalent) +/-1.0 diopters of their planned refraction within 90 days of surgery Ⓑ M
* ✻ **G9521** Total number of emergency department visits and inpatient hospitalizations less than two in the past 12 months Ⓑ M
* ✻ **G9522** Total number of emergency department visits and inpatient hospitalizations equal to or greater than two in the past 12 months or patient not screened, reason not given Ⓑ M
* ~~G9523 Patient discontinued from hemodialysis or peritoneal dialysis~~ ✖
* ~~G9524 Patient was referred to hospice care~~ ✖
* ~~G9525 Documentation of patient reason(s) for not referring to hospice care (e.g., patient declined, other patient reasons)~~ ✖
* ~~G9526 Patient was not referred to hospice care, reason not given~~ ✖
* ✻ **G9529** Patient with minor blunt head trauma had an appropriate indication(s) for a head CT Ⓑ M
* ✻ **G9530** Patient presented within a minor blunt head trauma and had a head CT ordered for trauma by an emergency care provider Ⓑ M
* ✻ **G9531** Patient has documentation of ventricular shunt, brain tumor, multisystem trauma, or is currently taking an antiplatelet medication including: abciximab, anagrelide, cangrelor, cilostazol, clopidogrel, dipyridamole, eptifibatide, prasugrel, ticlopidine, ticagrelor, tirofiban, or vorapaxar Ⓑ M
* ~~G9532 Patient had a head CT for trauma ordered by someone other than an emergency care provider, or was ordered for a reason other than trauma~~ ✖
* ✻ **G9533** Patient with minor blunt head trauma did not have an appropriate indication(s) for a head CT Ⓑ M
* ⮌ ✻ **G9537** Imaging needed as part of a clinical trial; or other clinician ordered the study Ⓑ M
* ✻ **G9539** Intent for potential removal at time of placement Ⓑ M
* ✻ **G9540** Patient alive 3 months post procedure Ⓑ M
* ✻ **G9541** Filter removed within 3 months of placement Ⓑ M
* ✻ **G9542** Documented re-assessment for the appropriateness of filter removal within 3 months of placement Ⓑ M
* ✻ **G9543** Documentation of at least two attempts to reach the patient to arrange a clinical re-assessment for the appropriateness of filter removal within 3 months of placement Ⓑ M
* ✻ **G9544** Patients that do not have the filter removed, documented re-assessment for the appropriateness of filter removal, or documentation of at least two attempts to reach the patient to arrange a clinical re-assessment for the appropriateness of filter removal within 3 months of placement Ⓑ M
* ✻ **G9547** Cystic renal lesion that is simple appearing (Bosniak I or II), or adrenal lesion less than or equal to 1.0 cm or adrenal lesion greater than 1.0 cm but less than or equal to 4.0 cm classified as likely benign by unenhanced CT or washout protocol CT, or MRI with in- and opposed-phase sequences or other equivalent institutional imaging protocols Ⓑ M
* ✻ **G9548** Final reports for imaging studies stating no follow-up imaging is recommended Ⓑ M
* ✻ **G9549** Documentation of medical reason(s) that follow-up imaging is indicated (e.g., patient has lymphadenopathy, signs of metastasis or an active diagnosis or history of cancer, and other medical reason(s)) Ⓑ M
* ⮌ ✻ **G9550** Final reports for imaging studies with follow-up imaging recommended, or final reports that do not include a specific recommendation of no follow-up Ⓑ M

* G9551 Final reports for imaging studies without an incidentally found lesion noted M
* G9552 Incidental thyroid nodule <1.0 cm noted in report M
* G9553 Prior thyroid disease diagnosis M
* G9554 Final reports for CT, CTA, MRI or MRA of the chest or neck or ultrasound of the neck with follow-up imaging recommended M
* G9555 Documentation of medical reason(s) for recommending follow up imaging (e.g., patient has multiple endocrine neoplasia, patient has cervical lymphadenopathy, other medical reason(s)) M
* G9556 Final reports for CT, CTA, MRI or MRA of the chest or neck or ultrasound of the neck with follow-up imaging not recommended M
* G9557 Final reports for CT, CTA, MRI or MRA studies of the chest or neck or ultrasound of the neck without an incidentally found thyroid nodule <1.0 cm noted or no nodule found M

~~G9558 Patient treated with a beta-lactam antibiotic as definitive therapy~~ ✖

~~G9559 Documentation of medical reason(s) for not prescribing a beta-lactam antibiotic (e.g., allergy, intolerance to beta-lactam antibiotics)~~ ✖

~~G9560 Patient not treated with a beta-lactam antibiotic as definitive therapy, reason not given~~ ✖

* G9561 Patients prescribed opiates for longer than six weeks M
* G9562 Patients who had a follow-up evaluation conducted at least every three months during opioid therapy M
* G9563 Patients who did not have a follow-up evaluation conducted at least every three months during opioid therapy M

~~G9573 Adult patients 18 years of age or older with major depression or dysthymia who did not reach remission at six months as demonstrated by a six month (+/-60 days) PHQ-9 or PHQ-9m score of less than five~~ ✖

~~G9574 Adult patients 18 years of age or older with major depression or dysthymia who did not reach remission at six months as demonstrated by a six month (+/-60 days) PHQ-9 or PHQ-9m score of less than five; either PHQ-9 or PHQ-9m score was not assessed or is greater than or equal to five~~ ✖

* G9577 Patients prescribed opiates for longer than six weeks M
* G9578 Documentation of signed opioid treatment agreement at least once during opioid therapy M
* G9579 No documentation of signed an opioid treatment agreement at least once during opioid therapy M
* G9580 Door to puncture time of less than 2 hours M
* G9582 Door to puncture time of greater than 2 hours, no reason given M
* G9583 Patients prescribed opiates for longer than 6 weeks M
* G9584 Patient evaluated for risk of misuse of opiates by using a brief validated instrument (e.g., opioid risk tool, SOAPP-R) or patient interviewed at least once during opioid therapy M
* G9585 Patient not evaluated for risk of misuse of opiates by using a brief validated instrument (e.g., opioid risk tool, SOAPP-R) or patient not interviewed at least once during opioid therapy M
* G9593 Pediatric patient with minor blunt head trauma classified as low risk according to the pecarn Prediction Rules A M
* G9594 Patient presented with a minor blunt head trauma and had a head CT ordered for trauma by an emergency care provider M
* G9595 Patient has documentation of ventricular shunt, brain tumor, or coagulopathy M
* G9596 Pediatric patient had a head CT for trauma ordered by someone other than an emergency care provider, or was ordered for a reason other than trauma A M
* G9597 Pediatric patient with minor blunt head trauma not classified as low risk according to the pecarn Prediction Rules A M
* G9598 Aortic aneurysm 5.5-5.9 cm maximum diameter on centerline formatted CT or minor diameter on axial formatted CT M
* G9599 Aortic aneurysm 6.0 cm or greater maximum diameter on centerline formatted CT or minor diameter on axial formatted CT M

~~G9600 Symptomatic AAAS that required urgent/emergent (non-elective) repair~~ ✖

~~G9601 Patient discharge to home no later than post-operative day #7~~ ✖

▶ New ↻ Revised ✔ Reinstated ~~deleted~~ Deleted ⊘ Not covered or valid by Medicare
Special coverage instructions * Carrier discretion Ⓑ Bill Part B MAC Ⓔ Bill DME MAC

~~G9602 Patient not discharged to home by post-operative day #7~~ ✖

✻ **G9603** Patient survey score improved from baseline following treatment M

✻ **G9604** Patient survey results not available M

✻ **G9605** Patient survey score did not improve from baseline following treatment M

✻ **G9606** Intraoperative cystoscopy performed to evaluate for lower tract injury M

✻ **G9607** Documented medical reasons for not performing intraoperative cystoscopy (e.g., urethral pathology precluding cystoscopy, any patient who has a congenital or acquired absence of the urethra) or in the case of patient death M

✻ **G9608** Intraoperative cystoscopy not performed to evaluate for lower tract injury M

✻ **G9609** Documentation of an order for anti-platelet agents M

✻ **G9610** Documentation of medical reason(s) in the patient's record for not ordering anti-platelet agents M

✻ **G9611** Order for anti-platelet agents was not documented in the patient's record, reason not given M

✻ **G9612** Photodocumentation of two or more cecal landmarks to establish a complete examination M

✻ **G9613** Documentation of post-surgical anatomy (e.g., right hemicolectomy, ileocecal resection, etc.) M

✻ **G9614** Photodocumentation of less than two cecal landmarks (i.e., no cecal landmarks or only one cecal landmark) to establish a complete examination M

~~G9615 Preoperative assessment documented~~ ✖

~~G9616 Documentation of reason(s) for not documenting a preoperative assessment (e.g., patient with a gynecologic or other pelvic malignancy noted at the time of surgery)~~ ✖

~~G9617 Preoperative assessment not documented, reason not given~~ ✖

✻ **G9618** Documentation of screening for uterine malignancy or those that had an ultrasound and/or endometrial sampling of any kind M

✻ **G9620** Patient not screened for uterine malignancy, or those that have not had an ultrasound and/or endometrial sampling of any kind, reason not given M

✻ **G9621** Patient identified as an unhealthy alcohol user when screened for unhealthy alcohol use using a systematic screening method and received brief counseling M

✻ **G9622** Patient not identified as an unhealthy alcohol user when screened for unhealthy alcohol use using a systematic screening method M

✻ **G9623** Documentation of medical reason(s) for not screening for unhealthy alcohol use (e.g., limited life expectancy, other medical reasons) M

✻ **G9624** Patient not screened for unhealthy alcohol use using a systematic screening method or patient did not receive brief counseling if identified as an unhealthy alcohol user, reason not given M

✻ **G9625** Patient sustained bladder injury at the time of surgery or discovered subsequently up to 30 days post-surgery M

✻ **G9626** Documented medical reason for reporting bladder injury (e.g., gynecologic or other pelvic malignancy documented, concurrent surgery involving bladder pathology, injury that occurs during urinary incontinence procedure, patient death from non-medical causes not related to surgery, patient died during procedure without evidence of bladder injury) M

✻ **G9627** Patient did not sustain bladder injury at the time of surgery nor discovered subsequently up to 30 days post-surgery M

✻ **G9628** Patient sustained bowel injury at the time of surgery or discovered subsequently up to 30 days post-surgery M

✻ **G9629** Documented medical reasons for not reporting bowel injury (e.g., gynecologic or other pelvic malignancy documented, planned (e.g., not due to an unexpected bowel injury) resection and/or re-anastomosis of bowel, or patient death from non-medical causes not related to surgery, patient died during procedure without evidence of bowel injury) M

✻ **G9630** Patient did not sustain a bowel injury at the time of surgery nor discovered subsequently up to 30 days post-surgery M

* G9631 Patient sustained ureter injury at the time of surgery or discovered subsequently up to 30 days post-surgery B M
* G9632 Documented medical reasons for not reporting ureter injury (e.g., gynecologic or other pelvic malignancy documented, concurrent surgery involving bladder pathology, injury that occurs during a urinary incontinence procedure, patient death from non-medical causes not related to surgery, patient died during procedure without evidence of ureter injury) B M
* G9633 Patient did not sustain ureter injury at the time of surgery nor discovered subsequently up to 30 days post-surgery B M
* G9634 Health-related quality of life assessed with tool during at least two visits and quality of life score remained the same or improved B M
* G9635 Health-related quality of life not assessed with tool for documented reason(s) (e.g., patient has a cognitive or neuropsychiatric impairment that impairs his/her ability to complete the HRQOL survey, patient has the inability to read and/or write in order to complete the HRQOL questionnaire) B M
* G9636 Health-related quality of life not assessed with tool during at least two visits or quality of life score declined B M
* G9637 At least two orders for the same high-risk medications B M
* G9638 At least two orders for the same high-risk medications not ordered B M
* G9639 Major amputation or open surgical bypass not required within 48 hours of the index endovascular lower extremity revascularization procedure B M
* G9640 Documentation of planned hybrid or staged procedure B M
* G9641 Major amputation or open surgical bypass required within 48 hours of the index endovascular lower extremity revascularization procedure B M
* G9642 Current smoker (e.g., cigarette, cigar, pipe, e-cigarette or marijuana) B M
* G9643 Elective surgery B M
* G9644 Patients who abstained from smoking prior to anesthesia on the day of surgery or procedure B M
* G9645 Patients who did not abstain from smoking prior to anesthesia on the day of surgery or procedure B M
* G9646 Patients with 90 day MRS score of 0 to 2 B M
* G9647 Patients in whom MRS score could not be obtained at 90 day follow-up B M
* G9648 Patients with 90 day MRS score greater than 2 B M
* G9649 Psoriasis assessment tool documented meeting any one of the specified benchmarks (e.g., PGA; 5-point or 6-point scale), body surface area (BSA), psoriasis area and severity index (PASI) and/or dermatology life quality index) (DLQI)) B M
* G9651 Psoriasis assessment tool documented not meeting any one of the specified benchmarks (e.g., (pga; 5-point or 6-point scale), body surface area (bsa), psoriasis area and severity index (pasi) and/or dermatology life quality index) (dlqi)) or psoriasis assessment tool not documented B M
* G9654 Monitored anesthesia care (mac) B M
* G9655 A transfer of care protocol or handoff tool/checklist that includes the required key handoff elements is used B M
* G9656 Patient transferred directly from anesthetizing location to PACU or other non-ICU location B M
* G9658 A transfer of care protocol or handoff tool/checklist that includes the required key handoff elements is not used B M
* G9659 Patients greater than 86 years of age who underwent a screening colonoscopy and did not have a history of colorectal cancer or valid medical reason for the colonoscopy, including: iron deficiency anemia, lower gastrointestinal bleeding, Crohn disease (i.e., regional enteritis), familial adenomatous polyposis, Lynch syndrome (i.e., hereditary non-polyposis colorectal cancer), inflammatory bowel disease, ulcerative colitis, abnormal finding of gastrointestinal tract, or changes in bowel habits B M

▶ New ⟲ Revised ✔ Reinstated ~~deleted~~ Deleted ⊘ Not covered or valid by Medicare
Special coverage instructions * Carrier discretion B Bill Part B MAC B Bill DME MAC

G9660 Documentation of medical reason(s) for a colonoscopy performed on a patient greater than or equal to 86 years of age (e.g., iron deficiency anemia, lower gastrointestinal bleeding, Crohn disease (i.e., regional enteritis), familial history of adenomatous polyposis, Lynch syndrome (i.e., hereditary non-polyposis colorectal cancer), inflammatory bowel disease, ulcerative colitis, abnormal finding of gastrointestinal tract, or changes in bowel habits) M

G9661 Patients greater than or equal to 86 years of age who received a colonoscopy for an assessment of signs/ symptoms of GI tract illness, and/or because the patient meets high risk criteria, and/or to follow-up on previously diagnosed advance lesions M

G9662 Previously diagnosed or have an active diagnosis of clinical ascvd M

G9663 Any fasting or direct ldl-c laboratory test result >=190 mg/dL M

G9664 Patients who are currently statin therapy users or received an order (prescription) for statin therapy M

G9665 Patients who are not currently statin therapy users or did not receive an order (prescription) for statin therapy M

G9666 Patient's highest fasting or direct ldl-c laboratory test result of in the measurement period or two years prior to the beginning of the measurement period is 70-189 mg/dl M

G9674 Patients with clinical ascvd diagnosis M

G9675 Patients who have ever had a fasting or direct laboratory result of ldl-c = 190 mg/dl M

G9676 Patients aged 40 to 75 years at the beginning of the measurement period with type 1 or type 2 diabetes and with an ldl-c result of 70-189 mg/dl recorded as the highest fasting or direct laboratory test result in the measurement year or during the two years prior to the beginning of the measurement period M

G9678 Oncology care model (OCM) monthly enhanced oncology services (MEOS) payment for OCM enhanced services. G9678 payments may only be made to OCM practitioners for ocm beneficiaries for the furnishment of enhanced services as defined in the OCM participation agreement Qp Qh B

G9679 This code is for onsite acute care treatment of a nursing facility resident with pneumonia; may only be billed once per day per beneficiary B

G9680 This code is for onsite acute care treatment of a nursing facility resident with CHF; may only be billed once per day per beneficiary B

G9681 This code is for onsite acute care treatment of a resident with COPD or asthma; may only be billed once per day per beneficiary B

G9682 This code is for the onsite acute care treatment a nursing facility resident with a skin infection; may only be billed once per day per beneficiary B

G9683 Facility service(s) for the onsite acute care treatment of a nursing facility resident with fluid or electrolyte disorder. (May only be billed once per day per beneficiary). This service is for a demonstration project. B

G9684 This code is for the onsite acute care treatment of a nursing facility resident for a UTI; may only be billed once per day per beneficiary B

G9685 Physician service or other qualified health care professional for the evaluation and management of a beneficiary's acute change in condition in a nursing facility. This service is for a demonstration project. M

G9687 Hospice services provided to patient any time during the measurement period M

G9688 Patients using hospice services any time during the measurement period M

G9689 Patient admitted for performance of elective carotid intervention M

G9690 Patient receiving hospice services any time during the measurement period M

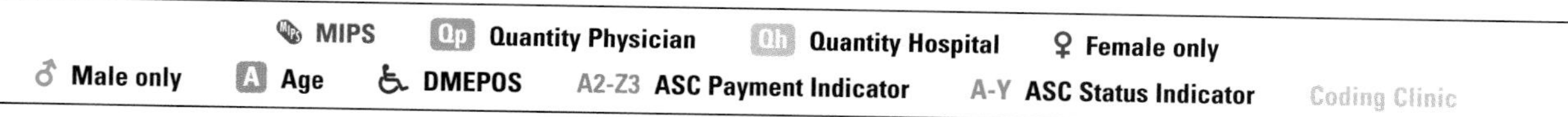

MIPS
Qp Quantity Physician
Qh Quantity Hospital
Female only
Male only
A Age
DMEPOS
A2-Z3 ASC Payment Indicator
A-Y ASC Status Indicator
Coding Clinic

* G9691 Patient had hospice services any time during the measurement period M

* G9692 Hospice services received by patient any time during the measurement period M

* G9693 Patient use of hospice services any time during the measurement period M

* G9694 Hospice services utilized by patient any time during the measurement period M

* G9695 Long-acting inhaled bronchodilator prescribed M

* G9696 Documentation of medical reason(s) for not prescribing a long-acting inhaled bronchodilator M

* G9697 Documentation of patient reason(s) for not prescribing a long-acting inhaled bronchodilator M

* G9698 Documentation of system reason(s) for not prescribing a long-acting inhaled bronchodilator M

* G9699 Long-acting inhaled bronchodilator not prescribed, reason not otherwise specified M

* G9700 Patients who use hospice services any time during the measurement period M

~~G9701 Children who are taking antibiotics in the 30 days prior to the date of the encounter during which the diagnosis was established~~

* G9702 Patients who use hospice services any time during the measurement period M

* G9703 Episodes where the patient is taking antibiotics (table 1) in the 30 days prior to the episode date M

* G9704 AJCC breast cancer stage I: T1 mic or T1a documented M

* G9705 AJCC breast cancer stage I: T1b (tumor >0.5 cm but <=1 cm in greatest dimension) documented M

* G9706 Low (or very low) risk of recurrence, prostate cancer M

* G9707 Patient received hospice services any time during the measurement period M

* G9708 Women who had a bilateral mastectomy or who have a history of a bilateral mastectomy or for whom there is evidence of a right and a left unilateral mastectomy M

* G9709 Hospice services used by patient any time during the measurement period M

* G9710 Patient was provided hospice services any time during the measurement period M

* G9711 Patients with a diagnosis or past history of total colectomy or colorectal cancer M

* G9712 Documentation of medical reason(s) for prescribing or dispensing antibiotic (e.g., intestinal infection, pertussis, bacterial infection, Lyme disease, otitis media, acute sinusitis, acute pharyngitis, acute tonsillitis, chronic sinusitis, infection of the pharynx/larynx/tonsils/adenoids, prostatitis, cellulitis/ mastoiditis/bone infections, acute lymphadenitis, impetigo, skin staph infections, pneumonia, gonococcal infections/venereal disease/syphilis, chlamydia, inflammatory diseases, female reproductive organs), infections of the kidney, cystitis/UTI, acne, HIV disease/asymptomatic HIV, cystic fibrosis, disorders of the immune system, malignancy neoplasms, chronic bronchitis, emphysema, bronchiectasis, extrinsic allergic alveolitis, chronic airway obstruction, chronic obstructive asthma, pneumoconiosis and other lung disease due to external agents, other diseases of the respiratory system, and tuberculosis M

* G9713 Patients who use hospice services any time during the measurement period M

* G9714 Patient is using hospice services any time during the measurement period M

* G9715 Patients who use hospice services any time during the measurement period M

* G9716 BMI is documented as being outside of normal parameters, follow-up plan is not completed for documented reason M

* G9717 Documentation stating the patient has had a diagnosis of depression or has had a diagnosis bipolar disorder M

* G9718 Hospice services for patient provided any time during the measurement period M

* G9719 Patient is not ambulatory, bed ridden, immobile, confined to chair, wheelchair bound, dependent on helper pushing wheelchair, independent in wheelchair or minimal help in wheelchair M

* G9720 Hospice services for patient occurred any time during the measurement period M

New | Revised | Reinstated | ~~deleted~~ Deleted | Not covered or valid by Medicare
Special coverage instructions | * Carrier discretion | Bill Part B MAC | Bill DME MAC

✱ **G9721** Patient not ambulatory, bed ridden, immobile, confined to chair, wheelchair bound, dependent on helper pushing wheelchair, independent in wheelchair or minimal help in wheelchair M

✱ **G9722** Documented history of renal failure or baseline serum creatinine > = 4.0 mg/dl; renal transplant recipients are not considered to have preoperative renal failure, unless, since transplantation the CR has been or is 4.0 or higher M

✱ **G9723** Hospice services for patient received any time during the measurement period M

✱ **G9724** Patients who had documentation of use of anticoagulant medications overlapping the measurement year M

✱ **G9725** Patients who use hospice services any time during the measurement period M

✱ **G9726** Patient refused to participate M

✱ **G9727** Patient unable to complete the LEPF prom at initial evaluation and/or discharge due to blindness, illiteracy, severe mental incapacity or language incompatibility and an adequate proxy is not available M

✱ **G9728** Patient refused to participate M

✱ **G9729** Patient unable to complete the LEPF prom at initial evaluation and/or discharge due to blindness, illiteracy, severe mental incapacity or language incompatibility and an adequate proxy is not available M

✱ **G9730** Patient refused to participate M

✱ **G9731** Patient unable to complete the LEPF prom at initial evaluation and/or discharge due to blindness, illiteracy, severe mental incapacity or language incompatibility and an adequate proxy is not available M

✱ **G9732** Patient refused to participate M

✱ **G9733** Patient unable to complete the low back FS prom at initial evaluation and/or discharge due to blindness, illiteracy, severe mental incapacity or language incompatibility and an adequate proxy is not available M

✱ **G9734** Patient refused to participate M

✱ **G9735** Patient unable to complete the shoulder FS prom at initial evaluation and/or discharge due to blindness, illiteracy, severe mental incapacity or language incompatibility and an adequate proxy is not available M

✱ **G9736** Patient refused to participate M

✱ **G9737** Patient unable to complete the elbow/wrist/hand FS prom at initial evaluation and/or discharge due to blindness, illiteracy, severe mental incapacity or language incompatibility and an adequate proxy is not available M

~~G9738 Patient refused to participate~~ ✖

~~G9739 Patient unable to complete the general orthopedic FS prom at initial evaluation and/or discharge due to blindness, illiteracy, severe mental incapacity or language incompatibility and an adequate proxy is not available~~ ✖

✱ **G9740** Hospice services given to patient any time during the measurement period M

✱ **G9741** Patients who use hospice services any time during the measurement period M

✱ **G9744** Patient not eligible due to active diagnosis of hypertension M

✱ **G9745** Documented reason for not screening or recommending a follow-up for high blood pressure M

✱ **G9746** Patient has mitral stenosis or prosthetic heart valves or patient has transient or reversible cause of AF (e.g., pneumonia, hyperthyroidism, pregnancy, cardiac surgery) M

~~G9747 Patient is undergoing palliative dialysis with a catheter~~ ✖

~~G9748 Patient approved by a qualified transplant program and scheduled to receive a living donor kidney transplant~~ ✖

~~G9749 Patient is undergoing palliative dialysis with a catheter~~ ✖

~~G9750 Patient approved by a qualified transplant program and scheduled to receive a living donor kidney transplant~~ ✖

✱ **G9751** Patient died at any time during the 24-month measurement period M

✱ **G9752** Emergency surgery M

✱ **G9753** Documentation of medical reason for not conducting a search for DICOM format images for prior patient CT imaging studies completed at non-affiliated external healthcare facilities or entities within the past 12 months that are available through a secure, authorized, media-free, shared archive (e.g., trauma, acute myocardial infarction, stroke, aortic aneurysm where time is of the essence) M

* G9754 A finding of an incidental pulmonary nodule M

* G9755 Documentation of medical reason(s) for not including a recommended interval and modality for follow-up or for no follow-up, and source of recommendations (e.g., patients with unexplained fever, immunocompromised patients who are at risk for infection) M

* G9756 Surgical procedures that included the use of silicone oil M

* G9757 Surgical procedures that included the use of silicone oil M

* G9758 Patient in hospice at any time during the measurement period M

~~G9759 History of preoperative posterior capsule rupture~~ ✖

* G9760 Patients who use hospice services any time during the measurement period M

* G9761 Patients who use hospice services any time during the measurement period M

* G9762 Patient had at least two HPV vaccines (with at least 146 days between the two) or three HPV vaccines on or between the patient's 9th and 13th birthdays M

* G9763 Patient did not have at least two HPV vaccines (with at least 146 days between the two) or three HPV vaccines on or between the patient's 9th and 13th birthdays M

* G9764 Patient has been treated with systemic medication for psoriasis vulgaris M

* G9765 Documentation that the patient declined change in medication or alternative therapies were unavailable, has documented contraindications, or has not been treated with systemic for at least six consecutive months (e.g., experienced adverse effects or lack of efficacy with all other therapy options) in order to achieve better disease control as measured by PGA, BSA, PASI, or DLQI M

* G9766 Patients who are transferred from one institution to another with a known diagnosis of CVA for endovascular stroke treatment M

* G9767 Hospitalized patients with newly diagnosed CVA considered for endovascular stroke treatment M

* G9768 Patients who utilize hospice services any time during the measurement period M

* G9769 Patient had a bone mineral density test in the past two years or received osteoporosis medication or therapy in the past 12 months M

* G9770 Peripheral nerve block (PNB) M

* G9771 At least 1 body temperature measurement equal to or greater than 35.5 degrees Celsius (or 95.9 degrees Fahrenheit) achieved within the 30 minutes immediately before or the 15 minutes immediately after anesthesia end time M

* G9772 Documentation of medical reason(s) for not achieving at least 1 body temperature measurement equal to or greater than 35.5 degrees Celsius (or 95.9 degrees Fahrenheit) within the 30 minutes immediately before or the 15 minutes immediately after anesthesia end time (e.g., emergency cases, intentional hypothermia, etc.) M

* G9773 At least 1 body temperature measurement equal to or greater than 35.5 degrees Celsius (or 95.9 degrees Fahrenheit) not achieved within the 30 minutes immediately before or the 15 minutes immediately after anesthesia end time, reason not given M

* G9774 Patients who have had a hysterectomy M

* G9775 Patient received at least 2 prophylactic pharmacologic anti-emetic agents of different classes preoperatively and/or intraoperatively M

* G9776 Documentation of medical reason for not receiving at least 2 prophylactic pharmacologic anti-emetic agents of different classes preoperatively and/or intraoperatively (e.g., intolerance or other medical reason) M

* G9777 Patient did not receive at least 2 prophylactic pharmacologic anti-emetic agents of different classes preoperatively and/or intraoperatively M

* G9778 Patients who have a diagnosis of pregnancy M

* G9779 Patients who are breastfeeding M

* G9780 Patients who have a diagnosis of rhabdomyolysis M

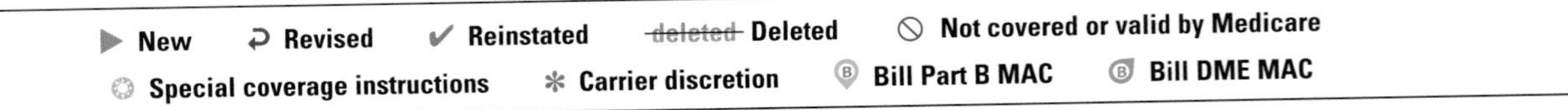

▶ New
Revised
✓ Reinstated
~~deleted~~ Deleted
Not covered or valid by Medicare
Special coverage instructions
* Carrier discretion
Bill Part B MAC
Bill DME MAC

* **G9781** Documentation of medical reason(s) for not currently being a statin therapy user or receive an order (prescription) for statin therapy (e.g., patient with adverse effect, allergy or intolerance to statin medication therapy, patients who are receiving palliative care or hospice care, patients with active liver disease or hepatic disease or insufficiency, and patients with end stage renal disease [ESRD]) M
* **G9782** History of or active diagnosis of familial or pure hypercholesterolemia M
* **G9783** Documentation of patients with diabetes who have a most recent fasting or direct LDL-C laboratory test result <70 mg/dl and are not taking statin therapy M
* **G9784** Pathologists/dermatopathologists providing a second opinion on a biopsy M
* **G9785** Pathology report diagnosing cutaneous basal cell carcinoma, squamous cell carcinoma, or melanoma (to include in situ disease) sent from the pathologist/dermatopathologist to the biopsying clinician for review within 7 days from the time when the tissue specimen was received by the pathologist M
* **G9786** Pathology report diagnosing cutaneous basal cell carcinoma, squamous cell carcinoma, or melanoma (to include in situ disease) was not sent from the pathologist/dermatopathologist to the biopsying clinician for review within 7 days from the time when the tissue specimen was received by the pathologist M
* **G9787** Patient alive as of the last day of the measurement year M
* **G9788** Most recent bp is less than or equal to 140/90 mm hg M
* **G9789** Blood pressure recorded during inpatient stays, emergency room visits, urgent care visits, and patient self-reported BP's (home and health fair BP results) M
* **G9790** Most recent BP is greater than 140/90 mm hg, or blood pressure not documented M
* **G9791** Most recent tobacco status is tobacco free M
* **G9792** Most recent tobacco status is not tobacco free M
* **G9793** Patient is currently on a daily aspirin or other antiplatelet M
* **G9794** Documentation of medical reason(s) for not on a daily aspirin or other antiplatelet (e.g., history of gastrointestinal bleed, intra-cranial bleed, idiopathic thrombocytopenic purpura (ITP), gastric bypass or documentation of active anticoagulant use during the measurement period) M
* **G9795** Patient is not currently on a daily aspirin or other antiplatelet M
* **G9796** Patient is currently on a statin therapy M
* **G9797** Patient is not on a statin therapy M

~~G9798 Discharge(s) for AMI between July 1 of the year prior measurement period year to June 30 of the measurement period~~ ✖

~~G9799 Patients with a medication dispensing event indicator of a history of asthma any time during the patient's history through the end of the measure period~~ ✖

~~G9800 Patients who are identified as having an intolerance or allergy to beta-blocker therapy~~ ✖

~~G9801 Hospitalizations in which the patient was transferred directly to a non-acute care facility for any diagnosis~~ ✖

~~G9802 Patients who use hospice services any time during the measurement period~~ ✖

~~G9803 Patient prescribed at least a 135 day treatment within the 180-day course of treatment with beta-blockers post discharge for AMI~~ ✖

~~G9804 Patient was not prescribed at least a 135 day treatment within the 180-day course of treatment with beta-blockers post discharge for AMI~~ ✖

* **G9805** Patients who use hospice services any time during the measurement period M
* **G9806** Patients who received cervical cytology or an HPV test M
* **G9807** Patients who did not receive cervical cytology or an HPV test M
* **G9808** Any patients who had no asthma controller medications dispensed during the measurement year M
* **G9809** Patients who use hospice services any time during the measurement period M
* **G9810** Patient achieved a pDC of at least 75% for their asthma controller medication M

MIPS | Op Quantity Physician | Oh Quantity Hospital | ♀ Female only | ♂ Male only | A Age | DMEPOS | A2-Z3 ASC Payment Indicator | A-Y ASC Status Indicator | Coding Clinic

* G9811 Patient did not achieve a pDC of at least 75% for their asthma controller medication M
* G9812 Patient died including all deaths occurring during the hospitalization in which the operation was performed, even if after 30 days, and those deaths occurring after discharge from the hospital, but within 30 days of the procedure M
* G9813 Patient did not die within 30 days of the procedure or during the index hospitalization M

~~G9814 Death occurring during the index acute care hospitalization~~

~~G9815 Death did not occur during the index acute care hospitalization~~

~~G9816 Death occurring after discharge from the hospital but within 30 days post procedure~~

~~G9817 Death did not occur after discharge from the hospital within 30 days post procedure~~

* G9818 Documentation of sexual activity M
* G9819 Patients who use hospice services any time during the measurement period M
* G9820 Documentation of a chlamydia screening test with proper follow-up M
* G9821 No documentation of a chlamydia screening test with proper follow-up M
* G9822 Women who had an endometrial ablation procedure during the year prior to the index date (exclusive of the index date) M
* G9823 Endometrial sampling or hysteroscopy with biopsy and results documented M
* G9824 Endometrial sampling or hysteroscopy with biopsy and results not documented M

~~G9825 HER-2/neu negative or undocumented/unknown~~

~~G9826 Patient transferred to practice after initiation of chemotherapy~~

~~G9827 HER2-targeted therapies not administered during the initial course of treatment~~

~~G9828 HER2-targeted therapies administered during the initial course of treatment~~

~~G9829 Breast adjuvant chemotherapy administered~~

* G9830 HER-2/neu positive M
* G9831 AJCC stage at breast cancer diagnosis = II or III M
* G9832 AJCC stage at breast cancer diagnosis = I (Ia or Ib) and T-stage at breast cancer diagnosis does not equal = T1, T1a, T1b M

~~G9833 Patient transfer to practice after initiation of chemotherapy~~

~~G9834 Patient has metastatic disease at diagnosis~~

~~G9835 Trastuzumab administered within 12 months of diagnosis~~

~~G9836 Reason for not administering trastuzumab documented (e.g., patient declined, patient died, patient transferred, contraindication or other clinical exclusion, neoadjuvant chemotherapy or radiation not complete)~~

~~G9837 Trastuzumab not administered within 12 months of diagnosis~~

* G9838 Patient has metastatic disease at diagnosis M
* G9839 Anti-EGFR monoclonal antibody therapy M
* G9840 Ras (KRas and NRas) gene mutation testing performed before initiation of anti-EGFR MoAb M
* G9841 Ras (KRas and NRas) gene mutation testing not performed before initiation of anti-EGFR MoAb M
* G9842 Patient has metastatic disease at diagnosis M
* G9843 Ras (KRas and NRas) gene mutation M
* G9844 Patient did not receive anti-EGFR monoclonal antibody therapy M
* G9845 Patient received anti-EGFR monoclonal antibody therapy M
* G9846 Patients who died from cancer M
* G9847 Patient received chemotherapy in the last 14 days of life M
* G9848 Patient did not receive chemotherapy in the last 14 days of life M

~~G9849 Patients who died from cancer~~

~~G9850 Patient had more than one emergency department visit in the last 30 days of life~~

~~G9851 Patient had one or less emergency department visits in the last 30 days of life~~

* G9852 Patients who died from cancer M

* **G9853** Patient admitted to the ICU in the last 30 days of life M
* **G9854** Patient was not admitted to the ICU in the last 30 days of life M

~~G9855 Patients who died from cancer~~ ✖

~~G9856 Patient was not admitted to hospice~~ ✖

~~G9857 Patient admitted to hospice~~ ✖

* **G9858** Patient enrolled in hospice M
* **G9859** Patients who died from cancer M
* **G9860** Patient spent less than three days in hospice care M
* **G9861** Patient spent greater than or equal to three days in hospice care M
* **G9862** Documentation of medical reason(s) for not recommending at least a 10 year follow-up interval (e.g., inadequate prep, familial or personal history of colonic polyps, patient had no adenoma and age is = 66 years old, or life expectancy <10 years old, other medical reasons) M
* **G9873** First Medicare diabetes prevention program (MDPP) core session was attended by an MDPP beneficiary under the MDPP expanded model (EM). A core session is an MDPP service that: (1) is furnished by an MDPP supplier during months 1 through 6 of the MDPP services period; (2) is approximately 1 hour in length; and (3) adheres to a CDC-approved DPP curriculum for core sessions. M
* **G9874** Four total Medicare diabetes prevention program (MDPP) core sessions were attended by an MDPP beneficiary under the mdpp expanded model (EM). A core session is an MDPP service that: (1) is furnished by an MDPP supplier during months 1 through 6 of the MDPP services period; (2) is approximately 1 hour in length; and (3) adheres to a CDC-approved DPP curriculum for core sessions. M
* **G9875** Nine total Medicare diabetes prevention program (MDPP) core sessions were attended by an MDPP beneficiary under the MDPP expanded model (EM). A core session is an MDPP service that: (1) is furnished by an MDPP supplier during months 1 through 6 of the MDPP services period; (2) is approximately 1 hour in length; and (3) adheres to a CDC-approved DPP curriculum for core sessions. M
* **G9876** Two Medicare diabetes prevention program (MDPP) core maintenance sessions (MS) were attended by an MDPP beneficiary in months (mo) 7-9 under the mdpp expanded model (EM). A core maintenance session is an MDPP service that: (1) is furnished by an MDPP supplier during months 7 through 12 of the MDPP services period; (2) is approximately 1 hour in length; and (3) adheres to a CDC-approved DPP curriculum for maintenance sessions. The beneficiary did not achieve at least 5% weight loss (WL) from his/her baseline weight, as measured by at least one in-person weight measurement at a core maintenance session in months 7-9. M
* **G9877** Two Medicare diabetes prevention program (MDPP) core maintenance sessions (MS) were attended by an MDPP beneficiary in months (mo) 10-12 under the MDPP expanded model (EM). A core maintenance session is an MDPP service that: (1) is furnished by an MDPP supplier during months 7 through 12 of the MDPP services period; (2) is approximately 1 hour in length; and (3) adheres to a CDC-approved DPP curriculum for maintenance sessions. The beneficiary did not achieve at least 5% weight loss (WL) from his/her baseline weight, as measured by at least one in-person weight measurement at a core maintenance session in months 10-12. M
* **G9878** Two Medicare diabetes prevention program (MDPP) core maintenance sessions (MS) were attended by an MDPP beneficiary in months (mo) 7-9 under the MDPP expanded model (EM). A core maintenance session is an MDPP service that: (1) is furnished by an MDPP supplier during months 7 through 12 of the MDPP services period; (2) is approximately 1 hour in length; and (3) adheres to a CDC-approved DPP curriculum for maintenance sessions. The beneficiary achieved at least 5% weight loss (WL) from his/her baseline weight, as measured by at least one in-person weight measurement at a core maintenance session in months 7-9. M

* **G9879** Two Medicare diabetes prevention program (MDPP) core maintenance sessions (MS) were attended by an MDPP beneficiary in months (mo) 10-12 under the MDPP expanded model (EM). A core maintenance session is an MDPP service that: (1) is furnished by an MDPP supplier during months 7 through 12 of the MDPP services period; (2) is approximately 1 hour in length; and (3) adheres to a CDC-approved DPP curriculum for maintenance sessions. The beneficiary achieved at least 5% weight loss (WL) from his/her baseline weight, as measured by at least one in-person weight measurement at a core maintenance session in months 10-12. M

* **G9880** The MDPP beneficiary achieved at least 5% weight loss (WL) from his/her baseline weight in months (mo) 1-12 of the MDPP services period under the MDPP expanded model (EM). This is a one-time payment available when a beneficiary first achieves at least 5% weight loss from baseline as measured by an in-person weight measurement at a core session or core maintenance session. M

* **G9881** The MDPP beneficiary achieved at least 9% weight loss (WL) from his/her baseline weight in months (mo) 1-24 under the MDPP expanded model (EM). This is a one-time payment available when a beneficiary first achieves at least 9% weight loss from baseline as measured by an in-person weight measurement at a core session, core maintenance session, or ongoing maintenance session. M

* **G9882** Two Medicare diabetes prevention program (MDPP) ongoing maintenance sessions (MS) were attended by an MDPP beneficiary in months (mo) 13-15 under the MDPP expanded model (EM). An ongoing maintenance session is an MDPP service that: (1) is furnished by an MDPP supplier during months 13 through 24 of the MDPP services period; (2) is approximately 1 hour in length; and (3) adheres to a CDC-approved DPP curriculum for maintenance sessions. The beneficiary maintained at least 5% weight loss (WL) from his/her baseline weight, as measured by at least one in-person weight measurement at an ongoing maintenance session in months 13-15. M

* **G9883** Two Medicare diabetes prevention program (MDPP) ongoing maintenance sessions (MS) were attended by an MDPP beneficiary in months (mo) 16-18 under the MDPP expanded model (EM). An ongoing maintenance session is an MDPP service that: (1) is furnished by an MDPP supplier during months 13 through 24 of the MDPP services period; (2) is approximately 1 hour in length; and (3) adheres to a CDC-approved DPP curriculum for maintenance sessions. The beneficiary maintained at least 5% weight loss (WL) from his/her baseline weight, as measured by at least one in-person weight measurement at an ongoing maintenance session in months 16-18. M

* **G9884** Two Medicare diabetes prevention program (MDPP) ongoing maintenance sessions (MS) were attended by an MDPP beneficiary in months (mo) 19-21 under the MDPP expanded model (EM). An ongoing maintenance session is an MDPP service that: (1) is furnished by an MDPP supplier during months 13 through 24 of the MDPP services period; (2) is approximately 1 hour in length; and (3) adheres to a CDC-approved DPP curriculum for maintenance sessions. The beneficiary maintained at least 5% weight loss (WL) from his/her baseline weight, as measured by at least one in-person weight measurement at an ongoing maintenance session in months 19-21. M

* **G9885** Two Medicare diabetes prevention program (MDPP) ongoing maintenance sessions (MS) were attended by an MDPP beneficiary in months (mo) 22-24 under the MDPP expanded model (EM). An ongoing maintenance session is an MDPP service that: (1) is furnished by an MDPP supplier during months 13 through 24 of the MDPP services period; (2) is approximately 1 hour in length; and (3) adheres to a CDC-approved DPP curriculum for maintenance sessions. The beneficiary maintained at least 5% weight loss (WL) from his/her baseline weight, as measured by at least one in-person weight measurement at an ongoing maintenance session in months 22-24. M

Note: The following codes do not imply that codes in other sections are necessarily covered.

Quality Measures: Miscellaneous

* **G9890** Bridge payment: a one-time payment for the first Medicare diabetes prevention program (MDPP) core session, core maintenance session, or ongoing maintenance session furnished by an MDPP supplier to an MDPP beneficiary during months 1-24 of the MDPP expanded model (EM) who has previously received MDPP services from a different MDPP supplier under the MDPP expanded model. A supplier may only receive one bridge payment per MDPP beneficiary. M
* **G9891** MDPP session reported as a line-item on a claim for a payable MDPP expanded model (EM) HCPCS code for a session furnished by the billing supplier under the MDPP expanded model and counting toward achievement of the attendance performance goal for the payable MDPP expanded model HCPCS code (this code is for reporting purposes only) M
* **G9890** Dilated macular exam performed, including documentation of the presence or absence of macular thickening or geographic atrophy or hemorrhage and the level of macular degeneration severity M
* **G9891** Documentation of medical reason(s) for not performing a dilated macular examination M
* **G9892** Documentation of patient reason(s) for not performing a dilated macular examination M
* **G9893** Dilated macular exam was not performed, reason not otherwise specified M
* **G9894** Androgen deprivation therapy prescribed/administered in combination with external beam radiotherapy to the prostate M
* **G9895** Documentation of medical reason(s) for not prescribing/administering androgen deprivation therapy in combination with external beam radiotherapy to the prostate (e.g., salvage therapy) M
* **G9896** Documentation of patient reason(s) for not prescribing/administering androgen deprivation therapy in combination with external beam radiotherapy to the prostate M
* **G9897** Patients who were not prescribed/administered androgen deprivation therapy in combination with external beam radiotherapy to the prostate, reason not given M
* **G9898** Patient age 66 or older in institutional special needs plans (SNP) or residing in long-term care with pos code 32, 33, 34, 54, or 56 for more than 90 consecutive days during the measurement period M
* **G9899** Screening, diagnostic, film, digital or digital breast tomosynthesis (3D) mammography results documented and reviewed M
* **G9900** Screening, diagnostic, film, digital or digital breast tomosynthesis (3D) mammography results were not documented and reviewed, reason not otherwise specified M
* **G9901** Patient age 66 or older in institutional special needs plans (SNP) or residing in long-term care with pos code 32, 33, 34, 54, or 56 for more than 90 consecutive days during the measurement period M
* **G9902** Patient screened for tobacco use and identified as a tobacco user M
* **G9903** Patient screened for tobacco use and identified as a tobacco non-user M
* **G9904** Documentation of medical reason(s) for not screening for tobacco use (e.g., limited life expectancy, other medical reason) M
* **G9905** Patient not screened for tobacco use, reason not given M
* **G9906** Patient identified as a tobacco user received tobacco cessation intervention (counseling and/or pharmacotherapy) M
* **G9907** Documentation of medical reason(s) for not providing tobacco cessation intervention (e.g., limited life expectancy, other medical reason) M
* **G9908** Patient identified as tobacco user did not receive tobacco cessation intervention (counseling and/or pharmacotherapy), reason not given M

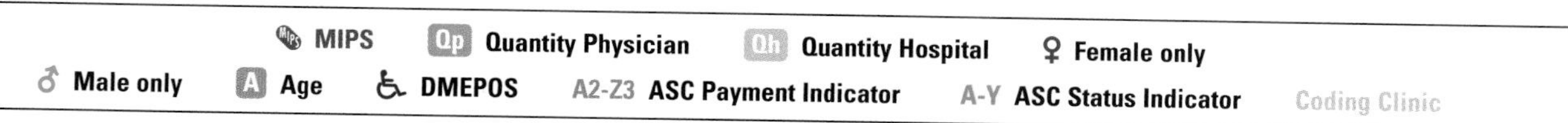
MIPS
Qp Quantity Physician
Qh Quantity Hospital
♀ Female only
♂ Male only
A Age
DMEPOS
A2-Z3 ASC Payment Indicator
A-Y ASC Status Indicator
Coding Clinic

✻ **G9909** Documentation of medical reason(s) for not providing tobacco cessation intervention if identified as a tobacco user (e.g., limited life expectancy, other medical reason) Ⓑ M

⊋ ✻ **G9910** Patients age 66 or older in institutional special needs plans (SNP) or residing in long-term care with pos code 32, 33, 34, 54, or 56 for more than 90 consecutive days during the measurement period Ⓑ M

✻ **G9911** Clinically node negative (t1n0m0 or t2n0m0) invasive breast cancer before or after neoadjuvant systemic therapy Ⓑ M

✻ **G9912** Hepatitis B virus (HBV) status assessed and results interpreted prior to initiating anti-TNF (tumor necrosis factor) therapy Ⓑ M

✻ **G9913** Hepatitis B virus (HBV) status not assessed and results interpreted prior to initiating anti-TNF (tumor necrosis factor) therapy, reason not given Ⓑ M

✻ **G9914** Patient receiving an anti-TNF agent Ⓑ M

✻ **G9915** No record of HBV results documented Ⓑ M

✻ **G9916** Functional status performed once in the last 12 months Ⓑ M

✻ **G9917** Documentation of advanced stage dementia and caregiver knowledge is limited Ⓑ M

✻ **G9918** Functional status not performed, reason not otherwise specified Ⓑ M

✻ **G9919** Screening performed and positive and provision of recommendations Ⓑ M

✻ **G9920** Screening performed and negative Ⓑ M

✻ **G9921** No screening performed, partial screening performed or positive screen without recommendations and reason is not given or otherwise specified Ⓑ M

✻ **G9922** Safety concerns screen provided and if positive then documented mitigation recommendations Ⓑ M

✻ **G9923** Safety concerns screen provided and negative Ⓑ M

~~G9924 Documentation of medical reason(s) for not providing safety concerns screen or for not providing recommendations, orders or referrals for positive screen (e.g., patient in palliative care, other medical reason)~~ ✖

✻ **G9925** Safety concerns screening not provided, reason not otherwise specified Ⓑ M

✻ **G9926** Safety concerns screening positive screen is without provision of mitigation recommendations, including but not limited to referral to other resources Ⓑ M

✻ **G9927** Documentation of system reason(s) for not prescribing warfarin or another FDA-approved anticoagulation due to patient being currently enrolled in a clinical trial related to af/atrial flutter treatment Ⓑ M

✻ **G9928** Warfarin or another FDA-approved anticoagulant not prescribed, reason not given Ⓑ M

✻ **G9929** Patient with transient or reversible cause of AF (e.g., pneumonia, hyperthyroidism, pregnancy, cardiac surgery) Ⓑ M

✻ **G9930** Patients who are receiving comfort care only Ⓑ M

⊋ ✻ **G9931** Documentation of CHA2DS2-VASc risk score of 0 or 1 for men; or 0, 1, or 2 for women Ⓑ M

✻ **G9932** Documentation of patient reason(s) for not having records of negative or managed positive TB screen (e.g., patient does not return for mantoux (ppd) skin test evaluation) Ⓑ M

~~G9933 Adenoma(s) or colorectal cancer detected during screening colonoscopy~~ ✖

~~G9934 Documentation that neoplasm detected is only diagnosed as traditional serrated adenoma, sessile serrated polyp, or sessile serrated adenoma~~ ✖

~~G9935 Adenoma(s) or colorectal cancer not detected during screening colonoscopy~~ ✖

~~G9936 Surveillance colonoscopy - personal history of colonic polyps, colon cancer, or other malignant neoplasm of rectum, rectosigmoid junction, and anus~~ ✖

~~G9937 Diagnostic colonoscopy~~ ✖

⊋ ✻ **G9938** Patients age 66 or older in institutional special needs plans (SNP) or residing in long-term care with POS code 32, 33, 34, 54, or 56 for more than 90 consecutive days during the six months prior to the measurement period through December 31 of the measurement period Ⓑ M

✻ **G9939** Pathologist/dermatopathologist is the same clinician who performed the biopsy Ⓑ M

▶ New ⊋ Revised ✔ Reinstated ~~deleted~~ Deleted ⊘ Not covered or valid by Medicare
Special coverage instructions ✻ Carrier discretion Ⓑ Bill Part B MAC Ⓓ Bill DME MAC

✻ **G9940** Documentation of medical reason(s) for not on a statin (e.g., pregnancy, in vitro fertilization, clomiphene rx, ESRD, cirrhosis, muscular pain and disease during the measurement period or prior year) M

✻ **G9942** Patient had any additional spine procedures performed on the same date as the lumbar discectomy/laminectomy M

✻ **G9943** Back pain was not measured by the visual analog scale (VAS) within three months preoperatively and at three months (6-20 weeks) postoperatively M

✻ **G9945** Patient had cancer, acute fracture or infection related to the lumbar spine or patient had neuromuscular, idiopathic or congenital lumbar scoliosis M

✻ **G9946** Back pain was not measured by the visual analog scale (VAS) within three months preoperatively and at one year (9 to 15 months) postoperatively M

✻ **G9948** Patient had any additional spine procedures performed on the same date as the lumbar discectomy/laminectomy M

✻ **G9949** Leg pain was not measured by the visual analog scale (VAS) at three months (6 to 20 weeks) postoperatively M

✻ **G9954** Patient exhibits 2 or more risk factors for post-operative vomiting M

✻ **G9955** Cases in which an inhalational anesthetic is used only for induction M

✻ **G9956** Patient received combination therapy consisting of at least two prophylactic pharmacologic anti-emetic agents of different classes preoperatively and/or intraoperatively M

✻ **G9957** Documentation of medical reason for not receiving combination therapy consisting of at least two prophylactic pharmacologic anti-emetic agents of different classes preoperatively and/or intraoperatively (e.g., intolerance or other medical reason) M

✻ **G9958** Patient did not receive combination therapy consisting of at least two prophylactic pharmacologic anti-emetic agents of different classes preoperatively and/or intraoperatively M

✻ **G9959** Systemic antimicrobials not prescribed M

✻ **G9960** Documentation of medical reason(s) for prescribing systemic antimicrobials M

✻ **G9961** Systemic antimicrobials prescribed M

✻ **G9962** Embolization endpoints are documented separately for each embolized vessel and ovarian artery angiography or embolization performed in the presence of variant uterine artery anatomy M

✻ **G9963** Embolization endpoints are not documented separately for each embolized vessel or ovarian artery angiography or embolization not performed in the presence of variant uterine artery anatomy M

✻ **G9964** Patient received at least one well-child visit with a PCP during the performance period M

✻ **G9965** Patient did not receive at least one well-child visit with a PCP during the performance period M

~~G9966 Children who were screened for risk of developmental, behavioral and social delays using a standardized tool with interpretation and report~~ ✖

~~G9967 Children who were not screened for risk of developmental, behavioral and social delays using a standardized tool with interpretation and report~~ ✖

✻ **G9968** Patient was referred to another provider or specialist during the performance period M

✻ **G9969** Provider who referred the patient to another provider received a report from the provider to whom the patient was referred M

✻ **G9970** Provider who referred the patient to another provider did not receive a report from the provider to whom the patient was referred M

✻ **G9974** Dilated macular exam performed, including documentation of the presence or absence of macular thickening or geographic atrophy or hemorrhage and the level of macular degeneration severity M

✻ **G9975** Documentation of medical reason(s) for not performing a dilated macular examination M

✻ **G9976** Documentation of patient reason(s) for not performing a dilated macular examination M

MIPS | Qp Quantity Physician | Qh Quantity Hospital | ♀ Female only | ♂ Male only | A Age | DMEPOS | A2-Z3 ASC Payment Indicator | A-Y ASC Status Indicator | Coding Clinic

✻ **G9977** Dilated macular exam was not performed, reason not otherwise specified Ⓑ M

✻ **G9978** Remote in-home visit for the evaluation and management of a new patient for use only in a Medicare-approved bundled payments for care improvement advanced (BCPI advanced) model episode of care, which requires these 3 key components: a problem focused history; a problem focused examination; and straightforward medical decision making, furnished in real time using interactive audio and video technology. Counseling and coordination of care with other physicians, other qualified health care professionals or agencies are provided consistent with the nature of the problem(s) and the needs of the patient or the family or both. Usually, the presenting problem(s) are self limited or minor. Typically, 10 minutes are spent with the patient or family or both via real time, audio and video intercommunications technology. Ⓑ B

✻ **G9979** Remote in-home visit for the evaluation and management of a new patient for use only in a Medicare-approved bundled payments for care improvement advanced (BCPI advanced) model episode of care, which requires these 3 key components: an expanded problem focused history; an expanded problem focused examination; straightforward medical decision making, furnished in real time using interactive audio and video technology. Counseling and coordination of care with other physicians, other qualified health care professionals or agencies are provided consistent with the nature of the problem(s) and the needs of the patient or the family or both. Usually, the presenting problem(s) are of low to moderate severity. Typically, 20 minutes are spent with the patient or family or both via real time, audio and video intercommunications technology. Ⓑ B

✻ **G9980** Remote in-home visit for the evaluation and management of a new patient for use only in a Medicare-approved bundled payments for care improvement advanced (BCPI advanced) model episode of care, which requires these 3 key components: a detailed history; a detailed examination; medical decision making of low complexity, furnished in real time using interactive audio and video technology. Counseling and coordination of care with other physicians, other qualified health care professionals or agencies are provided consistent with the nature of the problem(s) and the needs of the patient or the family or both. Usually, the presenting problem(s) are of moderate severity. Typically, 30 minutes are spent with the patient or family or both via real time, audio and video intercommunications technology. Ⓑ B

✻ **G9981** Remote in-home visit for the evaluation and management of a new patient for use only in a Medicare-approved bundled payments for care improvement advanced (BCPI advanced) model episode of care, which requires these 3 key components: a comprehensive history; a comprehensive examination; medical decision making of moderate complexity, furnished in real time using interactive audio and video technology. Counseling and coordination of care with other physicians, other qualified health care professionals or agencies are provided consistent with the nature of the problem(s) and the needs of the patient or the family or both. Usually, the presenting problem(s) are of moderate to high severity. Typically, 45 minutes are spent with the patient or family or both via real time, audio and video intercommunications technology. Ⓑ B

* **G9982** Remote in-home visit for the evaluation and management of a new patient for use only in a Medicare-approved bundled payments for care improvement advanced (BCPI advanced) model episode of care, which requires these 3 key components: a comprehensive history; a comprehensive examination; medical decision making of high complexity, furnished in real time using interactive audio and video technology. Counseling and coordination of care with other physicians, other qualified health care professionals or agencies are provided consistent with the nature of the problem(s) and the needs of the patient or the family or both. Usually, the presenting problem(s) are of moderate to high severity. Typically, 60 minutes are spent with the patient or family or both via real time, audio and video intercommunications technology. B

* **G9983** Remote in-home visit for the evaluation and management of an established patient for use only in a Medicare-approved bundled payments for care improvement advanced (BCPI advanced) model episode of care, which requires at least 2 of the following 3 key components: a problem focused history; a problem focused examination; straightforward medical decision making, furnished in real time using interactive audio and video technology. Counseling and coordination of care with other physicians, other qualified health care professionals or agencies are provided consistent with the nature of the problem(s) and the needs of the patient or the family or both. Usually, the presenting problem(s) are self limited or minor. Typically, 10 minutes are spent with the patient or family or both via real time, audio and video intercommunications technology. B

* **G9984** Remote in-home visit for the evaluation and management of an established patient for use only in a Medicare-approved bundled payments for care improvement advanced (BCPI advanced) model episode of care, which requires at least 2 of the following 3 key components: an expanded problem focused history; an expanded problem focused examination; medical decision making of low complexity, furnished in real time using interactive audio and video technology. Counseling and coordination of care with other physicians, other qualified health care professionals or agencies are provided consistent with the nature of the problem(s) and the needs of the patient or the family or both. Usually, the presenting problem(s) are of low to moderate severity. Typically, 15 minutes are spent with the patient or family or both via real time, audio and video intercommunications technology. B

* **G9985** Remote in-home visit for the evaluation and management of an established patient for use only in a Medicare-approved bundled payments for care improvement advanced (BCPI advanced) model episode of care, which requires at least 2 of the following 3 key components: a detailed history; a detailed examination; medical decision making of moderate complexity, furnished in real time using interactive audio and video technology. Counseling and coordination of care with other physicians, other qualified health care professionals or agencies are provided consistent with the nature of the problem(s) and the needs of the patient or the family or both. Usually, the presenting problem(s) are of moderate to high severity. Typically, 25 minutes are spent with the patient or family or both via real time, audio and video intercommunications technology. B

✻ **G9986** Remote in-home visit for the evaluation and management of an established patient for use only in a Medicare-approved bundled payments for care improvement advanced (BCPI advanced) model episode of care, which requires at least 2 of the following 3 key components: a comprehensive history; a comprehensive examination; medical decision making of high complexity, furnished in real time using interactive audio and video technology. Counseling and coordination of care with other physicians, other qualified health care professionals or agencies are provided consistent with the nature of the problem(s) and the needs of the patient or the family or both. Usually, the presenting problem(s) are of moderate to high severity. Typically, 40 minutes are spent with the patient or family or both via real time, audio and video intercommunications technology. Ⓑ B

✻ **G9987** Bundled payments for care improvement advanced (BCPI advanced) model home visit for patient assessment performed by clinical staff for an individual not considered homebound, including, but not necessarily limited to patient assessment of clinical status, safety/fall prevention, functional status/ambulation, medication reconciliation/management, compliance with orders/plan of care, performance of activities of daily living, and ensuring beneficiary connections to community and other services; for use only for a BCPI advanced model episode of care; may not be billed for a 30-day period covered by a transitional care management code. Ⓑ B

BEHAVIORAL HEALTH AND/OR SUBSTANCE ABUSE TREATMENT SERVICES (H0001-H9999)

NOTE: Used by Medicaid state agencies because no national code exists to meet the reporting needs of these agencies.

⊘ **H0001** Alcohol and/or drug assessment

⊘ **H0002** Behavioral health screening to determine eligibility for admission to treatment program

⊘ **H0003** Alcohol and/or drug screening; laboratory analysis of specimens for presence of alcohol and/or drugs

⊘ **H0004** Behavioral health counseling and therapy, per 15 minutes

⊘ **H0005** Alcohol and/or drug services; group counseling by a clinician

⊘ **H0006** Alcohol and/or drug services; case management

⊘ **H0007** Alcohol and/or drug services; crisis intervention (outpatient)

⊘ **H0008** Alcohol and/or drug services; sub-acute detoxification (hospital inpatient)

⊘ **H0009** Alcohol and/or drug services; acute detoxification (hospital inpatient)

⊘ **H0010** Alcohol and/or drug services; sub-acute detoxification (residential addiction program inpatient)

⊘ **H0011** Alcohol and/or drug services; acute detoxification (residential addiction program inpatient)

⊘ **H0012** Alcohol and/or drug services; sub-acute detoxification (residential addiction program outpatient)

⊘ **H0013** Alcohol and/or drug services; acute detoxification (residential addiction program outpatient)

⊘ **H0014** Alcohol and/or drug services; ambulatory detoxification

⊘ **H0015** Alcohol and/or drug services; intensive outpatient (treatment program that operates at least 3 hours/day and at least 3 days/week and is based on an individualized treatment plan), including assessment, counseling; crisis intervention, and activity therapies or education

⊘ **H0016** Alcohol and/or drug services; medical/somatic (medical intervention in ambulatory setting)

⊘ **H0017** Behavioral health; residential (hospital residential treatment program), without room and board, per diem

⊘ **H0018** Behavioral health; short-term residential (non-hospital residential treatment program), without room and board, per diem

⊘ **H0019** Behavioral health; long-term residential (non-medical, non-acute care in a residential treatment program where stay is typically longer than 30 days), without room and board, per diem

⊘ **H0020** Alcohol and/or drug services; methadone administration and/or service (provision of the drug by a licensed program)

⊘ **H0021** Alcohol and/or drug training service (for staff and personnel not employed by providers)

⊘ **H0022** Alcohol and/or drug intervention service (planned facilitation)

⊘ **H0023** Behavioral health outreach service (planned approach to reach a targeted population)

⊘ **H0024** Behavioral health prevention information dissemination service (one-way direct or non-direct contact with service audiences to affect knowledge and attitude)

⊘ **H0025** Behavioral health prevention education service (delivery of services with target population to affect knowledge, attitude and/or behavior)

⊘ **H0026** Alcohol and/or drug prevention process service, community-based (delivery of services to develop skills of impactors)

⊘ **H0027** Alcohol and/or drug prevention environmental service (broad range of external activities geared toward modifying systems in order to mainstream prevention through policy and law)

⊘ **H0028** Alcohol and/or drug prevention problem identification and referral service (e.g., student assistance and employee assistance programs), does not include assessment

⊘ **H0029** Alcohol and/or drug prevention alternatives service (services for populations that exclude alcohol and other drug use, e.g., alcohol-free social events)

⊘ **H0030** Behavioral health hotline service

⊘ **H0031** Mental health assessment, by non-physician

⊘ **H0032** Mental health service plan development by non-physician

⊘ **H0033** Oral medication administration, direct observation

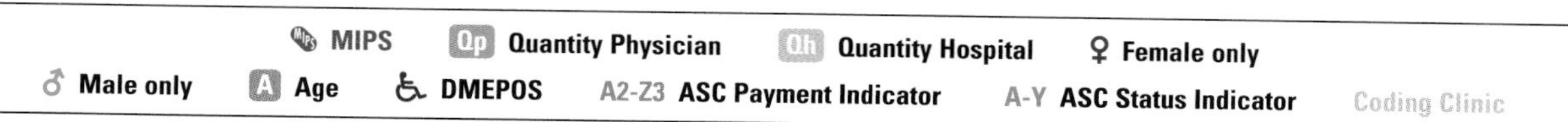

MIPS
Qp Quantity Physician
Qh Quantity Hospital
♀ Female only
♂ Male only
A Age
DMEPOS
A2-Z3 ASC Payment Indicator
A-Y ASC Status Indicator
Coding Clinic

H0034 Medication training and support, per 15 minutes

H0035 Mental health partial hospitalization, treatment, less than 24 hours

H0036 Community psychiatric supportive treatment, face-to-face, per 15 minutes

H0037 Community psychiatric supportive treatment program, per diem

H0038 Self-help/peer services, per 15 minutes

H0039 Assertive community treatment, face-to-face, per 15 minutes

H0040 Assertive community treatment program, per diem

H0041 Foster care, child, non-therapeutic, per diem A

H0042 Foster care, child, non-therapeutic, per month A

H0043 Supported housing, per diem

H0044 Supported housing, per month

H0045 Respite care services, not in the home, per diem

H0046 Mental health services, not otherwise specified

H0047 Alcohol and/or other drug abuse services, not otherwise specified

H0048 Alcohol and/or other drug testing: collection and handling only, specimens other than blood

H0049 Alcohol and/or drug screening

H0050 Alcohol and/or drug services, brief intervention, per 15 minutes

H1000 Prenatal care, at-risk assessment ♀

H1001 Prenatal care, at-risk enhanced service; antepartum management ♀

H1002 Prenatal care, at-risk enhanced service; care coordination ♀

H1003 Prenatal care, at-risk enhanced service; education ♀

H1004 Prenatal care, at-risk enhanced service; follow-up home visit ♀

H1005 Prenatal care, at-risk enhanced service package (includes H1001-H1004) ♀

H1010 Non-medical family planning education, per session

H1011 Family assessment by licensed behavioral health professional for state defined purposes

H2000 Comprehensive multidisciplinary evaluation

H2001 Rehabilitation program, per 1/2 day

H2010 Comprehensive medication services, per 15 minutes

H2011 Crisis intervention service, per 15 minutes

H2012 Behavioral health day treatment, per hour

H2013 Psychiatric health facility service, per diem

H2014 Skills training and development, per 15 minutes

H2015 Comprehensive community support services, per 15 minutes

H2016 Comprehensive community support services, per diem

H2017 Psychosocial rehabilitation services, per 15 minutes

H2018 Psychosocial rehabilitation services, per diem

H2019 Therapeutic behavioral services, per 15 minutes

H2020 Therapeutic behavioral services, per diem

H2021 Community-based wrap-around services, per 15 minutes

H2022 Community-based wrap-around services, per diem

H2023 Supported employment, per 15 minutes

H2024 Supported employment, per diem

H2025 Ongoing support to maintain employment, per 15 minutes

H2026 Ongoing support to maintain employment, per diem

H2027 Psychoeducational service, per 15 minutes

H2028 Sexual offender treatment service, per 15 minutes

H2029 Sexual offender treatment service, per diem

H2030 Mental health clubhouse services, per 15 minutes

H2031 Mental health clubhouse services, per diem

H2032 Activity therapy, per 15 minutes

H2033 Multisystemic therapy for juveniles, per 15 minutes A

H2034 Alcohol and/or drug abuse halfway house services, per diem

H2035 Alcohol and/or other drug treatment program, per hour

H2036 Alcohol and/or other drug treatment program, per diem

H2037 Developmental delay prevention activities, dependent child of client, per 15 minutes A

▶ New ⮌ Revised ✔ Reinstated ~~deleted~~ Deleted ⊘ Not covered or valid by Medicare
Special coverage instructions * Carrier discretion Bill Part B MAC Bill DME MAC

DRUGS OTHER THAN CHEMOTHERAPY DRUGS (J0100-J8999)

Injection

	Code	Description	
○	**J0120**	Injection, tetracycline, up to 250 mg Qp Qh *Other: Achromycin* *IOM: 100-02, 15, 50*	N1 N
✻	**J0121**	Injection, omadacycline, 1 mg	K2 G
✻	**J0122**	Injection, eravacycline, 1 mg	K2 K
✻	**J0129**	Injection, abatacept, 10 mg (Code may be used for Medicare when drug administered under the direct supervision of a physician, not for use when drug is self-administered) Qp Qh *Other: Orencia*	K2 K
○	**J0130**	Injection, abciximab, 10 mg Qp Qh *Other: ReoPro* *IOM: 100-02, 15, 50*	N1 N
✻	**J0131**	Injection, acetaminophen, 10 mg Qp Qh *Other: Ofirmev* Coding Clinic: 2012, Q1, P9	N1 N
✻	**J0132**	Injection, acetylcysteine, 100 mg Qp Qh *Other: Acetadote*	N1 N
✻	**J0133**	Injection, acyclovir, 5 mg Qp Qh	N1 N
✻	**J0135**	Injection, adalimumab, 20 mg Qp Qh *Other: Humira* *IOM: 100-02, 15, 50*	K2 K
○	**J0153**	Injection, adenosine, 1 mg (not to be used to report any adenosine phosphate compounds) Qp Qh *Other: Adenocard, Adenoscan*	N1 N
○	**J0171**	Injection, adrenalin, epinephrine, 0.1 mg Qp Qh *Other: AUVI-Q, Sus-Phrine* *IOM: 100-02, 15, 50* Coding Clinic: 2011, Q1, P8	N1 N
✻	**J0178**	Injection, aflibercept, 1 mg Qp Qh *Other: Eylea*	K2 K
✻	**J0179**	Injection, brolucizumab-dbll, 1 mg	K2 K
✻	**J0180**	Injection, agalsidase beta, 1 mg Qp Qh *Other: Fabrazyme* *IOM: 100-02, 15, 50*	K2 K
✻	**J0185**	Injection, aprepitant, 1 mg *Other: Emend*	G
○	**J0190**	Injection, biperiden lactate, per 5 mg Qp Qh *Other: Akineton* *IOM: 100-02, 15, 50*	E2
○	**J0200**	Injection, alatrofloxacin mesylate, 100 mg Qp Qh *Other: Trovan* *IOM: 100-02, 15, 50*	E2
✻	**J0202**	Injection, alemtuzumab, 1 mg Qp Qh *Other: Lemtrada*	K2 K
○	**J0205**	Injection, alglucerase, per 10 units Qp Qh *Other: Ceredase* *IOM: 100-02, 15, 50*	E2
○	**J0207**	Injection, amifostine, 500 mg Qp Qh *Other: Ethyol* *IOM: 100-02, 15, 50*	K2 K
○	**J0210**	Injection, methyldopate HCL, up to 250 mg Qp Qh *Other: Aldomet* *IOM: 100-02, 15, 50*	N1 N
✻	**J0215**	Injection, alefacept, 0.5 mg Qp Qh	E2
✻	**J0220**	Injection, alglucosidase alfa, not otherwise specified, 10 mg Qp Qh Coding Clinic: 2013: Q2, P5; 2012, Q1, P9	K2 K
✻	**J0221**	Injection, alglucosidase alfa, (lumizyme), 10 mg Qp Qh Coding Clinic: 2013: Q2, P5	K2 K
✻	**J0222**	Injection, patisiran, 0.1 mg	K2 G
▶	**J0223**	Injection, givosiran, 0.5 mg	K2
○	**J0256**	Injection, alpha 1-proteinase inhibitor (human), not otherwise specified, 10 mg Qp Qh *Other: Prolastin, Zemaira* *IOM: 100-02, 15, 50* Coding Clinic: 2012, Q1, P9	K2 K

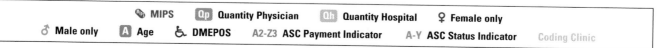

J0257 Injection, alpha 1 proteinase inhibitor (human), (glassia), 10 mg Qp Qh K2 K

IOM: 100-02, 15, 50

Coding Clinic: 2012, Q1, P8

J0270 Injection, alprostadil, per 1.25 mcg (Code may be used for Medicare when drug administered under the direct supervision of a physician, not for use when drug is self-administered) Qp Qh B

Other: Caverject, Prostaglandin E1, Prostin VR Pediatric

IOM: 100-02, 15, 50

J0275 Alprostadil urethral suppository (Code may be used for Medicare when drug administered under the direct supervision of a physician, not for use when drug is self-administered) Qp Qh B

Other: Muse

IOM: 100-02, 15, 50

* **J0278** Injection, amikacin sulfate, 100 mg Qp Qh N1 N

J0280 Injection, aminophylline, up to 250 mg Qp Qh N1 N

IOM: 100-02, 15, 50

J0282 Injection, amiodarone hydrochloride, 30 mg Qp Qh N1 N

Other: Cordarone

IOM: 100-02, 15, 50

J0285 Injection, amphotericin B, 50 mg Qp Qh N1 N

Other: ABLC, Amphocin, Fungizone

IOM: 100-02, 15, 50

J0287 Injection, amphotericin B lipid complex, 10 mg Qp Qh K2 K

Other: Abelcet

IOM: 100-02, 15, 50

J0288 Injection, amphotericin B cholesteryl sulfate complex, 10 mg Qp Qh E2

IOM: 100-02, 15, 50

J0289 Injection, amphotericin B liposome, 10 mg Qp Qh K2 K

Other: AmBisome

IOM: 100-02, 15, 50

J0290 Injection, ampicillin sodium, 500 mg Qp Qh N1 N

Other: Omnipen-N, Polycillin-N, Totacillin-N

IOM: 100-02, 15, 50

* **J0291** Injection, plazomicin, 5 mg K2 G

J0295 Injection, ampicillin sodium/sulbactam sodium, per 1.5 gm Qp Qh N1 N

Other: Omnipen-N, Polycillin-N, Totacillin-N, Unasyn

IOM: 100-02, 15, 50

J0300 Injection, amobarbital, up to 125 mg Qp Qh K2 K

Other: Amytal

IOM: 100-02, 15, 50

J0330 Injection, succinylcholine chloride, up to 20 mg Qp Qh N1 N

Other: Anectine, Quelicin, Surostrin

IOM: 100-02, 15, 50

* **J0348** Injection, anidulafungin, 1 mg Qp Qh N1 N

Other: Eraxis

J0350 Injection, anistreplase, per 30 units Qp Qh E2

Other: Eminase

IOM: 100-02, 15, 50

J0360 Injection, hydralazine hydrochloride, up to 20 mg Qp Qh N1 N

Other: Apresoline

IOM: 100-02, 15, 50

* **J0364** Injection, apomorphine hydrochloride, 1 mg Qp Qh E2

J0365 Injection, aprotinin, 10,000 KIU Qp Qh E2

IOM: 100-02, 15, 50

J0380 Injection, metaraminol bitartrate, per 10 mg Qp Qh N1 N

Other: Aramine

IOM: 100-02, 15, 50

J0390 Injection, chloroquine hydrochloride, up to 250 mg Qp Qh N1 N

Benefit only for diagnosed malaria or amebiasis

Other: Aralen

IOM: 100-02, 15, 50

J0395 Injection, arbutamine HCL, 1 mg Qp Qh E2

IOM: 100-02, 15, 50

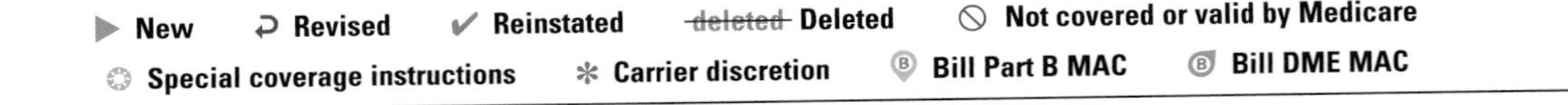

New
Revised
Reinstated
deleted Deleted
Not covered or valid by Medicare
Special coverage instructions
Carrier discretion
Bill Part B MAC
Bill DME MAC

✻ **J0400** Injection, aripiprazole, intramuscular, 0.25 mg Qp Qh K2 K

✻ **J0401** Injection, aripiprazole, extended release, 1 mg Qp Qh K2 K
Other: Abilify Maintena

J0456 Injection, azithromycin, 500 mg Qp Qh N1 N
Other: Zithromax
IOM: 100-02, 15, 50

J0461 Injection, atropine sulfate, 0.01 mg Qp Qh N1 N
IOM: 100-02, 15, 50

J0470 Injection, dimercaprol, per 100 mg Qp Qh K2 K
Other: BAL In Oil
IOM: 100-02, 15, 50

J0475 Injection, baclofen, 10 mg Qp Qh K2 K
Other: Gablofen, Lioresal
IOM: 100-02, 15, 50

J0476 Injection, baclofen 50 mcg for intrathecal trial Qp Qh K2 K
Other: Gablofen, Lioresal
IOM: 100-02, 15, 50

J0480 Injection, basiliximab, 20 mg Qp Qh K2 K
Other: Simulect
IOM: 100-02, 15, 50

✻ **J0485** Injection, belatacept, 1 mg Qp Qh K2 K
Other: Nulojix

✻ **J0490** Injection, belimumab, 10 mg Qp Qh K2 K
Other: Benlysta
Coding Clinic: 2012, Q1, P9

J0500 Injection, dicyclomine HCL, up to 20 mg Qp Qh N1 N
Other: Antispas, Bentyl, Dibent, Dilomine, Di-Spaz, Neoquess, Or-Tyl, Spasmoject
IOM: 100-02, 15, 50

J0515 Injection, benztropine mesylate, per 1 mg Qp Qh N1 N
Other: Cogentin
IOM: 100-02, 15, 50

✻ **J0517** Injection, benralizumab, 1 mg G
Other: Fasenra

J0520 Injection, bethanechol chloride, myotonachol or urecholine, up to 5 mg Qp Qh E2
IOM: 100-02, 15, 50

✻ **J0558** Injection, penicillin G benzathine and penicillin G procaine,100,000 units Qp Qh N1 N
Other: Bicillin C-R
Coding Clinic: 2011, Q1, P8

J0561 Injection, penicillin G benzathine, 100,000 units Qp Qh K2 K
Other: Bicillin L-A, Permapen
IOM: 100-02, 15, 50
Coding Clinic: 2013: Q2, P3; 2011, Q1, P8

✻ **J0565** Injection, bezlotoxumab, 10 mg K2 G

✻ **J0567** Injection, cerliponase alfa, 1 mg G
Other: Brineura

✻ **J0570** Buprenorphine implant, 74.2 mg Qp Qh K2 G
Other: Probuphine System Kit
Coding Clinic: 2017, Q1, P9

J0571 Buprenorphine, oral, 1 mg Qp Qh E1

J0572 Buprenorphine/naloxone, oral, less than or equal to 3 mg buprenorphine Qp Qh E1

J0573 Buprenorphine/naloxone, oral, greater than 3 mg, but less than or equal to 6 mg buprenorphine Qp Qh E1

J0574 Buprenorphine/naloxone, oral, greater than 6 mg, but less than or equal to 10 mg buprenorphine Qp Qh E1

J0575 Buprenorphine/naloxone, oral, greater than 10 mg buprenorphine Qp Qh E1

✻ **J0583** Injection, bivalirudin, 1 mg Qp Qh N1 N
Other: Angiomax

✻ **J0584** Injection, burosumab-twza 1 mg K
Other: Crysvita

J0585 Injection, onabotulinumtoxinaA, 1 unit Qp Qh K2 K
Other: Botox, Botox Cosmetic, Oculinum
IOM: 100-02, 15, 50

✻ **J0586** Injection, abobotulinumtoxinaA, 5 units Qp Qh K2 K

J0587 Injection, rimabotulinumtoxinB, 100 units Qp Qh K2 K
Other: Myobloc, Nplate
IOM: 100-02, 15, 50

MIPS Qp Quantity Physician Qh Quantity Hospital ♀ Female only
♂ Male only A Age DMEPOS A2-Z3 ASC Payment Indicator A-Y ASC Status Indicator Coding Clinic

✻ **J0588** Injection, incobotulinumtoxin A, 1 unit Ⓑ Ⓓ Qp Qh K2 K
Other: Xeomin
Coding Clinic: 2012, Q1, P9

▶ **J0591** Injection, deoxycholic acid, 1 mg E1

⚙ **J0592** Injection, buprenorphine hydrochloride, 0.1 mg Ⓑ Ⓓ Qp Qh N1 N
Other: Buprenex
IOM: 100-02, 15, 50

✻ **J0593** Injection, lanadelumab-flyo, 1 mg (Code may be used for Medicare when drug administered under direct supervision of a physician, not for use when drug is self-administered) K2 K

✻ **J0594** Injection, busulfan, 1 mg Ⓑ Ⓓ Qp Qh K2 K
Other: Myleran

✻ **J0595** Injection, butorphanol tartrate, 1 mg Ⓑ Ⓓ Qp Qh N1 N

✻ **J0596** Injection, C1 esterase inhibitor (recombinant), ruconest, 10 units Ⓑ Ⓓ Qp Qh K2 K

✻ **J0597** Injection, C-1 esterase inhibitor (human), Berinert, 10 units Ⓑ Ⓓ Qp Qh K2 K
Coding Clinic: 2011, Q1, P7

✻ **J0598** Injection, C1 esterase inhibitor (human), cinryze, 10 units Ⓑ Ⓓ Qp Qh K2 K

✻ **J0599** Injection, c-1 esterase inhibitor (human), (haegarda), 10 units G
Other: Berinert

⚙ **J0600** Injection, edetate calcium disodium, up to 1000 mg Ⓑ Ⓓ Qp Qh K2 K
Other: Calcium Disodium Versenate
IOM: 100-02, 15, 50

⚙ **J0604** Cinacalcet, oral, 1 mg, (for ESRD on dialysis) B

⚙ **J0606** Injection, etelcalcetide, 0.1 mg K2 K

⚙ **J0610** Injection, calcium gluconate, per 10 ml Ⓑ Ⓓ Qp Qh N1 N
Other: Kaleinate
IOM: 100-02, 15, 50

⚙ **J0620** Injection, calcium glycerophosphate and calcium lactate, per 10 ml Ⓑ Ⓓ Qp Qh N1 N
Other: Calphosan
MCM: 2049
IOM: 100-02, 15, 50

⚙ **J0630** Injection, calcitonin (salmon), up to 400 units Ⓑ Ⓓ Qp Qh K2 K
Other: Calcimar, Calcitonin-salmon, Miacalcin
IOM: 100-02, 15, 50

⚙ **J0636** Injection, calcitriol, 0.1 mcg Ⓑ Ⓓ Qp Qh N1 N
Non-dialysis use
Other: Calcijex
IOM: 100-02, 15, 50

✻ **J0637** Injection, caspofungin acetate, 5 mg Ⓑ Ⓓ Qp Qh K2 K
Other: Cancidas, Caspofungin

✻ **J0638** Injection, canakinumab, 1 mg Ⓑ Ⓓ Qp Qh K2 K
Other: Ilaris

⚙ **J0640** Injection, leucovorin, calcium, per 50 mg Ⓑ Ⓓ Qp Qh N1 N
Other: Wellcovorin
IOM: 100-02, 15, 50
Coding Clinic: 2009, Q1, P10

⚙ **J0641** Injection, levoleucovorin, not otherwise specified, 0.5 mg Ⓑ Ⓓ Qp Qh K2 K
Part of treatment regimen for osteosarcoma

✻ **J0642** Injection, levoleucovorin, (khapzory), 0.5 mg K2 G

⚙ **J0670** Injection, mepivacaine HCL, per 10 ml Ⓑ Ⓓ Qp Qh N1 N
Other: Carbocaine, Isocaine HCl, Polocaine
IOM: 100-02, 15, 50

⚙ **J0690** Injection, cefezolin sodium, 500 mg Ⓑ Ⓓ Qp Qh N1 N
Other: Ancef, Kefzol, Zolicef
IOM: 100-02, 15, 50

▶ **J0691** Injection, lefamulin, 1 mg K2 G

✻ **J0692** Injection, cefepime HCL, 500 mg Ⓑ Ⓓ Qp Qh N1 N
Other: Maxipime

▶ **J0693** Injection, cefiderocol, 5 mg K2 G

⚙ **J0694** Injection, cefoxitin sodium, 1 gm Ⓑ Ⓓ Qp Qh N1 N
Other: Mefoxin
IOM: 100-02, 15, 50,
Cross Reference Q0090

✻ **J0695** Injection, ceftolozane 50 mg and tazobactam25 mg Ⓑ Ⓓ Qp Qh K2 K
Other: Zerbaxa

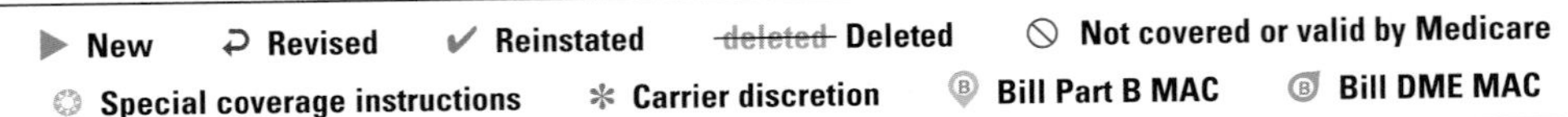
▶ New
↩ Revised
✔ Reinstated
~~deleted~~ Deleted
⦸ Not covered or valid by Medicare
⚙ Special coverage instructions
✻ Carrier discretion
Ⓑ Bill Part B MAC
Ⓓ Bill DME MAC

J0696 Injection, ceftriaxone sodium, per 250 mg Qp Qh N1 N
Other: Rocephin
IOM: 100-02, 15, 50

J0697 Injection, sterile cefuroxime sodium, per 750 mg Qp Qh N1 N
Other: Kefurox, Zinacef
IOM: 100-02, 15, 50

J0698 Injection, cefotaxime sodium, per gm Qp Qh N1 N
Other: Claforan
IOM: 100-02, 15, 50

J0702 Injection, betamethasone acetate 3 mg and betamethasone sodium phosphate 3 mg Qp Qh N1 N
Other: Betameth, Celestone Soluspan, Selestoject
IOM: 100-02, 15, 50
Coding Clinic: 2018, Q4, P6

* **J0706** Injection, caffeine citrate, 5 mg Qp Qh N1 N
Other: Cafcit, Cipro IV, Ciprofloxacin

J0710 Injection, cephapirin sodium, up to 1 gm Qp Qh E2
Other: Cefadyl
IOM: 100-02, 15, 50

* **J0712** Injection, ceftaroline fosamil, 10 mg Qp Qh K2 K
Other: Teflaro
Coding Clinic: 2012, Q1, P9

J0713 Injection, ceftazidime, per 500 mg Qp Qh N1 N
Other: Fortaz, Tazicef
IOM: 100-02, 15, 50

* **J0714** Injection, ceftazidime and avibactam, 0.5 g/0.125 g Qp Qh K2 K

J0715 Injection, ceftizoxime sodium, per 500 mg Qp Qh N1 N
IOM: 100-02, 15, 50

* **J0716** Injection, centruroides immune F(ab)2, up to 120 milligrams Qp Qh K2 K
Other: Anascorp

* **J0717** Injection, certolizumab pegol, 1 mg (Code may be used for Medicare when drug administered under the direct supervision of a physician, not for use when drug is self-administered) Qp Qh K2 K
Other: Cimzia

J0720 Injection, chloramphenicol sodium succinate, up to 1 gm Qp Qh N1 N
Other: Chloromycetin Sodium Succinate
IOM: 100-02, 15, 50

J0725 Injection, chorionic gonadotropin, per 1,000 USP units Qp Qh N1 N
Other: A.P.L., Chorex-5, Chorex-10, Chorignon, Choron-10, Chorionic Gonadotropin, Choron 10, Corgonject-5, Follutein, Glukor, Gonic, Novarel, Pregnyl, Profasi HP
IOM: 100-02, 15, 50

J0735 Injection, clonidine hydrochloride (HCL), 1 mg Qp Qh N1 N
Other: Duraclon
IOM: 100-02, 15, 50

J0740 Injection, cidofovir, 375 mg Qp Qh K2 K
Other: Vistide
IOM: 100-02, 15, 50

▶ **J0742** Injection, imipenem 4 mg, cilastatin 4 mg and relebactam 2 mg K2 G

J0743 Injection, cilastatin sodium; imipenem, per 250 mg Qp Qh N1 N
Other: Primaxin
IOM: 100-02, 15, 50

* **J0744** Injection, ciprofloxacin for intravenous infusion, 200 mg Qp Qh N1 N

J0745 Injection, codeine phosphate, per 30 mg Qp Qh N1 N
IOM: 100-02, 15, 50

J0770 Injection, colistimethate sodium, up to 150 mg Qp Qh N1 N
Other: Coly-Mycin M
IOM: 100-02, 15, 50

* **J0775** Injection, collagenase, clostridium histolyticum, 0.01 mg Qp Qh K2 K
Other: Xiaflex
Coding Clinic: 2011, Q1, P7

J0780 Injection, prochlorperazine, up to 10 mg Qp Qh N1 N
Other: Compa-Z, Compazine, Cotranzine, Ultrazine-10
IOM: 100-02, 15, 50

▶ **J0791** Injection, crizanlizumab-tmca, 5 mg K2 G

MIPS | Qp Quantity Physician | Qh Quantity Hospital | ♀ Female only
♂ Male only | A Age | DMEPOS | A2-Z3 ASC Payment Indicator | A-Y ASC Status Indicator | Coding Clinic

J0795 Injection, corticorelin ovine triflutate, 1 mcg Qp Qh K2 K
Other: Acthrel
IOM: 100-02, 15, 50

J0800 Injection, corticotropin, up to 40 units Qp Qh K2 K
Other: ACTH, Acthar
IOM: 100-02, 15, 50

* **J0834** Injection, cosyntropin, 0.25 mg Qp Qh N1 N

* **J0840** Injection, crotalidae polyvalent immune fab (ovine), up to 1 gram Qp Qh K2 K
Other: Crofab
Coding Clinic: 2012, Q1, P9

* **J0841** Injection, crotalidae immune f(ab')2 (equine), 120 mg K
Other: Anavip

J0850 Injection, cytomegalovirus immune globulin intravenous (human), per vial Qp Qh K2 K
Prophylaxis to prevent cytomegalovirus disease associated with transplantation of kidney, lung, liver, pancreas, and heart.
Other: Cytogam
IOM: 100-02, 15, 50

* **J0875** Injection, dalbavancin, 5 mg Qp Qh K2 K
Other: Dalvance

* **J0878** Injection, daptomycin, 1 mg Qp Qh K2 K
Other: Cubicin

J0881 Injection, darbepoetin alfa, 1 mcg (non-ESRD use) Qp Qh K2 K
Other: Aranesp

J0882 Injection, darbepoetin alfa, 1 mcg (for ESRD on dialysis) Qp Qh K2 K
Other: Aranesp
IOM: 100-02, 6, 10; 100-04, 4, 240

J0883 Injection, argatroban, 1 mg (for non-ESRD use) Qp Qh K2 K
IOM: 100-02, 15, 50

J0884 Injection, argatroban, 1 mg (for ESRD on dialysis) Qp Qh K2 K
IOM: 100-02, 15, 50

J0885 Injection, epoetin alfa, (for non-ESRD use), 1000 units Qp Qh K2 K
Other: Epogen, Procrit
IOM: 100-02, 15, 50
Coding Clinic: 2006, Q2, P5

J0887 Injection, epoetin beta, 1 mcg, (for ESRD on dialysis) Qp Qh N1 N
Other: Mircera

J0888 Injection, epoetin beta, 1 mcg, (for non-ESRD use) Qp Qh K2 K
Other: Mircera

* **J0890** Injection, peginesatide, 0.1 mg (for ESRD on dialysis) Qp Qh E1
Other: Omontys

* **J0894** Injection, decitabine, 1 mg Qp Qh K2 K
Indicated for treatment of myelodysplastic syndromes (MDS)
Other: Dacogen

J0895 Injection, deferoxamine mesylate, 500 mg Qp Qh N1 N
Other: Desferal, Desferal mesylate
IOM: 100-02, 15, 50,
Cross Reference Q0087

▶ **J0896** Injection, luspatercept-aamt, 0.25 mg K2 G

* **J0897** Injection, denosumab, 1 mg Qp Qh K2 K
Other: Prolia, Xgeva
Coding Clinic: 2016, Q1, P5; 2012, Q1, P9

J0945 Injection, brompheniramine maleate, per 10 mg Qp Qh N1 N
Other: Codimal-A, Cophene-B, Dehist, Histaject, Nasahist B, ND Stat, Oraminic II, Sinusol-B
IOM: 100-02, 15, 50

J1000 Injection, depo-estradiol cypionate, up to 5 mg Qp Qh N1 N
Other: DepGynogen, Depogen, Dura-Estrin, Estra-D, Estro-Cyp, Estroject LA, Estronol-LA
IOM: 100-02, 15, 50

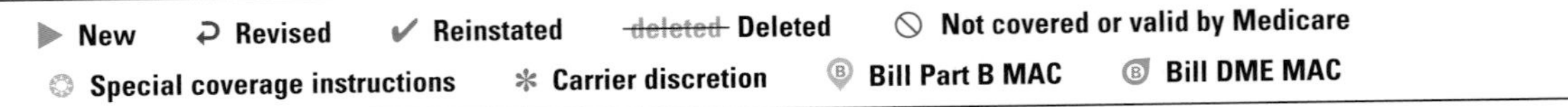
▶ New
Revised
✔ Reinstated
~~deleted~~ Deleted
Not covered or valid by Medicare
Special coverage instructions
* Carrier discretion
Bill Part B MAC
Bill DME MAC

J1020 Injection, methylprednisolone acetate, 20 mg Qp Qh N1 N

Other: DepMedalone, Depoject, Depo-Medrol, Depopred, D-Med 80, Duralone, Medralone, M-Prednisol, Rep-Pred

IOM: 100-02, 15, 50

Coding Clinic: 2019, Q3, P14; 2018, Q4, P5-6; 2005, Q3, P10

J1030 Injection, methylprednisolone acetate, 40 mg Qp Qh N1 N

Other: DepMedalone, Depoject, Depo-Medrol, Depropred, D-Med 80, Duralone, Medralone, M-Prednisol, Rep-Pred

IOM: 100-02, 15, 50

Coding Clinic: 2019, Q3, P14; 2018, Q4, P6; 2005, Q3, P10

J1040 Injection, methylprednisolone acetate, 80 mg Qp Qh N1 N

Other: DepMedalone, Depoject, Depo-Medrol, Depropred, D-Med 80, Duralone, Medralone, M-Prednisol, Rep-Pred

IOM: 100-02, 15, 50

Coding Clinic: 2018, Q4, P6

* **J1050** Injection, medroxyprogesterone acetate, 1 mg Qp Qh N1 N

Other: Depo-Provera Contraceptive

J1071 Injection, testosterone cypionate, 1 mg Qp Qh N1 N

Other: Andro-Cyp, Andro/Fem, Andronaq-LA, Andronate, De-Comberol, DepAndro, DepAndrogyn, Depotest, Depo-Testadiol, Depo-Testosterone, Depotestrogen, Duratest, Duratestrin, Menoject LA, Testa-C, Testadiate-Depo, Testaject-LA, Test-Estro Cypionates, Testoject-LA

Coding Clinic: 2015, Q2, P7

J1094 Injection, dexamethasone acetate, 1 mg Qp Qh N1 N

Other: Dalalone LA, Decadron LA, Decaject LA, Dexacen-LA-8, Dexasone L.A., Dexone-LA, Solurex LA

IOM: 100-02, 15, 50

J1095 Injection, dexamethasone 9%

* **J1096** Dexamethasone, lacrimal ophthalmic insert, 0.1 mg K2 G

* **J1097** Phenylephrine 10.16 mg/ml and ketorolac 2.88 mg/ml ophthalmic irrigation solution, 1 ml K2 G

J1100 Injection, dexamethasone sodium phosphate, 1 mg Qp Qh N1 N

Other: Dalalone, Decadron Phosphate, Decaject, Dexacen-4, Dexone, Hexadrol Phosphate, Solurex

IOM: 100-02, 15, 50

J1110 Injection, dihydroergotamine mesylate, per 1 mg Qp Qh K2 K

Other: D.H.E. 45

IOM: 100-02, 15, 50

J1120 Injection, acetazolamide sodium, up to 500 mg Qp Qh N1 N

Other: Diamox

IOM: 100-02, 15, 50

* **J1130** Injection, diclofenac sodium, 0.5 mg Qp Qh K2 K

Coding Clinic: 2017, Q1, P9

J1160 Injection, digoxin, up to 0.5 mg Qp Qh N1 N

Other: Lanoxin

IOM: 100-02, 15, 50

J1162 Injection, digoxin immune Fab (ovine), per vial Qp Qh K2 K

Other: DigiFab

IOM: 100-02, 15, 50

J1165 Injection, phenytoin sodium, per 50 mg Qp Qh N1 N

Other: Dilantin

IOM: 100-02, 15, 50

J1170 Injection, hydromorphone, up to 4 mg Qp Qh N1 N

Other: Dilaudid

IOM: 100-02, 15, 50

J1180 Injection, dyphylline, up to 500 mg Qp Qh E2

Other: Dilor, Lufyllin

IOM: 100-02, 15, 50

J1190 Injection, dexrazoxane hydrochloride, per 250 mg Qp Qh K2 K

Other: Totect, Zinecard

IOM: 100-02, 15, 50

J1200 Injection, diphenhydramine HCL, up to 50 mg Qp Qh N1 N

Other: Bena-D, Benadryl, Benahist, Ben-Allergin, Benoject, Chlorothiazide sodium, Dihydrex, Diphenacen-50, Hyrexin-50, Nordryl, Wehdryl

IOM: 100-02, 15, 50

▶ **J1201** Injection, cetirizine hydrochloride, 0.5 mg K2 G

⊛ **J1205** Injection, chlorothiazide sodium, per 500 mg Ⓑ Ⓓ Op Oh N1 N
Other: Diuril
IOM: 100-02, 15, 50

⊛ **J1212** Injection, DMSO, dimethyl sulfoxide, 50%, 50 ml Ⓑ Ⓓ Op Oh K2 K
Other: Rimso-50
IOM: 100-02, 15, 50; 100-03, 4, 230.12

⊛ **J1230** Injection, methadone HCL, up to 10 mg Ⓑ Ⓓ Op Oh N1 N
Other: Dolophine HCl
MCM: 2049
IOM: 100-02, 15, 50

⊛ **J1240** Injection, dimenhydrinate, up to 50 mg Ⓑ Ⓓ Op Oh N1 N
Other: Dinate, Dommanate, Dramamine, Dramanate, Dramilin, Dramocen, Dramoject, Dymenate, Hydrate, Marmine, Wehamine
IOM: 100-02, 15, 50

⊛ **J1245** Injection, dipyridamole, per 10 mg Ⓑ Ⓓ Op Oh N1 N
Other: Persantine
IOM: 100-04, 15, 50; 100-04, 12, 30.6

⊛ **J1250** Injection, dobutamine HCL, per 250 mg Ⓑ Ⓓ Op Oh N1 N
Other: Dobutrex
IOM: 100-02, 15, 50

⊛ **J1260** Injection, dolasetron mesylate, 10 mg Ⓑ Ⓓ Op Oh N1 N
Other: Anzemet
IOM: 100-02, 15, 50

✻ **J1265** Injection, dopamine HCL, 40 mg Ⓑ Ⓓ Op Oh N1 N

✻ **J1267** Injection, doripenem, 10 mg Ⓑ Ⓓ Op Oh N1 N
Other: Donbax, Doribax

✻ **J1270** Injection, doxercalciferol, 1 mcg Ⓑ Ⓓ Op Oh N1 N
Other: Hectorol

✻ **J1290** Injection, ecallantide, 1 mg Ⓑ Ⓓ Op Oh K2 K
Other: Kalbitor
Coding Clinic: 2011, Q1, P7

✻ **J1300** Injection, eculizumab, 10 mg Ⓑ Ⓓ Op Oh K2 K
Other: Soliris

✻ **J1301** Injection, edaravone, 1 mg Ⓑ G
Other: Radicava

✻ **J1303** Injection, ravulizumab-cwvz, 10 mg K2 G

⊛ **J1320** Injection, amitriptyline HCL, up to 20 mg Ⓑ Ⓓ Op Oh N1 N
Other: Elavil, Enovil
IOM: 100-02, 15, 50

✻ **J1322** Injection, elosulfase alfa, 1 mg Ⓑ Ⓓ Op Oh K2 K

✻ **J1324** Injection, enfuvirtide, 1 mg Ⓑ Ⓓ Op Oh E2

⊛ **J1325** Injection, epoprostenol, 0.5 mg Ⓑ Ⓓ Op Oh N1 N
Other: Flolan, Veletri
IOM: 100-02, 15, 50

⊛ **J1327** Injection, eptifibatide, 5 mg Ⓑ Ⓓ Op Oh K2 K
Other: Integrilin
IOM: 100-02, 15, 50

⊛ **J1330** Injection, ergonovine maleate, up to 0.2 mg Ⓑ Ⓓ Op Oh N1 N
Benefit limited to obstetrical diagnosis
IOM: 100-02, 15, 50

✻ **J1335** Injection, ertapenem sodium, 500 mg Ⓑ Ⓓ Op Oh N1 N
Other: Invanz

⊛ **J1364** Injection, erythromycin lactobionate, per 500 mg Ⓑ Ⓓ Op Oh K2 K
IOM: 100-02, 15, 50

⊛ **J1380** Injection, estradiol valerate, up to 10 mg Ⓑ Ⓓ Op Oh N1 N
Other: Delestrogen, Dioval, Duragen, Estra-L, Gynogen L.A., L.A.E. 20, Valergen
IOM: 100-02, 15, 50
Coding Clinic: 2011, Q1, P8

⊛ **J1410** Injection, estrogen conjugated, per 25 mg Ⓑ Ⓓ Op Oh K2 K
Other: Premarin
IOM: 100-02, 15, 50

✻ **J1428** Injection, eteplirsen, 10 mg K2 G

▶ **J1429** Injection, golodirsen, 10 mg K2 G

⊛ **J1430** Injection, ethanolamine oleate, 100 mg Ⓑ Ⓓ Op Oh K2 K
Other: Ethamolin
IOM: 100-02, 15, 50

J1435 Injection, estrone, per 1 mg Qp Qh E2
Other: Estronol, Kestrone 5, Theelin Aqueous
IOM: 100-02, 15, 50

J1436 Injection, etidronate disodium, per 300 mg Qp Qh E1
Other: Didronel
IOM: 100-02, 15, 50

J1437 Injection, ferric derisomaltose, 10 mg K2 G

J1438 Injection, etanercept, 25 mg (Code may be used for Medicare when drug administered under the direct supervision of a physician, not for use when drug is self-administered) Qp Qh K2 K
Other: Enbrel
IOM: 100-02, 15, 50

* **J1439** Injection, ferric carboxymaltose, 1 mg Qp Qh K2 K
Other: Injectafer

J1442 Injection, filgrastim (G-CSF), excludes biosimilars, 1 mcg Qp Qh K2 K
Other: Neupogen

* **J1443** Injection, ferric pyrophosphate citrate solution, 0.1 mg of iron Qp Qh N1 N

J1444 Injection, ferric pyrophosphate citrate powder, 0.1 mg of iron N

J1447 Injection, TBO-filgrastim, 1 mcg Qp Qh K2 K
Other: GRANIX
IOM: 100-02, 15, 50

J1450 Injection, fluconazole, 200 mg Qp Qh N1 N
Other: Diflucan
IOM: 100-02, 15, 50

J1451 Injection, fomepizole, 15 mg Qp Qh K2 K
IOM: 100-02, 15, 50

J1452 Injection, fomivirsen sodium, intraocular, 1.65 mg Qp Qh E2
IOM: 100-02, 15, 50

* **J1453** Injection, fosaprepitant, 1 mg Qp Qh K2 K
Prevents chemotherapy-induced nausea and vomiting
Other: Emend

* **J1454** Injection, fosnetupitant 235 mg and palonosetron 0.25 mg G
Other: Akynzeo and Aloxi

J1455 Injection, foscarnet sodium, per 1000 mg Qp Qh K2 K
Other: Foscavir
IOM: 100-02, 15, 50

* **J1457** Injection, gallium nitrate, 1 mg Qp Qh E2

* **J1458** Injection, galsulfase, 1 mg Qp Qh K2 K
Other: Naglazyme

* **J1459** Injection, immune globulin (Privigen), intravenous, non-lyophilized (e.g., liquid), 500 mg Qp Qh K2 K

J1460 Injection, gamma globulin, intramuscular, 1 cc Qp Qh K2 K
Other: Gammar, GamaSTAN
IOM: 100-02, 15, 50
Coding Clinic: 2011, Q1, P8

* **J1555** Injection, immune globulin (cuvitru), 100 mg K2 K

* **J1556** Injection, immune globulin (Bivigam), 500 mg Qp Qh K2 K

* **J1557** Injection, immune globulin, (gammaplex), intravenous, non-lyophilized (e.g., liquid), 500 mg Qp Qh K2 K
Coding Clinic: 2012, Q1, P9

J1558 Injection, immune globulin (xembify), 100 mg K2 G

* **J1559** Injection, immune globulin (hizentra), 100 mg Qp Qh K2 K
Coding Clinic: 2011, Q1, P6

J1560 Injection, gamma globulin, intramuscular, over 10 cc Qp Qh K2 K
Other: Gammar, GamaSTAN
IOM: 100-02, 15, 50

J1561 Injection, immune globulin, (Gamunex-C/Gammaked), non-lyophilized (e.g., liquid), 500 mg Qp Qh K2 K
IOM: 100-02, 15, 50
Coding Clinic: 2012, Q1, P9

* **J1562** Injection, immune globulin (Vivaglobin), 100 mg Qp Qh E2

MIPS | Qp Quantity Physician | Qh Quantity Hospital | ♀ Female only | ♂ Male only | A Age | DMEPOS | A2-Z3 ASC Payment Indicator | A-Y ASC Status Indicator | Coding Clinic

J1566 Injection, immune globulin, intravenous, lyophilized (e.g., powder), not otherwise specified, 500 mg Qp Qh K2 K
Other: Carimune, Gammagard S/D, Polygam
IOM: 100-02, 15, 50

* **J1568** Injection, immune globulin, (Octagam), intravenous, non-lyophilized (e.g., liquid), 500 mg Qp Qh K2 K

J1569 Injection, immune globulin, (Gammagard Liquid), non-lyophilized (e.g., liquid), 500 mg Qp Qh K2 K
IOM: 100-02, 15, 50

J1570 Injection, ganciclovir sodium, 500 mg Qp Qh N1 N
Other: Cytovene
IOM: 100-02, 15, 50

J1571 Injection, hepatitis B immune globulin (HepaGam B), intramuscular, 0.5 ml Qp Qh K2 K
IOM: 100-02, 15, 50
Coding Clinic: 2008, Q3, P7-8

J1572 Injection, immune globulin, (flebogamma/flebogamma DIF) intravenous, non-lyophilized (e.g., liquid), 500 mg Qp Qh K2 K
IOM: 100-02, 15, 50

* **J1573** Injection, hepatitis B immune globulin (HepaGam B), intravenous, 0.5 ml Qp Qh K2 K
Coding Clinic: 2008, Q3, P8

* **J1575** Injection, immune globulin/ hyaluronidase (HYQVIA), 100 mg immunoglobulin Qp Qh K2 K

J1580 Injection, Garamycin, gentamicin, up to 80 mg Qp Qh N1 N
Other: Gentamicin Sulfate, Jenamicin
IOM: 100-02, 15, 50

J1595 Injection, glatiramer acetate, 20 mg Qp Qh K2 K
Other: Copaxone
IOM: 100-02, 15, 50

* **J1599** Injection, immune globulin, intravenous, non-lyophilized (e.g., liquid), not otherwise specified, 500 mg Qp Qh N1 N
Coding Clinic: 2011, P1, Q6

J1600 Injection, gold sodium thiomalate, up to 50 mg Qp Qh E2
Other: Myochrysine
IOM: 100-02, 15, 50

* **J1602** Injection, golimumab, 1 mg for intravenous use Qp Qh K2 K
Other: Simponi Aria

J1610 Injection, glucagon hydrochloride, per 1 mg Qp Qh K2 K
Other: GlucaGen, Glucagon Emergency
IOM: 100-02, 15, 50

J1620 Injection, gonadorelin hydrochloride, per 100 mcg Qp Qh E2
Other: Factrel
IOM: 100-02, 15, 50

J1626 Injection, granisetron hydrochloride, 100 mcg Qp Qh N1 N
Other: Kytril
IOM: 100-02, 15, 50

* **J1627** Injection, granisetron, extended-release, 0.1 mg K2 G

* **J1628** Injection, guselkumab, 1 mg G
Other: Tremfya

J1630 Injection, haloperidol, up to 5 mg Qp Qh N1 N
Other: Haldol, Haloperidol Lactate
IOM: 100-02, 15, 50

J1631 Injection, haloperidol decanoate, per 50 mg Qp Qh N1 N
IOM: 100-02, 15, 50

▶ **J1632** Injection, brexanolone, 1 mg K2 G

J1640 Injection, hemin, 1 mg Qp Qh K2 K
Other: Panhematin
IOM: 100-02, 15, 50

J1642 Injection, heparin sodium (heparin lock flush), per 10 units Qp Qh N1 N
Other: Hep-Lock U/P, Vasceze
IOM: 100-02, 15, 50

J1644 Injection, heparin sodium, per 1000 units Qp Qh N1 N
Other: Heparin Sodium (Porcine), Liquaemin Sodium
IOM: 100-02, 15, 50

J1645 Injection, dalteparin sodium, per 2500 IU Qp Qh N1 N
Other: Fragmin
IOM: 100-02, 15, 50

* **J1650** Injection, enoxaparin sodium, 10 mg Qp Qh N1 N
Other: Lovenox

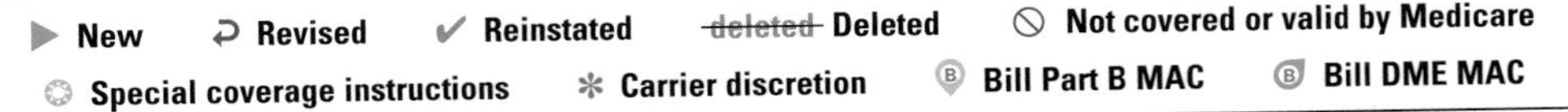
New
Revised
Reinstated
deleted Deleted
Not covered or valid by Medicare
Special coverage instructions
Carrier discretion
Bill Part B MAC
Bill DME MAC

J1652 Injection, fondaparinux sodium, 0.5 mg Qp Qh N1 N
Other: Arixtra
IOM: 100-02, 15, 50

* **J1655** Injection, tinzaparin sodium, 1000 IU Qp Qh N1 N
Other: Innohep

J1670 Injection, tetanus immune globulin, human, up to 250 units Qp Qh K2 K
Indicated for transient protection against tetanus post-exposure to tetanus (Z23).
Other: Hyper-Tet
IOM: 100-02, 15, 50

J1675 Injection, histrelin acetate, 10 mcg Qp Qh B
IOM: 100-02, 15, 50

J1700 Injection, hydrocortisone acetate, up to 25 mg Qp Qh N1 N
Other: Hydrocortone Acetate
IOM: 100-02, 15, 50

J1710 Injection, hydrocortisone sodium phosphate, up to 50 mg Qp Qh N1 N
Other: A-hydroCort, Hydrocortone phosphate, Solu-Cortef
IOM: 100-02, 15, 50

J1720 Injection, hydrocortisone sodium succinate, up to 100 mg Qp Qh N1 N
Other: A-HydroCort, Solu-Cortef
IOM: 100-02, 15, 50

* **J1726** Injection, hydroxyprogesterone caproate (makena), 10 mg K2 K

* **J1729** Injection, hydroxyprogesterone caproate, not otherwise specified, 10 mg N1 N

J1730 Injection, diazoxide, up to 300 mg Qp Qh E2
Other: Hyperstat
IOM: 100-02, 15, 50

▶ **J1738** Injection, meloxicam, 1 mg K2 G

* **J1740** Injection, ibandronate sodium, 1 mg Qp Qh K2 K
Other: Boniva

* **J1741** Injection, ibuprofen, 100 mg Qp Qh N1 N
Other: Caldolor

J1742 Injection, ibutilide fumarate, 1 mg Qp Qh K2 K
Other: Corvert
IOM: 100-02, 15, 50

* **J1743** Injection, idursulfase, 1 mg Qp Qh K2 K
Other: Elaprase

* **J1744** Injection, icatibant, 1 mg Qp Qh K2 K
Other: Firazyr

J1745 Injection, infliximab, excludes biosimilar, 10 mg Qp Qh K2 K
Report total number of 10 mg increments administered
For biosimilar, Inflectra, report Q5102
Other: Remicade
IOM: 100-02, 15, 50

* **J1746** Injection, ibalizumab-uiyk, 10 mg K
Other: Trogarzo

J1750 Injection, iron dextran, 50 mg Qp Qh K2 K
Other: Dexferrum, Imferon, Infed
IOM: 100-02, 15, 50

* **J1756** Injection, iron sucrose, 1 mg Qp Qh N1 N
Other: Venofer

J1786 Injection, imiglucerase, 10 units Qp Qh K2 K
Other: Cerezyme
IOM: 100-02, 15, 50
Coding Clinic: 2011, Q1, P8

J1790 Injection, droperidol, up to 5 mg Qp Qh N1 N
Other: Inapsine
IOM: 100-02, 15, 50

J1800 Injection, propranolol HCL, up to 1 mg Qp Qh N1 N
Other: Inderal
IOM: 100-02, 15, 50

J1810 Injection, droperidol and fentanyl citrate, up to 2 ml ampule Qp Qh E1
Other: Innovar
IOM: 100-02, 15, 50

MIPS | Qp Quantity Physician | Qh Quantity Hospital | ♀ Female only
♂ Male only | A Age | DMEPOS | A2-Z3 ASC Payment Indicator | A-Y ASC Status Indicator | Coding Clinic

J1815 Injection, insulin, per 5 units Qp Qh N1 N

Other: Humalog, Humulin, Lantus, Novolin, Novolog

IOM: 100-02, 15, 50; 100-03, 4, 280.14

* **J1817** Insulin for administration through DME (i.e., insulin pump) per 50 units Qp Qh N1 N

Other: Apidra Solostar, Insulin Lispro, Humalog, Humulin, Novolin, Novolog

▶ **J1823** Injection, inebilizumab-cdon, 1 mg K2 G

* **J1826** Injection, interferon beta-1a, 30 mcg K2 K

Other: Avonex

Coding Clinic: 2011, Q2, P9; Q1, P8

J1830 Injection, interferon beta-1b, 0.25 mg (Code may be used for Medicare when drug administered under the direct supervision of a physician, not for use when drug is self-administered) Qp Qh K2 K

Other: Betaseron

IOM: 100-02, 15, 50

* **J1833** Injection, isavuconazonium, 1 mg Qp Qh K2 K

* **J1835** Injection, itraconazole, 50 mg Qp Qh E2

Other: Sporanox

J1840 Injection, kanamycin sulfate, up to 500 mg Qp Qh N1 N

Other: Kantrex, Klebcil

IOM: 100-02, 15, 50

J1850 Injection, kanamycin sulfate, up to 75 mg Qp Qh N1 N

Other: Kantrex, Klebcil

IOM: 100-02, 15, 50

Coding Clinic: 2013: Q2, P3

J1885 Injection, ketorolac tromethamine, per 15 mg Qp Qh N1 N

Other: Toradol

IOM: 100-02, 15, 50

J1890 Injection, cephalothin sodium, up to 1 gram Qp Qh N1 N

Other: Keflin

IOM: 100-02, 15, 50

* **J1930** Injection, lanreotide, 1 mg Qp Qh K2 K

Treats acromegaly and symptoms caused by neuroendocrine tumors

Other: Somatuline Depot

* **J1931** Injection, laronidase, 0.1 mg Qp Qh K2 K

Other: Aldurazyme

J1940 Injection, furosemide, up to 20 mg Qp Qh N1 N

Other: Furomide M.D., Lasix

MCM: 2049

IOM: 100-02, 15, 50

* **J1943** Injection, aripiprazole lauroxil, (aristada initio), 1 mg K2 G

* **J1944** Injection, aripiprazole lauroxil, (aristada), 1 mg K2 K

J1945 Injection, lepirudin, 50 mg Qp Qh E2

IOM: 100-02, 15, 50

J1950 Injection, leuprolide acetate (for depot suspension), per 3.75 mg Qp Qh K2 K

Other: Lupron, Lupron Depot, Lupron Depot-Ped

IOM: 100-02, 15, 50

Coding Clinic: 2019, Q2, P11-12

* **J1953** Injection, levetiracetam, 10 mg Qp Qh N1 N

Other: Keppra

J1955 Injection, levocarnitine, per 1 gm Qp Qh B

Other: Carnitor

IOM: 100-02, 15, 50

J1956 Injection, levofloxacin, 250 mg Qp Qh N1 N

Other: Levaquin

IOM: 100-02, 15, 50

J1960 Injection, levorphanol tartrate, up to 2 mg Qp Qh N1 N

Other: Levo-Dromoran

MCM: 2049

IOM: 100-02, 15, 50

J1980 Injection, hyoscyamine sulfate, up to 0.25 mg Qp Qh N1 N

Other: Levsin

IOM: 100-02, 15, 50

▶ New ↩ Revised ✓ Reinstated ~~deleted~~ Deleted ⊘ Not covered or valid by Medicare
Special coverage instructions * Carrier discretion Bill Part B MAC Bill DME MAC

J1990 Injection, chlordiazepoxide HCL, up to 100 mg Qp Qh N1 N
Other: Librium
IOM: 100-02, 15, 50

J2001 Injection, lidocaine HCL for intravenous infusion, 10 mg Qp Qh N1 N
Other: Caine-1, Caine-2, Dilocaine, L-Caine, Lidocaine in D5W, Lidoject, Nervocaine, Nulicaine, Xylocaine
IOM: 100-02, 15, 50

J2010 Injection, lincomycin HCL, up to 300 mg Qp Qh N1 N
Other: Lincocin
IOM: 100-02, 15, 50

* **J2020** Injection, linezolid, 200 mg Qp Qh N1 N
Other: Zyvox

J2060 Injection, lorazepam, 2 mg Qp Qh N1 N
Other: Ativan
IOM: 100-02, 15, 50

* **J2062** Loxapine for inhalation, 1 mg K
Other: Adasuve

J2150 Injection, mannitol, 25% in 50 ml Qp Qh N1 N
Other: Aridol
MCM: 2049
IOM: 100-02, 15, 50

* **J2170** Injection, mecasermin, 1 mg Qp Qh N1 N
Other: Increlex

J2175 Injection, meperidine hydrochloride, per 100 mg Qp Qh N1 N
Other: Demerol
IOM: 100-02, 15, 50

J2180 Injection, meperidine and promethazine HCL, up to 50 mg Qp Qh N1 N
Other: Mepergan
IOM: 100-02, 15, 50

* **J2182** Injection, mepolizumab, 1 mg Qp Qh K2 G

* **J2185** Injection, meropenem, 100 mg Qp Qh N1 N
Other: Merrem

* **J2186** Inj., meropenem, vaborbactam G
Other: Vabomere
Medicare Statute 1833(t)

J2210 Injection, methylergonovine maleate, up to 0.2 mg Qp Qh N1 N
Benefit limited to obstetrical diagnoses for prevention and control of post-partum hemorrhage
Other: Methergine
IOM: 100-02, 15, 50

* **J2212** Injection, methylnaltrexone, 0.1 mg Qp Qh N1 N
Other: Relistor

* **J2248** Injection, micafungin sodium, 1 mg Qp Qh N1 N
Other: Mycamine

J2250 Injection, midazolam hydrochloride, per 1 mg Qp Qh N1 N
Other: Versed
IOM: 100-02, 15, 50

J2260 Injection, milrinone lactate, 5 mg Qp Qh N1 N
Other: Primacor
IOM: 100-02, 15, 50

* **J2265** Injection, minocycline hydrochloride, 1 mg Qp Qh K2 K
Other: Minocine

J2270 Injection, morphine sulfate, up to 10 mg Qp Qh N1 N
Other: Astramorph PF, Duramorph
IOM: 100-02, 15, 50
Coding Clinic: 2013, Q2, P4

J2274 Injection, morphine sulfate, preservative-free for epidural or intrathecal use, 10 mg Qp Qh N1 N
Other: Duramorph, Infumorph
IOM: 100-03, 4, 280.1; 100-02, 15, 50

J2278 Injection, ziconotide, 1 mcg Qp Qh K2 K
Other: Prialt

* **J2280** Injection, moxifloxacin, 100 mg Qp Qh N1 N
Other: Avelox

J2300 Injection, nalbuphine hydrochloride, per 10 mg Qp Qh N1 N
Other: Nubain
IOM: 100-02, 15, 50

J2310 Injection, naloxone hydrochloride, per 1 mg Qp Qh N1 N
Other: Narcan
IOM: 100-02, 15, 50

MIPS Qp Quantity Physician Qh Quantity Hospital ♀ Female only
♂ Male only A Age DMEPOS A2-Z3 ASC Payment Indicator A-Y ASC Status Indicator Coding Clinic

✻ **J2315** Injection, naltrexone, depot form, 1 mg Ⓑ Ⓓ Qp Qh K2 K
Other: Vivitrol

◌ **J2320** Injection, nandrolone decanoate, up to 50 mg Ⓑ Ⓓ Qp Qh K2 K
Other: Anabolin LA 100, Androlone, Deca-Durabolin, Decolone, Hybolin Decanoate, Nandrobolic LA, Neo-Durabolic
IOM: 100-02, 15, 50
Coding Clinic: 2011, Q1, P8

✻ **J2323** Injection, natalizumab, 1 mg Ⓑ Ⓓ Qp Qh K2 K
Other: Tysabri

◌ **J2325** Injection, nesiritide, 0.1 mg Ⓑ Ⓓ Qp Qh K2 K
Other: Natrecor
IOM: 100-02, 15, 50

✻ **J2326** Injection, nusinersen, 0.1 mg K2 G
Coding Clinic: 2020, Q1, P11

✻ **J2350** Injection, ocrelizumab, 1 mg K2 G

✻ **J2353** Injection, octreotide, depot form for intramuscular injection, 1 mg Ⓑ Ⓓ Qp Qh K2 K
Other: Sandostatin LAR Depot

✻ **J2354** Injection, octreotide, non-depot form for subcutaneous or intravenous injection, 25 mcg Ⓑ Ⓓ Qp Qh N1 N
Other: Sandostatin LAR Depot

◌ **J2355** Injection, oprelvekin, 5 mg Ⓑ Ⓓ Qp Qh K2 K
Other: Neumega
IOM: 100-02, 15, 50

✻ **J2357** Injection, omalizumab, 5 mg Ⓑ Ⓓ Qp Qh K2 K
Other: Xolair

✻ **J2358** Injection, olanzapine, long-acting, 1 mg Ⓑ Ⓓ Qp Qh N1 N
Other: Zyprexa Relprevv
Coding Clinic: 2011, Q1, P6

◌ **J2360** Injection, orphenadrine citrate, up to 60 mg Ⓑ Ⓓ Qp Qh N1 N
Other: Antiflex, Banflex, Flexoject, Flexon, K-Flex, Myolin, Neocyten, Norflex, O-Flex, Orphenate
IOM: 100-02, 15, 50

◌ **J2370** Injection, phenylephrine HCL, up to 1 ml Ⓑ Ⓓ Qp Qh N1 N
Other: Neo-Synephrine
IOM: 100-02, 15, 50

◌ **J2400** Injection, chloroprocaine hydrochloride, per 30 ml Ⓑ Ⓓ Qp Qh N1 N
Other: Nesacaine, Nesacaine-MPF
IOM: 100-02, 15, 50

◌ **J2405** Injection, ondansetron hydrochloride, per 1 mg Ⓑ Ⓓ Qp Qh N1 N
Other: Zofran
IOM: 100-02, 15, 50

◌ **J2407** Injection, oritavancin, 10 mg Ⓑ Ⓓ Qp Qh K2 K
Other: Orbactiv
IOM: 100-02, 15, 50

◌ **J2410** Injection, oxymorphone HCL, up to 1 mg Ⓑ Ⓓ Qp Qh N1 N
Other: Numorphan, Opana
IOM: 100-02, 15, 50

✻ **J2425** Injection, palifermin, 50 mcg Ⓑ Ⓓ Qp Qh K2 K
Other: Kepivance

✻ **J2426** Injection, paliperidone palmitate extended release, 1 mg Ⓑ Ⓓ Qp Qh K2 K
Other: Invega Sustenna
Coding Clinic: 2011, Q1, P7

◌ **J2430** Injection, pamidronate disodium, per 30 mg Ⓑ Ⓓ Qp Qh N1 N
Other: Aredia
IOM: 100-02, 15, 50

◌ **J2440** Injection, papaverine HCL, up to 60 mg Ⓑ Ⓓ Qp Qh N1 N
IOM: 100-02, 15, 50

◌ **J2460** Injection, oxytetracycline HCL, up to 50 mg Ⓑ Ⓓ Qp Qh E2
Other: Terramycin IM
IOM: 100-02, 15, 50

✻ **J2469** Injection, palonosetron HCL, 25 mcg Ⓑ Ⓓ Qp Qh K2 K
Example: 0.25 mgm dose = 10 units
Example of use is acute, delayed, nausea and vomiting due to chemotherapy
Other: Aloxi

◌ **J2501** Injection, paricalcitol, 1 mcg Ⓑ Ⓓ Qp Qh N1 N
Other: Zemplar
IOM: 100-02, 15, 50

▶ New ⤾ Revised ✔ Reinstated ~~deleted~~ Deleted ⊘ Not covered or valid by Medicare
◌ Special coverage instructions ✻ Carrier discretion Ⓑ Bill Part B MAC Ⓓ Bill DME MAC

* **J2502** Injection, pasireotide long acting, 1 mg Qp Qh K2 K
  Other: Signifor LAR

* **J2503** Injection, pegaptanib sodium, 0.3 mg Qp Qh K2 K
  Other: Macugen

J2504 Injection, pegademase bovine, 25 IU Qp Qh K2 K
  Other: Adagen
  IOM: 100-02, 15, 50

* **J2505** Injection, pegfilgrastim, 6 mg Qp Qh K2 K
  Report 1 unit per 6 mg.
  Other: Neulasta

* **J2507** Injection, pegloticase, 1 mg Qp Qh K2 K
  Other: Krystexxa
  Coding Clinic: 2012, Q1, P9

J2510 Injection, penicillin G procaine, aqueous, up to 600,000 units Qp Qh N1 N
  Other: Crysticillin, Duracillin AS, Pfizerpen AS, Wycillin
  IOM: 100-02, 15, 50

J2513 Injection, pentastarch, 10% solution, 100 ml Qp Qh E2
  IOM: 100-02, 15, 50

J2515 Injection, pentobarbital sodium, per 50 mg Qp Qh K2 K
  Other: Nembutal sodium solution
  IOM: 100-02, 15, 50

J2540 Injection, penicillin G potassium, up to 600,000 units Qp Qh N1 N
  Other: Pfizerpen-G
  IOM: 100-02, 15, 50

J2543 Injection, piperacillin sodium/tazobactam sodium, 1 gram/0.125 grams (1.125 grams) Qp Qh N1 N
  Other: Zosyn
  IOM: 100-02, 15, 50

J2545 Pentamidine isethionate, inhalation solution, FDA-approved final product, non-compounded, administered through DME, unit dose form, per 300 mg Qp Qh B
  Other: Nebupent

* **J2547** Injection, peramivir, 1 mg Qp Qh K2 K

J2550 Injection, promethazine HCL, up to 50 mg Qp Qh N1 N
  Administration of phenergan suppository considered part of E/M encounter
  Other: Anergan, Phenazine, Phenergan, Prorex, Prothazine, V-Gan
  IOM: 100-02, 15, 50

J2560 Injection, phenobarbital sodium, up to 120 mg Qp Qh N1 N
  Other: Luminal Sodium
  IOM: 100-02, 15, 50

* **J2562** Injection, plerixafor, 1 mg Qp Qh K2 K
  FDA approved for non-Hodgkin lymphoma and multiple myeloma in 2008.
  Other: Mozobil

J2590 Injection, oxytocin, up to 10 units Qp Qh N1 N
  Other: Pitocin, Syntocinon
  IOM: 100-02, 15, 50

J2597 Injection, desmopressin acetate, per 1 mcg Qp Qh K2 K
  Other: DDAVP
  IOM: 100-02, 15, 50

J2650 Injection, prednisolone acetate, up to 1 ml Qp Qh N1 N
  Other: Key-Pred, Predalone, Predcor, Predicort, Predoject
  IOM: 100-02, 15, 50

J2670 Injection, tolazoline HCL, up to 25 mg Qp Qh N1 N
  Other: Priscoline HCl
  IOM: 100-02, 15, 50

J2675 Injection, progesterone, per 50 mg Qp Qh N1 N
  Other: Gesterol 50, Progestaject
  IOM: 100-02, 15, 50

J2680 Injection, fluphenazine decanoate, up to 25 mg Qp Qh N1 N
  Other: Prolixin Decanoate
  MCM: 2049
  IOM: 100-02, 15, 50

J2690 Injection, procainamide HCL, up to 1 gm Qp Qh ♀ N1 N
  Benefit limited to obstetrical diagnoses
  Other: Pronestyl, Prostaphlin
  IOM: 100-02, 15, 50

J2700 Injection, oxacillin sodium, up to 250 mg Qp Qh N1 N
Other: Bactocill
IOM: 100-02, 15, 50

J2704 Injection, propofol, 10 mg Qp Qh N1 N
Other: Diprivan

J2710 Injection, neostigmine methylsulfate, up to 0.5 mg Qp Qh N1 N
Other: Prostigmin
IOM: 100-02, 15, 50

J2720 Injection, protamine sulfate, per 10 mg Qp Qh N1 N
IOM: 100-02, 15, 50

J2724 Injection, protein C concentrate, intravenous, human, 10 IU Qp Qh K2 K
Other: Ceprotin

J2725 Injection, protirelin, per 250 mcg Qp Qh E2
Other: Relefact TRH, Thypinone
IOM: 100-02, 15, 50

J2730 Injection, pralidoxime chloride, up to 1 gm Qp Qh N1 N
Other: Protopam Chloride
IOM: 100-02, 15, 50

J2760 Injection, phentolamine mesylate, up to 5 mg Qp Qh K2 K
Other: Regitine
IOM: 100-02, 15, 50

J2765 Injection, metoclopramide HCL, up to 10 mg Qp Qh N1 N
Other: Reglan
IOM: 100-02, 15, 50

J2770 Injection, quinupristin/dalfopristin, 500 mg (150/350) Qp Qh K2 K
Other: Synercid
IOM: 100-02, 15, 50

J2778 Injection, ranibizumab, 0.1 mg Qp Qh K2 K
May be reported for exudative senile macular degeneration (wet AMD) with 67028 (RT or LT)
Other: Lucentis

J2780 Injection, ranitidine hydrochloride, 25 mg Qp Qh N1 N
Other: Zantac
IOM: 100-02, 15, 50

J2783 Injection, rasburicase, 0.5 mg Qp Qh K2 K
Other: Elitek

J2785 Injection, regadenoson, 0.1 mg Qp Qh N1 N
One billing unit equal to 0.1 mg of regadenoson
Other: Lexiscan

J2786 Injection, reslizumab, 1 mg Qp Qh K2 G
Coding Clinic: 2016, Q4, P9

J2787 Riboflavin 5'-phosphate, ophthalmic solution, up to 3 mL
Other: Photrexa Viscous

J2788 Injection, Rho D immune globulin, human, minidose, 50 mcg (250 IU) Qp Qh N1 N
Other: HypRho-D, MicRhoGAM, Rhesonativ, RhoGam
IOM: 100-02, 15, 50

J2790 Injection, Rho D immune globulin, human, full dose, 300 mcg (1500 IU) Qp Qh N1 N
Administered to pregnant female to prevent hemolistic disease of newborn. Report 90384 to private payer
Other: Gamulin Rh, Hyperrho S/D, HypRho-D, Rhesonativ, RhoGAM
IOM: 100-02, 15, 50

J2791 Injection, Rho(D) immune globulin (human), (Rhophylac), intramuscular or intravenous, 100 IU Qp Qh N1 N
Agent must be billed per 100 IU in both physician office and hospital outpatient settings
Other: HypRho-D
IOM: 100-02, 15, 50

J2792 Injection, Rho D immune globulin intravenous, human, solvent detergent, 100 IU Qp Qh K2 K
Other: Gamulin Rh, Hyperrho S/D, WinRHo-SDF
IOM: 100-02, 15, 50

J2793 Injection, rilonacept, 1 mg Qp Qh K2 K
Other: Arcalyst
IOM: 100-02, 15, 50

J2794 Injection, risperidone (risperdal consta), 0.5 mg Qp Qh K2 K
Other: Risperdal Costa

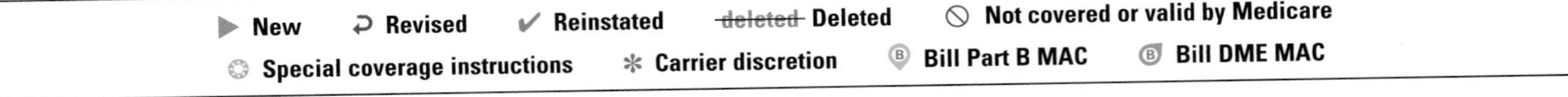

New
Revised
Reinstated
~~deleted~~ Deleted
Not covered or valid by Medicare
Special coverage instructions
Carrier discretion
Bill Part B MAC
Bill DME MAC

✻ **J2795** Injection, ropivacaine hydrochloride, 1 mg Qp Qh N1 N
Other: Naropin

✻ **J2796** Injection, romiplostim, 10 mcg Qp Qh K2 K
Stimulates bone marrow megakarocytes to produce platelets (i.e., ITP)
Other: Nplate

J2797 Injection, rolapitant, 0.5 mg G
Other: Varubi

✻ **J2798** Injection, risperidone, (perseris), 0.5 mg K2 G

J2800 Injection, methocarbamol, up to 10 ml Qp Qh N1 N
Other: Robaxin
IOM: 100-02, 15, 50

✻ **J2805** Injection, sincalide, 5 mcg Qp Qh N1 N
Other: Kinevac

J2810 Injection, theophylline, per 40 mg Qp Qh N1 N
IOM: 100-02, 15, 50

J2820 Injection, sargramostim (GM-CSF), 50 mcg Qp Qh K2 K
Other: Leukine, Prokine
IOM: 100-02, 15, 50

✻ **J2840** Injection, sebelipase alfa, 1 mg Qp Qh K2 G

J2850 Injection, secretin, synthetic, human, 1 mcg Qp Qh K2 K
Other: Chirhostim
IOM: 100-02, 15, 50

✻ **J2860** Injection, siltuximab, 10 mg Qp Qh K2 K

J2910 Injection, aurothioglucose, up to 50 mg Qp Qh E2
Other: Solganal
IOM: 100-02, 15, 50

J2916 Injection, sodium ferric gluconate complex in sucrose injection, 12.5 mg Qp Qh N1 N
Other: Ferrlecit, Nulecit
IOM: 100-02, 15, 50

J2920 Injection, methylprednisolone sodium succinate, up to 40 mg Qp Qh N1 N
Other: A-MethaPred, Solu-Medrol
IOM: 100-02, 15, 50

J2930 Injection, methylprednisolone sodium succinate, up to 125 mg Qp Qh N1 N
Other: A-MethaPred, Solu-Medrol
IOM: 100-02, 15, 50

J2940 Injection, somatrem, 1 mg Qp Qh E2
IOM: 100-02, 15, 50,
Medicare Statute 1861s2b

J2941 Injection, somatropin, 1 mg Qp Qh K2 K
Other: Genotropin, Humatrope, Nutropin, Omnitrope, Saizen, Serostim, Zorbtive
IOM: 100-02, 15, 50,
Medicare Statute 1861s2b

J2950 Injection, promazine HCL, up to 25 mg Qp Qh N1 N
Other: Prozine-50, Sparine
IOM: 100-02, 15, 50

J2993 Injection, reteplase, 18.1 mg Qp Qh K2 K
Other: Retavase
IOM: 100-02, 15, 50

J2995 Injection, streptokinase, per 250,000 IU Qp Qh N1 N
Bill 1 unit for each 250,000 IU
Other: Kabikinase, Streptase
IOM: 100-02, 15, 50

J2997 Injection, alteplase recombinant, 1 mg Qp Qh K2 K
Thrombolytic agent, treatment of occluded catheters. Bill units of 1 mg administered.
Other: Activase, Cathflo Activase
IOM: 100-02, 15, 50
Coding Clinic: 2014, Q1, P4

J3000 Injection, streptomycin, up to 1 gm Qp Qh N1 N
IOM: 100-02, 15, 50

J3010 Injection, fentanyl citrate, 0.1 mg Qp Qh N1 N
Other: Sublimaze
IOM: 100-02, 15, 50

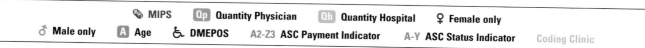

MIPS Qp Quantity Physician Qh Quantity Hospital ♀ Female only
♂ Male only A Age DMEPOS A2-Z3 ASC Payment Indicator A-Y ASC Status Indicator Coding Clinic

J3030 Injection, sumatriptan succinate, 6 mg (Code may be used for Medicare when drug administered under the direct supervision of a physician, not for use when drug is self-administered) Ⓑ Ⓓ Qp Qh N1 N

Other: Imitrex, Sumarel Dosepro

IOM: 100-02, 15, 150

✻ **J3031** Injection, fremanezumab-vfrm, 1 mg (Code may be used for Medicare when drug administered under the direct supervision of a physician, not for use when drug is self-administered) K2 G

▶ **J3032** Injection, eptinezumab-jjmr, 1 mg K2 G

✻ **J3060** Injection, taliglucerase alfa, 10 units Ⓑ Ⓓ Qp Qh K2 K

Other: Elelyso

J3070 Injection, pentazocine, 30 mg Ⓑ Ⓓ Qp Qh K2 K

Other: Talwin

IOM: 100-02, 15, 50

✻ **J3090** Injection, tedizolid phosphate, 1 mg Ⓑ Ⓓ Qp Qh K2 K

Other: Sivextro

✻ **J3095** Injection, televancin, 10 mg Ⓑ Ⓓ Qp Qh K2 K

Prescribed for the treatment of adults with complicated skin and skin structure infections (cSSSI) of the following Gram-positive microorganisms: Staphylococcus aureus; Streptococcus pyogenes, Streptococcus agalactiae, Streptococcus anginosusgroup. Separately payable under the ASC payment system.

Other: Vibativ

Coding Clinic: 2011, Q1, P7

✻ **J3101** Injection, tenecteplase, 1 mg Ⓑ Ⓓ Qp Qh K2 K

Other: TNKase

J3105 Injection, terbutaline sulfate, up to 1 mg Ⓑ Ⓓ Qp Qh N1 N

Other: Brethine

IOM: 100-02, 15, 50

J3110 Injection, teriparatide, 10 mcg Ⓑ Ⓓ Qp Qh B

✻ **J3111** Injection, romosozumab-aqqg, 1 mg K2 G

J3121 Injection, testosterone enanthate, 1 mg Ⓑ Ⓓ Qp Qh N1 N

Other: Andrest 90-4, Andro L.A. 200, Andro-Estro 90-4, Androgyn L.A, Andropository 100, Andryl 200, Deladumone, Deladumone OB, Delatest, Delatestadiol, Delatestryl, Ditate-DS, Dua-Gen L.A., Duoval P.A., Durathate-200, Estra-Testrin, Everone, TEEV, Testadiate, Testone LA, Testradiol 90/4, Testrin PA, Valertest

J3145 Injection, testosterone undecanoate, 1 mg Ⓑ Ⓓ Qp Qh K2 K

J3230 Injection, chlorpromazine HCL, up to 50 mg Ⓑ Ⓓ Qp Qh N1 N

Other: Ormazine, Thorazine

IOM: 100-02, 15, 50

J3240 Injection, thyrotropin alfa, 0.9 mg provided in 1.1 mg vial Ⓑ Ⓓ Qp Qh K2 K

Other: Thyrogen

IOM: 100-02, 15, 50

▶ **J3241** Injection, teprotumumab-trbw, 10 mg K2 G

✻ **J3243** Injection, tigecycline, 1 mg Ⓑ Ⓓ Qp Qh K2 K

✻ **J3245** Injection, tildrakizumab, 1 mg Ⓑ Ⓓ E2

Other: Ilumya

✻ **J3246** Injection, tirofiban HCL, 0.25 mg Ⓑ Ⓓ Qp Qh K2 K

Other: Aggrastat

J3250 Injection, trimethobenzamide HCL, up to 200 mg Ⓑ Ⓓ Qp Qh N1 N

Other: Arrestin, Ticon, Tigan, Tiject 20

IOM: 100-02, 15, 50

J3260 Injection, tobramycin sulfate, up to 80 mg Ⓑ Ⓓ Qp Qh N1 N

Other: Nebcin

IOM: 100-02, 15, 50

✻ **J3262** Injection, tocilizumab, 1 mg Ⓑ Ⓓ Qp Qh K2 K

Indicated for the treatment of adult patients with moderately to severely active rheumatoid arthritis (RA) who have had an inadequate response to one or more tumor necrosis factor (TNF) antagonist therapies.

Other: Actemra

Coding Clinic: 2011, Q1, P7

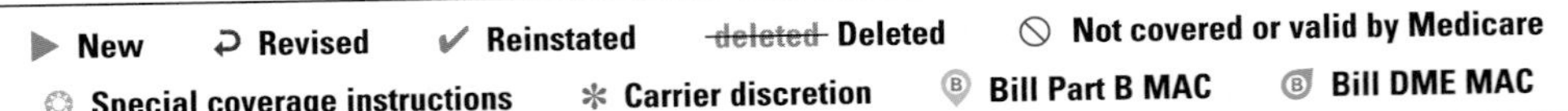
▶ New
Revised
✔ Reinstated
~~deleted~~ Deleted
Not covered or valid by Medicare
Special coverage instructions
✻ Carrier discretion
Bill Part B MAC
Bill DME MAC

J3265 Injection, torsemide, 10 mg/ml Qp Qh N1 N
Other: Demadex
IOM: 100-02, 15, 50

J3280 Injection, thiethylperazine maleate, up to 10 mg Qp Qh E2
Other: Norzine, Torecan
IOM: 100-02, 15, 50

*** J3285** Injection, treprostinil, 1 mg Qp Qh K2 K
Other: Remodulin

J3300 Injection, triamcinolone acetonide, preservative free, 1 mg Qp Qh K2 K
Other: Cenacort A-40, Kenaject-40, Kenalog, Triam-A, Triesence, Tri-Kort, Trilog

J3301 Injection, triamcinolone acetonide, not otherwise specified, 10 mg Qp Qh N1 N
Other: Cenacort A-40, Kenaject-40, Kenalog, Triam A, Triesence, Tri-Kort, Trilog
IOM: 100-02, 15, 50
Coding Clinic: 2018, Q4, P7; 2013, Q2, P4

J3302 Injection, triamcinolone diacetate, per 5 mg Qp Qh N1 N
Other: Amcort, Aristocort , Cenacort Forte, Trilone
IOM: 100-02, 15, 50

J3303 Injection, triamcinolone hexacetonide, per 5 mg Qp Qh N1 N
Other: Aristospan
IOM: 100-02, 15, 50

J3304 Injection, triamcinolone acetonide, preservative-free, extended-release, microsphere formulation, 1 mg G
Other: Zilretta

J3305 Injection, trimetrexate glucuronate, per 25 mg Qp Qh E2
Other: NeuTrexin
IOM: 100-02, 15, 50

J3310 Injection, perphenazine, up to 5 mg Qp Qh N1 N
Other: Trilafon
IOM: 100-02, 15, 50

J3315 Injection, triptorelin pamoate, 3.75 mg Qp Qh K2 K
Other: Trelstar
IOM: 100-02, 15, 50

J3316 Injection, triptorelin, extended-release, 3.75 mg G
Other: Trelstar, Trelstar Depot, Trelstar LA

J3320 Injection, spectinomycin dihydrochloride, up to 2 gm Qp Qh E2
Other: Trobicin
IOM: 100-02, 15, 50

J3350 Injection, urea, up to 40 gm Qp Qh N1 N
Other: Ureaphil
IOM: 100-02, 15, 50

J3355 Injection, urofollitropin, 75 IU Qp Qh E2
Other: Bravelle, Metrodin
IOM: 100-02, 15, 50

*** J3357** Ustekinumab, for subcutaneous injection, 1 mg Qp Qh K2 K
Other: Stelara
Coding Clinic: 2017, Q1, P3; 2016, Q4, P10; 2011, Q1, P7

*** J3358** Ustekinumab, for intravenous injection, 1 mg K2 G
Cross Reference Q9989

J3360 Injection, diazepam, up to 5 mg Qp Qh N1 N
Other: Valium, Zetran
IOM: 100-02, 15, 50
Coding Clinic: 2007, Q2, P6-7

J3364 Injection, urokinase, 5000 IU vial Qp Qh N1 N
Other: Abbokinase
IOM: 100-02, 15, 50

J3365 Injection, IV, urokinase, 250,000 IU vial Qp Qh E2
Other: Abbokinase
IOM: 100-02, 15, 50,
Cross Reference Q0089

J3370 Injection, vancomycin HCL, 500 mg Qp Qh N1 N
Other: Vancocin, Vancoled
IOM: 100-02, 15, 50; 100-03, 4, 280.14

J3380 Injection, vedolizumab, 1 mg B D Qp Qh K2 K
Other: Entyvio

✻ J3385 Injection, velaglucerase alfa, 100 units B D Qp Qh K2 K
Enzyme replacement therapy in Gaucher Disease that results from a specific enzyme deficiency in the body, caused by a genetic mutation received from both parents. Type 1 is the most prevalent Ashkenazi Jewish genetic disease, occurring in one in every 1,000.
Other: VPRIV
Coding Clinic: 2011, Q1, P7

J3396 Injection, verteporfin, 0.1 mg B D Qp Qh K2 K
Other: Visudyne
IOM: 100-03, 1, 80.2; 100-03, 1, 80.3

✻ J3397 Injection, vestronidase alfa-vjbk, 1 mg B D K
Other: Mepsevii

✻ J3398 Injection, voretigene neparvovec-rzyl, 1 billion vector genomes B D G
Other: Luxturna

▶ J3399 Injection, onasemnogene abeparvovec-xioi, per treatment, up to 5x10^15 vector genomes K

J3400 Injection, triflupromazine HCL, up to 20 mg B D Qp Qh E2
Other: Vesprin
IOM: 100-02, 15, 50

J3410 Injection, hydroxyzine HCL, up to 25 mg B D Qp Qh N1 N
Other: Hyzine-50, Vistaject 25, Vistaril
IOM: 100-02, 15, 50

✻ J3411 Injection, thiamine HCL, 100 mg B D Qp Qh N1 N

✻ J3415 Injection, pyridoxine HCL, 100 mg B D Qp Qh N1 N

J3420 Injection, vitamin B-12 cyanocobalamin, up to 1000 mcg B D Qp Qh N1 N
Medicare carriers may have local coverage decisions regarding vitamin B12 injections that provide reimbursement only for patients with certain types of anemia and other conditions.
Other: Berubigen, Betalin 12, Cobex, Redisol, Rubramin PC, Sytobex
IOM: 100-02, 15, 50; 100-03, 2, 150.6

J3430 Injection, phytonadione (vitamin K), per 1 mg B D Qp Qh N1 N
Other: AquaMephyton, Konakion, Menadione, Synkavite, Vitamin K1
IOM: 100-02, 15, 50

J3465 Injection, voriconazole, 10 mg B D Qp Qh K2 K
Other: VFEND
IOM: 100-02, 15, 50

J3470 Injection, hyaluronidase, up to 150 units B D Qp Qh N1 N
Other: Amphadase, Wydase
IOM: 100-02, 15, 50

J3471 Injection, hyaluronidase, ovine, preservative free, per 1 USP unit (up to 999 USP units) B D Qp Qh N1 N
Other: Vitrase

J3472 Injection, hyaluronidase, ovine, preservative free, per 1000 USP units B D Qp Qh N1 N

J3473 Injection, hyaluronidase, recombinant, 1 USP unit B D Qp Qh N1 N
Other: Hylenex
IOM: 100-02, 15, 50

J3475 Injection, magnesium sulfate, per 500 mg B D Qp Qh N1 N
IOM: 100-02, 15, 50

J3480 Injection, potassium chloride, per 2 meq B D Qp Qh N1 N
IOM: 100-02, 15, 50

J3485 Injection, zidovudine, 10 mg B D Qp Qh N1 N
Other: Retrovir
IOM: 100-02, 15, 50

✻ J3486 Injection, ziprasidone mesylate, 10 mg B D Qp Qh N1 N
Other: Geodon

✻ J3489 Injection, zoledronic acid, 1 mg B D Qp Qh N1 N
Other: Reclast, Zometra

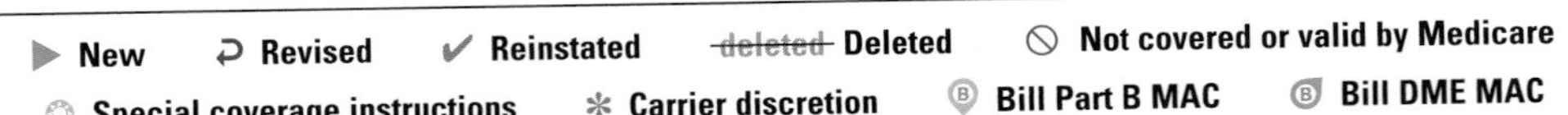
▶ New
Revised
✔ Reinstated
~~deleted~~ Deleted
Not covered or valid by Medicare
Special coverage instructions
✻ Carrier discretion
Bill Part B MAC
Bill DME MAC

J3490 Unclassified drugs N1 N

Bill on paper. Bill one unit. Identify drug and total dosage in "Remarks" field.

Other: Acthib, Aminocaproic Acid, Baciim, Bacitracin, Benzocaine, Bumetanide, Bupivacaine, Cefotetan, Ciprofloxacin, Cleocin Phosphate, Clindamycin, Cortisone Acetate Micronized, Definity, Diprivan, Doxy, Engerix-B, Ethanolamine, Famotidine, Ganirelix, Gonal-F, Hyaluronic Acid, Marcaine, Metronidazole, Nafcillin, Naltrexone, Ovidrel, Pegasys, Peg-Intron, Penicillin G Sodium, Propofol, Protonix, Recombivax, Rifadin, Rifampin, Sensorcaine-MPF, Smz-TMP, Sufentanil Citrate, Testopel Pellets, Testosterone, Treanda, Valcyte, Veritas Collagen Matrix

IOM: 100-02, 15, 50

Coding Clinic: 2017, Q1, P1-3, P8; 2014, Q2, P6; 2013, Q2, P3-4

J3520 Edetate disodium, per 150 mg Qp Qh E1

Other: Chealamide, Disotate, Endrate ethylenediamine-tetra-acetic

IOM: 100-03, 1, 20.21; 100-03, 1, 20.22

J3530 Nasal vaccine inhalation Qp Qh N1 N

IOM: 100-02, 15, 50

J3535 Drug administered through a metered dose inhaler E1

Other: Ipratropium bromide

IOM: 100-02, 15, 50

J3570 Laetrile, amygdalin, vitamin B-17 E1

IOM: 100-03, 1, 30.7

* **J3590** Unclassified biologics N1 N

Bill on paper. Bill one unit. Identify drug and total dosage in "Remarks" field.

Coding Clinic: 2017, Q1, P1-3; 2016, Q4, P10

* **J3591** Unclassified drug or biological used for ESRD on dialysis B

J7030 Infusion, normal saline solution, 1000 cc Qp Qh N1 N

Other: Sodium Chloride

IOM: 100-02, 15, 50

J7040 Infusion, normal saline solution, sterile (500 ml = 1 unit) Qp Qh N1 N

Other: Sodium Chloride

IOM: 100-02, 15, 50

J7042 5% dextrose/normal saline (500 ml = 1 unit) Qp Qh N1 N

Other: Dextrose-Nacl

IOM: 100-02, 15, 50

J7050 Infusion, normal saline solution, 250 cc Qp Qh N1 N

Other: Sodium Chloride

IOM: 100-02, 15, 50

J7060 5% dextrose/water (500 ml = 1 unit) Qp Qh N1 N

IOM: 100-02, 15, 50

J7070 Infusion, D 5 W, 1000 cc Qp Qh N1 N

Other: Dextrose

IOM: 100-02, 15, 50

J7100 Infusion, dextran 40, 500 ml Qp Qh N1 N

Other: Gentran, LMD, Rheomacrodex

IOM: 100-02, 15, 50

J7110 Infusion, dextran 75, 500 ml Qp Qh N1 N

Other: Gentran 75

IOM: 100-02, 15, 50

J7120 Ringer's lactate infusion, up to 1000 cc Qp Qh N1 N

Replacement fluid or electrolytes.

Other: Potassium Chloride

IOM: 100-02, 15, 50

J7121 5% dextrose in lactated ringers infusion, up to 1000 cc Qp Qh N1 N

IOM: 100-02, 15, 50

J7131 Hypertonic saline solution, 1 ml Qp Qh N1 N

IOM: 100-02, 15, 50

Coding Clinic: 2012, Q1, P9

Clotting Factors

▶ * **J7169** Injection, coagulation factor xa (recombinant), inactivated-zhzo (andexxa), 10 mg K2 G

* **J7170** Injection, emicizumab-kxwh, 0.5 mg G

Other: Hemlibra

* **J7175** Injection, Factor X, (human), 1 IU Qp Qh K2 K

Coding Clinic: 2017, Q1, P9

MIPS | Qp Quantity Physician | Qh Quantity Hospital | ♀ Female only
♂ Male only | A Age | DMEPOS | A2-Z3 ASC Payment Indicator | A-Y ASC Status Indicator | Coding Clinic

* J7177 Injection, human fibrinogen concentrate (fibryga), 1 mg (B) K
* J7178 Injection, human fibrinogen concentrate, not otherwise specified, 1 mg (B) Qp Qh K2 K
  Other: Riastap
* J7179 Injection, von Willebrand factor (recombinant), (vonvendi), 1 IU VWF:RCo (B) Qp Qh K2 G
  Coding Clinic: 2017, Q1, P9
* J7180 Injection, factor XIII (antihemophilic factor, human), 1 IU (B) Qp Qh K2 K
  Other: Corifact
  Coding Clinic: 2012, Q1, P8
* J7181 Injection, factor XIII a-subunit, (recombinant), per IU (B) Qp Qh K2 K
* J7182 Injection, factor VIII, (antihemophilic factor, recombinant), (novoeight), per IU (B) Qp Qh K2 K
* J7183 Injection, von Willebrand factor complex (human), wilate, 1 IU VWF:RCo (B) Qp Qh K2 K
  IOM: 100-02, 15, 50
  Coding Clinic: 2012, Q1, P9
* J7185 Injection, Factor VIII (antihemophilic factor, recombinant) (Xyntha), per IU (B) Qp Qh K2 K
* J7186 Injection, anti-hemophilic factor VIII/von Willebrand factor complex (human), per factor VIII IU (B) Qp Qh K2 K
  Other: Alphanate
  IOM: 100-02, 15, 50
* J7187 Injection, von Willebrand factor complex (HUMATE-P), per IU VWF:RCo (B) Qp Qh K2 K
  Other: Humate-P Low Dilutent
  IOM: 100-02, 15, 50
* J7188 Injection, factor VIII (antihemophilic factor, recombinant), (obizur), per IU (B) Qp Qh K2 K
  IOM: 100-02, 15, 50
* J7189 Factor VIIa (anti-hemophilic factor, recombinant), (novoseven rt), per 1 mcg (B) Qp Qh K2 K
  Other: NovoSeven
  IOM: 100-02, 15, 50
* J7190 Factor VIII anti-hemophilic factor, human, per IU (B) Qp Qh K2 K
  Other: Alphanate/von Willebrand factor complex, Hemofil M, Koate DVI, Koate-HP, Kogenate, Monoclate-P, Recombinate
  IOM: 100-02, 15, 50
* J7191 Factor VIII, anti-hemophilic factor (porcine), per IU (B) Qp Qh E2
  Other: Hyate:C, Koate-HP, Kogenate, Monoclate-P, Recombinate
  IOM: 100-02, 15, 50
* J7192 Factor VIII (anti-hemophilic factor, recombinant) per IU, not otherwise specified (B) Qp Qh K2 K
  Other: Advate, Helixate FS, Kogenate FS, Koate-HP, Recombinate, Xyntha
  IOM: 100-02, 15, 50
* J7193 Factor IX (anti-hemophilic factor, purified, non-recombinant) per IU (B) Qp Qh K2 K
  Other: AlphaNine SD, Mononine, Proplex
  IOM: 100-02, 15, 50
* J7194 Factor IX, complex, per IU (B) Qp Qh K2 K
  Other: Bebulin, Konyne-80, Profilnine Heat-treated, Profilnine SD, Proplex SX-T, Proplex T
  IOM: 100-02, 15, 50
* J7195 Injection, Factor IX (anti-hemophilic factor, recombinant) per IU, not otherwise specified (B) Qp Qh K2 K
  Other: Benefix, Profiline, Proplex T
  IOM: 100-02, 15, 50
* J7196 Injection, antithrombin recombinant, 50 IU (B) Qp Qh E2
  Other: ATryn, Feiba VH Immuno
  Coding Clinic: 2011, Q1, P6
* J7197 Anti-thrombin III (human), per IU (B) Qp Qh K2 K
  Other: Thrombate III
  IOM: 100-02, 15, 50
* J7198 Anti-inhibitor, per IU (B) Qp Qh K2 K
  Diagnosis examples: D66 Congenital Factor VIII disorder; D67 Congenital Factor IX disorder; D68.0 VonWillebrand's disease
  Other: Autoplex T, Feiba NF, Hemophilia clotting factors
  IOM: 100-02, 15, 50; 100-03, 2, 110.3

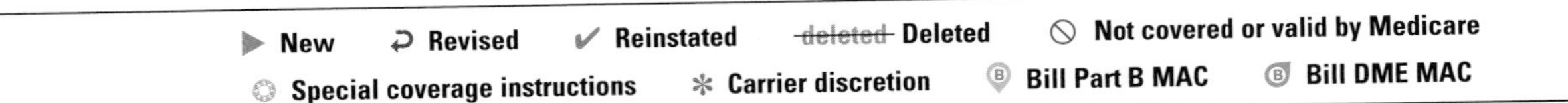
▶ New ↩ Revised ✔ Reinstated ~~deleted~~ Deleted ⊘ Not covered or valid by Medicare
Special coverage instructions * Carrier discretion (B) Bill Part B MAC (E) Bill DME MAC

J7199 Hemophilia clotting factor, not otherwise classified B

Other: Autoplex T

IOM: 100-02, 15, 50; 100-03, 2, 110.3

J7200 Injection, factor IX, (antihemophilic factor, recombinant), rixubis, per IU Qp Qh K2 K

IOM: 100-02, 15, 50

J7201 Injection, factor IX, fc fusion protein (recombinant), alprolix, 1 IU Qp Qh K2 K

IOM: 100-02, 15, 50

J7202 Injection, Factor IX, albumin fusion protein, (recombinant), idelvion, 1 IU Qp Qh K2 G

Coding Clinic: 2016, Q4, P9

J7203 Injection factor ix, (antihemophilic factor, recombinant), glycopegylated, (rebinyn), 1 iu G

Other: Profilnine SD, Bebulin VH, Bebulin, Proplex T

J7204 Injection, factor viii, antihemophilic factor (recombinant), (esperoct), glycopegylated-exei, per iu K2 G

J7205 Injection, factor VIII Fc fusion protein (recombinant), per IU Qp Qh K2 K

Other: Eloctate

J7207 Injection, Factor VIII, (antihemophilic factor, recombinant), PEGylated, 1 IU Qp Qh K2 G

Other: Adynovate

J7208 Injection, Factor VIII, (antihemophilic factor, recombinant), pegylated-aucl, (jivi), 1 i.u. K2 G

* J7209 Injection, Factor VIII, (antihemophilic factor, recombinant), (Nuwiq), 1 IU Qp Qh K2 G

* J7210 Injection, Factor VIII, (antihemophilic factor, recombinant), (afstyla), 1 i.u. K2 G

* J7211 Injection, Factor VIII, (antihemophilic factor, recombinant), (kovaltry), 1 i.u. K2 K

J7212 Factor viia (antihemophilic factor, recombinant)-jncw (sevenfact), 1 microgram K2 K

Contraceptives

J7296 Levonorgestrel-releasing intrauterine contraceptive system (Kyleena), 19.5 mg ♀ E1

Medicare Statute 1862(a)(1)

Cross Reference Q9984

J7297 Levonorgestrel-releasing intrauterine contraceptive system (Liletta), 52 mg Qp Qh ♀ E1

Medicare Statute 1862(a)(1)

J7298 Levonorgestrel-releasing intrauterine contraceptive system (Mirena), 52 mg Qp Qh ♀ E1

Medicare Statute 1862(a)(1)

J7300 Intrauterine copper contraceptive ♀ E1

Report IUD insertion with 58300. Bill usual and customary charge.

Other: Paragard T 380 A

Medicare Statute 1862a1

J7301 Levonorgestrel-releasing intrauterine contraceptive system (Skyla), 13.5 mg Qp Qh ♀ E1

Medicare Statute 1862(a)(1)

J7303 Contraceptive supply, hormone containing vaginal ring, each ♀ E1

Medicare Statute 1862.1

J7304 Contraceptive supply, hormone containing patch, each ♀ E1

Only billed by Family Planning Clinics

Medicare Statute 1862.1

J7306 Levonorgestrel (contraceptive) implant system, including implants and supplies ♀ E1

J7307 Etonogestrel (contraceptive) implant system, including implant and supplies ♀ E1

Aminolevulinic Acid HCL

* J7308 Aminolevulinic acid HCL for topical administration, 20%, single unit dosage form (354 mg) Qp Qh K2 K

Other: Levulan Kerastick

J7309 Methyl aminolevulinate (MAL) for topical administration, 16.8%, 1 gram Qp Qh N1 N

Other: Metvixia

Coding Clinic: 2011, Q1, P6

Ganciclovir

J7310 Ganciclovir, 4.5 mg, long-acting implant Ⓑ Qp Qh E2
IOM: 100-02, 15, 50

Ophthalmic Drugs

* **J7311** Injection, fluocinolone acetonide, intravitreal implant (retisert), 0.01 mg Ⓑ Qp Qh K2 K
Treatment of chronic noninfectious posterior segment uveitis
Other: Retisert

* **J7312** Injection, dexamethasone, intravitreal implant, 0.1 mg Ⓑ Qp Qh K2 K
To bill for Ozurdex services submit the following codes: J7312 and 67028 with the modifier -22 (for the increased work difficulty and increased risk). Indicated for the treatment of macular edema occurring after branch retinal vein occlusion (BRVO) or central retinal vein occlusion (CRVO) and non-infectious uveitis affecting the posterior segment of the eye.
Other: Ozurdex
Coding Clinic: 2011, Q1, P7

* **J7313** Injection, fluocinolone acetonide, intravitreal implant (iluvien), 0.01 mg Ⓑ Qp Qh K2 K
Other: Iluvien

* **J7314** Injection, fluocinolone acetonide, intravitreal implant (yutiq), 0.01 mg K2 G

* **J7315** Mitomycin, ophthalmic, 0.2 mg Ⓑ Qp Qh N1 N
Other: Mitosol, Mutamycin
Coding Clinic: 2016, Q4, P8; 2014, Q2, P6

* **J7316** Injection, ocriplasmin, 0.125 mg Ⓑ Qp Qh K2 K
Other: Jetrea

Hyaluronan

* **J7318** Hyaluronan or derivative, durolane, for intra-articular injection, 1 mg Ⓑ G
Other: Morisu

* **J7320** Hyaluronan or derivitive, genvisc 850, for intra-articular injection, 1 mg Ⓑ Qp Qh K2 K

Revised * **J7321** Hyaluronan or derivative, Hyalgan, Supartz, for intra-articular injection, per dose Ⓑ Qp Qh K2 K
Therapeutic goal is to restore visco-elasticity of synovial hyaluronan, thereby decreasing pain, improving mobility and restoring natural protective functions of hyaluronan in joint

* **J7322** Hyaluronan or derivative, hymovis, for intra-articular injection, 1 mg Ⓑ Qp Qh K2 G

* **J7323** Hyaluronan or derivative, Euflexxa, for intra-articular injection, per dose Ⓑ Qp Qh K2 K

* **J7324** Hyaluronan or derivative, Orthovisc, for intra-articular injection, per dose Ⓑ Qp Qh K2 K

* **J7325** Hyaluronan or derivative, Synvisc or Synvisc-One, for intra-articular injection, 1 mg Ⓑ Qp Qh K2 K

* **J7326** Hyaluronan or derivative, Gel-One, for intra-articular injection, per dose Ⓑ Qp Qh K2 K
Coding Clinic: 2012, Q1, P8

* **J7327** Hyaluronan or derivative, monovisc, for intra-articular injection, per dose Ⓑ Qp Qh K2 K

* **J7328** Hyaluronan or derivative, gelsyn-3, for intra-articular injection, 0.1 mg Ⓑ Qp Qh K2 G

* **J7329** Hyaluronan or derivative, trivisc, for intra-articular injection, 1 mg Ⓑ E2

Miscellaneous Drugs

* **J7330** Autologous cultured chondrocytes, implant Ⓑ Qp Qh B
Other: Carticel
Coding Clinic: 2010, Q4, P3

* **J7331** Hyaluronan or derivative, synojoynt, for intra-articular injection, 1 mg Ⓓ K

* **J7332** Hyaluronan or derivative, triluron, for intra-articular injection, 1 mg Ⓓ K

▶ * **J7333** Hyaluronan or derivative, visco-3, for intra-articular injection, per dose N1 N

* **J7336** Capsaicin 8% patch, per square centimeter Ⓑ Qp Qh K2 K
Other: Qutenza

* **J7340** Carbidopa 5 mg/levodopa 20 mg enteral suspension, 100 ml Ⓑ Ⓓ Qp Qh K2 K
Other: Duopa

▶ New ↻ Revised ✔ Reinstated ~~deleted~~ Deleted ⊘ Not covered or valid by Medicare
⊛ Special coverage instructions * Carrier discretion Ⓑ Bill Part B MAC Ⓓ Bill DME MAC

* J7342 Instillation, ciprofloxacin otic suspension, 6 mg Qp Qh K2 G

J7345 Aminolevulinic acid HCL for topical administration, 10% gel, 10 mg K2 G

▶ J7351 Injection, bimatoprost, intracameral implant, 1 microgram K2 G

▶ J7352 Afamelanotide implant, 1 mg K2 K

* J7401 Mometasone furoate sinus implant, 10 micrograms N

Immunosuppressive Drugs (Includes Non-injectibles)

J7500 Azathioprine, oral, 50 mg Qp Qh N1 N

Other: Azasan, Imuran

IOM: 100-02, 15, 50

J7501 Azathioprine, parenteral, 100 mg Qp Qh K2 K

Other: Imuran

IOM: 100-02, 15, 50

J7502 Cyclosporine, oral, 100 mg Qp Qh N1 N

Other: Gengraf, Neoral, Sandimmune

IOM: 100-02, 15, 50

J7503 Tacrolimus, extended release, (Envarsus XR), oral, 0.25 mg Qp Qh K2 G

IOM: 100-02, 15, 50

J7504 Lymphocyte immune globulin, antithymocyte globulin, equine, parenteral, 250 mg Qp Qh K2 K

Other: Atgam

IOM: 100-02, 15, 50; 100-03, 2, 110.3

J7505 Muromonab-CD3, parenteral, 5 mg Qp Qh K2 K

Other: Monoclonal antibodies (parenteral)

IOM: 100-02, 15, 50

J7507 Tacrolimus, immediate release, oral, 1 mg Qp Qh N1 N

Other: Prograf

IOM: 100-02, 15, 50

J7508 Tacrolimus, extended release, (Astagraf XL), oral, 0.1 mg Qp Qh N1 N

IOM: 100-02, 15, 50

J7509 Methylprednisolone oral, per 4 mg Qp Qh N1 N

Other: Medrol

IOM: 100-02, 15, 50

J7510 Prednisolone oral, per 5 mg Qp Qh N1 N

Other: Delta-Cortef, Flo-Pred, Orapred

IOM: 100-02, 15, 50

* J7511 Lymphocyte immune globulin, antithymocyte globulin, rabbit, parenteral, 25 mg Qp Qh K2 K

Other: Thymoglobulin

J7512 Prednisone, immediate release or delayed release, oral, 1 mg Qp Qh N1 N

Other: Cyclosporine

IOM: 100-02, 15, 50

J7513 Daclizumab, parenteral, 25 mg Qp Qh E2

Other: Zenapax

IOM: 100-02, 15, 50

* J7515 Cyclosporine, oral, 25 mg Qp Qh N1 N

Other: Gengraf, Neoral, Sandimmune

* J7516 Cyclosporin, parenteral, 250 mg Qp Qh N1 N

Other: Sandimmune

* J7517 Mycophenolate mofetil, oral, 250 mg Qp Qh N1 N

Other: CellCept

J7518 Mycophenolic acid, oral, 180 mg Qp Qh N1 N

Other: Myfortic

IOM: 100-04, 4, 240; 100-4, 17, 80.3.1

J7520 Sirolimus, oral, 1 mg Qp Qh N1 N

Other: Rapamune

IOM: 100-02, 15, 50

J7525 Tacrolimus, parenteral, 5 mg Qp Qh K2 K

Other: Prograf

IOM: 100-02, 15, 50

J7527 Everolimus, oral, 0.25 mg Qp Qh N1 N

Other: Zortress

IOM: 100-02, 15, 50

J7599 Immunosuppressive drug, not otherwise classified N1 N

Bill on paper. Bill one unit. Identify drug and total dosage in "Remarks" field.

IOM: 100-02, 15, 50

Inhalation Solutions

✻ **J7604** Acetylcysteine, inhalation solution, compounded product, administered through DME, unit dose form, per gram Ⓑ Ⓓ Qp Qh M

Other: Mucomyst (unit dose form), Mucosol

✻ **J7605** Arformoterol, inhalation solution, FDA approved final product, non-compounded, administered through DME, unit dose form, 15 mcg Ⓑ Ⓓ Qp Qh M

Maintenance treatment of bronchoconstriction in patients with chronic obstructive pulmonary disease (COPD).

Other: Brovana

✻ **J7606** Formoterol fumarate, inhalation solution, FDA approved final product, non-compounded, administered through DME, unit dose form, 20 mcg Ⓑ Ⓓ Qp Qh M

Other: Perforomist

✻ **J7607** Levalbuterol, inhalation solution, compounded product, administered through DME, concentrated form, 0.5 mg Ⓑ Ⓓ Qp Qh M

◎ **J7608** Acetylcysteine, inhalation solution, FDA-approved final product, non-compounded, administered through DME, unit dose form, per gram Ⓑ Ⓓ Qp Qh M

Other: Mucomyst, Mucosol

✻ **J7609** Albuterol, inhalation solution, compounded product, administered through DME, unit dose, 1 mg Ⓑ Ⓓ Qp Qh M

Patient's home, medications—such as albuterol when administered through a nebulizer—are considered DME and are payable under Part B.

Other: Proventil, Ventolin, Xopenex

✻ **J7610** Albuterol, inhalation solution, compounded product, administered through DME, concentrated form, 1 mg Ⓑ Ⓓ Qp Qh M

Other: Proventil, Ventolin, Xopenex

◎ **J7611** Albuterol, inhalation solution, FDA-approved final product, non-compounded, administered through DME, concentrated form, 1 mg Ⓑ Ⓓ Qp Qh M

Report once for each milligram administered. For example, 2 mg of concentrated albuterol (usually diluted with saline), reported with J7611×2.

Other: Proventil, Ventolin, Xopenex

◎ **J7612** Levalbuterol, inhalation solution, FDA-approved final product, non-compounded, administered through DME, concentrated form, 0.5 mg Ⓑ Ⓓ Qp Qh M

Other: Xopenex

◎ **J7613** Albuterol, inhalation solution, FDA-approved final product, non-compounded, administered through DME, unit dose, 1 mg Ⓑ Ⓓ Qp Qh M

Other: Accuneb, Proventil, Ventolin, Xopenex

◎ **J7614** Levalbuterol, inhalation solution, FDA-approved final product, non-compounded, administered through DME, unit dose, 0.5 mg Ⓑ Ⓓ Qp Qh M

Other: Xopenex

✻ **J7615** Levalbuterol, inhalation solution, compounded product, administered through DME, unit dose, 0.5 mg Ⓑ Ⓓ Qp Qh M

◎ **J7620** Albuterol, up to 2.5 mg and ipratropium bromide, up to 0.5 mg,FDA-approved final product, non-compounded, administered through DME Ⓑ Ⓓ Qp Qh M

Other: DuoNeb

✻ **J7622** Beclomethasone, inhalation solution, compounded product, administered through DME, unit dose form, per mg Ⓑ Ⓓ Qp Qh M

✻ **J7624** Betamethasone, inhalation solution, compounded product, administered through DME, unit dose form, per mg Ⓑ Ⓓ Qp Qh M

✻ **J7626** Budesonide inhalation solution, FDA-approved final product, non-compounded, administered through DME, unit dose form, up to 0.5 mg Ⓑ Ⓓ Qp Qh M

Other: Pulmicort

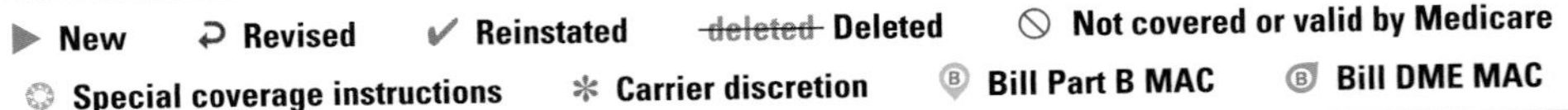

▶ New
↩ Revised
✔ Reinstated
~~deleted~~ Deleted
⊘ Not covered or valid by Medicare
◎ Special coverage instructions
✻ Carrier discretion
Ⓑ Bill Part B MAC
Ⓓ Bill DME MAC

* **J7627** Budesonide, inhalation solution, compounded product, administered through DME, unit dose form, up to 0.5 mg Qp Qh M

Other: Pulmicort Respules

J7628 Bitolterol mesylate, inhalation solution, compounded product, administered through DME, concentrated form, per milligram Qp Qh M

Other: Tornalate

J7629 Bitolterol mesylate, inhalation solution, compounded product, administered through DME, unit dose form, per milligram Qp Qh M

Other: Tornalate

J7631 Cromolyn sodium, inhalation solution, FDA-approved final product, non-compounded, administered through DME, unit dose form, per 10 mg Qp Qh M

Other: Intal

* **J7632** Cromolyn sodium, inhalation solution, compounded product, administered through DME, unit dose form, per 10 mg Qp Qh M

Other: Intal

* **J7633** Budesonide, inhalation solution, FDA-approved final product, non-compounded, administered through DME, concentrated form, per 0.25 mg Qp Qh M

Other: Pulmicort Respules

* **J7634** Budesonide, inhalation solution, compounded product, administered through DME, concentrated form, per 0.25 mg Qp Qh M

Other: Pulmicort Respules

J7635 Atropine, inhalation solution, compounded product, administered through DME, concentrated form, per milligram Qp Qh M

J7636 Atropine, inhalation solution, compounded product, administered through DME, unit dose form, per milligram Qp Qh M

J7637 Dexamethasone, inhalation solution, compounded product, administered through DME, concentrated form, per milligram Qp Qh M

J7638 Dexamethasone, inhalation solution, compounded product, administered through DME, unit dose form, per milligram Qp Qh M

J7639 Dornase alfa, inhalation solution, FDA-approved final product, non-compounded, administered through DME, unit dose form, per milligram Qp Qh M

Other: Pulmozyme

* **J7640** Formoterol, inhalation solution, compounded product, administered through DME, unit dose form, 12 mcg Qp Qh E1

* **J7641** Flunisolide, inhalation solution, compounded product, administered through DME, unit dose, per milligram Qp Qh M

J7642 Glycopyrrolate, inhalation solution, compounded product, administered through DME, concentrated form, per milligram Qp Qh M

J7643 Glycopyrrolate, inhalation solution, compounded product, administered through DME, unit dose form, per milligram Qp Qh M

J7644 Ipratropium bromide, inhalation solution, FDA-approved final product, non-compounded, administered through DME, unit dose form, per milligram Qp Qh M

Other: Atrovent

* **J7645** Ipratropium bromide, inhalation solution, compounded product, administered through DME, unit dose form, per milligram Qp Qh M

Other: Atrovent

* **J7647** Isoetharine HCL, inhalation solution, compounded product, administered through DME, concentrated form, per milligram Qp Qh M

Other: Bronkosol

J7648 Isoetharine HCL, inhalation solution, FDA-approved final product, non-compounded, administered through DME, concentrated form, per milligram Qp Qh M

Other: Bronkosol

J7649 Isoetharine HCL, inhalation solution, FDA-approved final product, non-compounded, administered through DME, unit dose form, per milligram Qp Qh M

Other: Bronkosol

* **J7650** Isoetharine HCL, inhalation solution, compounded product, administered through DME, unit dose form, per milligram Qp Qh M

Other: Bronkosol

✻ J7657 Isoproterenol HCL, inhalation solution, compounded product, administered through DME, concentrated form, per milligram Qp Qh M

Other: Isuprel

J7658 Isoproterenol HCL inhalation solution, FDA-approved final product, non-compounded, administered through DME, concentrated form, per milligram Qp Qh M

Other: Isuprel

J7659 Isoproterenol HCL, inhalation solution, FDA-approved final product, non-compounded, administered through DME, unit dose form, per milligram Qp Qh M

Other: Isuprel

✻ J7660 Isoproterenol HCL, inhalation solution, compounded product, administered through DME, unit dose form, per milligram Qp Qh M

Other: Isuprel

✻ J7665 Mannitol, administered through an inhaler, 5 mg Qp Qh N1 N

Other: Aridol

✻ J7667 Metaproterenol sulfate, inhalation solution, compounded product, concentrated form, per 10 mg Qp Qh M

Other: Alupent, Metaprel

J7668 Metaproterenol sulfate, inhalation solution, FDA-approved final product, non-compounded, administered through DME, concentrated form, per 10 mg Qp Qh M

Other: Alupent, Metaprel

J7669 Metaproterenol sulfate, inhalation solution, FDA-approved final product, non-compounded, administered through DME, unit dose form, per 10 mg Qp Qh M

Other: Alupent, Metaprel

✻ J7670 Metaproterenol sulfate, inhalation solution, compounded product, administered through DME, unit dose form, per 10 mg Qp Qh M

Other: Alupent, Metaprel

✻ J7674 Methacholine chloride administered as inhalation solution through a nebulizer, per 1 mg Qp Qh N1 N

Other: Provocholine

✻ J7676 Pentamidine isethionate, inhalation solution, compounded product, administered through DME, unit dose form, per 300 mg Qp Qh M

Other: NebuPent, Pentam

✻ J7677 Revefenacin inhalation solution, FDA-approved final product, non-compounded, administered through DME, 1 microgram M

J7680 Terbutaline sulfate, inhalation solution, compounded product, administered through DME, concentrated form, per milligram Qp Qh M

Other: Brethine

J7681 Terbutaline sulfate, inhalation solution, compounded product, administered through DME, unit dose form, per milligram Qp Qh M

Other: Brethine

J7682 Tobramycin, inhalation solution, FDA-approved final product, non-compounded unit dose form, administered through DME, per 300 mg Qp Qh M

Other: Bethkis, Kitabis PAK, Tobi

J7683 Triamcinolone, inhalation solution, compounded product, administered through DME, concentrated form, per milligram Qp Qh M

J7684 Triamcinolone, inhalation solution, compounded product, administered through DME, unit dose form, per milligram Qp Qh M

Other: Triamcinolone acetonide

✻ J7685 Tobramycin, inhalation solution, compounded product, administered through DME, unit dose form, per 300 mg Qp Qh M

Other: Tobi

✻ J7686 Treprostinil, inhalation solution, FDA-approved final product, non-compounded, administered through DME, unit dose form, 1.74 mg Qp Qh M

Other: Tyvaso

Not Otherwise Classified/Specified

J7699 NOC drugs, inhalation solution administered through DME M

Other: Gentamicin Sulfate

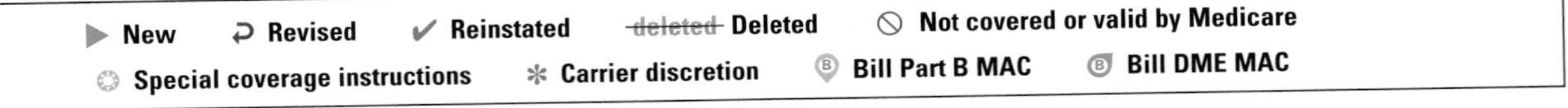
New
Revised
Reinstated
deleted Deleted
Not covered or valid by Medicare
Special coverage instructions
Carrier discretion
Bill Part B MAC
Bill DME MAC

J7799 NOC drugs, other than inhalation drugs, administered through DME N1 N

Bill on paper. Bill one unit and identify drug and total dosage in the "Remark" field.

Other: Cuvitru, Epinephrine, Mannitol, Osmitrol, Phenylephrine, Resectisol, Sodium chloride

IOM: 100-02, 15, 110.3

J7999 Compounded drug, not otherwise classified N1 N

Coding Clinic: 2017, Q1, P1-2; 2016, Q4, P8

J8498 Antiemetic drug, rectal/suppository, not otherwise specified B

Other: Compazine, Compro, Phenadoz, Phenergan, Prochlorperazine, Promethazine, Promethegan

Medicare Statute 1861(s)2t

J8499 Prescription drug, oral, non chemotherapeutic, NOS E1

Other: Acyclovir, Calcitrol, Cromolyn Sodium, OFEV, Valganciclovir HCL, Zovirax

IOM: 100-02, 15, 50

Coding Clinic: 2013, Q2, P4

Oral Anti-Cancer Drugs

J8501 Aprepitant, oral, 5 mg Qp Qh K2 K

Other: Emend

J8510 Busulfan; oral, 2 mg Qp Qh N1 N

Other: Myleran

IOM: 100-02, 15, 50; 100-04, 4, 240; 100-04, 17, 80.1.1

J8515 Cabergoline, oral, 0.25 mg E1

IOM: 100-02, 15, 50; 100-04, 4, 240

J8520 Capecitabine, oral, 150 mg Qp Qh N1 N

Other: Xeloda

IOM: 100-02, 15, 50; 100-04, 4, 240; 100-04, 17, 80.1.1

J8521 Capecitabine, oral, 500 mg Qp Qh N1 N

Other: Xeloda

IOM: 100-02, 15, 50; 100-04, 4, 240; 100-04, 17, 80.1.1

J8530 Cyclophosphamide; oral, 25 mg Qp Qh N1 N

Other: Cytoxan

IOM: 100-02, 15, 50; 100-04, 4, 240; 100-04, 17, 80.1.1

J8540 Dexamethasone, oral, 0.25 mg Qp Qh N1 N

Other: Decadron, Dexone, Dexpak, Locort

Medicare Statute 1861(s)2t

J8560 Etoposide; oral, 50 mg Qp Qh K2 K

Other: VePesid

IOM: 100-02, 15, 50; 100-04, 4, 230.1; 100-04, 4, 240; 100-04, 17, 80.1.1

* **J8562** Fludarabine phosphate, oral, 10 mg Qp Qh E2

Other: Fludara, Oforta

Coding Clinic: 2011, Q1, P9

J8565 Gefitinib, oral, 250 mg E2

Other: Iressa

J8597 Antiemetic drug, oral, not otherwise specified N1 N

Medicare Statute 1861(s)2t

J8600 Melphalan; oral, 2 mg Qp Qh N1 N

Other: Alkeran

IOM: 100-02, 15, 50; 100-04, 4, 240; 100-04, 17, 80.1.1

J8610 Methotrexate; oral, 2.5 mg Qp Qh N1 N

Other: Rheumatrex, Trexall

IOM: 100-02, 15, 50; 100-04, 4, 240; 100-04, 17, 80.1.1

* **J8650** Nabilone, oral, 1 mg Qp Qh E2

J8655 Netupitant 300 mg and palonosetron 0.5 mg, oral Qp Qh K2 K

Other: Akynzeo

Coding Clinic: 2015, Q4, P4

J8670 Rolapitant, oral, 1 mg Qp Qh K2 K

Other: Varubi

J8700 Temozolomide, oral, 5 mg Qp Qh N1 N

Other: Temodar

IOM: 100-02, 15, 50; 100-04, 4, 240

* **J8705** Topotecan, oral, 0.25 mg Qp Qh K2 K

Treatment for ovarian and lung cancers, etc. Report J9350 (Topotecan, 4 mg) for intravenous version

Other: Hycamtin

MIPS
Qp Quantity Physician
Qh Quantity Hospital
♀ Female only
♂ Male only
A Age
DMEPOS
A2-Z3 ASC Payment Indicator
A-Y ASC Status Indicator
Coding Clinic

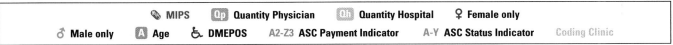

J8999 Prescription drug, oral, chemotherapeutic, NOS — B

Other: Anastrozole, Arimidex, Aromasin, Droxia, Erivedge, Flutamide, Gleevec, Hydrea, Hydroxyurea, Leukeran, Matulane, Megestrol Acetate, Mercaptopurine, Nolvadex, Tamoxifen Citrate

IOM: 100-02, 15, 50; 100-04, 4, 250; 100-04, 17, 80.1.1; 100-04, 17, 80.1.2

CHEMOTHERAPY DRUGS (J9000-J9999)

NOTE: These codes cover the cost of the chemotherapy drug only, not to include the administration

J9000 Injection, doxorubicin hydrochloride, 10 mg Qp Qh — N1 N

Other: Adriamycin, Rubex

IOM: 100-02, 15, 50

Coding Clinic: 2007, Q4, P5

J9015 Injection, aldesleukin, per single use vial Qp Qh — K2 K

Other: Proleukin

IOM: 100-02, 15, 50

* J9017 Injection, arsenic trioxide, 1 mg Qp Qh — K2 K

Other: Trisenox

J9019 Injection, asparaginase (Erwinaze), 1,000 IU Qp Qh — K2 K

IOM: 100-02, 15, 50

J9020 Injection, asparaginase, not otherwise specified 10,000 units Qp Qh — N1 N

IOM: 100-02, 15, 50

* J9022 Injection, atezolizumab, 10 mg — K2 G

* J9023 Injection, avelumab, 10 mg — K2 G

* J9025 Injection, azacitidine, 1 mg Qp Qh — K2 K

* J9027 Injection, clofarabine, 1 mg Qp Qh — K2 K

Other: Clolar

J9030 BCG live intravesical instillation, 1 mg — K2 K

* J9032 Injection, belinostat, 10 mg Qp Qh — K2 K

Other: Beleodaq

* J9033 Injection, bendamustine HCL (treanda), 1 mg Qp Qh — K2 K

Treatment for form of non-Hodgkin's lymphoma; standard administration time is as an intravenous infusion over 30 minutes

Other: Treanda

* J9034 Injection, bendamustine HCL (bendeka), 1 mg Qp Qh — K2 G

Coding Clinic: 2017, Q1, P10

* J9035 Injection, bevacizumab, 10 mg Qp Qh — K2 K

For malignant neoplasm of breast, considered J9207.

Other: Avastin

Coding Clinic: 2013, Q3, P9, Q2, P8

* J9036 Injection, bendamustine hydrochloride, (belrapzo/bendamustine), 1 mg — K2 G

* J9039 Injection, blinatumomab, 1 mcg Qp Qh — K2 K

Other: Blincyto

J9040 Injection, bleomycin sulfate, 15 units Qp Qh — N1 N

Other: Blenoxane

IOM: 100-02, 15, 50

* J9041 Injection, bortezomib (velcade), 0.1 mg Qp Qh — K2 K

Other: Velcade

* J9042 Injection, brentuximab vedotin, 1 mg Qp Qh — K2 K

Other: Adcetris

* J9043 Injection, cabazitaxel, 1 mg Qp Qh — K2 K

Other: Jevtana

Coding Clinic: 2012, Q1, P9

* J9044 Injection, bortezomib, not otherwise specified, 0.1 mg — K

Other: Velcade

J9045 Injection, carboplatin, 50 mg Qp Qh — N1 N

Other: Paraplatin

IOM: 100-02, 15, 50

* J9047 Injection, carfilzomib, 1 mg Qp Qh — K2 K

Other: Kyprolis

J9050 Injection, carmustine, 100 mg Qp Qh — K2 K

Other: BiCNU

IOM: 100-02, 15, 50

Code	Description	Indicators
* J9055	Injection, cetuximab, 10 mg Qp Qh *Other: Erbitux*	K2 K
* J9057	Injection, copanlisib, 1 mg *Other: Aliqopa*	G
J9060	Injection, cisplatin, powder or solution, 10 mg Qp Qh *Other: Plantinol AQ* *IOM: 100-02, 15, 50* Coding Clinic: 2013, Q2, P6; 2011, Q1, P8	N1 N
J9065	Injection, cladribine, per 1 mg Qp Qh *Other: Leustatin* *IOM: 100-02, 15, 50*	K2 K
J9070	Cyclophosphamide, 100 mg Qp Qh *Other: Cytoxan, Neosar* *IOM: 100-02, 15, 50* Coding Clinic: 2011, Q1, P8-9	K2 K
* J9098	Injection, cytarabine liposome, 10 mg Qp Qh *Other: DepoCyt*	K2 K
J9100	Injection, cytarabine, 100 mg Qp Qh *Other: Cytosar-U* *IOM: 100-02, 15, 50* Coding Clinic: 2011, Q1, P9	N1 N
* J9118	Injection, calaspargase pegol-mknl, 10 units	E2
* J9119	Injection, cemiplimab-rwlc, 1 mg	K2 G
J9120	Injection, dactinomycin, 0.5 mg Qp Qh *Other: Cosmegen* *IOM: 100-02, 15, 50*	K2 K
J9130	Dacarbazine, 100 mg Qp Qh *Other: DTIC-Dome* *IOM: 100-02, 15, 50* Coding Clinic: 2011, Q1, P9	N1 N
▶ J9144	Injection, daratumumab, 10 mg and hyaluronidase-fihj	K2 G
J9145	Injection, daratumumab, 10 mg Qp Qh *Other: Darzalex* *IOM: 100-02, 15, 50*	K2 G
J9150	Injection, daunorubicin, 10 mg Qp Qh *Other: Cerubidine* *IOM: 100-02, 15, 50*	K2 K
J9151	Injection, daunorubicin citrate, liposomal formulation, 10 mg Qp Qh *Other: Daunoxome* *IOM: 100-02, 15, 50*	E2
* J9153	njection, liposomal, 1 mg daunorubicin and 2.27 mg cytarabine *Other: Vyxeos*	G
* J9155	Injection, degarelix, 1 mg Qp Qh Report 1 unit for every 1 mg. *Other: Firmagon*	K2 K
* J9160	Injection, denileukin diftitox, 300 mcg Qp Qh	E2
J9165	Injection, diethylstilbestrol diphosphate, 250 mg Qp Qh *Other: Stilphostrol* *IOM: 100-02, 15, 50*	E2
J9171	Injection, docetaxel, 1 mg Qp Qh Report 1 unit for every 1 mg. *Other: Docefrez, Taxotere* *IOM: 100-02, 15, 50* Coding Clinic: 2012, Q1, P9	K2 K
* J9173	Injection, durvalumab, 10 mg *Other: Imfinzi*	G
J9175	Injection, Elliott's B solution, 1 ml Qp Qh *IOM: 100-02, 15, 50*	N1 N
* J9176	Injection, elotuzumab, 1 mg Qp Qh *Other: Empliciti*	K2 G
▶ J9177	Injection, enfortumab vedotin-ejfv, 0.25 mg	K2 G
* J9178	Injection, epirubicin HCL, 2 mg Qp Qh *Other: Ellence*	N1 N
* J9179	Injection, eribulin mesylate, 0.1 mg Qp Qh *Other: Halaven*	K2 K
J9181	Injection, etoposide, 10 mg Qp Qh *Other: Etopophos, Toposar*	N1 N
J9185	Injection, fludarabine phosphate, 50 mg Qp Qh *Other: Fludara* *IOM: 100-02, 15, 50*	K2 K

MIPS · Qp Quantity Physician · Qh Quantity Hospital · ♀ Female only · ♂ Male only · A Age · DMEPOS · A2-Z3 ASC Payment Indicator · A-Y ASC Status Indicator · Coding Clinic

J9190 Injection, fluorouracil, 500 mg Ⓑ Ⓔ Qp Qh N1 N
Other: Adrucil
IOM: 100-02, 15, 50

▶ **J9198** Injection, gemcitabine hydrochloride, (infugem), 100 mg K2 G

~~J9199 Injection, gemcitabine hydrochloride (infugem), 200 mg~~ ✖

J9200 Injection, floxuridine, 500 mg Ⓑ Ⓔ Qp Qh N1 N
Other: FUDR
IOM: 100-02, 15, 50

J9201 Injection, gemcitabine hydrochloride, not otherwise specified, 200 mg Ⓑ Ⓔ Qp Qh N1 N
Other: Gemzar
IOM: 100-02, 15, 50

J9202 Goserelin acetate implant, per 3.6 mg Ⓑ Ⓔ Qp Qh K2 K
Other: Zoladex
IOM: 100-02, 15, 50

✻ **J9203** Injection, gemtuzumab ozogamicin, 0.1 mg K2 G

✻ **J9204** Injection, mogamulizumab-kpkc, 1 mg K2 G

J9205 Injection, irinotecan liposome, 1 mg Qp Qh K2 G
Other: ONIVYDE
IOM: 100-02, 15, 50

J9206 Injection, irinotecan, 20 mg Ⓑ Ⓔ Qp Qh N1 N
Other: Camptosar
IOM: 100-02, 15, 50

✻ **J9207** Injection, ixabepilone, 1 mg Ⓑ Ⓔ Qp Qh K2 K
Other: Ixempra Kit

J9208 Injection, ifosfamide, 1 gm Ⓑ Ⓔ Qp Qh N1 N
Other: Ifex
IOM: 100-02, 15, 50

J9209 Injection, mesna, 200 mg Ⓑ Ⓔ Qp Qh N1 N
Other: Mesnex
IOM: 100-02, 15, 50

✻ **J9210** Injection, emapalumab-lzsg, 1 mg K2 G

J9211 Injection, idarubicin hydrochloride, 5 mg Ⓑ Ⓔ Qp Qh K2 K
Other: Idamycin PFS
IOM: 100-02, 15, 50

J9212 Injection, interferon alfacon-1, recombinant, 1 mcg Ⓑ Ⓔ Qp Qh N1 N
Other: Amgen, Infergen
IOM: 100-02, 15, 50

J9213 Injection, interferon, alfa-2a, recombinant, 3 million units Ⓑ Ⓔ Qp Qh N1 N
Other: Roferon-A
IOM: 100-02, 15, 50

J9214 Injection, interferon, alfa-2b, recombinant, 1 million units Ⓑ Ⓔ Qp Qh K2 K
Other: Intron-A
IOM: 100-02, 15, 50

J9215 Injection, interferon, alfa-n3 (human leukocyte derived), 250,000 IU Ⓑ Ⓔ Qp Qh E2
Other: Alferon N
IOM: 100-02, 15, 50

J9216 Injection, interferon, gamma-1B, 3 million units Ⓑ Ⓔ Qp Qh K2 K
Other: Actimmune
IOM: 100-02, 15, 50

J9217 Leuprolide acetate (for depot suspension), 7.5 mg Ⓑ Ⓔ Qp Qh K2 K
Other: Eligard, Lupron Depot
IOM: 100-02, 15, 50
Coding Clinic: 2019, Q2, P11; 2015, Q3, P3

J9218 Leuprolide acetate, per 1 mg Ⓑ Ⓔ Qp Qh K2 K
Other: Lupron
IOM: 100-02, 15, 50
Coding Clinic: 2019, Q2, P11; 2015, Q3, P3

J9219 Leuprolide acetate implant, 65 mg Ⓑ Ⓔ Qp Qh E2
Other: Viadur
IOM: 100-02, 15, 50

▶ **J9223** Injection, lurbinectedin, 0.1 mg K2 G

J9225 Histrelin implant (Vantas), 50 mg Ⓑ Ⓔ Qp Qh K2 K
IOM: 100-02, 15, 50

▶ New ↻ Revised ✓ Reinstated ~~deleted~~ Deleted ⊘ Not covered or valid by Medicare
Special coverage instructions ✻ Carrier discretion Ⓑ Bill Part B MAC Ⓔ Bill DME MAC

J9226 Histrelin implant (Supprelin LA), 50 mg Qp Qh K2 K
Other: Vantas
IOM: 100-02, 15, 50

J9227 Injection, isatuximab-irfc, 10 mg K2 G

* **J9228** Injection, ipilimumab, 1 mg Qp Qh K2 K
Other: Yervoy
Coding Clinic: 2012, Q1, P9

* **J9229** Injection, inotuzumab ozogamicin, 0.1 mg G
Other: Besponsa

J9230 Injection, mechlorethamine hydrochloride, (nitrogen mustard), 10 mg Qp Qh K2 K
Other: Mustargen
IOM: 100-02, 15, 50

J9245 Injection, melphalan hydrochloride, not otherwise specified, 50 mg Qp Qh K2 K

J9246 Injection, melphalan (evomela), 1 mg K2 K
Other: Alkeran, Evomela
IOM: 100-02, 15, 50

J9250 Methotrexate sodium, 5 mg Qp Qh N1 N
Other: Folex
IOM: 100-02, 15, 50

J9260 Methotrexate sodium, 50 mg Qp Qh N1 N
Other: Folex
IOM: 100-02, 15, 50

* **J9261** Injection, nelarabine, 50 mg Qp Qh K2 K
Other: Arranon

* **J9262** Injection, omacetaxine mepesuccinate, 0.01 mg Qp Qh K2 K
Other: Synribo

* **J9263** Injection, oxaliplatin, 0.5 mg Qp Qh N1 N
Eloxatin, platinum-based anticancer drug that destroys cancer cells
Other: Eloxatin
Coding Clinic: 2009, Q1, P10

* **J9264** Injection, paclitaxel protein-bound particles, 1 mg K2 K
Other: Abraxane

J9266 Injection, pegaspargase, per single dose vial Qp Qh K2 K
Other: Oncaspar
IOM: 100-02, 15, 50

J9267 Injection, paclitaxel, 1 mg Qp Qh N1 N
Other: Taxol

J9268 Injection, pentostatin, 10 mg Qp Qh K2 K
Other: Nipent
IOM: 100-02, 15, 50

* **J9269** Injection, tagraxofusp-erzs, 10 micrograms K2 G

J9270 Injection, plicamycin, 2.5 mg Qp Qh N1 N
Other: Mithracin
IOM: 100-02, 15, 50

* **J9271** Injection, pembrolizumab, 1 mg Qp Qh K2 K
Other: Keytruda

J9280 Injection, mitomycin, 5 mg Qp Qh K2 K
Other: Mitosol, Mutamycin
IOM: 100-02, 15, 50
Coding Clinic: 2016, Q4, P8; 2014, Q2, P6; 2011, Q1, P9

J9281 Mitomycin pyelocalyceal instillation, 1 mg K2 G

* **J9285** Injection, olaratumab, 10 mg K2 G

J9293 Injection, mitoxantrone hydrochloride, per 5 mg Qp Qh K2 K
Other: Novantrone
IOM: 100-02, 15, 50

* **J9295** Injection, necitumumab, 1 mg Qp Qh K2 G
Other: Portrazza

J9299 Injection, nivolumab, 1 mg Qp Qh K2 K
Other: Opdivo

* **J9301** Injection, obinutuzumab, 10 mg Qp Qh K2 K
Other: Gazyva

* **J9302** Injection, ofatumumab, 10 mg Qp Qh K2 K
Other: Arzerra
Coding Clinic: 2011, Q1, P7

MIPS Qp Quantity Physician Qh Quantity Hospital ♀ Female only
♂ Male only A Age DMEPOS A2-Z3 ASC Payment Indicator A-Y ASC Status Indicator Coding Clinic

↩ * **J9303** Injection, panitumumab, not otherwise specified, 10 mg B D Qp Qh K2 K
Other: Vectibix

▶ * **J9304** Injection, pemetrexed (pemfexy), 10 mg K5 E2

* **J9305** Injection, pemetrexed, 10 mg B D Qp Qh K2 K
Other: Alimta

* **J9306** Injection, pertuzumab, 1 mg B D Qp Qh K2 K
Other: Perjeta

* **J9307** Injection, pralatrexate, 1 mg B D Qp Qh K2 K
Other: Folotyn
Coding Clinic: 2011, Q1, P7

* **J9308** Injection, ramucirumab, 5 mg B D Qp Qh K2 K
Other: Cyramza

* **J9309** Injection, polatuzumab vedotin-piiq, 1 mg K2 G

○ **J9311** Injection, rituximab 10 mg and hyaluronidase G
Other: Rituxan

○ **J9312** Injection, rituximab, 10 mg K
Other: Rituxan

* **J9313** Injection, moxetumomab pasudotox-tdfk, 0.01 mg K2 G

* **J9315** Injection, romidepsin, 1 mg B D Qp Qh K2 K
Other: Istodax
Coding Clinic: 2011, Q1, P7

▶ **J9316** Injection, pertuzumab, trastuzumab, and hyaluronidase-zzxf, per 10 mg K2 G

▶ **J9317** Injection, sacituzumab govitecan-hziy, 2.5 mg K2 G

○ **J9320** Injection, streptozocin, 1 gram B D Qp Qh K2 K
Other: Zanosar
IOM: 100-02, 15, 50

* **J9325** Injection, talimogene laherparepvec, per 1 million plaque forming units Qp Qh K2 G
Other: Imlygic
Coding Clinic: 2019, Q2, P12

* **J9328** Injection, temozolomide, 1 mg B D Qp Qh K2 K
Intravenous formulation, not for oral administration
Other: Temodar

* **J9330** Injection, temsirolimus, 1 mg B D Qp Qh K2 K
Treatment for advanced renal cell carcinoma; standard administration is intravenous infusion greater than 30-60 minutes
Other: Torisel

○ **J9340** Injection, thiotepa, 15 mg B D Qp Qh K2 K
Other: Tepadina, Triethylene thio Phosphoramide/T
IOM: 100-02, 15, 50

* **J9351** Injection, topotecan, 0.1 mg B D Qp Qh N1 N
Other: Hycamtin
Coding Clinic: 2011, Q1, P9

* **J9352** Injection, trabectedin, 0.1 mg Qp Qh K2 G
Other: Yondelis

* **J9354** Injection, ado-trastuzumab emtansine, 1 mg B D Qp Qh K2 K
Other: Kadcyla

* **J9355** Injection, trastuzumab, excludes biosimilar, 10 mg B D Qp Qh K2 K
Other: Herceptin

* **J9356** Injection, trastuzumab, 10 mg and hyaluronidase-oysk K2 G

○ **J9357** Injection, valrubicin, intravesical, 200 mg B D Qp Qh K2 K
Other: Valstar
IOM: 100-02, 15, 50

▶ **J9358** Injection, fam-trastuzumab deruxtecan-nxki, 1 mg K2 G

○ **J9360** Injection, vinblastine sulfate, 1 mg B D Qp Qh N1 N
Other: Alkaban-AQ, Velban, Velsar
IOM: 100-02, 15, 50

○ **J9370** Vincristine sulfate, 1 mg B D Qp Qh N1 N
Other: Oncovin, Vincasar PFS
IOM: 100-02, 15, 50
Coding Clinic: 2011, Q1, P9

* **J9371** Injection, vincristine sulfate liposome, 1 mg B D Qp Qh K2 K

○ **J9390** Injection, vinorelbine tartrate, 10 mg B D Qp Qh N1 N
Other: Navelbine
IOM: 100-02, 15, 50

* **J9395** Injection, fulvestrant, 25 mg Qp Qh K2 K

  Other: Faslodex

* **J9400** Injection, ziv-aflibercept, 1 mg Qp Qh K2 K

  Other: Zaltrap

J9600 Injection, porfimer sodium, 75 mg Qp Qh K2 K

Other: Photofrin

IOM: 100-02, 15, 50

J9999 Not otherwise classified, antineoplastic drugs N1 N

Bill on paper, bill one unit, and identify drug and total dosage in "Remarks" field. Include invoice of cost or NDC number in "Remarks" field.

Other: Imlygic, Yondelis

IOM: 100-02, 15, 50; 100-03, 2, 110.2

Coding Clinic: 2017, Q1, P3; 2013, Q2, P3

MIPS | Qp Quantity Physician | Qh Quantity Hospital | ♀ Female only | ♂ Male only | A Age | DMEPOS | A2-Z3 ASC Payment Indicator | A-Y ASC Status Indicator | Coding Clinic

TEMPORARY CODES ASSIGNED TO DME REGIONAL CARRIERS (K0000-K9999)

Note: This section contains national codes assigned by CMS on a temporary basis and for the exclusive use of the durable medical equipment regional carriers (DMERC).

Wheelchairs and Accessories

* **K0001** Standard wheelchair
  Capped rental
* **K0002** Standard hemi (low seat) wheelchair
  Capped rental
* **K0003** Lightweight wheelchair
  Capped rental
* **K0004** High strength, lightweight wheelchair
  Capped rental
* **K0005** Ultralightweight wheelchair
  Capped rental. Inexpensive and routinely purchased DME
* **K0006** Heavy duty wheelchair
  Capped rental
* **K0007** Extra heavy duty wheelchair
  Capped rental
* **K0008** Custom manual wheelchair/base
* **K0009** Other manual wheelchair/base
  Not otherwise classified
* **K0010** Standard - weight frame motorized/power wheelchair
  Capped rental. Codes K0010-K0014 are not for manual wheelchairs with add-on power packs. Use the appropriate code for the manual wheelchair base provided (K0001-K0009) and code K0460.
* **K0011** Standard - weight frame motorized/power wheelchair with programmable control parameters for speed adjustment, tremor dampening, acceleration control and braking
  Capped rental. A patient who requires a power wheelchair usually is totally nonambulatory and has severe weakness of the upper extremities due to a neurologic or muscular disease/condition.
* **K0012** Lightweight portable motorized/power wheelchair
  Capped rental
* **K0013** Custom motorized/power wheelchair base
* **K0014** Other motorized/power wheelchair base
  Capped rental
* **K0015** Detachable, non-adjustable height armrest, replacement only, each
  Inexpensive and routinely purchased DME
* **K0017** Detachable, adjustable height armrest, base, replacement only, each
  Inexpensive and routinely purchased DME
* **K0018** Detachable, adjustable height armrest, upper portion, replacement only, each
  Inexpensive and routinely purchased DME
* **K0019** Arm pad, replacement only, each
  Inexpensive and routinely purchased DME
* **K0020** Fixed, adjustable height armrest, pair
  Inexpensive and routinely purchased DME
* **K0037** High mount flip-up footrest, each
  Inexpensive and routinely purchased DME
* **K0038** Leg strap, each
  Inexpensive and routinely purchased DME
* **K0039** Leg strap, H style, each
  Inexpensive and routinely purchased DME

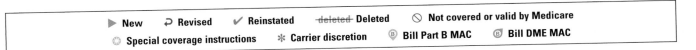

New
Revised
Reinstated
deleted Deleted
Not covered or valid by Medicare
Special coverage instructions
Carrier discretion
Bill Part B MAC
Bill DME MAC

* **K0040** Adjustable angle footplate, each Qp Qh Y
Inexpensive and routinely purchased DME

* **K0041** Large size footplate, each Qp Qh Y
Inexpensive and routinely purchased DME

* **K0042** Standard size footplate, replacement only, each Qp Qh Y
Inexpensive and routinely purchased DME

* **K0043** Footrest, lower extension tube, replacement only, each Qp Qh Y
Inexpensive and routinely purchased DME

* **K0044** Footrest, upper hanger bracket, replacement only, each Qp Qh Y
Inexpensive and routinely purchased DME

* **K0045** Footrest, complete assembly, replacement only, each Qp Qh Y
Inexpensive and routinely purchased DME

* **K0046** Elevating legrest, lower extension tube, replacement only, each Qp Qh Y
Inexpensive and routinely purchased DME

* **K0047** Elevating legrest, upper hanger bracket, replacement only, each Qp Qh Y
Inexpensive and routinely purchased DME

* **K0050** Ratchet assembly, replacement only Qp Qh Y
Inexpensive and routinely purchased DME

* **K0051** Cam release assembly, footrest or legrests, replacement only, each Qp Qh Y
Inexpensive and routinely purchased DME

* **K0052** Swing-away, detachable footrests, replacement only, each Qp Qh Y
Inexpensive and routinely purchased DME

* **K0053** Elevating footrests, articulating (telescoping), each Qp Qh Y
Inexpensive and routinely purchased DME

* **K0056** Seat height less than 17" or equal to or greater than 21" for a high strength, lightweight, or ultralightweight wheelchair Qp Qh Y
Inexpensive and routinely purchased DME

* **K0065** Spoke protectors, each Qp Qh Y
Inexpensive and routinely purchased DME

* **K0069** Rear wheel assembly, complete, with solid tire, spokes or molded, replacement only, each Qp Qh Y
Inexpensive and routinely purchased DME

* **K0070** Rear wheel assembly, complete, with pneumatic tire, spokes or molded, replacement only, each Qp Qh Y
Inexpensive and routinely purchased DME

* **K0071** Front caster assembly, complete, with pneumatic tire, replacement only, each Qp Qh Y
Caster assembly includes a caster fork (E2396), wheel rim, and tire.
Inexpensive and routinely purchased DME

* **K0072** Front caster assembly, complete, with semi-pneumatic tire, replacement only, each Qp Qh Y
Inexpensive and routinely purchased DME

* **K0073** Caster pin lock, each Qp Qh Y
Inexpensive and routinely purchased DME

* **K0077** Front caster assembly, complete, with solid tire, replacement only, each Qp Qh Y

* **K0098** Drive belt for power wheelchair, replacement only Y
Inexpensive and routinely purchased DME

* **K0105** IV hanger, each Qp Qh Y
Inexpensive and routinely purchased DME

* **K0108** Wheelchair component or accessory, not otherwise specified Y

K0195 Elevating leg rests, pair (for use with capped rental wheelchair base) Qp Qh Y
Medically necessary replacement items are covered if rollabout chair or transport chair covered
IOM: 100-03, 4, 280.1

MIPS | Qp Quantity Physician | Qh Quantity Hospital | ♀ Female only
♂ Male only | A Age | DMEPOS | A2-Z3 ASC Payment Indicator | A-Y ASC Status Indicator | Coding Clinic

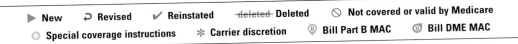

Infusion Pump, Supplies, and Batteries

K0455 Infusion pump used for uninterrupted parenteral administration of medication (e.g., epoprostenol or treprostinol) Ⓔ Op Qh ♿ Y

An EIP may also be referred to as an external insulin pump, ambulatory pump, or mini-infuser. CMN/DIF required. Frequent and substantial service DME.

IOM: 100-03, 1, 50.3

K0462 Temporary replacement for patient owned equipment being repaired, any type Ⓔ Op Qh Y

Only report for maintenance and service for an item for which initial claim was paid. The term power mobility device (PMD) includes power operated vehicles (POVs) and power wheelchairs (PWCs). Not otherwise classified.

IOM: 100-04, 20, 40.1

K0552 Supplies for external non-insulin drug infusion pump, syringe type cartridge, sterile, each Ⓔ Qh ♿ Y

Supplies

IOM: 100-03, 1, 50.3

K0553 Supply allowance for therapeutic continuous glucose monitor (CGM), includes all supplies and accessories, 1 month supply = 1 unit of service Ⓔ ♿ Y

K0554 Receiver (monitor), dedicated, for use with therapeutic glucose continuous monitor system Ⓔ ♿ Y

* **K0601** Replacement battery for external infusion pump owned by patient, silver oxide, 1.5 volt, each Ⓔ Qh ♿ Y

Inexpensive and routinely purchased DME

* **K0602** Replacement battery for external infusion pump owned by patient, silver oxide, 3 volt, each Ⓔ Op Qh ♿ Y

Inexpensive and routinely purchased DME

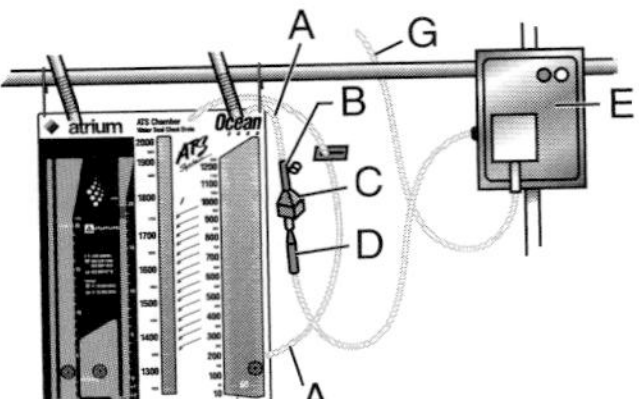
A
G
B
C
D
E
A
atrium
Ocean

Figure 18 Infusion pump.

* **K0603** Replacement battery for external infusion pump owned by patient, alkaline, 1.5 volt, each Ⓔ Qh ♿ Y

Inexpensive and routinely purchased DME

* **K0604** Replacement battery for external infusion pump owned by patient, lithium, 3.6 volt, each Ⓔ Qh ♿ Y

Inexpensive and routinely purchased DME

* **K0605** Replacement battery for external infusion pump owned by patient, lithium, 4.5 volt, each Ⓔ Op Qh ♿ Y

Inexpensive and routinely purchased DME

Defibrillator and Accessories

* **K0606** Automatic external defibrillator, with integrated electrocardiogram analysis, garment type Ⓔ Op Qh ♿ Y

Capped rental

* **K0607** Replacement battery for automated external defibrillator, garment type only, each Ⓔ Op Qh ♿ Y

Inexpensive and routinely purchased DME

* **K0608** Replacement garment for use with automated external defibrillator, each Ⓔ Op Qh ♿ Y

Inexpensive and routinely purchased DME

* **K0609** Replacement electrodes for use with automated external defibrillator, garment type only, each Ⓔ Op Qh ♿ Y

Supplies

Miscellaneous

* **K0669** Wheelchair accessory, wheelchair seat or back cushion, does not meet specific code criteria or no written coding verification from DME PDAC Ⓔ Y

Inexpensive and routinely purchased DME

* **K0672** Addition to lower extremity orthosis, removable soft interface, all components, replacement only, each Ⓔ Op ♿ A

Prosthetics/Orthotics

▶ New ⤺ Revised ✓ Reinstated ~~deleted~~ Deleted ⊘ Not covered or valid by Medicare
Special coverage instructions * Carrier discretion Ⓑ Bill Part B MAC Ⓔ Bill DME MAC

✻ **K0730** Controlled dose inhalation drug delivery system Ⓑ Qp Qh ♿ Y
Inexpensive and routinely purchased DME

✻ **K0733** Power wheelchair accessory, 12 to 24 amp hour sealed lead acid battery, each (e.g., gel cell, absorbed glassmat) Ⓑ Qp Qh ♿ Y
Inexpensive and routinely purchased DME

✻ **K0738** Portable gaseous oxygen system, rental; home compressor used to fill portable oxygen cylinders; includes portable containers, regulator, flowmeter, humidifier, cannula or mask, and tubing Ⓑ Qp Qh ♿ Y
Oxygen and oxygen equipment

✻ **K0739** Repair or nonroutine service for durable medical equipment other than oxygen equipment requiring the skill of a technician, labor component, per 15 minutes Ⓑ Y

⊘ **K0740** Repair or nonroutine service for oxygen equipment requiring the skill of a technician, labor component, per 15 minutes Ⓑ Qp Qh E1

✻ **K0743** Suction pump, home model, portable, for use on wounds Ⓑ Qp Qh Y

✻ **K0744** Absorptive wound dressing for use with suction pump, home model, portable, pad size 16 square inches or less Ⓑ Qp A

✻ **K0745** Absorptive wound dressing for use with suction pump, home model, portable, pad size more than 16 square inches but less than or equal to 48 square inches Ⓑ Qp A

✻ **K0746** Absorptive wound dressing for use with suction pump, home model, portable, pad size greater than 48 square inches Ⓑ Qp A

Power Mobility Devices

✻ **K0800** Power operated vehicle, group 1 standard, patient weight capacity up to and including 300 pounds Ⓑ Qp Qh ♿ Y
Power mobility device (PMD) includes power operated vehicles (POVs) and power wheelchairs (PWCs). Inexpensive and routinely purchased DME

✻ **K0801** Power operated vehicle, group 1 heavy duty, patient weight capacity 301 to 450 pounds Ⓑ Qp Qh ♿ Y
Inexpensive and routinely purchased DME

✻ **K0802** Power operated vehicle, group 1 very heavy duty, patient weight capacity 451 to 600 pounds Ⓑ Qp Qh ♿ Y
Inexpensive and routinely purchased DME

✻ **K0806** Power operated vehicle, group 2 standard, patient weight capacity up to and including 300 pounds Ⓑ Qp Qh ♿ Y
Inexpensive and routinely purchased DME

✻ **K0807** Power operated vehicle, group 2 heavy duty, patient weight capacity 301 to 450 pounds Ⓑ Qp Qh ♿ Y
Inexpensive and routinely purchased DME

✻ **K0808** Power operated vehicle, group 2 very heavy duty, patient weight capacity 451 to 600 pounds Ⓑ Qp Qh ♿ Y
Inexpensive and routinely purchased DME

✻ **K0812** Power operated vehicle, not otherwise classified Ⓑ Qp Qh Y
Not otherwise classified.

✻ **K0813** Power wheelchair, group 1 standard, portable, sling/solid seat and back, patient weight capacity up to and including 300 pounds Ⓑ Qp Qh ♿ Y
Capped rental

✻ **K0814** Power wheelchair, group 1 standard, portable, captains chair, patient weight capacity up to and including 300 pounds Ⓑ Qp Qh ♿ Y
Capped rental

✻ **K0815** Power wheelchair, group 1 standard, sling/solid seat and back, patient weight capacity up to and including 300 pounds Ⓑ Qp Qh ♿ Y
Capped rental

✻ **K0816** Power wheelchair, group 1 standard, captains chair, patient weight capacity up to and including 300 pounds Ⓑ Qp Qh ♿ Y
Capped rental

✻ **K0820** Power wheelchair, group 2 standard, portable, sling/solid seat/back, patient weight capacity up to and including 300 pounds Y
Capped rental

✻ **K0821** Power wheelchair, group 2 standard, portable, captains chair, patient weight capacity up to and including 300 pounds Y
Capped rental

✻ **K0822** Power wheelchair, group 2 standard, sling/solid seat/back, patient weight capacity up to and including 300 pounds Y
Capped rental

✻ **K0823** Power wheelchair, group 2 standard, captains chair, patient weight capacity up to and including 300 pounds Y
Capped rental

✻ **K0824** Power wheelchair, group 2 heavy duty, sling/solid seat/back, patient weight capacity 301 to 450 pounds Y
Capped rental

✻ **K0825** Power wheelchair, group 2 heavy duty, captains chair, patient weight capacity 301 to 450 pounds Y
Capped rental

✻ **K0826** Power wheelchair, group 2 very heavy duty, sling/solid seat/back, patient weight capacity 451 to 600 pounds Y
Capped rental

✻ **K0827** Power wheelchair, group 2 very heavy duty, captains chair, patient weight capacity 451 to 600 pounds Y
Capped rental

✻ **K0828** Power wheelchair, group 2 extra heavy duty, sling/solid seat/back, patient weight capacity 601 pounds or more Y
Capped rental

✻ **K0829** Power wheelchair, group 2 extra heavy duty, captains chair, patient weight 601 pounds or more Y
Capped rental

✻ **K0830** Power wheelchair, group 2 standard, seat elevator, sling/solid seat/back, patient weight capacity up to and including 300 pounds Y
Capped rental

✻ **K0831** Power wheelchair, group 2 standard, seat elevator, captains chair, patient weight capacity up to and including 300 pounds Y

✻ **K0835** Power wheelchair, group 2 standard, single power option, sling/solid seat/back, patient weight capacity up to and including 300 pounds Y
Capped rental

✻ **K0836** Power wheelchair, group 2 standard, single power option, captains chair, patient weight capacity up to and including 300 pounds Y
Capped rental

✻ **K0837** Power wheelchair, group 2 heavy duty, single power option, sling/solid seat/back, patient weight capacity 301 to 450 pounds Y
Capped rental

✻ **K0838** Power wheelchair, group 2 heavy duty, single power option, captains chair, patient weight capacity 301 to 450 pounds Y
Capped rental

✻ **K0839** Power wheelchair, group 2 very heavy duty, single power option, sling/solid seat/back, patient weight capacity 451 to 600 pounds Y
Capped rental

✻ **K0840** Power wheelchair, group 2 extra heavy duty, single power option, sling/solid seat/back, patient weight capacity 601 pounds or more Y
Capped rental

✻ **K0841** Power wheelchair, group 2 standard, multiple power option, sling/solid seat/back, patient weight capacity up to and including 300 pounds Y
Capped rental

✻ **K0842** Power wheelchair, group 2 standard, multiple power option, captains chair, patient weight capacity up to and including 300 pounds Y
Capped rental

✻ **K0843** Power wheelchair, group 2 heavy duty, multiple power option, sling/solid seat/back, patient weight capacity 301 to 450 pounds Y
Capped rental

✻ **K0848** Power wheelchair, group 3 standard, sling/solid seat/back, patient weight capacity up to and including 300 pounds Y
Capped rental

* **K0849** Power wheelchair, group 3 standard, captains chair, patient weight capacity up to and including 300 pounds Ⓑ Qp Qh ♿ Y
Capped rental

* **K0850** Power wheelchair, group 3 heavy duty, sling/solid seat/back, patient weight capacity 301 to 450 pounds Ⓑ Qp Qh ♿ Y
Capped rental

* **K0851** Power wheelchair, group 3 heavy duty, captains chair, patient weight capacity 301 to 450 pounds Ⓑ Qp Qh ♿ Y
Capped rental

* **K0852** Power wheelchair, group 3 very heavy duty, sling/solid seat/back, patient weight capacity 451 to 600 pounds Ⓑ Qp Qh ♿ Y
Capped rental

* **K0853** Power wheelchair, group 3 very heavy duty, captains chair, patient weight capacity 451 to 600 pounds Ⓑ Qp Qh ♿ Y
Capped rental

* **K0854** Power wheelchair, group 3 extra heavy duty, sling/solid seat/back, patient weight capacity 601 pounds or more Ⓑ Qp Qh ♿ Y
Capped rental

* **K0855** Power wheelchair, group 3 extra heavy duty, captains chair, patient weight capacity 601 pounds or more Ⓑ Qp Qh ♿ Y
Capped rental

* **K0856** Power wheelchair, group 3 standard, single power option, sling/solid seat/back, patient weight capacity up to and including 300 pounds Ⓑ Qp Qh ♿ Y
Capped rental

* **K0857** Power wheelchair, group 3 standard, single power option, captains chair, patient weight capacity up to and including 300 pounds Ⓑ Qp Qh ♿ Y
Capped rental

* **K0858** Power wheelchair, group 3 heavy duty, single power option, sling/solid seat/back, patient weight 301 to 450 pounds Ⓑ Qp Qh ♿ Y
Capped rental

* **K0859** Power wheelchair, group 3 heavy duty, single power option, captains chair, patient weight capacity 301 to 450 pounds Ⓑ Qp Qh ♿ Y
Capped rental

* **K0860** Power wheelchair, group 3 very heavy duty, single power option, sling/solid seat/back, patient weight capacity 451 to 600 pounds Ⓑ Qp Qh ♿ Y
Capped rental

* **K0861** Power wheelchair, group 3 standard, multiple power option, sling/solid seat/back, patient weight capacity up to and including 300 pounds Ⓑ Qp Qh ♿ Y
Capped rental

* **K0862** Power wheelchair, group 3 heavy duty, multiple power option, sling/solid seat/back, patient weight capacity 301 to 450 pounds Ⓑ Qp Qh ♿ Y
Capped rental

* **K0863** Power wheelchair, group 3 very heavy duty, multiple power option, sling/solid seat/back, patient weight capacity 451 to 600 pounds Ⓑ Qp Qh ♿ Y
Capped rental

* **K0864** Power wheelchair, group 3 extra heavy duty, multiple power option, sling/solid seat/back, patient weight capacity 601 pounds or more Ⓑ Qp Qh ♿ Y
Capped rental

* **K0868** Power wheelchair, group 4 standard, sling/solid seat/back, patient weight capacity up to and including 300 pounds Ⓑ Qp Qh Y
Capped rental

* **K0869** Power wheelchair, group 4 standard, captains chair, patient weight capacity up to and including 300 pounds Ⓑ Qp Qh Y
Capped rental

* **K0870** Power wheelchair, group 4 heavy duty, sling/solid seat/back, patient weight capacity 301 to 450 pounds Ⓑ Qp Qh Y
Capped rental

* **K0871** Power wheelchair, group 4 very heavy duty, sling/solid seat/back, patient weight capacity 451 to 600 pounds Ⓑ Qp Qh Y
Capped rental

* **K0877** Power wheelchair, group 4 standard, single power option, sling/solid seat/back, patient weight capacity up to and including 300 pounds Ⓑ Qp Qh Y
Capped rental

* K0878 Power wheelchair, group 4 standard, single power option, captains chair, patient weight capacity up to and including 300 pounds Ⓑ Qp Qh Y
  Capped rental

* K0879 Power wheelchair, group 4 heavy duty, single power option, sling/solid seat/back, patient weight capacity 301 to 450 pounds Ⓑ Qp Qh Y
  Capped rental

* K0880 Power wheelchair, group 4 very heavy duty, single power option, sling/solid seat/back, patient weight 451 to 600 pounds Ⓑ Qp Qh Y
  Capped rental

* K0884 Power wheelchair, group 4 standard, multiple power option, sling/solid seat/back, patient weight capacity up to and including 300 pounds Ⓑ Qp Qh Y
  Capped rental

* K0885 Power wheelchair, group 4 standard, multiple power option, captains chair, patient weight capacity up to and including 300 pounds Ⓑ Qp Qh Y
  Capped rental

* K0886 Power wheelchair, group 4 heavy duty, multiple power option, sling/solid seat/back, patient weight capacity 301 to 450 pounds Ⓑ Qp Qh Y
  Capped rental

* K0890 Power wheelchair, group 5 pediatric, single power option, sling/solid seat/back, patient weight capacity up to and including 125 pounds Ⓑ Qp Qh A Y
  Capped rental

* K0891 Power wheelchair, group 5 pediatric, multiple power option, sling/solid seat/back, patient weight capacity up to and including 125 pounds Ⓑ Qp Qh A Y
  Capped rental

* K0898 Power wheelchair, not otherwise classified Ⓑ Qp Qh Y

* K0899 Power mobility device, not coded by DME PDAC or does not meet criteria Ⓑ Y

Customized DME: Other than Wheelchair

K0900 Customized durable medical equipment, other than wheelchair Ⓑ Qp Qh Y

Devices

* K1001 Electronic positional obstructive sleep apnea treatment, with sensor, includes all components and accessories, any type Ⓑ Y

⊘ K1002 Cranial electrotherapy stimulation (CES) system, includes all supplies and accessories, any type Ⓑ E1

* K1003 Whirlpool tub, walk-in, portable Ⓑ Y

* K1004 Low frequency ultrasonic diathermy treatment device for home use, includes all components and accessories Ⓑ Y

* K1005 Disposable collection and storage bag for breast milk, any size, any type, each Ⓑ Y

▶ * K1006 Suction pump, home model, portable or stationary, electric, any type, for use with external urine management system Y

▶ * K1007 Bilateral hip, knee, ankle, foot device, powered, includes pelvic component, single or double upright(s), knee joints any type, with or without ankle joints any type, includes all components and accessories, motors, microprocessors, sensors Y

▶ * K1009 Speech volume modulation system, any type, including all components and accessories Y

▶ * K1010 Indwelling intraurethral drainage device with valve, patient inserted, replacement only, each Y

▶ * K1011 Activation device for intraurethral drainage device with valve, replacement only, each Y

▶ * K1012 Charger and base station for intraurethral activation device, replacement only Y

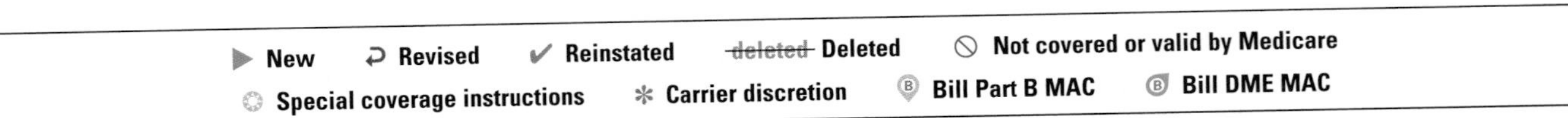
▶ New
Revised
✔ Reinstated
deleted Deleted
⊘ Not covered or valid by Medicare
Special coverage instructions
* Carrier discretion
Bill Part B MAC
Ⓑ Bill DME MAC

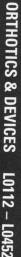

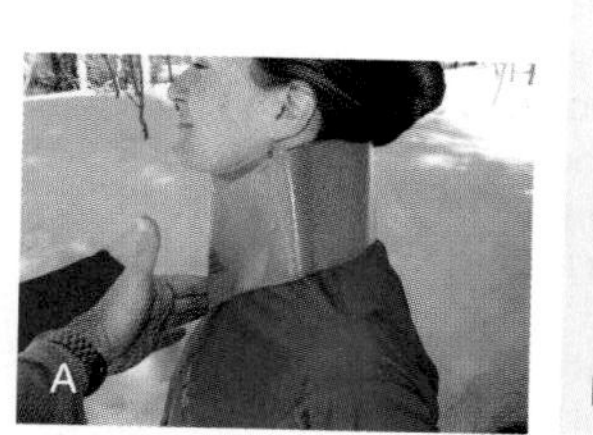
A

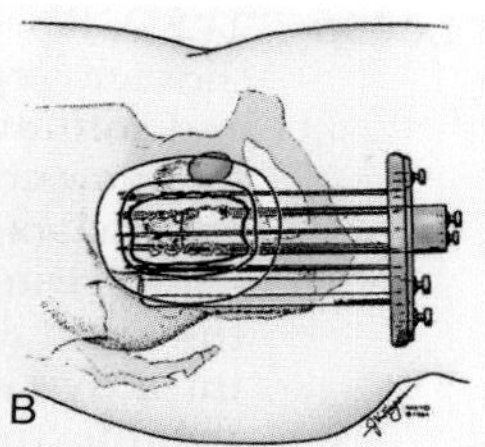
B

Figure 19 (A) Flexible cervical collar. (B) Adjustable cervical collar.

ORTHOTICS & DEVICES (L0112-L4631)

Note: DMEPOS fee schedule https://www.cms.gov/Medicare/Medicare-Fee-for-Service-Payment/DMEPOSFeeSched/DMEPOS-Fee-Schedule.html

Cervical Orthotics

* **L0112** Cranial cervical orthosis, congenital torticollis type, with or without soft interface material, adjustable range of motion joint, custom fabricated Qp Qh A
* **L0113** Cranial cervical orthosis, torticollis type, with or without joint, with or without soft interface material, prefabricated, includes fitting and adjustment Qp Qh A
* **L0120** Cervical, flexible, non-adjustable, prefabricated, off-the-shelf (foam collar) Qp Qh A

  Cervical orthoses including soft and rigid devices may be used as nonoperative management for cervical trauma
* **L0130** Cervical, flexible, thermoplastic collar, molded to patient Qp Qh A
* **L0140** Cervical, semi-rigid, adjustable (plastic collar) Qp Qh A
* **L0150** Cervical, semi-rigid, adjustable molded chin cup (plastic collar with mandibular/occipital piece) Qp Qh A
* **L0160** Cervical, semi-rigid, wire frame occipital/mandibular support, prefabricated, off-the-shelf Qp Qh A
* **L0170** Cervical, collar, molded to patient model Qp Qh A
* **L0172** Cervical, collar, semi-rigid thermoplastic foam, two-piece, prefabricated, off-the-shelf Qp Qh A
* **L0174** Cervical, collar, semi-rigid, thermoplastic foam, two piece with thoracic extension, prefabricated, off-the-shelf Qp Qh A

Multiple Post Collar: Cervical

* **L0180** Cervical, multiple post collar, occipital/mandibular supports, adjustable Qp Qh A
* **L0190** Cervical, multiple post collar, occipital/mandibular supports, adjustable cervical bars (SOMI, Guilford, Taylor types) Qp Qh A
* **L0200** Cervical, multiple post collar, occipital/mandibular supports, adjustable cervical bars, and thoracic extension Qp Qh A

Thoracic Rib Belt

* **L0220** Thoracic, rib belt, custom fabricated Qp Qh A

Thoracic-Lumbar-Sacral Orthotics

* **L0450** TLSO, flexible, provides trunk support, upper thoracic region, produces intracavitary pressure to reduce load on the intervertebral disks with rigid stays or panel(s), includes shoulder straps and closures, prefabricated, off-the-shelf Qp Qh A

  Used to immobilize specified area of spine, and is generally worn under clothing
* **L0452** TLSO, flexible, provides trunk support, upper thoracic region, produces intracavitary pressure to reduce load on the intervertebral disks with rigid stays or panel(s), includes shoulder straps and closures, custom fabricated Qp Qh A

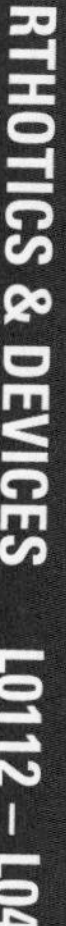
ORTHOTICS & DEVICES L0112 – L0452

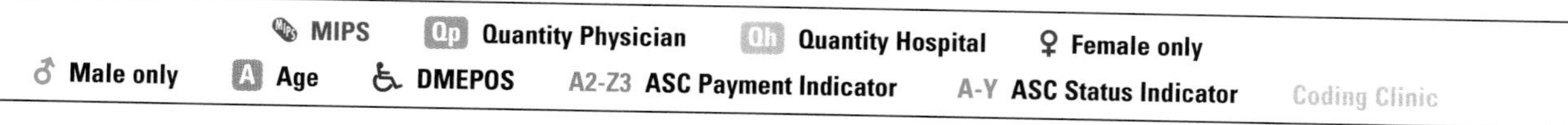
MIPS
Qp Quantity Physician
Qh Quantity Hospital
♀ Female only
♂ Male only
A Age
DMEPOS
A2-Z3 ASC Payment Indicator
A-Y ASC Status Indicator
Coding Clinic

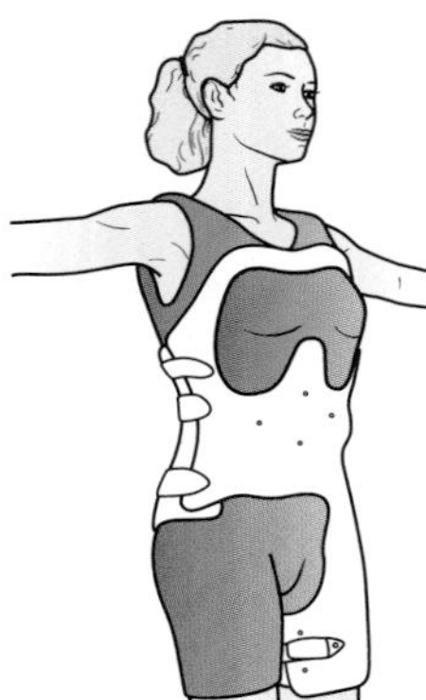

Figure 20 Thoracic-lumbar-sacral-orthosis (TLSO).

✻ **L0454** TLSO flexible, provides trunk support, extends from sacrococcygeal junction to above T-9 vertebra, restricts gross trunk motion in the sagittal plane, produces intracavitary pressure to reduce load on the intervertebral disks with rigid stays or panel(s), includes shoulder straps and closures, prefabricated item that has been trimmed, bent, molded, assembled, or otherwise customized to fit a specific patient by an individual with expertise Ⓔ Qp Qh ♿ A

Used to immobilize specified areas of spine; and is generally designed to be worn under clothing; not specifically designed for patients in wheelchairs

✻ **L0455** TLSO, flexible, provides trunk support, extends from sacrococcygeal junction to above T-9 vertebra, restricts gross trunk motion in the sagittal plane, produces intracavitary pressure to reduce load on the intervertebral disks with rigid stays or panel(s), includes shoulder straps and closures, prefabricated, off-the-shelf Ⓔ Qp Qh ♿ A

✻ **L0456** TLSO, flexible, provides trunk support, thoracic region, rigid posterior panel and soft anterior apron, extends from the sacrococcygeal junction and terminates just inferior to the scapular spine, restricts gross trunk motion in the sagittal plane, produces intracavitary pressure to reduce load on the intervertebral disks, includes straps and closures, prefabricated item that has been trimmed, bent, molded, assembled, or otherwise customized to fit a specific patient by an individual with expertise Ⓔ Qp Qh ♿ A

✻ **L0457** TLSO, flexible, provides trunk support, thoracic region, rigid posterior panel and soft anterior apron, extends from the sacrococcygeal junction and terminates just inferior to the scapular spine, restricts gross trunk motion in the sagittal plane, produces intracavitary pressure to reduce load on the intervertebral disks, includes straps and closures, prefabricated, off-the-shelf Ⓔ Qp Qh ♿ A

✻ **L0458** TLSO, triplanar control, modular segmented spinal system, two rigid plastic shells, posterior extends from the sacrococcygeal junction and terminates just inferior to the scapular spine, anterior extends from the symphysis pubis to the xiphoid, soft liner, restricts gross trunk motion in the sagittal, coronal, and transverse planes, lateral strength is provided by overlapping plastic and stabilizing closures, includes straps and closures, prefabricated, includes fitting and adjustment Ⓔ Qp Qh ♿ A

To meet Medicare's definition of body jacket, orthosis has to have rigid plastic shell that circles trunk with overlapping edges and stabilizing closures, and entire circumference of shell must be made of same rigid material.

✻ **L0460** TLSO, triplanar control, modular segmented spinal system, two rigid plastic shells, posterior extends from the sacrococcygeal junction and terminates just inferior to the scapular spine, anterior extends from the symphysis pubis to the sternal notch, soft liner, restricts gross trunk motion in the sagittal, coronal, and transverse planes, lateral strength is provided by overlapping plastic and stabilizing closures, includes straps and closures, prefabricated item that has been trimmed, bent, molded, assembled, or otherwise customized to fit a specific patient by an individual with expertise Ⓑ Qp Qh ♿ A

✻ **L0462** TLSO, triplanar control, modular segmented spinal system, three rigid plastic shells, posterior extends from the sacrococcygeal junction and terminates just inferior to the scapular spine, anterior extends from the symphysis pubis to the sternal notch, soft liner, restricts gross trunk motion in the sagittal, coronal, and transverse planes, lateral strength is provided by overlapping plastic and stabilizing closures, includes straps and closures, prefabricated, includes fitting and adjustment Ⓑ Qp Qh ♿ A

✻ **L0464** TLSO, triplanar control, modular segmented spinal system, four rigid plastic shells, posterior extends from sacrococcygeal junction and terminates just inferior to scapular spine, anterior extends from symphysis pubis to the sternal notch, soft liner, restricts gross trunk motion in sagittal, coronal, and transverse planes, lateral strength is provided by overlapping plastic and stabilizing closures, includes straps and closures, prefabricated, includes fitting and adjustment Ⓑ Qp Qh ♿ A

✻ **L0466** TLSO, sagittal control, rigid posterior frame and flexible soft anterior apron with straps, closures and padding, restricts gross trunk motion in sagittal plane, produces intracavitary pressure to reduce load on intervertebral disks, prefabricated item that has been trimmed, bent, molded, assembled, or otherwise customized to fit a specific patient by an individual with expertise Ⓑ Qp Qh ♿ A

✻ **L0467** TLSO, sagittal control, rigid posterior frame and flexible soft anterior apron with straps, closures and padding, restricts gross trunk motion in sagittal plane, produces intracavitary pressure to reduce load on intervertebral disks, prefabricated, off-the-shelf Ⓑ Qp Qh ♿ A

✻ **L0468** TLSO, sagittal-coronal control, rigid posterior frame and flexible soft anterior apron with straps, closures and padding, extends from sacrococcygeal junction over scapulae, lateral strength provided by pelvic, thoracic, and lateral frame pieces, restricts gross trunk motion in sagittal, and coronal planes, produces intracavitary pressure to reduce load on intervertebral disks, prefabricated item that has been trimmed, bent, molded, assembled, or otherwise customized to fit a specific patient by an individual with expertise Ⓑ Qp Qh ♿ A

✻ **L0469** TLSO, sagittal-coronal control, rigid posterior frame and flexible soft anterior apron with straps, closures and padding, extends from sacrococcygeal junction over scapulae, lateral strength provided by pelvic, thoracic, and lateral frame pieces, restricts gross trunk motion in sagittal and coronal planes, produces intracavitary pressure to reduce load on intervertebral disks, prefabricated, off-the-shelf Ⓑ Qp Qh ♿ A

✻ **L0470** TLSO, triplanar control, rigid posterior frame and flexible soft anterior apron with straps, closures and padding, extends from sacrococcygeal junction to scapula, lateral strength provided by pelvic, thoracic, and lateral frame pieces, rotational strength provided by subclavicular extensions, restricts gross trunk motion in sagittal, coronal, and transverse planes, provides intracavitary pressure to reduce load on the intervertebral disks, includes fitting and shaping the frame, prefabricated, includes fitting and adjustment Ⓑ Qp Qh ♿ A

✻ **L0472** TLSO, triplanar control, hyperextension, rigid anterior and lateral frame extends from symphysis pubis to sternal notch with two anterior components (one pubic and one sternal), posterior and lateral pads with straps and closures, limits spinal flexion, restricts gross trunk motion in sagittal, coronal, and transverse planes, includes fitting and shaping the frame, prefabricated, includes fitting and adjustment Ⓑ Qp Qh ♿ A

✻ **L0480** TLSO, triplanar control, one piece rigid plastic shell without interface liner, with multiple straps and closures, posterior extends from sacrococcygeal junction and terminates just inferior to scapular spine, anterior extends from symphysis pubis to sternal notch, anterior or posterior opening, restricts gross trunk motion in sagittal, coronal, and transverse planes, includes a carved plaster or CAD-CAM model, custom fabricated Ⓑ Qp Qh ♿ A

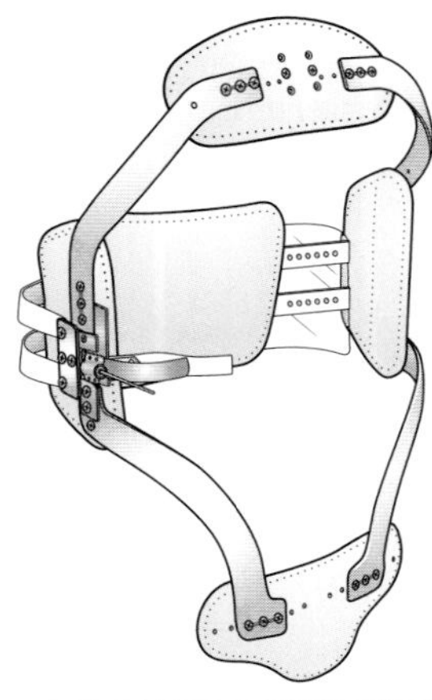

Figure 21 Thoracic-lumbar-sacral orthosis (TLSO) Jewett flexion control.

✻ **L0482** TLSO, triplanar control, one piece rigid plastic shell with interface liner, multiple straps and closures, posterior extends from sacrococcygeal junction and terminates just inferior to scapular spine, anterior extends from symphysis pubis to sternal notch, anterior or posterior opening, restricts gross trunk motion in sagittal, coronal, and transverse planes, includes a carved plaster or CAD-CAM model, custom fabricated Ⓑ Qp Qh ♿ A

✻ **L0484** TLSO, triplanar control, two piece rigid plastic shell without interface liner, with multiple straps and closures, posterior extends from sacrococcygeal junction and terminates just inferior to scapular spine, anterior extends from symphysis pubis to sternal notch, lateral strength is enhanced by overlapping plastic, restricts gross trunk motion in the sagittal, coronal, and transverse planes, includes a carved plaster or CAD-CAM model, custom fabricated Ⓑ Qp Qh ♿ A

✻ **L0486** TLSO, triplanar control, two piece rigid plastic shell with interface liner, multiple straps and closures, posterior extends from sacrococcygeal junction and terminates just inferior to scapular spine, anterior extends from symphysis pubis to sternal notch, lateral strength is enhanced by overlapping plastic, restricts gross trunk motion in the sagittal, coronal, and transverse planes, includes a carved plaster or CAD-CAM model, custom fabricated Ⓑ Qp Qh ♿ A

✻ **L0488** TLSO, triplanar control, one piece rigid plastic shell with interface liner, multiple straps and closures, posterior extends from sacrococcygeal junction and terminates just inferior to scapular spine, anterior extends from symphysis pubis to sternal notch, anterior or posterior opening, restricts gross trunk motion in sagittal, coronal, and transverse planes, prefabricated, includes fitting and adjustment Ⓑ Qp Qh ♿ A

▶ New ⤾ Revised ✓ Reinstated ~~deleted~~ Deleted ⊘ Not covered or valid by Medicare
Special coverage instructions ✻ Carrier discretion Ⓑ Bill Part B MAC Ⓑ Bill DME MAC

* **L0490** TLSO, sagittal-coronal control, one piece rigid plastic shell, with overlapping reinforced anterior, with multiple straps and closures, posterior extends from sacrococcygeal junction and terminates at or before the T-9 vertebra, anterior extends from symphysis pubis to xiphoid, anterior opening, restricts gross trunk motion in sagittal and coronal planes, prefabricated, includes fitting and adjustment Ⓔ Qp Qh ♿ A

* **L0491** TLSO, sagittal-coronal control, modular segmented spinal system, two rigid plastic shells, posterior extends from the sacrococcygeal junction and terminates just inferior to the scapular spine, anterior extends from the symphysis pubis to the xiphoid, soft liner, restricts gross trunk motion in the sagittal and coronal planes, lateral strength is provided by overlapping plastic and stabilizing closures, includes straps and closures, prefabricated, includes fitting and adjustment Ⓔ Qp Qh ♿ A

* **L0492** TLSO, sagittal-coronal control, modular segmented spinal system, three rigid plastic shells, posterior extends from the sacrococcygeal junction and terminates just inferior to the scapular spine, anterior extends from the symphysis pubis to the xiphoid, soft liner, restricts gross trunk motion in the sagittal and coronal planes, lateral strength is provided by overlapping plastic and stabilizing closures, includes straps and closures, prefabricated, includes fitting and adjustment Ⓔ Qp Qh ♿ A

Sacroilliac Orthotics

* **L0621** Sacroiliac orthosis, flexible, provides pelvic-sacral support, reduces motion about the sacroiliac joint, includes straps, closures, may include pendulous abdomen design, prefabricated, off-the-shelf Ⓔ Qp Qh ♿ A

* **L0622** Sacroiliac orthosis, flexible, provides pelvic-sacral support, reduces motion about the sacroiliac joint, includes straps, closures, may include pendulous abdomen design, custom fabricated Ⓔ Qp Qh ♿ A

Type of custom-fabricated device for which impression of specific body part is made (e.g., by means of plaster cast, or CAD-CAM [computer-aided design] technology); impression then used to make specific patient model

* **L0623** Sacroiliac orthosis, provides pelvic-sacral support, with rigid or semi-rigid panels over the sacrum and abdomen, reduces motion about the sacroiliac joint, includes straps, closures, may include pendulous abdomen design, prefabricated, off-the-shelf Ⓔ Qp Qh ♿ A

* **L0624** Sacroiliac orthosis, provides pelvic-sacral support, with rigid or semi-rigid panels placed over the sacrum and abdomen, reduces motion about the sacroiliac joint, includes straps, closures, may include pendulous abdomen design, custom fabricated Ⓔ Qp Qh ♿ A

Custom fitted

Lumbar Orthotics

* **L0625** Lumbar orthosis, flexible, provides lumbar support, posterior extends from L-1 to below L-5 vertebra, produces intracavitary pressure to reduce load on the intervertebral discs, includes straps, closures, may include pendulous abdomen design, shoulder straps, stays, prefabricated, off-the-shelf Ⓔ Qp Qh ♿ A

* **L0626** Lumbar orthosis, sagittal control, with rigid posterior panel(s), posterior extends from L-1 to below L-5 vertebra, produces intracavitary pressure to reduce load on the intervertebral discs, includes straps, closures, may include padding, stays, shoulder straps, pendulous abdomen design, prefabricated item that has been trimmed, bent, molded, assembled, or otherwise customized to fit a specific patient by an individual with expertise Ⓔ Qp Qh ♿ A

✻ **L0627** Lumbar orthosis, sagittal control, with rigid anterior and posterior panels, posterior extends from L-1 to below L-5 vertebra, produces intracavitary pressure to reduce load on the intervertebral discs, includes straps, closures, may include padding, shoulder straps, pendulous abdomen design, prefabricated item that has been trimmed, bent, molded, assembled, or otherwise customized to fit a specific patient by an individual with expertise Ⓑ Qp Qh ♿ A

Lumbar-Sacral Orthotics

✻ **L0628** Lumbar-sacral orthosis, flexible, provides lumbo-sacral support, posterior extends from sacrococcygeal junction to T-9 vertebra, produces intracavitary pressure to reduce load on the intervertebral discs, includes straps, closures, may include stays, shoulder straps, pendulous abdomen design, prefabricated, off-the-shelf Ⓑ Qp Qh ♿ A

✻ **L0629** Lumbar-sacral orthosis, flexible, provides lumbo-sacral support, posterior extends from sacrococcygeal junction to T-9 vertebra, produces intracavitary pressure to reduce load on the intervertebral discs, includes straps, closures, may include stays, shoulder straps, pendulous abdomen design, custom fabricated Ⓑ Qp Qh ♿ A

Custom fitted

✻ **L0630** Lumbar-sacral orthosis, sagittal control, with rigid posterior panel(s), posterior extends from sacrococcygeal junction to T-9 vertebra, produces intracavitary pressure to reduce load on the intervertebral discs, includes straps, closures, may include padding, stays, shoulder straps, pendulous abdomen design, prefabricated item that has been trimmed, bent, molded, assembled, or otherwise customized to fit a specific patient by an individual with expertise Ⓑ Qp Qh ♿ A

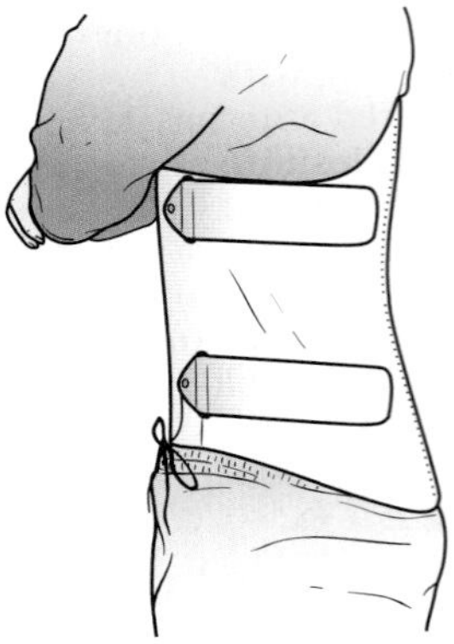

Figure 22 Lumbar-sacral orthosis.

✻ **L0631** Lumbar-sacral orthosis, sagittal control, with rigid anterior and posterior panels, posterior extends from sacrococcygeal junction to T-9 vertebra, produces intracavitary pressure to reduce load on the intervertebral discs, includes straps, closures, may include padding, shoulder straps, pendulous abdomen design, prefabricated item that has been trimmed, bent, molded, assembled, or otherwise customized to fit a specific patient by an individual with expertise Ⓑ Qp Qh ♿ A

✻ **L0632** Lumbar-sacral orthosis, sagittal control, with rigid anterior and posterior panels, posterior extends from sacrococcygeal junction to T-9 vertebra, produces intracavitary pressure to reduce load on the intervertebral discs, includes straps, closures, may include padding, shoulder straps, pendulous abdomen design, custom fabricated Ⓑ Qp Qh ♿ A

Custom fitted

✻ **L0633** Lumbar-sacral orthosis, sagittal-coronal control, with rigid posterior frame/panel(s), posterior extends from sacrococcygeal junction to T-9 vertebra, lateral strength provided by rigid lateral frame/panels, produces intracavitary pressure to reduce load on intervertebral discs, includes straps, closures, may include padding, stays, shoulder straps, pendulous abdomen design, prefabricated item that has been trimmed, bent, molded, assembled, or otherwise customized to fit a specific patient by an individual with expertise Ⓑ Qp Qh ♿ A

▶ New ↺ Revised ✓ Reinstated ~~deleted~~ Deleted ⊘ Not covered or valid by Medicare
Special coverage instructions ✻ Carrier discretion Ⓑ Bill Part B MAC Ⓑ Bill DME MAC

✻ **L0634** Lumbar-sacral orthosis, sagittal-coronal control, with rigid posterior frame/panel(s), posterior extends from sacrococcygeal junction to T-9 vertebra, lateral strength provided by rigid lateral frame/panel(s), produces intracavitary pressure to reduce load on intervertebral discs, includes straps, closures, may include padding, stays, shoulder straps, pendulous abdomen design, custom fabricated Ⓑ Qp Qh ♿ A

Custom fitted

✻ **L0635** Lumbar-sacral orthosis, sagittal-coronal control, lumbar flexion, rigid posterior frame/panel(s), lateral articulating design to flex the lumbar spine, posterior extends from sacrococcygeal junction to T-9 vertebra, lateral strength provided by rigid lateral frame/panel(s), produces intracavitary pressure to reduce load on intervertebral discs, includes straps, closures, may include padding, anterior panel, pendulous abdomen design, prefabricated, includes fitting and adjustment Ⓑ Qp Qh ♿ A

✻ **L0636** Lumbar sacral orthosis, sagittal-coronal control, lumbar flexion, rigid posterior frame/panels, lateral articulating design to flex the lumbar spine, posterior extends from sacrococcygeal junction to T-9 vertebra, lateral strength provided by rigid lateral frame/panels, produces intracavitary pressure to reduce load on intervertebral discs, includes straps, closures, may include padding, anterior panel, pendulous abdomen design, custom fabricated Ⓑ Qp Qh ♿ A

Custom fitted

✻ **L0637** Lumbar-sacral orthosis, sagittal-coronal control, with rigid anterior and posterior frame/panels, posterior extends from sacrococcygeal junction to T-9 vertebra, lateral strength provided by rigid lateral frame/panels, produces intracavitary pressure to reduce load on intervertebral discs, includes straps, closures, may include padding, shoulder straps, pendulous abdomen design, prefabricated item that has been trimmed, bent, molded, assembled, or otherwise customized to fit a specific patient by an individual with expertise Ⓑ Qp Qh ♿ A

✻ **L0638** Lumbar-sacral orthosis, sagittal-coronal control, with rigid anterior and posterior frame/panels, posterior extends from sacrococcygeal junction to T-9 vertebra, lateral strength provided by rigid lateral frame/panels, produces intracavitary pressure to reduce load on intervertebral discs, includes straps, closures, may include padding, shoulder straps, pendulous abdomen design, custom fabricated Ⓑ Qp Qh ♿ A

✻ **L0639** Lumbar-sacral orthosis, sagittal-coronal control, rigid shell(s)/panel(s), posterior extends from sacrococcygeal junction to T-9 vertebra, anterior extends from symphysis pubis to xyphoid, produces intracavitary pressure to reduce load on the intervertebral discs, overall strength is provided by overlapping rigid material and stabilizing closures, includes straps, closures, may include soft interface, pendulous abdomen design, prefabricated item that has been trimmed, bent, molded, assembled, or otherwise customized to fit a specific patient by an individual with expertise Ⓑ Qp Qh ♿ A

Characterized by rigid plastic shell that encircles trunk with overlapping edges and stabilizing closures and provides high degree of immobility

✻ **L0640** Lumbar-sacral orthosis, sagittal-coronal control, rigid shell(s)/panel(s), posterior extends from sacrococcygeal junction to T-9 vertebra, anterior extends from symphysis pubis to xyphoid, produces intracavitary pressure to reduce load on the intervertebral discs, overall strength is provided by overlapping rigid material and stabilizing closures, includes straps, closures, may include soft interface, pendulous abdomen design, custom fabricated Ⓑ Qp Qh ♿ A

Custom fitted

Lumbar Orthotics

✻ **L0641** Lumbar orthosis, sagittal control, with rigid posterior panel(s), posterior extends from L-1 to below L-5 vertebra, produces intracavitary pressure to reduce load on the intervertebral discs, includes straps, closures, may include padding, stays, shoulder straps, pendulous abdomen design, prefabricated, off-the-shelf Ⓑ Qp Qh ♿ A

* **L0642** Lumbar orthosis, sagittal control, with rigid anterior and posterior panels, posterior extends from L-1 to below L-5 vertebra, produces intracavitary pressure to reduce load on the intervertebral discs, includes straps, closures, may include padding, shoulder straps, pendulous abdomen design, prefabricated, off-the-shelf Ⓑ Qp Qh ♿ A

Lumbar-Sacral Orthotics

* **L0643** Lumbar-sacral orthosis, sagittal control, with rigid posterior panel(s), posterior extends from sacrococcygeal junction to T-9 vertebra, produces intracavitary pressure to reduce load on the intervertebral discs, includes straps, closures, may include padding, stays, shoulder straps, pendulous abdomen design, prefabricated, off-the-shelf Ⓑ Qp Qh ♿ A

* **L0648** Lumbar-sacral orthosis, sagittal control, with rigid anterior and posterior panels, posterior extends from sacrococcygeal junction to T-9 vertebra, produces intracavitary pressure to reduce load on the intervertebral discs, includes straps, closures, may include padding, shoulder straps, pendulous abdomen design, prefabricated, off-the-shelf Ⓑ Qp Qh ♿ A

* **L0649** Lumbar-sacral orthosis, sagittal-coronal control, with rigid posterior frame/panel(s), posterior extends from sacrococcygeal junction to T-9 vertebra, lateral strength provided by rigid lateral frame/panels, produces intracavitary pressure to reduce load on intervertebral discs, includes straps, closures, may include padding, stays, shoulder straps, pendulous abdomen design, prefabricated, off-the-shelf Ⓑ Qp Qh ♿ A

* **L0650** Lumbar-sacral orthosis, sagittal-coronal control, with rigid anterior and posterior frame/panel(s), posterior extends from sacrococcygeal junction to T-9 vertebra, lateral strength provided by rigid lateral frame/panel(s), produces intracavitary pressure to reduce load on intervertebral discs, includes straps, closures, may include padding, shoulder straps, pendulous abdomen design, prefabricated, off-the-shelf Ⓑ Qp Qh ♿ A

* **L0651** Lumbar-sacral orthosis, sagittal-coronal control, rigid shell(s)/panel(s), posterior extends from sacrococcygeal junction to T-9 vertebra, anterior extends from symphysis pubis to xyphoid, produces intracavitary pressure to reduce load on the intervertebral discs, overall strength is provided by overlapping rigid material and stabilizing closures, includes straps, closures, may include soft interface, pendulous abdomen design, prefabricated, off-the-shelf Ⓑ Qp Qh ♿ A

Cervical-Thoracic-Lumbar-Sacral

* **L0700** Cervical-thoracic-lumbar-sacral-orthoses (CTLSO), anterior-posterior-lateral control, molded to patient model (Minerva type) Ⓑ Qp Qh ♿ A

* **L0710** CTLSO, anterior-posterior-lateral-control, molded to patient model, with interface material (Minerva type) Ⓑ Qp Qh ♿ A

HALO Procedure

* **L0810** HALO procedure, cervical halo incorporated into jacket vest Ⓑ Qp Qh ♿ A

* **L0820** HALO procedure, cervical halo incorporated into plaster body jacket Ⓑ Qp Qh ♿ A

* **L0830** HALO procedure, cervical halo incorporated into Milwaukee type orthosis Ⓑ Qp Qh ♿ A

* **L0859** Addition to HALO procedure, magnetic resonance image compatible systems, rings and pins, any material Ⓑ Qp Qh ♿ A

* **L0861** Addition to HALO procedure, replacement liner/interface material Ⓑ Qp Qh ♿ A

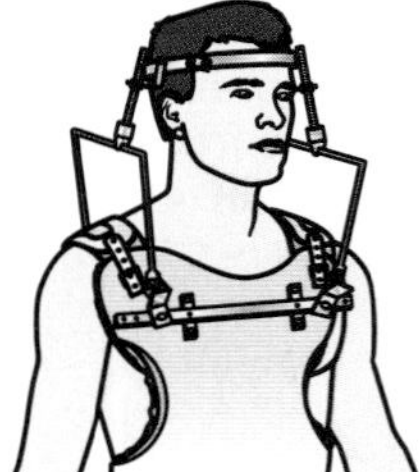

Figure 23 Halo device.

▶ New ⤾ Revised ✔ Reinstated ~~deleted~~ Deleted ⃠ Not covered or valid by Medicare
Special coverage instructions * Carrier discretion Ⓑ Bill Part B MAC Ⓑ Bill DME MAC

Additions to Spinal Orthotics

NOTE: TLSO - Thoraci-lumbar-sacral orthoses/ Spinal orthoses may be prefabricated, prefitted, or custom fabricated. Conservative treatment for back pain may include the use of spinal orthoses.

- * **L0970** TLSO, corset front Ⓑ Qp Qh ♿ A
- * **L0972** LSO, corset front Ⓑ Qp Qh ♿ A
- * **L0974** TLSO, full corset Ⓑ Qp Qh ♿ A
- * **L0976** LSO, full corset Ⓑ Qp Qh ♿ A
- * **L0978** Axillary crutch extension Ⓑ Qp Qh ♿ A
- * **L0980** Peroneal straps, prefabricated, off-the-shelf, pair Ⓑ Qp Qh ♿ A
- * **L0982** Stocking supporter grips, prefabricated, off-the-shelf, set of four (4) Ⓑ Qp Qh ♿ A

  Convenience item
- * **L0984** Protective body sock, prefabricated, off-the-shelf, each Ⓑ Qp Qh ♿ A

  Garment made of cloth or similar material that is worn under spinal orthosis and is not primarily medical in nature
- * **L0999** Addition to spinal orthosis, not otherwise specified Ⓑ A

Orthotic Devices: Scoliosis Procedures

NOTE: Orthotic care of scoliosis differs from other orthotic care in that the treatment is more dynamic in nature and uses ongoing continual modification of the orthosis to the patient's changing condition. This coding structure uses the proper names, or eponyms, of the procedures because they have historic and universal acceptance in the profession. It should be recognized that variations to the basic procedures described by the founders/ developers are accepted in various medical and orthotic practices throughout the country. All procedures include a model of patient when indicated.

- * **L1000** Cervical-thoracic-lumbar-sacral orthosis (CTLSO) (Milwaukee), inclusive of furnishing initial orthosis, including model Ⓑ Qp Qh ♿ A
- * **L1001** Cervical thoracic lumbar sacral orthosis, immobilizer, infant size, prefabricated, includes fitting and adjustment Ⓑ Qp Qh ♿ A

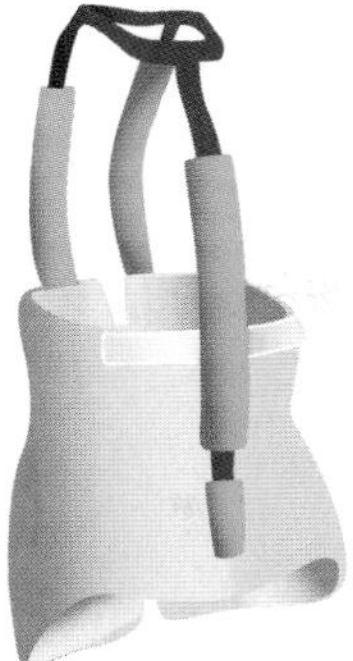

Figure 24 Milwaukee CTLSO.

- * **L1005** Tension based scoliosis orthosis and accessory pads, includes fitting and adjustment Ⓑ Qp Qh ♿ A
- * **L1010** Addition to cervical-thoracic-lumbar-sacral orthosis (CTLSO) or scoliosis orthosis, axilla sling Ⓑ Qp Qh ♿ A
- * **L1020** Addition to CTLSO or scoliosis orthosis, kyphosis pad Ⓑ Qp Qh ♿ A
- * **L1025** Addition to CTLSO or scoliosis orthosis, kyphosis pad, floating Ⓑ Qp Qh ♿ A
- * **L1030** Addition to CTLSO or scoliosis orthosis, lumbar bolster pad Ⓑ Qp Qh ♿ A
- * **L1040** Addition to CTLSO or scoliosis orthosis, lumbar or lumbar rib pad Ⓑ Qp Qh ♿ A
- * **L1050** Addition to CTLSO or scoliosis orthosis, sternal pad Ⓑ Qp Qh ♿ A
- * **L1060** Addition to CTLSO or scoliosis orthosis, thoracic pad Ⓑ Qp Qh ♿ A
- * **L1070** Addition to CTLSO or scoliosis orthosis, trapezius sling Ⓑ Qp Qh ♿ A
- * **L1080** Addition to CTLSO or scoliosis orthosis, outrigger Ⓑ Qp Qh ♿ A
- * **L1085** Addition to CTLSO or scoliosis orthosis, outrigger, bilateral with vertical extensions Ⓑ Qp Qh ♿ A
- * **L1090** Addition to CTLSO or scoliosis orthosis, lumbar sling Ⓑ Qp Qh ♿ A
- * **L1100** Addition to CTLSO or scoliosis orthosis, ring flange, plastic or leather Ⓑ Qp Qh ♿ A
- * **L1110** Addition to CTLSO or scoliosis orthosis, ring flange, plastic or leather, molded to patient model Ⓑ Qp Qh ♿ A
- * **L1120** Addition to CTLSO, scoliosis orthosis, cover for upright, each Ⓑ Qp Qh ♿ A

Thoracic-Lumbar-Sacral (Low Profile)

* **L1200** Thoracic-lumbar-sacral-orthosis (TLSO), inclusive of furnishing initial orthosis only Ⓑ Qp Qh ♿ A
* **L1210** Addition to TLSO, (low profile), lateral thoracic extension Ⓑ Qp Qh ♿ A
* **L1220** Addition to TLSO, (low profile), anterior thoracic extension Ⓑ Qp Qh ♿ A
* **L1230** Addition to TLSO, (low profile), Milwaukee type superstructure Ⓑ Qp Qh ♿ A
* **L1240** Addition to TLSO, (low profile), lumbar derotation pad Ⓑ Qp Qh ♿ A
* **L1250** Addition to TLSO, (low profile), anterior ASIS pad Ⓑ Qp Qh ♿ A
* **L1260** Addition to TLSO, (low profile), anterior thoracic derotation pad Ⓑ Qp Qh ♿ A
* **L1270** Addition to TLSO, (low profile), abdominal pad Ⓑ Qp Qh ♿ A
* **L1280** Addition to TLSO, (low profile), rib gusset (elastic), each Ⓑ Qp Qh ♿ A
* **L1290** Addition to TLSO, (low profile), lateral trochanteric pad Ⓑ Qp Qh ♿ A

Other Scoliosis Procedures

* **L1300** Other scoliosis procedure, body jacket molded to patient model Ⓑ Qp Qh ♿ A
* **L1310** Other scoliosis procedure, postoperative body jacket Ⓑ Qp Qh ♿ A
* **L1499** Spinal orthosis, not otherwise specified Ⓑ Qp Qh A

Orthotic Devices: Lower Limb (L1600-L3649)

Note: the procedures in L1600-L2999 are considered as base or basic procedures and may be modified by listing procedure from the Additions Sections and adding them to the base procedure.

Hip: Flexible

* **L1600** Hip orthosis, abduction control of hip joints, flexible, frejka type with cover, prefabricated item that has been trimmed, bent, molded, assembled, or otherwise customized to fit a specific patient by an individual with expertise Ⓑ Qp Qh ♿ A
* **L1610** Hip orthosis, abduction control of hip joints, flexible, (frejka cover only), prefabricated item that has been trimmed, bent, molded, assembled, or otherwise customized to fit a specific patient by an individual with expertise Ⓑ Qp Qh ♿ A
* **L1620** Hip orthosis, abduction control of hip joints, flexible, (Pavlik harness), prefabricated item that has been trimmed, bent, molded, assembled, or otherwise customized to fit a specific patient by an individual with expertise Ⓑ Qp Qh ♿ A
* **L1630** Hip orthosis, abduction control of hip joints, semi-flexible (Von Rosen type), custom-fabricated Ⓑ Qp Qh ♿ A
* **L1640** Hip orthosis, abduction control of hip joints, static, pelvic band or spreader bar, thigh cuffs, custom-fabricated Ⓑ Qp Qh ♿ A
* **L1650** Hip orthosis, abduction control of hip joints, static, adjustable, (Ilfled type), prefabricated, includes fitting and adjustment Ⓑ Qp Qh ♿ A
* **L1652** Hip orthosis, bilateral thigh cuffs with adjustable abductor spreader bar, adult size, prefabricated, includes fitting and adjustment, any type Ⓑ Qp Qh A ♿ A
* **L1660** Hip orthosis, abduction control of hip joints, static, plastic, prefabricated, includes fitting and adjustment Ⓑ Qp Qh ♿ A
* **L1680** Hip orthosis, abduction control of hip joints, dynamic, pelvic control, adjustable hip motion control, thigh cuffs (Rancho hip action type), custom fabrication Ⓑ Qp Qh ♿ A
* **L1685** Hip orthosis, abduction control of hip joint, postoperative hip abduction type, custom fabricated Ⓑ Qp Qh ♿ A
* **L1686** Hip orthosis, abduction control of hip joint, postoperative hip abduction type, prefabricated, includes fitting and adjustment Ⓑ Qp Qh ♿ A
* **L1690** Combination, bilateral, lumbo-sacral, hip, femur orthosis providing adduction and internal rotation control, prefabricated, includes fitting and adjustment Ⓑ Qp Qh ♿ A

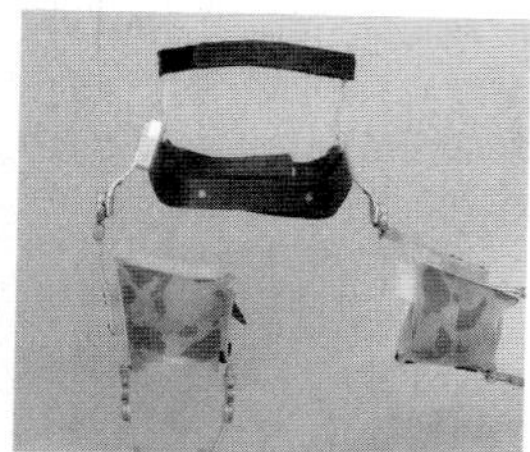

Figure 25 Thoracic-hip-knee-ankle orthosis (THKAO).

Legg Perthes

* **L1700** Legg-Perthes orthosis (Toronto type), custom-fabricated Qp Qh A
* **L1710** Legg-Perthes orthosis (Newington type), custom-fabricated Qp Qh A
* **L1720** Legg-Perthes orthosis, trilateral (Tachdjian type), custom-fabricated Qp Qh A
* **L1730** Legg-Perthes orthosis (Scottish Rite type), custom-fabricated Qp Qh A
* **L1755** Legg-Perthes orthosis (Patten bottom type), custom-fabricated Qp Qh A

Knee (KO)

* **L1810** Knee orthosis, elastic with joints, prefabricated item that has been trimmed, bent, molded, assembled, or otherwise customized to fit a specific patient by an individual with expertise Qp Qh A
* **L1812** Knee orthosis, elastic with joints, prefabricated, off-the-shelf Qp Qh A
* **L1820** Knee orthosis, elastic with condylar pads and joints, with or without patellar control, prefabricated, includes fitting and adjustment Qp Qh A

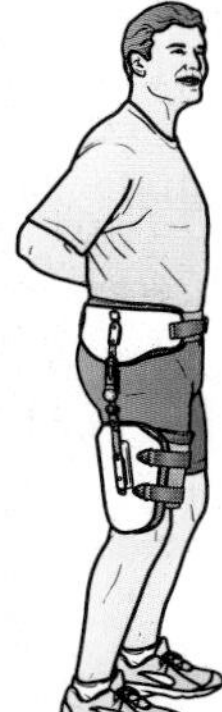

Figure 26 Hip orthosis.

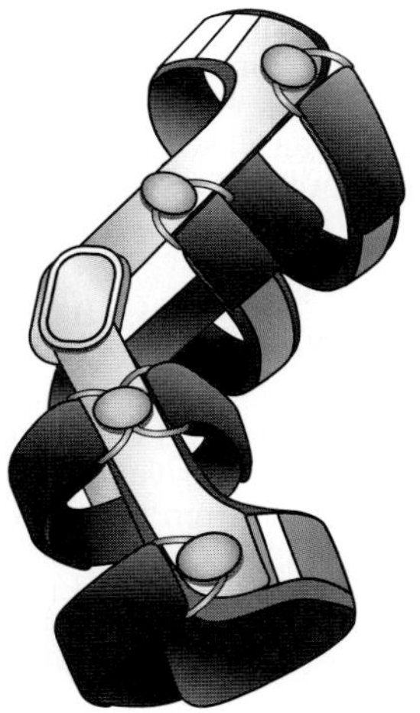

Figure 27 Knee orthosis.

* **L1830** Knee orthosis, immobilizer, canvas longitudinal, prefabricated, off-the-shelf Qp Qh A
* **L1831** Knee orthosis, locking knee joint(s), positional orthosis, prefabricated, includes fitting and adjustment Qp Qh A
* **L1832** Knee orthosis, adjustable knee joints (unicentric or polycentric), positional orthosis, rigid support, prefabricated item that has been trimmed, bent, molded, assembled, or otherwise customized to fit a specific patient by an individual with expertise Qp Qh A
* **L1833** Knee orthosis, adjustable knee joints (unicentric or polycentric), positional orthosis, rigid support, prefabricated, off-the-shelf Qp Qh A
* **L1834** Knee orthosis, without knee joint, rigid, custom-fabricated Qp Qh A
* **L1836** Knee orthosis, rigid, without joint(s), includes soft interface material, prefabricated, off-the-shelf Qp Qh A
* **L1840** Knee orthosis, derotation, medial-lateral, anterior cruciate ligament, custom fabricated Qp Qh A
* **L1843** Knee orthosis, single upright, thigh and calf, with adjustable flexion and extension joint (unicentric or polycentric), medial-lateral and rotation control, with or without varus/valgus adjustment, prefabricated item that has been trimmed, bent, molded, assembled, or otherwise customized to fit a specific patient by an individual with expertise Qp Qh A

* **L1844** Knee orthosis, single upright, thigh and calf, with adjustable flexion and extension joint (unicentric or polycentric), medial-lateral and rotation control, with or without varus/ valgus adjustment, custom fabricated Ⓑ Op Oh ♿ A

* **L1845** Knee orthosis, double upright, thigh and calf, with adjustable flexion and extension joint (unicentric or polycentric), medial-lateral and rotation control, with or without varus/valgus adjustment, prefabricated item that has been trimmed, bent, molded, assembled, or otherwise customized to fit a specific patient by an individual with expertise Ⓑ Op Oh ♿ A

* **L1846** Knee orthrosis, double upright, thigh and calf, with adjustable flexion and extension joint (unicentric or polycentric), medial-lateral and rotation control, with or without varus/ valgus adjustment, custom fabricated Ⓑ Op Oh ♿ A

* **L1847** Knee orthosis, double upright with adjustable joint, with inflatable air support chamber(s), prefabricated item that has been trimmed, bent, molded, assembled, or otherwise customized to fit a specific patient by an individual with expertise Ⓑ Op Oh ♿ A

* **L1848** Knee orthosis, double upright with adjustable joint, with inflatable air support chamber(s), prefabricated, off-the-shelf Ⓑ Op Oh ♿ A

* **L1850** Knee orthosis, Swedish type, prefabricated, off-the-shelf Ⓑ Op Oh ♿ A

* **L1851** Knee orthosis (KO), single upright, thigh and calf, with adjustable flexion and extension joint (unicentric or polycentric), medial-lateral and rotation control, with or without varus/valgus adjustment, prefabricated, off-the-shelf Op Oh ♿ A

* **L1852** Knee orthosis (KO), double upright, thigh and calf, with adjustable flexion and extension joint (unicentric or polycentric), medial-lateral and rotation control, with or without varus/valgus adjustment, prefabricated, off-the-shelf Op Oh ♿ A

* **L1860** Knee orthosis, modification of supracondylar prosthetic socket, custom fabricated (SK) Ⓑ Op Oh ♿ A

Ankle-Foot (AFO)

* **L1900** Ankle foot orthosis (AFO), spring wire, dorsiflexion assist calf band, custom-fabricated Ⓑ Op Oh ♿ A

* **L1902** Ankle orthosis, ankle gauntlet or similiar, with or without joints, prefabricated, off-the-shelf Ⓑ Op Oh ♿ A

* **L1904** Ankle orthosis, ankle gauntlet or similiar, with or without joints, custom fabricated Ⓑ Op Oh ♿ A

* **L1906** Ankle foot orthosis, multiligamentus ankle support, prefabricated, off-the-shelf Ⓑ Op Oh ♿ A

* **L1907** Ankle orthosis, supramalleolar with straps, with or without interface/pads, custom fabricated Ⓑ Op Oh ♿ A

* **L1910** Ankle foot orthosis, posterior, single bar, clasp attachment to shoe counter, prefabricated, includes fitting and adjustment Ⓑ Op Oh ♿ A

* **L1920** Ankle foot orthosis, single upright with static or adjustable stop (Phelps or Perlstein type), custom fabricated Ⓑ Op Oh ♿ A

* **L1930** Ankle foot orthosis, plastic or other material, prefabricated, includes fitting and adjustment Ⓑ Op Oh ♿ A

* **L1932** Ankle foot orthosis, rigid anterior tibial section, total carbon fiber or equal material, prefabricated, includes fitting and adjustment Ⓑ Op Oh ♿ A

* **L1940** Ankle foot orthosis, plastic or other material, custom fabricated Ⓑ Op Oh ♿ A

* **L1945** Ankle foot orthosis, plastic, rigid anterior tibial section (floor reaction), custom fabricated Ⓑ Op Oh ♿ A

* **L1950** Ankle foot orthosis, spiral (Institute of Rehabilitation Medicine type), plastic, custom fabricated Ⓑ Op Oh ♿ A

* **L1951** Ankle foot orthosis, spiral (Institute of Rehabilitative Medicine type), plastic or other material, prefabricated, includes fitting and adjustment Ⓑ Op Oh ♿ A

* **L1960** Ankle foot orthosis, posterior solid ankle, plastic, custom fabricated Ⓑ Op Oh ♿ A

* **L1970** Ankle foot orthosis, plastic, with ankle joint, custom fabricated Ⓑ Op Oh ♿ A

* **L1971** Ankle foot orthosis, plastic or other material with ankle joint, prefabricated, includes fitting and adjustment Ⓑ Op Oh ♿ A

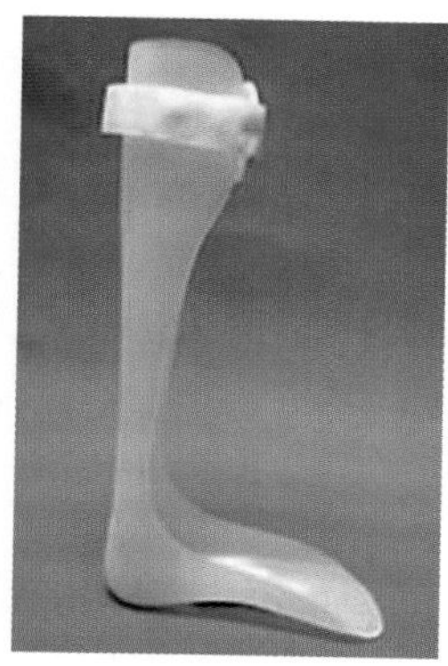

Figure 28 Ankle-foot orthosis (AFO).

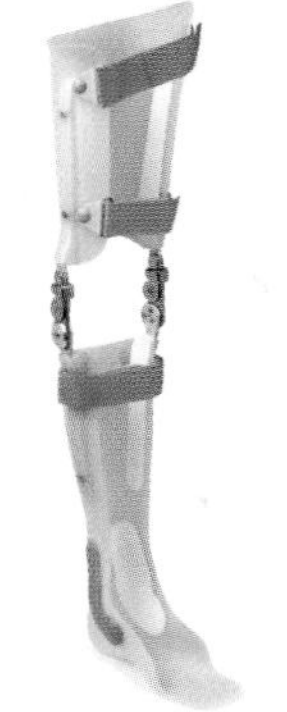

Figure 29 Knee-ankle-foot orthosis (KAFO).

* **L1980** Ankle foot orthosis, single upright free plantar dorsiflexion, solid stirrup, calf band/cuff (single bar 'BK' orthosis), custom fabricated Ⓑ Qp Qh ♿ A

* **L1990** Ankle foot orthosis, double upright free plantar dorsiflexion, solid stirrup, calf band/cuff (double bar 'BK' orthosis), custom fabricated Ⓑ Qp Qh ♿ A

Hip-Knee-Ankle-Foot (or Any Combination)

Note: L2000, L2020, and L2036 are base procedures to be used with any knee joint. L2010 and L2030 are to be used only with no knee joint.

* **L2000** Knee ankle foot orthosis, single upright, free knee, free ankle, solid stirrup, thigh and calf bands/cuffs (single bar 'AK' orthosis), custom-fabricated Ⓑ Qp Qh ♿ A

* **L2005** Knee ankle foot orthosis, any material, single or double upright, stance control, automatic lock and swing phase release, any type activation; includes ankle joint, any type, custom fabricated Ⓑ Qp Qh ♿ A

* **L2006** Knee ankle foot device, any material, single or double upright, swing and/or stance phase microprocessor control with adjustability, includes all components (e.g., sensors, batteries, charger), any type activation, with or without ankle joint(s), custom fabricated A

* **L2010** Knee ankle foot orthosis, single upright, free ankle, solid stirrup, thigh and calf bands/cuffs (single bar 'AK' orthosis), without knee joint, custom-fabricated Ⓑ Qp Qh ♿ A

* **L2020** Knee ankle foot orthosis, double upright, free knee, free ankle, solid stirrup, thigh and calf bands/cuffs (double bar 'AK' orthosis), custom fabricated Ⓑ Qp Qh ♿ A

* **L2030** Knee ankle foot orthosis, double upright, free ankle, solid stirrup, thigh and calf bands/cuffs (double bar 'AK' orthosis), without knee joint, custom fabricated Ⓑ Qp Qh ♿ A

* **L2034** Knee ankle foot orthosis, full plastic, single upright, with or without free motion knee, medial lateral rotation control, with or without free motion ankle, custom fabricated Ⓑ Qp Qh ♿ A

* **L2035** Knee ankle foot orthosis, full plastic, static (pediatric size), without free motion ankle, prefabricated, includes fitting and adjustment Ⓑ Qp Qh A ♿ A

* **L2036** Knee ankle foot orthosis, full plastic, double upright, with or without free motion knee, with or without free motion ankle, custom fabricated Ⓑ Qp Qh ♿ A

* **L2037** Knee ankle foot orthosis, full plastic, single upright, with or without free motion knee, with or without free motion ankle, custom fabricated Ⓑ Qp Qh ♿ A

* **L2038** Knee ankle foot orthosis, full plastic, with or without free motion knee, multi-axis ankle, custom fabricated Ⓑ Qp Qh ♿ A

Torsion Control: Hip-Knee-Ankle-Foot (TLSO)

* **L2040** Hip knee ankle foot orthosis, torsion control, bilateral rotation straps, pelvic band/belt, custom fabricated Ⓑ Qp Qh ♿ A

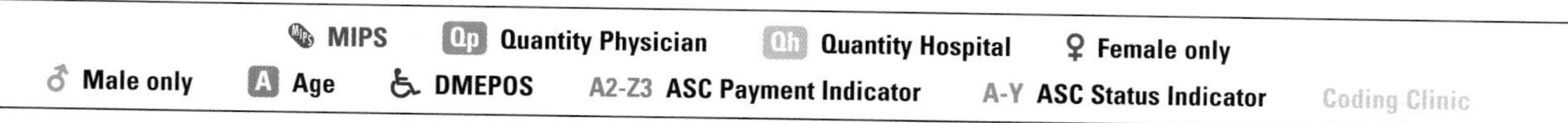

MIPS
Qp Quantity Physician
Qh Quantity Hospital
♀ Female only
♂ Male only
A Age
DMEPOS
A2-Z3 ASC Payment Indicator
A-Y ASC Status Indicator
Coding Clinic

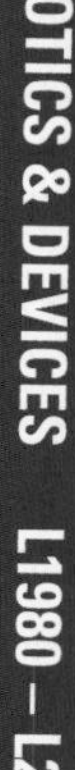

ORTHOTICS & DEVICES L1980 – L2040

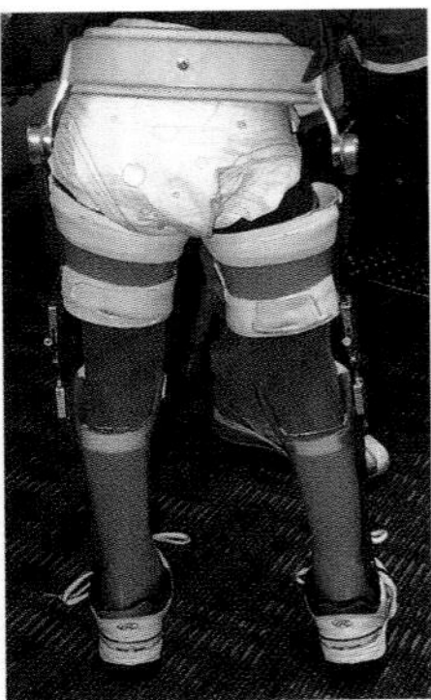

Figure 30 Hip-knee-ankle-foot orthosis (HKAFO).

* **L2050** Hip knee ankle foot orthosis, torsion control, bilateral torsion cables, hip joint, pelvic band/belt, custom fabricated Ⓑ Qp Qh ♿ A
* **L2060** Hip knee ankle foot orthosis, torsion control, bilateral torsion cables, ball bearing hip joint, pelvic band/belt, custom fabricated Ⓑ Qp Qh ♿ A
* **L2070** Hip knee ankle foot orthosis, torsion control, unilateral rotation straps, pelvic band/belt, custom fabricated Ⓑ Qp Qh ♿ A
* **L2080** Hip knee ankle foot orthosis, torsion control, unilateral torsion cable, hip joint, pelvic band/belt, custom fabricated Ⓑ Qp Qh ♿ A
* **L2090** Hip knee ankle foot orthosis, torsion control, unilateral torsion cable, ball bearing hip joint, pelvic band/belt, custom fabricated Ⓑ Qp Qh ♿ A

Fracture Orthotics: Ankle-Foot and Knee-Ankle-Foot

* **L2106** Ankle foot orthosis, fracture orthosis, tibial fracture cast orthosis, thermoplastic type casting material, custom fabricated Ⓑ Qp Qh ♿ A
* **L2108** Ankle foot orthosis, fracture orthosis, tibial fracture cast orthosis, custom fabricated Ⓑ Qp Qh ♿ A
* **L2112** Ankle foot orthosis, fracture orthosis, tibial fracture orthosis, soft, prefabricated, includes fitting and adjustment Ⓑ Qp Qh ♿ A
* **L2114** Ankle foot orthosis, fracture orthosis, tibial fracture orthosis, semi-rigid, prefabricated, includes fitting and adjustment Ⓑ Qp Qh ♿ A
* **L2116** Ankle foot orthosis, fracture orthosis, tibial fracture orthosis, rigid, prefabricated, includes fitting and adjustment Ⓑ Qp Qh ♿ A
* **L2126** Knee ankle foot orthosis, fracture orthosis, femoral fracture cast orthosis, thermoplastic type casting material, custom fabricated Ⓑ Qp Qh ♿ A
* **L2128** Knee ankle foot orthosis, fracture orthosis, femoral fracture cast orthosis, custom fabricated Ⓑ Qp Qh ♿ A
* **L2132** Knee ankle foot orthosis, femoral fracture cast orthosis, soft, prefabricated, includes fitting and adjustment Ⓑ Qp Qh ♿ A
* **L2134** Knee ankle foot orthosis, femoral fracture cast orthosis, semi-rigid, prefabricated, includes fitting and adjustment Ⓑ Qp Qh ♿ A
* **L2136** Knee ankle foot orthosis, fracture orthosis, femoral fracture cast orthosis, rigid, prefabricated, includes fitting and adjustment Ⓑ Qp Qh ♿ A

Additions to Fracture Orthotics

* **L2180** Addition to lower extremity fracture orthosis, plastic shoe insert with ankle joints Ⓑ Qp Qh ♿ A
* **L2182** Addition to lower extremity fracture orthosis, drop lock knee joint Ⓑ Qp Qh ♿ A
* **L2184** Addition to lower extremity fracture orthosis, limited motion knee joint Ⓑ Qp Qh ♿ A
* **L2186** Addition to lower extremity fracture orthosis, adjustable motion knee joint, Lerman type Ⓑ Qp Qh ♿ A
* **L2188** Addition to lower extremity fracture orthosis, quadrilateral brim Ⓑ Qp Qh ♿ A
* **L2190** Addition to lower extremity fracture orthosis, waist belt Ⓑ Qp Qh ♿ A
* **L2192** Addition to lower extremity fracture orthosis, hip joint, pelvic band, thigh flange, and pelvic belt Ⓑ Qp Qh ♿ A

Additions to Lower Extremity Orthotics

* **L2200** Addition to lower extremity, limited ankle motion, each joint Ⓑ Qp Qh ♿ A
* **L2210** Addition to lower extremity, dorsiflexion assist (plantar flexion resist), each joint Ⓑ Qp Qh ♿ A
* **L2220** Addition to lower extremity, dorsiflexion and plantar flexion assist/resist, each joint Ⓑ Qp Qh ♿ A
* **L2230** Addition to lower extremity, split flat caliper stirrups and plate attachment Ⓑ Qp Qh ♿ A

▶ New ↩ Revised ✔ Reinstated ~~deleted~~ Deleted ⊘ Not covered or valid by Medicare
Special coverage instructions * Carrier discretion Ⓑ Bill Part B MAC Ⓑ Bill DME MAC

✻ **L2232** Addition to lower extremity orthosis, rocker bottom for total contact ankle foot orthosis, for custom fabricated orthosis only Ⓑ Qp Qh ♿ A

✻ **L2240** Addition to lower extremity, round caliper and plate attachment Ⓑ Qp Qh ♿ A

✻ **L2250** Addition to lower extremity, foot plate, molded to patient model, stirrup attachment Ⓑ Qp Qh ♿ A

✻ **L2260** Addition to lower extremity, reinforced solid stirrup (Scott-Craig type) Ⓑ Qp Qh ♿ A

✻ **L2265** Addition to lower extremity, long tongue stirrup Ⓑ Qp Qh ♿ A

✻ **L2270** Addition to lower extremity, varus/valgus correction ('T') strap, padded/lined or malleolus pad Ⓑ Qp Qh ♿ A

✻ **L2275** Addition to lower extremity, varus/valgus correction, plastic modification, padded/lined Ⓑ Qp Qh ♿ A

✻ **L2280** Addition to lower extremity, molded inner boot Ⓑ Qp Qh ♿ A

✻ **L2300** Addition to lower extremity, abduction bar (bilateral hip involvement), jointed, adjustable Ⓑ Qp Qh ♿ A

✻ **L2310** Addition to lower extremity, abduction bar-straight Ⓑ Qp Qh ♿ A

✻ **L2320** Addition to lower extremity, non-molded lacer, for custom fabricated orthosis only Ⓑ Qp Qh ♿ A

✻ **L2330** Addition to lower extremity, lacer molded to patient model, for custom fabricated orthosis only Ⓑ Qp Qh ♿ A

Used whether closure is lacer or Velcro

✻ **L2335** Addition to lower extremity, anterior swing band Ⓑ Qp Qh ♿ A

✻ **L2340** Addition to lower extremity, pre-tibial shell, molded to patient model Ⓑ Qp Qh ♿ A

✻ **L2350** Addition to lower extremity, prosthetic type (BK) socket, molded to patient model, (used for 'PTB' and 'AFO' orthoses) Ⓑ Qp Qh ♿ A

✻ **L2360** Addition to lower extremity, extended steel shank Ⓑ Qp Qh ♿ A

✻ **L2370** Addition to lower extremity, Patten bottom Ⓑ Qp Qh ♿ A

✻ **L2375** Addition to lower extremity, torsion control, ankle joint and half solid stirrup Ⓑ Qp Qh ♿ A

✻ **L2380** Addition to lower extremity, torsion control, straight knee joint, each joint Ⓑ Qp Qh ♿ A

✻ **L2385** Addition to lower extremity, straight knee joint, heavy duty, each joint Ⓑ Qp ♿ A

✻ **L2387** Addition to lower extremity, polycentric knee joint, for custom fabricated knee ankle foot orthosis, each joint Ⓑ Qp ♿ A

✻ **L2390** Addition to lower extremity, offset knee joint, each joint Ⓑ Qp ♿ A

✻ **L2395** Addition to lower extremity, offset knee joint, heavy duty, each joint Ⓑ Qp ♿ A

✻ **L2397** Addition to lower extremity orthosis, suspension sleeve Ⓑ Qp ♿ A

Additions to Straight Knee or Offset Knee Joints

✻ **L2405** Addition to knee joint, drop lock, each Ⓑ Qp ♿ A

✻ **L2415** Addition to knee lock with integrated release mechanism (bail, cable, or equal), any material, each joint Ⓑ Qp ♿ A

✻ **L2425** Addition to knee joint, disc or dial lock for adjustable knee flexion, each joint Ⓑ Qp ♿ A

✻ **L2430** Addition to knee joint, ratchet lock for active and progressive knee extension, each joint Ⓑ Qp ♿ A

✻ **L2492** Addition to knee joint, lift loop for drop lock ring Ⓑ Qp ♿ A

Additions to Thigh/Weight Bearing Gluteal/Ischial Weight Bearing

✻ **L2500** Addition to lower extremity, thigh/weight bearing, gluteal/ischial weight bearing, ring Ⓑ Qp Qh ♿ A

✻ **L2510** Addition to lower extremity, thigh/weight bearing, quadri-lateral brim, molded to patient model Ⓑ Qp Qh ♿ A

✻ **L2520** Addition to lower extremity, thigh/weight bearing, quadri-lateral brim, custom fitted Ⓑ Qp Qh ♿ A

✻ **L2525** Addition to lower extremity, thigh/weight bearing, ischial containment/narrow M-L brim molded to patient model Ⓑ Qp Qh ♿ A

✻ **L2526** Addition to lower extremity, thigh/weight bearing, ischial containment/narrow M-L brim, custom fitted Ⓑ Qp Qh ♿ A

✻ **L2530** Addition to lower extremity, thigh-weight bearing, lacer, non-molded Ⓑ Qp Qh ♿ A

* **L2540** Addition to lower extremity, thigh/weight bearing, lacer, molded to patient model Ⓑ Op Oh ♿ A

* **L2550** Addition to lower extremity, thigh/weight bearing, high roll cuff Ⓑ Op Oh ♿ A

Additions to Pelvic and Thoracic Control

* **L2570** Addition to lower extremity, pelvic control, hip joint, Clevis type two position joint, each Ⓑ Op Oh ♿ A

* **L2580** Addition to lower extremity, pelvic control, pelvic sling Ⓑ Op Oh ♿ A

* **L2600** Addition to lower extremity, pelvic control, hip joint, Clevis type, or thrust bearing, free, each Ⓑ Op Oh ♿ A

* **L2610** Addition to lower extremity, pelvic control, hip joint, Clevis or thrust bearing, lock, each Ⓑ Op Oh ♿ A

* **L2620** Addition to lower extremity, pelvic control, hip joint, heavy duty, each Ⓑ Op Oh ♿ A

* **L2622** Addition to lower extremity, pelvic control, hip joint, adjustable flexion, each Ⓑ Op Oh ♿ A

* **L2624** Addition to lower extremity, pelvic control, hip joint, adjustable flexion, extension, abduction control, each Ⓑ Op Oh ♿ A

* **L2627** Addition to lower extremity, pelvic control, plastic, molded to patient model, reciprocating hip joint and cables Ⓑ Op Oh ♿ A

* **L2628** Addition to lower extremity, pelvic control, metal frame, reciprocating hip joint and cables Ⓑ Op Oh ♿ A

* **L2630** Addition to lower extremity, pelvic control, band and belt, unilateral Ⓑ Op Oh ♿ A

* **L2640** Addition to lower extremity, pelvic control, band and belt, bilateral Ⓑ Op Oh ♿ A

* **L2650** Addition to lower extremity, pelvic and thoracic control, gluteal pad, each Ⓑ Op Oh ♿ A

* **L2660** Addition to lower extremity, thoracic control, thoracic band Ⓑ Op Oh ♿ A

* **L2670** Addition to lower extremity, thoracic control, paraspinal uprights Ⓑ Op Oh ♿ A

* **L2680** Addition to lower extremity, thoracic control, lateral support uprights Ⓑ Op Oh ♿ A

General Additions

* **L2750** Addition to lower extremity orthosis, plating chrome or nickel, per bar Ⓑ Op ♿ A

* **L2755** Addition to lower extremity orthosis, high strength, lightweight material, all hybrid lamination/prepreg composite, per segment, for custom fabricated orthosis only Ⓑ Op ♿ A

* **L2760** Addition to lower extremity orthosis, extension, per extension, per bar (for lineal adjustment for growth) Ⓑ Op ♿ A

* **L2768** Orthotic side bar disconnect device, per bar Ⓑ Op ♿ A

* **L2780** Addition to lower extremity orthosis, non-corrosive finish, per bar Ⓑ Op ♿ A

* **L2785** Addition to lower extremity orthosis, drop lock retainer, each Ⓑ Op ♿ A

* **L2795** Addition to lower extremity orthosis, knee control, full kneecap Ⓑ Op Oh ♿ A

* **L2800** Addition to lower extremity orthosis, knee control, knee cap, medial or lateral pull, for use with custom fabricated orthosis only Ⓑ Op Oh ♿ A

* **L2810** Addition to lower extremity orthosis, knee control, condylar pad Ⓑ Op ♿ A

* **L2820** Addition to lower extremity orthosis, soft interface for molded plastic, below knee section Ⓑ Op Oh ♿ A

Only report if soft interface provided, either leather or other material

* **L2830** Addition to lower extremity orthosis, soft interface for molded plastic, above knee section Ⓑ Op Oh ♿ A

* **L2840** Addition to lower extremity orthosis, tibial length sock, fracture or equal, each Ⓑ Op ♿ A

* **L2850** Addition to lower extremity orthosis, femoral length sock, fracture or equal, each Ⓑ Op ♿ A

⊘ **L2861** Addition to lower extremity joint, knee or ankle, concentric adjustable torsion style mechanism for custom fabricated orthotics only, each Ⓑ Op Oh E1

* **L2999** Lower extremity orthoses, not otherwise specified Ⓑ A

▶ New ⤼ Revised ✔ Reinstated ~~deleted~~ Deleted ⊘ Not covered or valid by Medicare
Special coverage instructions * Carrier discretion Ⓑ Bill Part B MAC Ⓑ Bill DME MAC

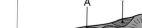

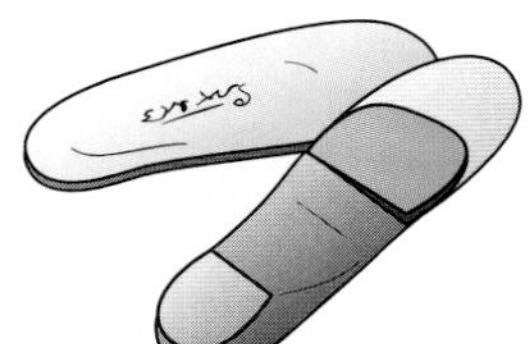

Figure 31 Foot inserts.

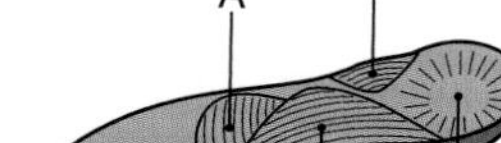
A
B
C
D
E

Figure 32 Arch support.

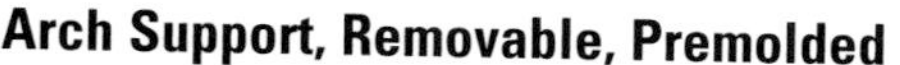

Foot (Orthopedic Shoes) (L3000-L3649)

Inserts

L3000 Foot, insert, removable, molded to patient model, 'UCB' type, Berkeley shell, each Qp Qh A

If both feet casted and supplied with an orthosis, bill L3000-LT and L3000-RT

IOM: 100-02, 15, 290

L3001 Foot, insert, removable, molded to patient model, Spenco, each Qp Qh A

IOM: 100-02, 15, 290

L3002 Foot, insert, removable, molded to patient model, Plastazote or equal, each Qp Qh A

IOM: 100-02, 15, 290

L3003 Foot, insert, removable, molded to patient model, silicone gel, each Qp Qh A

IOM: 100-02, 15, 290

L3010 Foot, insert, removable, molded to patient model, longitudinal arch support, each Qp Qh A

IOM: 100-02, 15, 290

L3020 Foot, insert, removable, molded to patient model, longitudinal/metatarsal support, each Qp Qh A

IOM: 100-02, 15, 290

L3030 Foot, insert, removable, formed to patient foot, each Qp Qh A

IOM: 100-02, 15, 290

* **L3031** Foot, insert/plate, removable, addition to lower extremity orthosis, high strength, lightweight material, all hybrid lamination/prepreg composite, each Qp Qh A

Arch Support, Removable, Premolded

L3040 Foot, arch support, removable, premolded, longitudinal, each Qp Qh A

IOM: 100-02, 15, 290

L3050 Foot, arch support, removable, premolded, metatarsal, each Qp Qh A

IOM: 100-02, 15, 290

L3060 Foot, arch support, removable, premolded, longitudinal/metatarsal, each Qp Qh A

IOM: 100-02, 15, 290

Arch Support, Non-removable, Attached to Shoe

L3070 Foot, arch support, non-removable attached to shoe, longitudinal, each Qp Qh A

IOM: 100-02, 15, 290

L3080 Foot, arch support, non-removable attached to shoe, metatarsal, each Qp Qh A

IOM: 100-02, 15, 290

L3090 Foot, arch support, non-removable attached to shoe, longitudinal/metatarsal, each Qp Qh A

IOM: 100-02, 15, 290

L3100 Hallus-valgus night dynamic splint, prefabricated, off-the-shelf Qp Qh A

IOM: 100-02, 15, 290

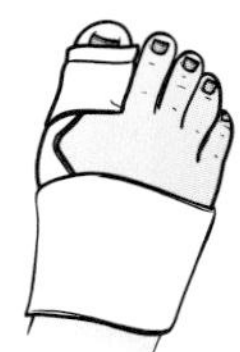

Figure 33 Hallux valgus splint.

MIPS | Qp Quantity Physician | Qh Quantity Hospital | ♀ Female only
♂ Male only | A Age | DMEPOS | A2-Z3 ASC Payment Indicator | A-Y ASC Status Indicator | Coding Clinic

Abduction and Rotation Bars

L3140 Foot, abduction rotation bar, including shoes Ⓑ Qp Qh ♿ A
IOM: 100-02, 15, 290

L3150 Foot, abduction rotation bar, without shoes Ⓑ Qp Qh ♿ A
IOM: 100-02, 15, 290

* **L3160** Foot, adjustable shoe-styled positioning device Ⓑ Qp Qh A

L3170 Foot, plastic, silicone or equal, heel stabilizer, prefabricated, off-the-shelf, each Ⓑ Qp Qh ♿ A
IOM: 100-02, 15, 290

Orthopedic Footwear

L3201 Orthopedic shoe, oxford with supinator or pronator, infant Ⓑ A A
IOM: 100-02, 15, 290

L3202 Orthopedic shoe, oxford with supinator or pronator, child Ⓑ A A
IOM: 100-02, 15, 290

L3203 Orthopedic shoe, oxford with supinator or pronator, junior Ⓑ A A
IOM: 100-02, 15, 290

L3204 Orthopedic shoe, hightop with supinator or pronator, infant Ⓑ A A
IOM: 100-02, 15, 290

L3206 Orthopedic shoe, hightop with supinator or pronator, child Ⓑ A A
IOM: 100-02, 15, 290

L3207 Orthopedic shoe, hightop with supinator or pronator, junior Ⓑ A A
IOM: 100-02, 15, 290

L3208 Surgical boot, infant, each Ⓑ A A
IOM: 100-02, 15, 100

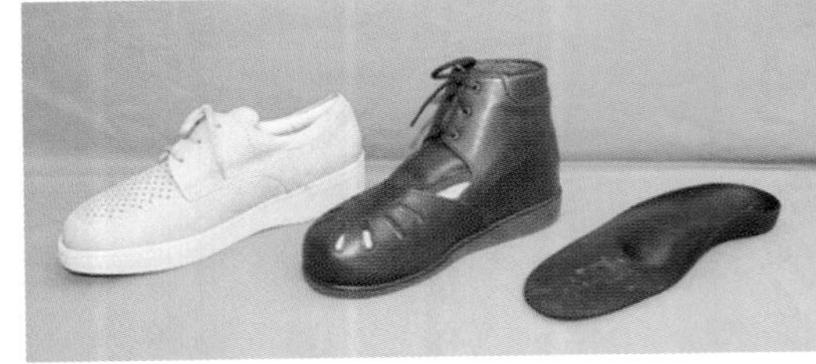

Figure 34 Molded custom shoe.

L3209 Surgical boot, each, child Ⓑ A A
IOM: 100-02, 15, 100

L3211 Surgical boot, each, junior Ⓑ A A
IOM: 100-02, 15, 100

L3212 Benesch boot, pair, infant Ⓑ A A
IOM: 100-02, 15, 100

L3213 Benesch boot, pair, child Ⓑ A A
IOM: 100-02, 15, 100

L3214 Benesch boot, pair, junior Ⓑ A A
IOM: 100-02, 15, 100

⃠ **L3215** Orthopedic footwear, ladies' shoe, oxford, each Ⓑ Qp Qh ♀ E1
Medicare Statute 1862a8

⃠ **L3216** Orthopedic footwear, ladies' shoe, depth inlay, each Ⓑ Qp Qh ♀ E1
Medicare Statute 1862a8

⃠ **L3217** Orthopedic footwear, ladies' shoe, hightop, depth inlay, each Ⓑ Qp Qh ♀ E1
Medicare Statute 1862a8

⃠ **L3219** Orthopedic footwear, men's shoe, oxford, each Ⓑ Qp Qh ♂ E1
Medicare Statute 1862a8

⃠ **L3221** Orthopedic footwear, men's shoe, depth inlay, each Ⓑ Qp Qh ♂ E1
Medicare Statute 1862a8

⃠ **L3222** Orthopedic footwear, men's shoe, hightop, depth inlay, each Ⓑ Qp Qh ♂ E1
Medicare Statute 1862a8

L3224 Orthopedic footwear, ladies' shoe, oxford, used as an integral part of a brace (orthosis) Ⓑ Qp Qh ♀ ♿ A
IOM: 100-02, 15, 290

L3225 Orthopedic footwear, men's shoe, oxford, used as an integral part of a brace (orthosis) Ⓑ Qp Qh ♂ ♿ A
IOM: 100-02, 15, 290

L3230 Orthopedic footwear, custom shoe, depth inlay, each Ⓑ Qp Qh A
IOM: 100-02, 15, 290

L3250 Orthopedic footwear, custom molded shoe, removable inner mold, prosthetic shoe, each Ⓑ Qp Qh A
IOM: 100-02, 15, 290

L3251 Foot, shoe molded to patient model, silicone shoe, each Ⓑ Qp Qh A
IOM: 100-02, 15, 290

L3252 Foot, shoe molded to patient model, Plastazote (or similar), custom fabricated, each Qp Qh A
IOM: 100-02, 15, 290

L3253 Foot, molded shoe Plastazote (or similar), custom fitted, each Qp Qh A
IOM: 100-02, 15, 290

L3254 Non-standard size or width A
IOM: 100-02, 15, 290

L3255 Non-standard size or length A
IOM: 100-02, 15, 290

L3257 Orthopedic footwear, additional charge for split size A
IOM: 100-02, 15, 290

L3260 Surgical boot/shoe, each E1
IOM: 100-02, 15, 100

* L3265 Plastazote sandal, each A

Shoe Lifts

L3300 Lift, elevation, heel, tapered to metatarsals, per inch Qp A
IOM: 100-02, 15, 290

L3310 Lift, elevation, heel and sole, Neoprene, per inch Qp A
IOM: 100-02, 15, 290

L3320 Lift, elevation, heel and sole, cork, per inch Qp A
IOM: 100-02, 15, 290

L3330 Lift, elevation, metal extension (skate) Qp Qh A
IOM: 100-02, 15, 290

L3332 Lift, elevation, inside shoe, tapered, up to one-half inch Qp Qh A
IOM: 100-02, 15, 290

L3334 Lift, elevation, heel, per inch Qp A
IOM: 100-02, 15, 290

Shoe Wedges

L3340 Heel wedge, SACH Qp Qh A
IOM: 100-02, 15, 290

L3350 Heel wedge Qp Qh A
IOM: 100-02, 15, 290

L3360 Sole wedge, outside sole Qp Qh A
IOM: 100-02, 15, 290

L3370 Sole wedge, between sole Qp Qh A
IOM: 100-02, 15, 290

L3380 Clubfoot wedge Qp Qh A
IOM: 100-02, 15, 290

L3390 Outflare wedge Qp Qh A
IOM: 100-02, 15, 290

L3400 Metatarsal bar wedge, rocker Qp Qh A
IOM: 100-02, 15, 290

L3410 Metatarsal bar wedge, between sole Qp Qh A
IOM: 100-02, 15, 290

L3420 Full sole and heel wedge, between sole Qp Qh A
IOM: 100-02, 15, 290

Shoe Heels

L3430 Heel, counter, plastic reinforced Qp Qh A
IOM: 100-02, 15, 290

L3440 Heel, counter, leather reinforced Qp Qh A
IOM: 100-02, 15, 290

L3450 Heel, SACH cushion type Qp Qh A
IOM: 100-02, 15, 290

L3455 Heel, new leather, standard Qp Qh A
IOM: 100-02, 15, 290

L3460 Heel, new rubber, standard Qp Qh A
IOM: 100-02, 15, 290

L3465 Heel, Thomas with wedge Qp Qh A
IOM: 100-02, 15, 290

L3470 Heel, Thomas extended to ball Qp Qh A
IOM: 100-02, 15, 290

L3480 Heel, pad and depression for spur Qp Qh A
IOM: 100-02, 15, 290

L3485 Heel, pad, removable for spur Qp Qh A
IOM: 100-02, 15, 290

Orthopedic Shoe Additions: Other

L3500 Orthopedic shoe addition, insole, leather Qp Qh A
IOM: 100-02, 15, 290

MIPS Qp Quantity Physician Qh Quantity Hospital ♀ Female only
♂ Male only A Age DMEPOS A2-Z3 ASC Payment Indicator A-Y ASC Status Indicator Coding Clinic

◌ **L3510** Orthopedic shoe addition, insole, rubber Ⓓ Op Oh ♿ A
IOM: 100-02, 15, 290

◌ **L3520** Orthopedic shoe addition, insole, felt covered with leather Ⓓ Op Oh ♿ A
IOM: 100-02, 15, 290

◌ **L3530** Orthopedic shoe addition, sole, half Ⓓ Op Oh ♿ A
IOM: 100-02, 15, 290

◌ **L3540** Orthopedic shoe addition, sole, full Ⓓ Op Oh ♿ A
IOM: 100-02, 15, 290

◌ **L3550** Orthopedic shoe addition, toe tap standard Ⓓ Op Oh ♿ A
IOM: 100-02, 15, 290

◌ **L3560** Orthopedic shoe addition, toe tap, horseshoe Ⓓ Op Oh ♿ A
IOM: 100-02, 15, 290

◌ **L3570** Orthopedic shoe addition, special extension to instep (leather with eyelets) Ⓓ Op Oh ♿ A
IOM: 100-02, 15, 290

◌ **L3580** Orthopedic shoe addition, convert instep to Velcro closure Ⓓ Op Oh ♿ A
IOM: 100-02, 15, 290

◌ **L3590** Orthopedic shoe addition, convert firm shoe counter to soft counter Ⓓ Op Oh ♿ A
IOM: 100-02, 15, 290

◌ **L3595** Orthopedic shoe addition, March bar Ⓓ Op Oh ♿ A
IOM: 100-02, 15, 290

Transfer or Replacement

◌ **L3600** Transfer of an orthosis from one shoe to another, caliper plate, existing Ⓓ Op Oh ♿ A
IOM: 100-02, 15, 290

◌ **L3610** Transfer of an orthosis from one shoe to another, caliper plate, new Ⓓ Op Oh ♿ A
IOM: 100-02, 15, 290

◌ **L3620** Transfer of an orthosis from one shoe to another, solid stirrup, existing Ⓓ Op Oh ♿ A
IOM: 100-02, 15, 290

◌ **L3630** Transfer of an orthosis from one shoe to another, solid stirrup, new Ⓓ Op Oh ♿ A
IOM: 100-02, 15, 290

◌ **L3640** Transfer of an orthosis from one shoe to another, Dennis Browne splint (Riveton), both shoes Ⓓ Op Oh ♿ A
IOM: 100-02, 15, 290

◌ **L3649** Orthopedic shoe, modification, addition or transfer, not otherwise specified Ⓓ A
IOM: 100-02, 15, 290

Orthotic Devices: Upper Limb

NOTE: The procedures in this section are considered as base or basic procedures and may be modified by listing procedures from the Additions section and adding them to the base procedure.

Shoulder

* **L3650** Shoulder orthosis, figure of eight design abduction restrainer, prefabricated, off-the-shelf Ⓓ Op Oh ♿ A

* **L3660** Shoulder orthosis, figure of eight design abduction restrainer, canvas and webbing, prefabricated, off-the-shelf Ⓓ Op Oh ♿ A

* **L3670** Shoulder orthosis, acromio/clavicular (canvas and webbing type), prefabricated, off-the-shelf Ⓓ Op Oh ♿ A

* **L3671** Shoulder orthosis, shoulder joint design, without joints, may include soft interface, straps, custom fabricated, includes fitting and adjustment Ⓓ Op Oh ♿ A

* **L3674** Shoulder orthosis, abduction positioning (airplane design), thoracic component and support bar, with or without nontorsion joint/turnbuckle, may include soft interface, straps, custom fabricated, includes fitting and adjustment Ⓓ Op Oh ♿ A

* **L3675** Shoulder orthosis, vest type abduction restrainer, canvas webbing type or equal, prefabricated, off-the-shelf Ⓓ Op Oh ♿ A

◌ **L3677** Shoulder orthosis, shoulder joint design, without joints, may include soft interface, straps, prefabricated item that has been trimmed, bent, molded, assembled, or otherwise customized to fit a specific patient by an individual with expertise Ⓓ Op Oh A

* **L3678** Shoulder orthosis, shoulder joint design, without joints, may include soft interface, straps, prefabricated, off-the-shelf Ⓓ Op Oh A

▶ New ↩ Revised ✔ Reinstated ~~deleted~~ Deleted ⃠ Not covered or valid by Medicare
◌ Special coverage instructions * Carrier discretion Ⓑ Bill Part B MAC Ⓓ Bill DME MAC

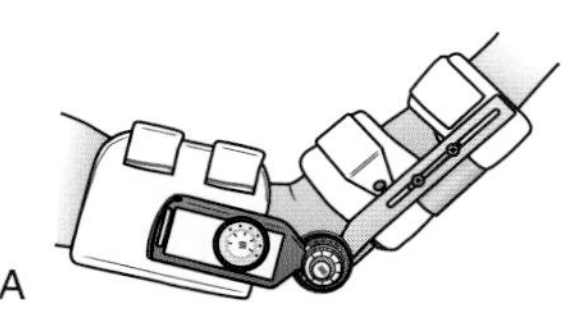
A
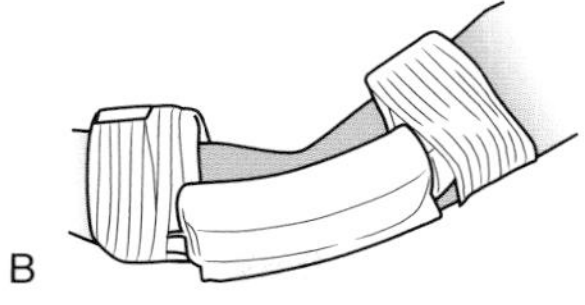
B

Figure 35 Elbow orthoses.

Elbow

✱ **L3702** Elbow orthosis, without joints, may include soft interface, straps, custom fabricated, includes fitting and adjustment Ⓑ Qp Qh ♿ A

✱ **L3710** Elbow orthosis, elastic with metal joints, prefabricated, off-the-shelf Ⓑ Qp Qh ♿ A

✱ **L3720** Elbow orthosis, double upright with forearm/arm cuffs, free motion, custom fabricated Ⓑ Qp Qh ♿ A

✱ **L3730** Elbow orthosis, double upright with forearm/arm cuffs, extension/flexion assist, custom fabricated Ⓑ Qp Qh ♿ A

✱ **L3740** Elbow orthosis, double upright with forearm/arm cuffs, adjustable position lock with active control, custom fabricated Ⓑ Qp Qh ♿ A

✱**L3760** Elbow orthosis (EO), with adjustable position locking joint(s), prefabricated, item that has been trimmed, bent, molded, assembled, or otherwise customized to fit a specific patient by an individual with expertise Ⓑ Qp Qh ♿ A

✱ **L3761** Elbow orthosis (EO), with adjustable position locking joint(s), prefabricated, off-the-shelf A

✱ **L3762** Elbow orthosis, rigid, without joints, includes soft interface material, prefabricated, off-the-shelf Ⓑ Qp Qh ♿ A

✱ **L3763** Elbow wrist hand orthosis, rigid, without joints, may include soft interface, straps, custom fabricated, includes fitting and adjustment Ⓑ Qp Qh ♿ A

✱ **L3764** Elbow wrist hand orthosis, includes one or more nontorsion joints, elastic bands, turnbuckles, may include soft interface, straps, custom fabricated, includes fitting and adjustment Ⓑ Qp Qh ♿ A

✱ **L3765** Elbow wrist hand finger orthosis, rigid, without joints, may include soft interface, straps, custom fabricated, includes fitting and adjustment Ⓑ Qp Qh ♿ A

✱ **L3766** Elbow wrist hand finger orthosis, includes one or more nontorsion joints, elastic bands, turnbuckles, may include soft interface, straps, custom fabricated, includes fitting and adjustment Ⓑ Qp Qh ♿ A

Wrist-Hand-Finger Orthosis (WHFO)

✱ **L3806** Wrist hand finger orthosis, includes one or more nontorsion joint(s), turnbuckles, elastic bands/springs, may include soft interface material, straps, custom fabricated, includes fitting and adjustment Ⓑ Qp Qh ♿ A

✱ **L3807** Wrist hand finger orthosis, without joint(s), prefabricated item that has been trimmed, bent, molded, assembled, or otherwise customized to fit a specific patient by an individual with expertise Ⓑ Qp Qh ♿ A

✱ **L3808** Wrist hand finger orthosis, rigid without joints, may include soft interface material; straps, custom fabricated, includes fitting and adjustment Ⓑ Qp Qh ♿ A

✱ **L3809** Wrist hand finger orthosis, without joint(s), prefabricated, off-the-shelf, any type Ⓑ Qp Qh ♿ A

⊘ **L3891** Addition to upper extremity joint, wrist or elbow, concentric adjustable torsion style mechanism for custom fabricated orthotics only, each Ⓑ Qp Qh E1

✱ **L3900** Wrist hand finger orthosis, dynamic flexor hinge, reciprocal wrist extension/flexion, finger flexion/extension, wrist or finger driven, custom fabricated Ⓑ Qp Qh ♿ A

✱ **L3901** Wrist hand finger orthosis, dynamic flexor hinge, reciprocal wrist extension/flexion, finger flexion/extension, cable driven, custom fabricated Ⓑ Qp Qh ♿ A

✱ **L3904** Wrist hand finger orthosis, external powered, electric, custom fabricated Ⓑ Qp Qh ♿ A

Other Upper Extremity Orthotics

* **L3905** Wrist hand orthosis, includes one or more nontorsion joints, elastic bands, turnbuckles, may include soft interface, straps, custom fabricated, includes fitting and adjustment Qp Qh A
* **L3906** Wrist hand orthosis, without joints, may include soft interface, straps, custom fabricated, includes fitting and adjustment Qp Qh A
* **L3908** Wrist hand orthosis, wrist extension control cock-up, non-molded, prefabricated, off-the-shelf Qp Qh A
* **L3912** Hand finger orthosis (HFO), flexion glove with elastic finger control, prefabricated, off-the-shelf Qp Qh A
* **L3913** Hand finger orthosis, without joints, may include soft interface, straps, custom fabricated, includes fitting and adjustment Qp Qh A
* **L3915** Wrist hand orthosis, includes one or more nontorsion joint(s), elastic bands, turnbuckles, may include soft interface, straps, prefabricated item that has been trimmed, bent, molded, assembled, or otherwise customized to fit a specific patient by an individual with expertise Qp Qh A
* **L3916** Wrist hand orthosis, includes one or more nontorsion joint(s), elastic bands, turnbuckles, may include soft interface, straps, prefabricated, off-the-shelf Qp Qh A
* **L3917** Hand orthosis, metacarpal fracture orthosis, prefabricated item that has been trimmed, bent, molded, assembled, or otherwise customized to fit a specific patient by an individual with expertise Qp Qh A
* **L3918** Hand orthosis, metacarpal fracture orthosis, prefabricated, off-the-shelf Qp Qh A
* **L3919** Hand orthosis, without joints, may include soft interface, straps, custom fabricated, includes fitting and adjustment Qp Qh A
* **L3921** Hand finger orthosis, includes one or more nontorsion joints, elastic bands, turnbuckles, may include soft interface, straps, custom fabricated, includes fitting and adjustment Qp Qh A
* **L3923** Hand finger orthosis, without joints, may include soft interface, straps, prefabricated item that has been trimmed, bent, molded, assembled, or otherwise customized to fit a specific patient by an individual with expertise Qp Qh A
* **L3924** Hand finger orthosis, without joints, may include soft interface, straps, prefabricated, off-the-shelf Qp Qh A
* **L3925** Finger orthosis, proximal interphalangeal (PIP)/distal interphalangeal (DIP), non torsion joint/spring, extension/flexion, may include soft interface material, prefabricated, off-the-shelf Qp Qh A
* **L3927** Finger orthosis, proximal interphalangeal (PIP)/distal interphalangeal (DIP), without joint/spring, extension/flexion (e.g., static or ring type), may include soft interface material, prefabricated, off-the-shelf Qp Qh A
* **L3929** Hand finger orthosis, includes one or more nontorsion joint(s), turnbuckles, elastic bands/springs, may include soft interface material, straps, prefabricated item that has been trimmed, bent, molded, assembled, or otherwise customized to fit a specific patient by an individual with expertise Qp Qh A
* **L3930** Hand finger orthosis, includes one or more nontorsion joint(s), turnbuckles, elastic bands/springs, may include soft interface material, straps, prefabricated, off-the-shelf Qp Qh A
* **L3931** Wrist hand finger orthosis, includes one or more nontorsion joint(s), turnbuckles, elastic bands/springs, may include soft interface material, straps, prefabricated, includes fitting and adjustment Qp Qh A
* **L3933** Finger orthosis, without joints, may include soft interface, custom fabricated, includes fitting and adjustment Qp Qh A
* **L3935** Finger orthosis, nontorsion joint, may include soft interface, custom fabricated, includes fitting and adjustment Qp Qh A
* **L3956** Addition of joint to upper extremity orthosis, any material, per joint Qp A

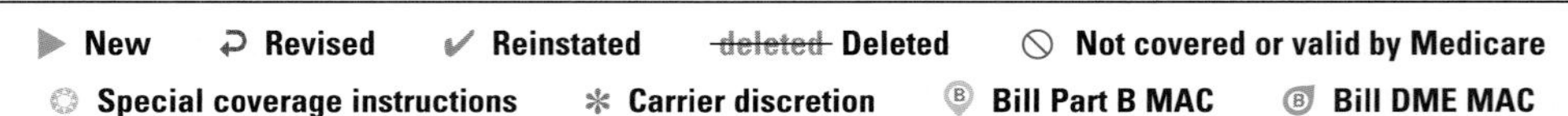
New
Revised
Reinstated
deleted Deleted
Not covered or valid by Medicare
Special coverage instructions
Carrier discretion
Bill Part B MAC
Bill DME MAC

Shoulder-Elbow-Wrist-Hand Orthotics (SEWHO) (L3960-L3973)

* **L3960** Shoulder elbow wrist hand orthosis, abduction positioning, airplane design, prefabricated, includes fitting and adjustment Ⓑ Qp Qh ♿ A
* **L3961** Shoulder elbow wrist hand orthosis, shoulder cap design, without joints, may include soft interface, straps, custom fabricated, includes fitting and adjustment Ⓑ Qp Qh ♿ A
* **L3962** Shoulder elbow wrist hand orthosis, abduction positioning, Erb's palsy design, prefabricated, includes fitting and adjustment Ⓑ Qp Qh ♿ A
* **L3967** Shoulder elbow wrist hand orthosis, abduction positioning (airplane design), thoracic component and support bar, without joints, may include soft interface, straps, custom fabricated, includes fitting and adjustment Ⓑ Qp Qh ♿ A
* **L3971** Shoulder elbow wrist hand orthosis, shoulder cap design, includes one or more nontorsion joints, elastic bands, turnbuckles, may include soft interface, straps, custom fabricated, includes fitting and adjustment Ⓑ Qp Qh ♿ A
* **L3973** Shoulder elbow wrist hand orthosis, abduction positioning (airplane design), thoracic component and support bar, includes one or more nontorsion joints, elastic bands, turnbuckles, may include soft interface, straps, custom fabricated, includes fitting and adjustment Ⓑ Qp Qh ♿ A

Shoulder-Elbow-Wrist-Hand-Finger Orthotics

* **L3975** Shoulder elbow wrist hand finger orthosis, shoulder cap design, without joints, may include soft interface, straps, custom fabricated, includes fitting and adjustment Ⓑ Qp Qh ♿ A
* **L3976** Shoulder elbow wrist hand finger orthosis, abduction positioning (airplane design), thoracic component and support bar, without joints, may include soft interface, straps, custom fabricated, includes fitting and adjustment Ⓑ Qp Qh ♿ A
* **L3977** Shoulder elbow wrist hand finger orthosis, shoulder cap design, includes one or more nontorsion joints, elastic bands, turnbuckles, may include soft interface, straps, custom fabricated, includes fitting and adjustment Ⓑ Qp Qh ♿ A
* **L3978** Shoulder elbow wrist hand finger orthosis, abduction positioning (airplane design), thoracic component and support bar, includes one or more nontorsion joints, elastic bands, turnbuckles, may include soft interface, straps, custom fabricated, includes fitting and adjustment Ⓑ Qp Qh ♿ A

Fracture Orthorics

* **L3980** Upper extremity fracture orthosis, humeral, prefabricated, includes fitting and adjustment Ⓑ Qp Qh ♿ A
* **L3981** Upper extremity fracture orthosis, humeral, prefabricated, includes shoulder cap design, with or without joints, forearm section, may include soft interface, straps, includes fitting and adjustments Ⓑ Qp Qh ♿ A
* **L3982** Upper extremity fracture orthosis, radius/ulnar, prefabricated, includes fitting and adjustment Ⓑ Qp Qh ♿ A
* **L3984** Upper extremity fracture orthosis, wrist, prefabricated, includes fitting and adjustment Ⓑ Qp Qh ♿ A
* **L3995** Addition to upper extremity orthosis, sock, fracture or equal, each Ⓑ Qp ♿ A
* **L3999** Upper limb orthosis, not otherwise specified Ⓑ A

Repairs

* **L4000** Replace girdle for spinal orthosis (CTLSO or SO) Ⓑ Qp Qh ♿ A
* **L4002** Replacement strap, any orthosis, includes all components, any length, any type Ⓑ Qp ♿ A
* **L4010** Replace trilateral socket brim Ⓑ Qp Qh ♿ A
* **L4020** Replace quadrilateral socket brim, molded to patient model Ⓑ Qp Qh ♿ A
* **L4030** Replace quadrilateral socket brim, custom fitted Ⓑ Qp Qh ♿ A
* **L4040** Replace molded thigh lacer, for custom fabricated orthosis only Ⓑ Qp Qh ♿ A
* **L4045** Replace non-molded thigh lacer, for custom fabricated orthosis only Ⓑ Qp Qh ♿ A
* **L4050** Replace molded calf lacer, for custom fabricated orthosis only Ⓑ Qp Qh ♿ A

MIPS | Qp Quantity Physician | Qh Quantity Hospital | ♀ Female only | ♂ Male only | A Age | ♿ DMEPOS | A2-Z3 ASC Payment Indicator | A-Y ASC Status Indicator | Coding Clinic

* **L4055** Replace non-molded calf lacer, for custom fabricated orthosis only A
* **L4060** Replace high roll cuff A
* **L4070** Replace proximal and distal upright for KAFO A
* **L4080** Replace metal bands KAFO, proximal thigh A
* **L4090** Replace metal bands KAFO-AFO, calf or distal thigh A
* **L4100** Replace leather cuff KAFO, proximal thigh A
* **L4110** Replace leather cuff KAFO-AFO, calf or distal thigh A
* **L4130** Replace pretibial shell A
* **L4205** Repair of orthotic device, labor component, per 15 minutes A

  IOM: 100-02, 15, 110.2
* **L4210** Repair of orthotic device, repair or replace minor parts A

  IOM: 100-02, 15, 110.2; 100-02, 15, 120

Ancillary Orthotic Services

* **L4350** Ankle control orthosis, stirrup style, rigid, includes any type interface (e.g., pneumatic, gel), prefabricated, off-the-shelf A
* **L4360** Walking boot, pneumatic and/or vacuum, with or without joints, with or without interface material, prefabricated item that has been trimmed, bent, molded, assembled, or otherwise customized to fit a specific patient by an individual with expertise A

  Noncovered when walking boots used primarily to relieve pressure, especially on sole of foot, or are used for patients with foot ulcers
* **L4361** Walking boot, pneumatic and/or vacuum, with or without joints, with or without interface material, prefabricated, off-the-shelf A
* **L4370** Pneumatic full leg splint, prefabricated, off-the-shelf A
* **L4386** Walking boot, non-pneumatic, with or without joints, with or without interface material, prefabricated item that has been trimmed, bent, molded, assembled, or otherwise customized to fit a specific patient by an individual with expertise A
* **L4387** Walking boot, non-pneumatic, with or without joints, with or without interface material, prefabricated, off-the-shelf A
* **L4392** Replacement, soft interface material, static AFO A
* **L4394** Replace soft interface material, foot drop splint A
* **L4396** Static or dynamic ankle foot orthosis, including soft interface material, adjustable for fit, for positioning, may be used for minimal ambulation, prefabricated item that has been trimmed, bent, molded, assembled, or otherwise customized to fit a specific patient by an individual with expertise A
* **L4397** Static or dynamic ankle foot orthosis, including soft interface material, adjustable for fit, for positioning, may be used for minimal ambulation, prefabricated, off-the-shelf A
* **L4398** Foot drop splint, recumbent positioning device, prefabricated, off-the-shelf A
* **L4631** Ankle foot orthosis, walking boot type, varus/valgus correction, rocker bottom, anterior tibial shell, soft interface, custom arch support, plastic or other material, includes straps and closures, custom fabricated A

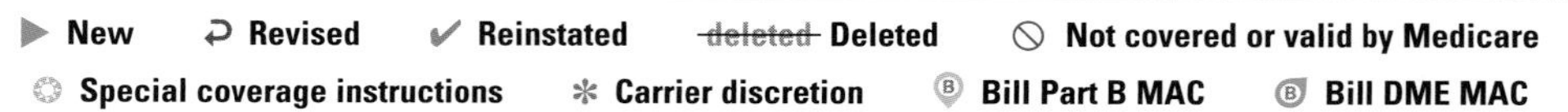
New
Revised
Reinstated
deleted Deleted
Not covered or valid by Medicare
Special coverage instructions
* Carrier discretion
Bill Part B MAC
Bill DME MAC

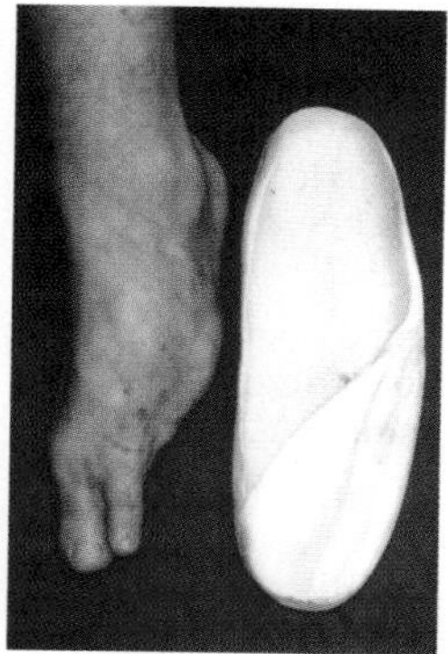

Figure 36 Partial foot.

PROSTHETICS (L5000-L9999)

Lower Limb (L5000-L5999)

Note: The procedures in this section are considered as base or basic proceduresand may be modified by listing items/procedures or special materials from the Additions section and adding them to the base procedure.

Partial Foot

L5000 Partial foot, shoe insert with longitudinal arch, toe filler Ⓑ Qp Qh ♿ A

IOM: 100-02, 15, 290

L5010 Partial foot, molded socket, ankle height, with toe filler Ⓑ Qp Qh ♿ A

IOM: 100-02, 15, 290

L5020 Partial foot, molded socket, tibial tubercle height, with toe filler Ⓑ Qp Qh ♿ A

IOM: 100-02, 15, 290

Ankle

* **L5050** Ankle, Symes, molded socket, SACH foot Ⓑ Qp Qh ♿ A

* **L5060** Ankle, Symes, metal frame, molded leather socket, articulated ankle/foot Ⓑ Qp Qh ♿ A

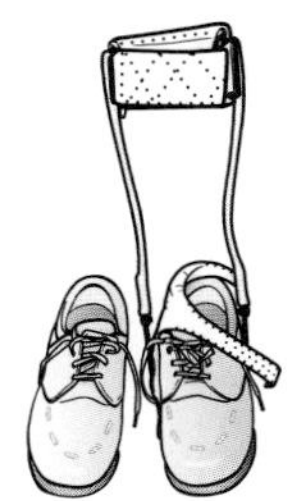

Figure 37 Ankle Symes.

Below Knee

* **L5100** Below knee, molded socket, shin, SACH foot Ⓑ Qp Qh ♿ A

* **L5105** Below knee, plastic socket, joints and thigh lacer, SACH foot Ⓑ Qp Qh ♿ A

Knee Disarticulation

* **L5150** Knee disarticulation (or through knee), molded socket, external knee joints, shin, SACH foot Ⓑ Qp Qh ♿ A

* **L5160** Knee disarticulation (or through knee), molded socket, bent knee configuration, external knee joints, shin, SACH foot Ⓑ Qp Qh ♿ A

Above Knee

* **L5200** Above knee, molded socket, single axis constant friction knee, shin, SACH foot Ⓑ Qp Qh ♿ A

* **L5210** Above knee, short prosthesis, no knee joint ('stubbies'), with foot blocks, no ankle joints, each Ⓑ Qp Qh ♿ A

* **L5220** Above knee, short prosthesis, no knee joint ('stubbies'), with articulated ankle/foot, dynamically aligned, each Ⓑ Qp Qh ♿ A

* **L5230** Above knee, for proximal femoral focal deficiency, constant friction knee, shin, SACH foot Ⓑ Qp Qh ♿ A

Hip Disarticulation

* **L5250** Hip disarticulation, Canadian type; molded socket, hip joint, single axis constant friction knee, shin, SACH foot Ⓑ Qp Qh ♿ A

* **L5270** Hip disarticulation, tilt table type; molded socket, locking hip joint, single axis constant friction knee, shin, SACH foot Ⓑ Qp Qh ♿ A

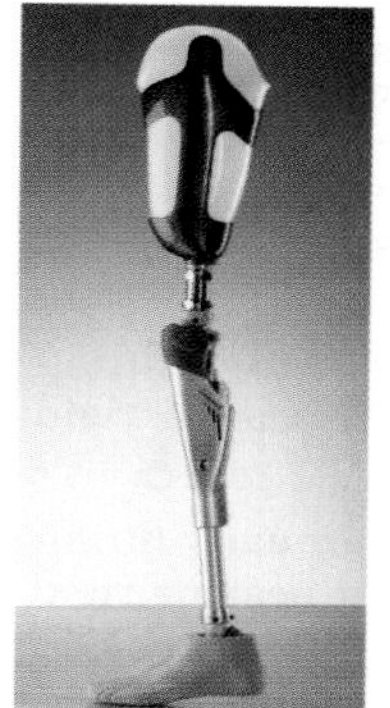

Figure 38 Above knee.

Hemipelvectomy

* **L5280** Hemipelvectomy, Canadian type; molded socket, hip joint, single axis constant friction knee, shin, SACH foot Ⓑ Qp Qh ♿ A

Endoskeletal

* **L5301** Below knee, molded socket, shin, SACH foot, endoskeletal system Ⓑ Qp Qh ♿ A
* **L5312** Knee disarticulation (or through knee), molded socket, single axis knee, pylon, sach foot, endoskeletal system Ⓑ Qp Qh ♿ A
* **L5321** Above knee, molded socket, open end, SACH foot, endoskeletal system, single axis knee Ⓑ Qp Qh ♿ A
* **L5331** Hip disarticulation, Canadian type, molded socket, endoskeletal system, hip joint, single axis knee, SACH foot Ⓑ Qp Qh ♿ A
* **L5341** Hemipelvectomy, Canadian type, molded socket, endoskeletal system, hip joint, single axis knee, SACH foot Ⓑ Qp Qh ♿ A

Immediate Postsurgical or Early Fitting Procedures

* **L5400** Immediate post surgical or early fitting, application of initial rigid dressing, including fitting, alignment, suspension, and one cast change, below knee Ⓑ Qp Qh ♿ A
* **L5410** Immediate post surgical or early fitting, application of initial rigid dressing, including fitting, alignment and suspension, below knee, each additional cast change and realignment Ⓑ Qp Qh ♿ A
* **L5420** Immediate post surgical or early fitting, application of initial rigid dressing, including fitting, alignment and suspension and one cast change 'AK' or knee disarticulation Ⓑ Qp Qh ♿ A
* **L5430** Immediate postsurgical or early fitting, application of initial rigid dressing, including fitting, alignment, and suspension, 'AK' or knee disarticulation, each additional cast change and realignment Ⓑ Qp Qh ♿ A
* **L5450** Immediate post surgical or early fitting, application of non-weight bearing rigid dressing, below knee Ⓑ Qp Qh ♿ A
* **L5460** Immediate post surgical or early fitting, application of non-weight bearing rigid dressing, above knee Ⓑ Qp Qh ♿ A

Initial Prosthesis

* **L5500** Initial, below knee 'PTB' type socket, non-alignable system, pylon, no cover, SACH foot, plaster socket, direct formed Ⓑ Qp Qh ♿ A
* **L5505** Initial, above knee-knee disarticulation, ischial level socket, non-alignable system, pylon, no cover, SACH foot, plaster socket, direct formed Ⓑ Qp Qh ♿ A

Preparatory Prosthesis

* **L5510** Preparatory, below knee 'PTB' type socket, non-alignable system, pylon, no cover, SACH foot, plaster socket, molded to model Ⓑ Qp Qh ♿ A
* **L5520** Preparatory, below knee 'PTB' type socket, non-alignable system, pylon, no cover, SACH foot, thermoplastic or equal, direct formed Ⓑ Qp Qh ♿ A
* **L5530** Preparatory, below knee 'PTB' type socket, non-alignable system, pylon, no cover, SACH foot, thermoplastic or equal, molded to model Ⓑ Qp Qh ♿ A
* **L5535** Preparatory, below knee 'PTB' type socket, non-alignable system, no cover, SACH foot, prefabricated, adjustable open end socket Ⓑ Qp Qh ♿ A
* **L5540** Preparatory, below knee 'PTB' type socket, non-alignable system, pylon, no cover, SACH foot, laminated socket, molded to model Ⓑ Qp Qh ♿ A
* **L5560** Preparatory, above knee - knee disarticulation, ischial level socket, non-alignable system, pylon, no cover, SACH foot, plaster socket, molded to model Ⓑ Qp Qh ♿ A
* **L5570** Preparatory, above knee - knee disarticulation, ischial level socket, non-alignable system, pylon, no cover, SACH foot, thermoplastic or equal, direct formed Ⓑ Qp Qh ♿ A
* **L5580** Preparatory, above knee - knee disarticulation, ischial level socket, non-alignable system, pylon, no cover, SACH foot, thermoplastic or equal, molded to model Ⓑ Qp Qh ♿ A
* **L5585** Preparatory, above knee - knee disarticulation, ischial level socket, non-alignable system, pylon, no cover, SACH foot, prefabricated adjustable open end socket Ⓑ Qp Qh ♿ A

✻ **L5590** Preparatory, above knee - knee disarticulation, ischial level socket, non-alignable system, pylon, no cover, SACH foot, laminated socket, molded to model Ⓑ Qp Qh ♿ A

✻ **L5595** Preparatory, hip disarticulation-hemipelvectomy, pylon, no cover, SACH foot, thermoplastic or equal, molded to patient model Ⓑ Qp Qh ♿ A

✻ **L5600** Preparatory, hip disarticulation-hemipelvectomy, pylon, no cover, SACH foot, laminated socket, molded to patient model Ⓑ Qp Qh ♿ A

Additions to Lower Extremity

✻ **L5610** Addition to lower extremity, endoskeletal system, above knee, hydracadence system Ⓑ Qp Qh ♿ A

✻ **L5611** Addition to lower extremity, endoskeletal system, above knee-knee disarticulation, 4 bar linkage, with friction swing phase control Ⓑ Qp Qh ♿ A

✻ **L5613** Addition to lower extremity, endoskeletal system, above knee-knee disarticulation, 4 bar linkage, with hydraulic swing phase control Ⓑ Qp Qh ♿ A

✻ **L5614** Addition to lower extremity, exoskeletal system, above knee-knee disarticulation, 4 bar linkage, with pneumatic swing phase control Ⓑ Qp Qh ♿ A

✻ **L5616** Addition to lower extremity, endoskeletal system, above knee, universal multiplex system, friction swing phase control Ⓑ Qp Qh ♿ A

✻ **L5617** Addition to lower extremity, quick change self-aligning unit, above knee or below knee, each Ⓑ Qp Qh ♿ A

Additions to Test Sockets

✻ **L5618** Addition to lower extremity, test socket, Symes Ⓑ Qp ♿ A

✻ **L5620** Addition to lower extremity, test socket, below knee Ⓑ Qp ♿ A

✻ **L5622** Addition to lower extremity, test socket, knee disarticulation Ⓑ Qp ♿ A

✻ **L5624** Addition to lower extremity, test socket, above knee Ⓑ Qp ♿ A

✻ **L5626** Addition to lower extremity, test socket, hip disarticulation Ⓑ Qp ♿ A

✻ **L5628** Addition to lower extremity, test socket, hemipelvectomy Ⓑ Qp Qh ♿ A

Additions to Socket Variations

✻ **L5629** Addition to lower extremity, below knee, acrylic socket Ⓑ Qp Qh ♿ A

✻ **L5630** Addition to lower extremity, Symes type, expandable wall socket Ⓑ Qp Qh ♿ A

✻ **L5631** Addition to lower extremity, above knee or knee disarticulation, acrylic socket Ⓑ Qp Qh ♿ A

✻ **L5632** Addition to lower extremity, Symes type, 'PTB' brim design socket Ⓑ Qp Qh ♿ A

✻ **L5634** Addition to lower extremity, Symes type, posterior opening (Canadian) socket Ⓑ Qp Qh ♿ A

✻ **L5636** Addition to lower extremity, Symes type, medial opening socket Ⓑ Qp Qh ♿ A

✻ **L5637** Addition to lower extremity, below knee, total contact Ⓑ Qp Qh ♿ A

✻ **L5638** Addition to lower extremity, below knee, leather socket Ⓑ Qp Qh ♿ A

✻ **L5639** Addition to lower extremity, below knee, wood socket Ⓑ Qp Qh ♿ A

✻ **L5640** Addition to lower extremity, knee disarticulation, leather socket Ⓑ Qp Qh ♿ A

✻ **L5642** Addition to lower extremity, above knee, leather socket Ⓑ Qp Qh ♿ A

✻ **L5643** Addition to lower extremity, hip disarticulation, flexible inner socket, external frame Ⓑ Qp Qh ♿ A

✻ **L5644** Addition to lower extremity, above knee, wood socket Ⓑ Qp Qh ♿ A

✻ **L5645** Addition to lower extremity, below knee, flexible inner socket, external frame Ⓑ Qp Qh ♿ A

✻ **L5646** Addition to lower extremity, below knee, air, fluid, gel or equal, cushion socket Ⓑ Qp Qh ♿ A

✻ **L5647** Addition to lower extremity, below knee, suction socket Ⓑ Qp Qh ♿ A

✻ **L5648** Addition to lower extremity, above knee, air, fluid, gel or equal, cushion socket Ⓑ Qp Qh ♿ A

✻ **L5649** Addition to lower extremity, ischial containment/narrow M-L socket Ⓑ Qp Qh ♿ A

✻ **L5650** Additions to lower extremity, total contact, above knee or knee disarticulation socket Ⓑ Qp Qh ♿ A

* **L5651** Addition to lower extremity, above knee, flexible inner socket, external frame Ⓑ Op Oh ♿ A

* **L5652** Addition to lower extremity, suction suspension, above knee or knee disarticulation socket Ⓑ Op Oh ♿ A

* **L5653** Addition to lower extremity, knee disarticulation, expandable wall socket Ⓑ Op Oh ♿ A

Additions to Socket Insert and Suspension

* **L5654** Addition to lower extremity, socket insert, Symes, (Kemblo, Pelite, Aliplast, Plastazote or equal) Ⓑ Op Oh ♿ A

* **L5655** Addition to lower extremity, socket insert, below knee (Kemblo, Pelite, Aliplast, Plastazote or equal) Ⓑ Op Oh ♿ A

* **L5656** Addition to lower extremity, socket insert, knee disarticulation (Kemblo, Pelite, Aliplast, Plastazote or equal) Ⓑ Op Oh ♿ A

* **L5658** Addition to lower extremity, socket insert, above knee (Kemblo, Pelite, Aliplast, Plastazote or equal) Ⓑ Op Oh ♿ A

* **L5661** Addition to lower extremity, socket insert, multi-durometer Symes Ⓑ Op Oh ♿ A

* **L5665** Addition to lower extremity, socket insert, multi-durometer, below knee Ⓑ Op Oh ♿ A

* **L5666** Addition to lower extremity, below knee, cuff suspension Ⓑ Op Oh ♿ A

* **L5668** Addition to lower extremity, below knee, molded distal cushion Ⓑ Op Oh ♿ A

* **L5670** Addition to lower extremity, below knee, molded supracondylar suspension ('PTS' or similar) Ⓑ Op Oh ♿ A

* **L5671** Addition to lower extremity, below knee/above knee suspension locking mechanism (shuttle, lanyard or equal), excludes socket insert Ⓑ Op Oh ♿ A

* **L5672** Addition to lower extremity, below knee, removable medial brim suspension Ⓑ Op Oh ♿ A

* **L5673** Addition to lower extremity, below knee/above knee, custom fabricated from existing mold or prefabricated, socket insert, silicone gel, elastomeric or equal, for use with locking mechanism Ⓑ Op ♿ A

* **L5676** Additions to lower extremity, below knee, knee joints, single axis, pair Ⓑ Op Oh ♿ A

* **L5677** Additions to lower extremity, below knee, knee joints, polycentric, pair Ⓑ Op Oh ♿ A

* **L5678** Additions to lower extremity, below knee, joint covers, pair Ⓑ Op Oh ♿ A

* **L5679** Addition to lower extremity, below knee/above knee, custom fabricated from existing mold or prefabricated, socket insert, silicone gel, elastomeric or equal, not for use with locking mechanism Ⓑ Op ♿ A

* **L5680** Addition to lower extremity, below knee, thigh lacer, non-molded Ⓑ Op Oh ♿ A

* **L5681** Addition to lower extremity, below knee/above knee, custom fabricated socket insert for congenital or atypical traumatic amputee, silicone gel, elastomeric or equal, for use with or without locking mechanism, initial only (for other than initial, use code L5673 or L5679) Ⓑ Op Oh ♿ A

* **L5682** Addition to lower extremity, below knee, thigh lacer, gluteal/ischial, molded Ⓑ Op Oh ♿ A

* **L5683** Addition to lower extremity, below knee/above knee, custom fabricated socket insert for other than congenital or atypical traumatic amputee, silicone gel, elastomeric, or equal, for use with or without locking mechanism, initial only (for other than initial, use code L5673 or L5679) Ⓑ Op Oh ♿ A

* **L5684** Addition to lower extremity, below knee, fork strap Ⓑ Op Oh ♿ A

* **L5685** Addition to lower extremity prosthesis, below knee, suspension/sealing sleeve, with or without valve, any material, each Ⓑ Op ♿ A

* **L5686** Addition to lower extremity, below knee, back check (extension control) Ⓑ Op Oh ♿ A

* **L5688** Addition to lower extremity, below knee, waist belt, webbing Ⓑ Op Oh ♿ A

* **L5690** Addition to lower extremity, below knee, waist belt, padded and lined Ⓑ Op Oh ♿ A

* **L5692** Addition to lower extremity, above knee, pelvic control belt, light Ⓑ Op Oh ♿ A

* **L5694** Addition to lower extremity, above knee, pelvic control belt, padded and lined Ⓑ Op Oh ♿ A

✱ **L5695** Addition to lower extremity, above knee, pelvic control, sleeve suspension, neoprene or equal, each Ⓑ Qp Qh ♿ A

✱ **L5696** Addition to lower extremity, above knee or knee disarticulation, pelvic joint Ⓑ Qp Qh ♿ A

✱ **L5697** Addition to lower extremity, above knee or knee disarticulation, pelvic band Ⓑ Qp Qh ♿ A

✱ **L5698** Addition to lower extremity, above knee or knee disarticulation, Silesian bandage Ⓑ Qp Qh ♿ A

✱ **L5699** All lower extremity prostheses, shoulder harness Ⓑ Qp Qh ♿ A

Replacement Sockets

✱ **L5700** Replacement, socket, below knee, molded to patient model Ⓑ Qp Qh ♿ A

✱ **L5701** Replacement, socket, above knee/knee disarticulation, including attachment plate, molded to patient model Ⓑ Qp Qh ♿ A

✱ **L5702** Replacement, socket, hip disarticulation, including hip joint, molded to patient model Ⓑ Qp Qh ♿ A

✱ **L5703** Ankle, Symes, molded to patient model, socket without solid ankle cushion heel (SACH) foot, replacement only Ⓑ Qp Qh ♿ A

Protective Covers

✱ **L5704** Custom shaped protective cover, below knee Ⓑ Qp Qh ♿ A

✱ **L5705** Custom shaped protective cover, above knee Ⓑ Qp Qh ♿ A

✱ **L5706** Custom shaped protective cover, knee disarticulation Ⓑ Qp Qh ♿ A

✱ **L5707** Custom shaped protective cover, hip disarticulation Ⓑ Qp Qh ♿ A

Additions to Exoskeletal–Knee-Shin System

✱ **L5710** Addition, exoskeletal knee-shin system, single axis, manual lock Ⓑ Qp Qh ♿ A

✱ **L5711** Additions exoskeletal knee-shin system, single axis, manual lock, ultra-light material Ⓑ Qp Qh ♿ A

✱ **L5712** Addition, exoskeletal knee-shin system, single axis, friction swing and stance phase control (safety knee) Ⓑ Qp Qh ♿ A

✱ **L5714** Addition, exoskeletal knee-shin system, single axis, variable friction swing phase control Ⓑ Qp Qh ♿ A

✱ **L5716** Addition, exoskeletal knee-shin system, polycentric, mechanical stance phase lock Ⓑ Qp Qh ♿ A

✱ **L5718** Addition, exoskeletal knee-shin system, polycentric, friction swing and stance phase control Ⓑ Qp Qh ♿ A

✱ **L5722** Addition, exoskeletal knee-shin system, single axis, pneumatic swing, friction stance phase control Ⓑ Qp Qh ♿ A

✱ **L5724** Addition, exoskeletal knee-shin system, single axis, fluid swing phase control Ⓑ Qp Qh ♿ A

✱ **L5726** Addition, exoskeletal knee-shin system, single axis, external joints, fluid swing phase control Ⓑ Qp Qh ♿ A

✱ **L5728** Addition, exoskeletal knee-shin system, single axis, fluid swing and stance phase control Ⓑ Qp Qh ♿ A

✱ **L5780** Addition, exoskeletal knee-shin system, single axis, pneumatic/hydra pneumatic swing phase control Ⓑ Qp Qh ♿ A

Vacuum Pumps

✱ **L5781** Addition to lower limb prosthesis, vacuum pump, residual limb volume management and moisture evacuation system Ⓑ Qp Qh ♿ A

✱ **L5782** Addition to lower limb prosthesis, vacuum pump, residual limb volume management and moisture evacuation system, heavy duty Ⓑ Qp Qh ♿ A

Component Modification

✱ **L5785** Addition, exoskeletal system, below knee, ultra-light material (titanium, carbon fiber, or equal) Ⓑ Qp Qh ♿ A

✱ **L5790** Addition, exoskeletal system, above knee, ultra-light material (titanium, carbon fiber, or equal) Ⓑ Qp Qh ♿ A

✱ **L5795** Addition, exoskeletal system, hip disarticulation, ultra-light material (titanium, carbon fiber, or equal) Ⓑ Qp Qh ♿ A

Endoskeletal

✱ **L5810** Addition, endoskeletal knee-shin system, single axis, manual lock Ⓑ Qp Qh ♿ A

✱ **L5811** Addition, endoskeletal knee-shin system, single axis, manual lock, ultralight material Ⓑ Qp Qh ♿ A

* L5812 Addition, endoskeletal knee-shin system, single axis, friction swing and stance phase control (safety knee) Ⓑ Qp Qh ♿ A

* L5814 Addition, endoskeletal knee-shin system, polycentric, hydraulic swing phase control, mechanical stance phase lock Ⓑ Qp Qh ♿ A

* L5816 Addition, endoskeletal knee-shin system, polycentric, mechanical stance phase lock Ⓑ Qp Qh ♿ A

* L5818 Addition, endoskeletal knee-shin system, polycentric, friction swing, and stance phase control Ⓑ Qp Qh ♿ A

* L5822 Addition, endoskeletal knee-shin system, single axis, pneumatic swing, friction stance phase control Ⓑ Qp Qh ♿ A

* L5824 Addition, endoskeletal knee-shin system, single axis, fluid swing phase control Ⓑ Qp Qh ♿ A

* L5826 Addition, endoskeletal knee-shin system, single axis, hydraulic swing phase control, with miniature high activity frame Ⓑ Qp Qh ♿ A

* L5828 Addition, endoskeletal knee-shin system, single axis, fluid swing and stance phase control Ⓑ Qp Qh ♿ A

* L5830 Addition, endoskeletal knee-shin system, single axis, pneumatic/swing phase control Ⓑ Qp Qh ♿ A

* L5840 Addition, endoskeletal knee/shin system, 4-bar linkage or multiaxial, pneumatic swing phase control Ⓑ Qp Qh ♿ A

* L5845 Addition, endoskeletal, knee-shin system, stance flexion feature, adjustable Ⓑ Qp Qh ♿ A

* L5848 Addition to endoskeletal, knee-shin system, fluid stance extension, dampening feature, with or without adjustability Ⓑ Qp Qh ♿ A

* L5850 Addition, endoskeletal system, above knee or hip disarticulation, knee extension assist Ⓑ Qp Qh ♿ A

* L5855 Addition, endoskeletal system, hip disarticulation, mechanical hip extension assist Ⓑ Qp Qh ♿ A

* L5856 Addition to lower extremity prosthesis, endoskeletal knee-shin system, microprocessor control feature, swing and stance phase; includes electronic sensor(s), any type Ⓑ Qp Qh ♿ A

* L5857 Addition to lower extremity prosthesis, endoskeletal knee-shin system, microprocessor control feature, swing phase only; includes electronic sensor(s), any type Ⓑ Qp Qh ♿ A

* L5858 Addition to lower extremity prosthesis, endoskeletal knee shin system, microprocessor control feature, stance phase only, includes electronic sensor(s), any type Ⓑ Qp Qh ♿ A

* L5859 Addition to lower extremity prosthesis, endoskeletal knee-shin system, powered and programmable flexion/extension assist control, includes any type motor(s) Ⓑ Qp Qh ♿ A

* L5910 Addition, endoskeletal system, below knee, alignable system Ⓑ Qp Qh ♿ A

* L5920 Addition, endoskeletal system, above knee or hip disarticulation, alignable system Ⓑ Qp Qh ♿ A

* L5925 Addition, endoskeletal system, above knee, knee disarticulation or hip disarticulation, manual lock Ⓑ Qp Qh ♿ A

* L5930 Addition, endoskeletal system, high activity knee control frame Ⓑ Qp Qh ♿ A

* L5940 Addition, endoskeletal system, below knee, ultra-light material (titanium, carbon fiber or equal) Ⓑ Qp Qh ♿ A

* L5950 Addition, endoskeletal system, above knee, ultra-light material (titanium, carbon fiber or equal) Ⓑ Qp Qh ♿ A

* L5960 Addition, endoskeletal system, hip disarticulation, ultra-light material (titanium, carbon fiber, or equal) Ⓑ Qp Qh ♿ A

* L5961 Addition, endoskeletal system, polycentric hip joint, pneumatic or hydraulic control, rotation control, with or without flexion, and/or extension control Ⓑ Qp Qh ♿ A

* L5962 Addition, endoskeletal system, below knee, flexible protective outer surface covering system Ⓑ Qp Qh ♿ A

* L5964 Addition, endoskeletal system, above knee, flexible protective outer surface covering system Ⓑ Qp Qh ♿ A

* L5966 Addition, endoskeletal system, hip disarticulation, flexible protective outer surface covering system Ⓑ Qp Qh ♿ A

▶ New ↻ Revised ✓ Reinstated ~~deleted~~ Deleted ⊘ Not covered or valid by Medicare
○ Special coverage instructions * Carrier discretion Ⓑ Bill Part B MAC Ⓑ Bill DME MAC

Additions to Ankle and/or Foot

* L5968 Addition to lower limb prosthesis, multiaxial ankle with swing phase active dorsiflexion feature Qp Qh A
* L5969 Addition, endoskeletal ankle-foot or ankle system, power assist, includes any type motor(s) Qp Qh A
* L5970 All lower extremity prostheses, foot, external keel, SACH foot Qp Qh A
* L5971 All lower extremity prosthesis, solid ankle cushion keel (SACH) foot, replacement only Qp Qh A
* L5972 All lower extremity prostheses (foot, flexible keel) Qp Qh A
* L5973 Endoskeletal ankle foot system, microprocessor controlled feature, dorsiflexion and/or plantar flexion control, includes power source Qh A
* L5974 All lower extremity prostheses, foot, single axis ankle/foot Qp Qh A
* L5975 All lower extremity prostheses, combination single axis ankle and flexible keel foot Qp Qh A
* L5976 All lower extremity prostheses, energy storing foot (Seattle Carbon Copy II or equal) Qp Qh A
* L5978 All lower extremity prostheses, foot, multiaxial ankle/foot Qp Qh A
* L5979 All lower extremity prostheses, multiaxial ankle, dynamic response foot, one piece system Qp Qh A
* L5980 All lower extremity prostheses, flex foot system Qp Qh A
* L5981 All lower extremity prostheses, flexwalk system or equal Qp Qh A
* L5982 All exoskeletal lower extremity prostheses, axial rotation unit Qp Qh A
* L5984 All endoskeletal lower extremity prostheses, axial rotation unit, with or without adjustability Qp Qh A
* L5985 All endoskeletal lower extremity prostheses, dynamic prosthetic pylon Qp Qh A
* L5986 All lower extremity prostheses, multiaxial rotation unit ('MCP' or equal) Qp Qh A
* L5987 All lower extremity prostheses, shank foot system with vertical loading pylon Qp Qh A
* L5988 Addition to lower limb prosthesis, vertical shock reducing pylon feature Qp Qh A
* L5990 Addition to lower extremity prosthesis, user adjustable heel height Qp Qh A
* L5999 Lower extremity prosthesis, not otherwise specified A

Upper Limb (L6000-L7600)

Note: The procedures in L6000-L6599 are considered as base or basic procedures and may be modified by listing procedures from the additions sections. The base procedures include only standard friction wrist and control cable system unless otherwise specified.

Partial Hand

* L6000 Partial hand, thumb remaining Qp Qh A
* L6010 Partial hand, little and/or ring finger remaining Qp Qh A
* L6020 Partial hand, no finger remaining Qp Qh A
* L6026 Transcarpal/metacarpal or partial hand disarticulation prosthesis, external power, self-suspended, inner socket with removable forearm section, electrodes and cables, two batteries, charger, myoelectric control of terminal device, excludes terminal device(s) Qp Qh A

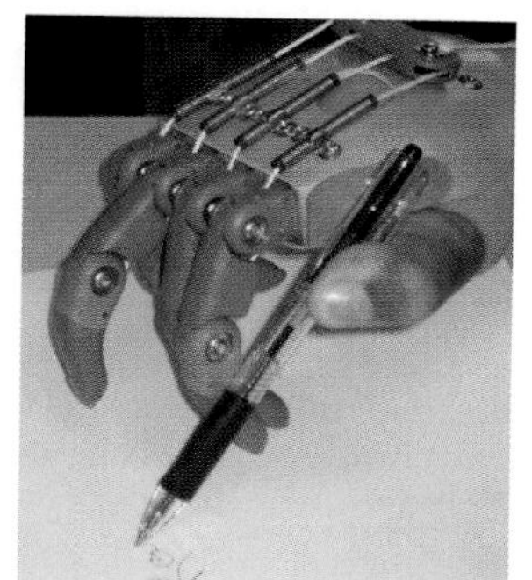

Figure 39 Partial hand.

Wrist Disarticulation

* L6050 Wrist disarticulation, molded socket, flexible elbow hinges, triceps pad Ⓑ Op Oh ♿ A
* L6055 Wrist disarticulation, molded socket with expandable interface, flexible elbow hinges, triceps pad Ⓑ Op Oh ♿ A

Below Elbow

* L6100 Below elbow, molded socket, flexible elbow hinge, triceps pad Ⓑ Op Oh ♿ A
* L6110 Below elbow, molded socket, (Muenster or Northwestern suspension types) Ⓑ Op Oh ♿ A
* L6120 Below elbow, molded double wall split socket, step-up hinges, half cuff Ⓑ Op Oh ♿ A
* L6130 Below elbow, molded double wall split socket, stump activated locking hinge, half cuff Ⓑ Op Oh ♿ A

Elbow Disarticulation

* L6200 Elbow disarticulation, molded socket, outside locking hinge, forearm Ⓑ Op Oh ♿ A
* L6205 Elbow disarticulation, molded socket with expandable interface, outside locking hinges, forearm Ⓑ Op Oh ♿ A

Above Elbow

* L6250 Above elbow, molded double wall socket, internal locking elbow, forearm Ⓑ Op Oh ♿ A

Shoulder Disarticulation

* L6300 Shoulder disarticulation, molded socket, shoulder bulkhead, humeral section, internal locking elbow, forearm Ⓑ Op Oh ♿ A
* L6310 Shoulder disarticulation, passive restoration (complete prosthesis) Ⓑ Op Oh ♿ A
* L6320 Shoulder disarticulation, passive restoration (shoulder cap only) Ⓑ Op Oh ♿ A

Interscapular Thoracic

* L6350 Interscapular thoracic, molded socket, shoulder bulkhead, humeral section, internal locking elbow, forearm Ⓑ Op Oh ♿ A
* L6360 Interscapular thoracic, passive restoration (complete prosthesis) Ⓑ Op Oh ♿ A
* L6370 Interscapular thoracic, passive restoration (shoulder cap only) Ⓑ Op Oh ♿ A

Immediate and Early Postsurgical Procedures

* L6380 Immediate post surgical or early fitting, application of initial rigid dressing, including fitting alignment and suspension of components, and one cast change, wrist disarticulation or below elbow Ⓑ Op Oh ♿ A
* L6382 Immediate post surgical or early fitting, application of initial rigid dressing including fitting alignment and suspension of components, and one cast change, elbow disarticulation or above elbow Ⓑ Op Oh ♿ A
* L6384 Immediate post surgical or early fitting, application of initial rigid dressing including fitting alignment and suspension of components, and one cast change, shoulder disarticulation or interscapular thoracic Ⓑ Op Oh ♿ A
* L6386 Immediate post surgical or early fitting, each additional cast change and realignment Ⓑ Op Oh ♿ A
* L6388 Immediate post surgical or early fitting, application of rigid dressing only Ⓑ Op Oh ♿ A

Molded Socket

* L6400 Below elbow, molded socket, endoskeletal system, including soft prosthetic tissue shaping Ⓑ Op Oh ♿ A
* L6450 Elbow disarticulation, molded socket, endoskeletal system, including soft prosthetic tissue shaping Ⓑ Op Oh ♿ A
* L6500 Above elbow, molded socket, endoskeletal system, including soft prosthetic tissue shaping Ⓑ Op Oh ♿ A
* L6550 Shoulder disarticulation, molded socket, endoskeletal system, including soft prosthetic tissue shaping Ⓑ Op Oh ♿ A
* L6570 Interscapular thoracic, molded socket, endoskeletal system, including soft prosthetic tissue shaping Ⓑ Op Oh ♿ A

Preparatory Prosthetic

* L6580 Preparatory, wrist disarticulation or below elbow, single wall plastic socket, friction wrist, flexible elbow hinges, figure of eight harness, humeral cuff, Bowden cable control, USMC or equal pylon, no cover, molded to patient model Ⓑ Qp Qh & A
* L6582 Preparatory, wrist disarticulation or below elbow, single wall socket, friction wrist, flexible elbow hinges, figure of eight harness, humeral cuff, Bowden cable control, USMC or equal pylon, no cover, direct formed Ⓑ Qp Qh & A
* L6584 Preparatory, elbow disarticulation or above elbow, single wall plastic socket, friction wrist, locking elbow, figure of eight harness, fair lead cable control, USMC or equal pylon, no cover, molded to patient model Ⓑ Qp Qh & A
* L6586 Preparatory, elbow disarticulation or above elbow, single wall socket, friction wrist, locking elbow, figure of eight harness, fair lead cable control, USMC or equal pylon, no cover, direct formed Ⓑ Qp Qh & A
* L6588 Preparatory, shoulder disarticulation or interscapular thoracic, single wall plastic socket, shoulder joint, locking elbow, friction wrist, chest strap, fair lead cable control, USMC or equal pylon, no cover, molded to patient model Ⓑ Qp Qh & A
* L6590 Preparatory, shoulder disarticulation or interscapular thoracic, single wall socket, shoulder joint, locking elbow, friction wrist, chest strap, fair lead cable control, USMC or equal pylon, no cover, direct formed Ⓑ Qp Qh & A

Additions to Upper Limb

Note: The following procedures/modifications/components may be added to other base procedures. The items in this section should reflect the additional complexity of each modification procedure, in addition to base procedure, at the time of the original order.

* L6600 Upper extremity additions, polycentric hinge, pair Ⓑ Qp Qh & A
* L6605 Upper extremity additions, single pivot hinge, pair Ⓑ Qp Qh & A
* L6610 Upper extremity additions, flexible metal hinge, pair Ⓑ Qp Qh & A
* L6611 Addition to upper extremity prosthesis, external powered, additional switch, any type Ⓑ Qp Qh & A
* L6615 Upper extremity addition, disconnect locking wrist unit Ⓑ Qp Qh & A
* L6616 Upper extremity addition, additional disconnect insert for locking wrist unit, each Ⓑ Qp Qh & A
* L6620 Upper extremity addition, flexion/extension wrist unit, with or without friction Ⓑ Qp Qh & A
* L6621 Upper extremity prosthesis addition, flexion/extension wrist with or without friction, for use with external powered terminal device Ⓑ Qp Qh & A
* L6623 Upper extremity addition, spring assisted rotational wrist unit with latch release Ⓑ Qp Qh & A
* L6624 Upper extremity addition, flexion/extension and rotation wrist unit Ⓑ Qp Qh & A
* L6625 Upper extremity addition, rotation wrist unit with cable lock Ⓑ Qp Qh & A
* L6628 Upper extremity addition, quick disconnect hook adapter, Otto Bock or equal Ⓑ Qp Qh & A
* L6629 Upper extremity addition, quick disconnect lamination collar with coupling piece, Otto Bock or equal Ⓑ Qp Qh & A
* L6630 Upper extremity addition, stainless steel, any wrist Ⓑ Qp Qh & A
* L6632 Upper extremity addition, latex suspension sleeve, each Ⓑ Qp & A
* L6635 Upper extremity addition, lift assist for elbow Ⓑ Qp Qh & A
* L6637 Upper extremity addition, nudge control elbow lock Ⓑ Qp Qh & A

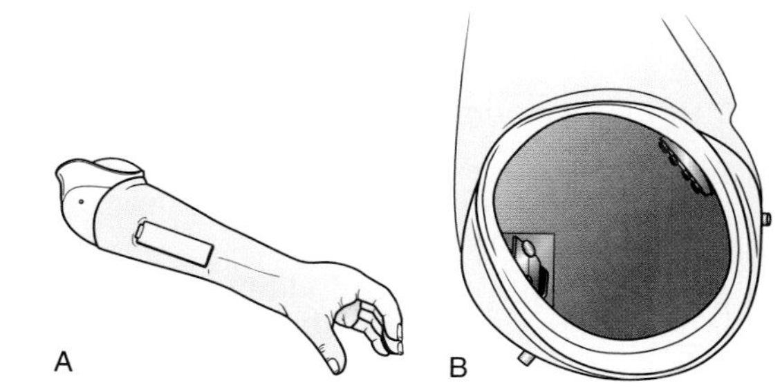
A
B

Figure 40 Upper extremity addition.

MIPS | Qp Quantity Physician | Qh Quantity Hospital | ♀ Female only
♂ Male only | A Age | & DMEPOS | A2-Z3 ASC Payment Indicator | A-Y ASC Status Indicator | Coding Clinic

* **L6638** Upper extremity addition to prosthesis, electric locking feature, only for use with manually powered elbow Ⓑ Qp Qh ♿ A
* **L6640** Upper extremity additions, shoulder abduction joint, pair Ⓑ Qp Qh ♿ A
* **L6641** Upper extremity addition, excursion amplifier, pulley type Ⓑ Qp Qh ♿ A
* **L6642** Upper extremity addition, excursion amplifier, lever type Ⓑ Qp Qh ♿ A
* **L6645** Upper extremity addition, shoulder flexion-abduction joint, each Ⓑ Qp Qh ♿ A
* **L6646** Upper extremity addition, shoulder joint, multipositional locking, flexion, adjustable abduction friction control, for use with body powered or external powered system Ⓑ Qp Qh ♿ A
* **L6647** Upper extremity addition, shoulder lock mechanism, body powered actuator Ⓑ Qp Qh ♿ A
* **L6648** Upper extremity addition, shoulder lock mechanism, external powered actuator Ⓑ Qp Qh ♿ A
* **L6650** Upper extremity addition, shoulder universal joint, each Ⓑ Qp Qh ♿ A
* **L6655** Upper extremity addition, standard control cable, extra Ⓑ Qp ♿ A
* **L6660** Upper extremity addition, heavy duty control cable Ⓑ Qp ♿ A
* **L6665** Upper extremity addition, Teflon, or equal, cable lining Ⓑ Qp ♿ A
* **L6670** Upper extremity addition, hook to hand, cable adapter Ⓑ Qp Qh ♿ A
* **L6672** Upper extremity addition, harness, chest or shoulder, saddle type Ⓑ Qp Qh ♿ A
* **L6675** Upper extremity addition, harness, (e.g., figure of eight type), single cable design Ⓑ Qp Qh ♿ A
* **L6676** Upper extremity addition, harness, (e.g., figure of eight type), dual cable design Ⓑ Qp Qh ♿ A
* **L6677** Upper extremity addition, harness, triple control, simultaneous operation of terminal device and elbow Ⓑ Qp Qh ♿ A
* **L6680** Upper extremity addition, test socket, wrist disarticulation or below elbow Ⓑ Qp ♿ A
* **L6682** Upper extremity addition, test socket, elbow disarticulation or above elbow Ⓑ Qp ♿ A
* **L6684** Upper extremity addition, test socket, shoulder disarticulation or interscapular thoracic Ⓑ Qp ♿ A
* **L6686** Upper extremity addition, suction socket Ⓑ Qp Qh ♿ A
* **L6687** Upper extremity addition, frame type socket, below elbow or wrist disarticulation Ⓑ Qp Qh ♿ A
* **L6688** Upper extremity addition, frame type socket, above elbow or elbow disarticulation Ⓑ Qp Qh ♿ A
* **L6689** Upper extremity addition, frame type socket, shoulder disarticulation Ⓑ Qp Qh ♿ A
* **L6690** Upper extremity addition, frame type socket, interscapular-thoracic Ⓑ Qp Qh ♿ A
* **L6691** Upper extremity addition, removable insert, each Ⓑ Qp ♿ A
* **L6692** Upper extremity addition, silicone gel insert or equal, each Ⓑ Qp ♿ A
* **L6693** Upper extremity addition, locking elbow, forearm counterbalance Ⓑ Qp Qh ♿ A
* **L6694** Addition to upper extremity prosthesis, below elbow/above elbow, custom fabricated from existing mold or prefabricated, socket insert, silicone gel, elastomeric or equal, for use with locking mechanism Ⓑ Qp Qh ♿ A
* **L6695** Addition to upper extremity prosthesis, below elbow/above elbow, custom fabricated from existing mold or prefabricated, socket insert, silicone gel, elastomeric or equal, not for use with locking mechanism Ⓑ Qp Qh ♿ A
* **L6696** Addition to upper extremity prosthesis, below elbow/above elbow, custom fabricated socket insert for congenital or atypical traumatic amputee, silicone gel, elastomeric or equal, for use with or without locking mechanism, initial only (for other than initial, use code L6694 or L6695) Ⓑ Qp Qh ♿ A
* **L6697** Addition to upper extremity prosthesis, below elbow/above elbow, custom fabricated socket insert for other than congenital or atypical traumatic amputee, silicone gel, elastomeric or equal, for use with or without locking mechanism, initial only (for other than initial, use code L6694 or L6695) Ⓑ Qp Qh ♿ A
* **L6698** Addition to upper extremity prosthesis, below elbow/above elbow, lock mechanism, excludes socket insert Ⓑ Qp Qh ♿ A

Terminal Devices (L6703-L6882)

* **L6703** Terminal device, passive hand/mitt, any material, any size Ⓑ Qp Qh ♿ A
* **L6704** Terminal device, sport/recreational/work attachment, any material, any size Ⓑ Qp Qh ♿ A
* **L6706** Terminal device, hook, mechanical, voluntary opening, any material, any size, lined or unlined Ⓑ Qp Qh ♿ A
* **L6707** Terminal device, hook, mechanical, voluntary closing, any material, any size, lined or unlined Ⓑ Qp Qh ♿ A
* **L6708** Terminal device, hand, mechanical, voluntary opening, any material, any size Ⓑ Qp Qh ♿ A
* **L6709** Terminal device, hand, mechanical, voluntary closing, any material, any size Ⓑ Qp Qh ♿ A
* **L6711** Terminal device, hook, mechanical, voluntary opening, any material, any size, lined or unlined, pediatric Ⓑ Qp Qh A ♿ A
* **L6712** Terminal device, hook, mechanical, voluntary closing, any material, any size, lined or unlined, pediatric Ⓑ Qp Qh A ♿ A
* **L6713** Terminal device, hand, mechanical, voluntary opening, any material, any size, pediatric Ⓑ Qp Qh A ♿ A
* **L6714** Terminal device, hand, mechanical, voluntary closing, any material, any size, pediatric Ⓑ Qp Qh A ♿ A
* **L6715** Terminal device, multiple articulating digit, includes motor(s), initial issue or replacement Ⓑ Qp Qh ♿ A
* **L6721** Terminal device, hook or hand, heavy duty, mechanical, voluntary opening, any material, any size, lined or unlined Ⓑ Qp Qh ♿ A

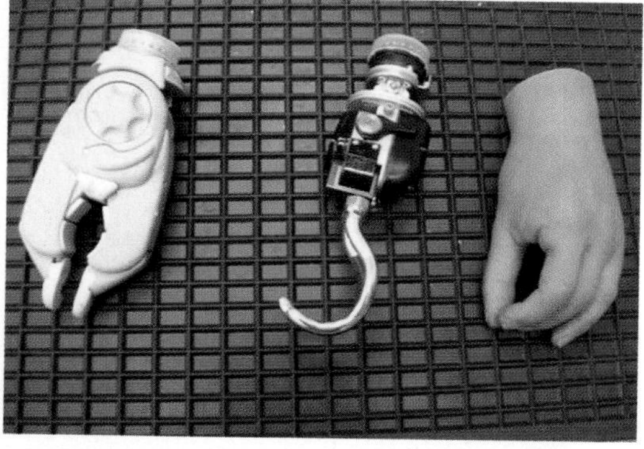

Figure 41 Terminal devices, hand and hook.

* **L6722** Terminal device, hook or hand, heavy duty, mechanical, voluntary closing, any material, any size, lined or unlined Ⓑ Qp Qh ♿ A

○ **L6805** Addition to terminal device, modifier wrist unit Ⓑ Qp Qh ♿ A

IOM: 100-02, 15, 120; 100-04, 3, 10.4

○ **L6810** Addition to terminal device, precision pinch device Ⓑ Qp Qh ♿ A

IOM: 100-02, 15, 120; 100-04, 3, 10.4

* **L6880** Electric hand, switch or myoelectric controlled, independently articulating digits, any grasp pattern or combination of grasp patterns, includes motor(s) Ⓑ Qp Qh ♿ A
* **L6881** Automatic grasp feature, addition to upper limb electric prosthetic terminal device Ⓑ Qp Qh ♿ A

○ **L6882** Microprocessor control feature, addition to upper limb prosthetic terminal device Ⓑ Qp Qh ♿ A

IOM: 100-02, 15, 120; 100-04, 3, 10.4

Replacement Sockets

* **L6883** Replacement socket, below elbow/wrist disarticulation, molded to patient model, for use with or without external power Ⓑ Qp Qh ♿ A
* **L6884** Replacement socket, above elbow/elbow disarticulation, molded to patient model, for use with or without external power Ⓑ Qp Qh ♿ A
* **L6885** Replacement socket, shoulder disarticulation/interscapular thoracic, molded to patient model, for use with or without external power Ⓑ Qp Qh ♿ A

Hand Restoration

* **L6890** Addition to upper extremity prosthesis, glove for terminal device, any material, prefabricated, includes fitting and adjustment Ⓑ Qp Qh ♿ A
* **L6895** Addition to upper extremity prosthesis, glove for terminal device, any material, custom fabricated Ⓑ Qp Qh ♿ A
* **L6900** Hand restoration (casts, shading and measurements included), partial hand, with glove, thumb or one finger remaining Ⓑ Qp Qh ♿ A
* **L6905** Hand restoration (casts, shading and measurements included), partial hand, with glove, multiple fingers remaining Ⓑ Qp Qh ♿ A

✻ **L6910** Hand restoration (casts, shading and measurements included), partial hand, with glove, no fingers remaining Ⓑ Qp Qh ♿ A

✻ **L6915** Hand restoration (shading, and measurements included), replacement glove for above Ⓑ Qp Qh ♿ A

External Power

✻ **L6920** Wrist disarticulation, external power, self-suspended inner socket, removable forearm shell, Otto Bock or equal switch, cables, two batteries and one charger, switch control of terminal device Ⓑ Qp Qh ♿ A

✻ **L6925** Wrist disarticulation, external power, self-suspended inner socket, removable forearm shell, Otto Bock or equal electrodes, cables, two batteries and one charger, myoelectronic control of terminal device Ⓑ Qp Qh ♿ A

✻ **L6930** Below elbow, external power, self-suspended inner socket, removable forearm shell, Otto Bock or equal switch, cables, two batteries and one charger, switch control of terminal device Ⓑ Qp Qh ♿ A

✻ **L6935** Below elbow, external power, self-suspended inner socket, removable forearm shell, Otto Bock or equal electrodes, cables, two batteries and one charger, myoelectronic control of terminal device Ⓑ Qp Qh ♿ A

✻ **L6940** Elbow disarticulation, external power, molded inner socket, removable humeral shell, outside locking hinges, forearm, Otto Bock or equal switch, cables, two batteries and one charger, switch control of terminal device Ⓑ Qp Qh ♿ A

✻ **L6945** Elbow disarticulation, external power, molded inner socket, removable humeral shell, outside locking hinges, forearm, Otto Bock or equal electrodes, cables, two batteries and one charger, myoelectronic control of terminal device Ⓑ Qp Qh ♿ A

✻ **L6950** Above elbow, external power, molded inner socket, removable humeral shell, internal locking elbow, forearm, Otto Bock or equal switch, cables, two batteries and one charger, switch control of terminal device Ⓑ Qp Qh ♿ A

✻ **L6955** Above elbow, external power, molded inner socket, removable humeral shell, internal locking elbow, forearm, Otto Bock or equal electrodes, cables, two batteries and one charger, myoelectronic control of terminal device Ⓑ Qp Qh ♿ A

✻ **L6960** Shoulder disarticulation, external power, molded inner socket, removable shoulder shell, shoulder bulkhead, humeral section, mechanical elbow, forearm, Otto Bock or equal switch, cables, two batteries and one charger, switch control of terminal device Ⓑ Qp Qh ♿ A

✻ **L6965** Shoulder disarticulation, external power, molded inner socket, removable shoulder shell, shoulder bulkhead, humeral section, mechanical elbow, forearm, Otto Bock or equal electrodes, cables, two batteries and one charger, myoelectronic control of terminal device Ⓑ Qp Qh ♿ A

✻ **L6970** Interscapular-thoracic, external power, molded inner socket, removable shoulder shell, shoulder bulkhead, humeral section, mechanical elbow, forearm, Otto Bock or equal switch, cables, two batteries and one charger, switch control of terminal device Ⓑ Qp Qh ♿ A

✻ **L6975** Interscapular-thoracic, external power, molded inner socket, removable shoulder shell, shoulder bulkhead, humeral section, mechanical elbow, forearm, Otto Bock or equal electrodes, cables, two batteries and one charger, myoelectronic control of terminal device Ⓑ Qp Qh ♿ A

Additions to Electronic Hand or Hook

✻ **L7007** Electric hand, switch or myoelectric controlled, adult Ⓑ Qp Qh A ♿ A

✻ **L7008** Electric hand, switch or myoelectric controlled, pediatric Ⓑ Qp Qh A ♿ A

✻ **L7009** Electric hook, switch or myoelectric controlled, adult Ⓑ Qp Qh A ♿ A

✻ **L7040** Prehensile actuator, switch controlled Ⓑ Qp Qh ♿ A

✻ **L7045** Electric hook, switch or myoelectric controlled, pediatric Ⓑ Qp Qh A ♿ A

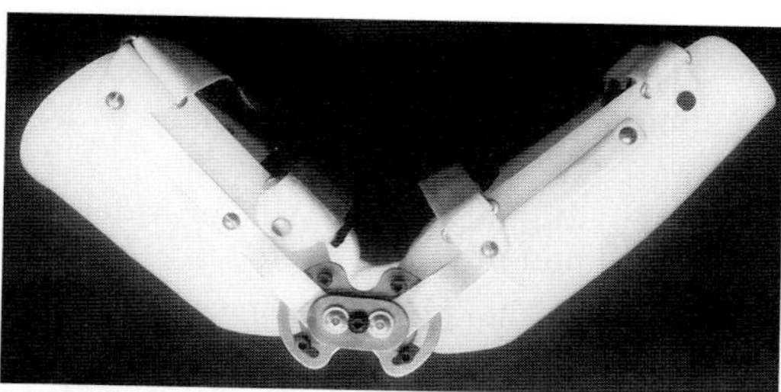

Figure 42 Electronic elbow.

Additions to Electronic Elbow

* L7170 Electronic elbow, Hosmer or equal, switch controlled Qp Qh A
* L7180 Electronic elbow, microprocessor sequential control of elbow and terminal device Qp Qh A
* L7181 Electronic elbow, microprocessor simultaneous control of elbow and terminal device Qp Qh A
* L7185 Electronic elbow, adolescent, Variety Village or equal, switch controlled Qp Qh A
* L7186 Electronic elbow, child, Variety Village or equal, switch controlled Qp Qh A A
* L7190 Electronic elbow, adolescent, Variety Village or equal, myoelectronically controlled Qp Qh A
* L7191 Electronic elbow, child, Variety Village or equal, myoelectronically controlled Qp Qh A A

Wrist

* L7259 Electronic wrist rotator, any type Qp Qh A

Battery Components

* L7360 Six volt battery, each Qp A
* L7362 Battery charger, six volt, each Qp Qh A
* L7364 Twelve volt battery, each Qp A
* L7366 Battery charger, twelve volt, each Qp Qh A
* L7367 Lithium ion battery, rechargeable, replacement Qp A
* L7368 Lithium ion battery charger, replacement only Qp Qh A

Additions

* L7400 Addition to upper extremity prosthesis, below elbow/wrist disarticulation, ultralight material (titanium, carbon fiber or equal) Qp Qh A
* L7401 Addition to upper extremity prosthesis, above elbow disarticulation, ultralight material (titanium, carbon fiber or equal) Qp Qh A
* L7402 Addition to upper extremity prosthesis, shoulder disarticulation/interscapular thoracic, ultralight material (titanium, carbon fiber or equal) Qp Qh A
* L7403 Addition to upper extremity prosthesis, below elbow/wrist disarticulation, acrylic material Qp Qh A
* L7404 Addition to upper extremity prosthesis, above elbow disarticulation, acrylic material Qp Qh A
* L7405 Addition to upper extremity prosthesis, shoulder disarticulation/interscapular thoracic, acrylic material Qp Qh A

Other/Repair

* L7499 Upper extremity prosthesis, not otherwise specified A
* L7510 Repair of prosthetic device, repair or replace minor parts Qp Qh A

  IOM: 100-02, 15, 110.2; 100-02, 15, 120; 100-04, 32, 100
* L7520 Repair prosthetic device, labor component, per 15 minutes A
* L7600 Prosthetic donning sleeve, any material, each E1

  Medicare Statute 1862(1)(a)

General

Prosthetic Socket Insert

* L7700 Gasket or seal, for use with prosthetic socket insert, any type, each A

Penile Prosthetics

* L7900 Male vacuum erection system Qp Qh ♂ E1

  Medicare Statute 1834a
* L7902 Tension ring, for vacuum erection device, any type, replacement only, each Qp Qh E1

  Medicare Statute 1834a

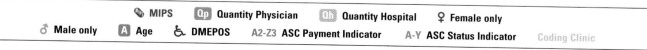

MIPS | Qp Quantity Physician | Qh Quantity Hospital | ♀ Female only | ♂ Male only | A Age | DMEPOS | A2-Z3 ASC Payment Indicator | A-Y ASC Status Indicator | Coding Clinic

Breast Prosthetics

- L8000 Breast prosthesis, mastectomy bra, without integrated breast prosthesis form, any size, any type Ⓑ Qp ♀ ♿ A
  IOM: 100-02, 15, 120
- L8001 Breast prosthesis, mastectomy bra, with integrated breast prosthesis form, unilateral, any size, any type Ⓑ Qp ♀ ♿ A
  IOM: 100-02, 15, 120
- L8002 Breast prosthesis, mastectomy bra, with integrated breast prosthesis form, bilateral, any size, any type Ⓑ Qp ♀ ♿ A
  IOM: 100-02, 15, 120
- L8010 Breast prosthesis, mastectomy sleeve Ⓑ ♀ A
  IOM: 100-02, 15, 120
- L8015 External breast prosthesis garment, with mastectomy form, post mastectomy Ⓑ Qp ♀ ♿ A
  IOM: 100-02, 15, 120
- L8020 Breast prosthesis, mastectomy form Ⓑ Qp ♀ ♿ A
  IOM: 100-02, 15, 120
- L8030 Breast prosthesis, silicone or equal, without integral adhesive Ⓑ Qp Qh ♀ ♿ A
  IOM: 100-02, 15, 120
- L8031 Breast prosthesis, silicone or equal, with integral adhesive Ⓑ Qp Qh ♿ A
  IOM: 100-02, 15, 120
- * L8032 Nipple prosthesis, prefabricated, reusable, any type, each Ⓑ Qp Qh ♿ A
- * L8033 Nipple prosthesis, custom fabricated, reusable, any material, any type, each A
- L8035 Custom breast prosthesis, post mastectomy, molded to patient model Ⓑ Qp Qh ♀ ♿ A
  IOM: 100-02, 15, 120
- * L8039 Breast prosthesis, not otherwise specified Ⓑ Qp Qh ♀ A

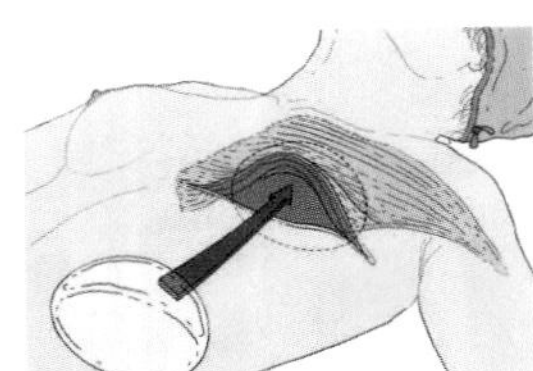

Figure 43 Implant breast prosthesis.

Nasal, Orbital, Auricular Prosthetics

- * L8040 Nasal prosthesis, provided by a non-physician Ⓑ Qp Qh ♿ A
- * L8041 Midfacial prosthesis, provided by a non-physician Ⓑ Qp Qh ♿ A
- * L8042 Orbital prosthesis, provided by a non-physician Ⓑ Qp Qh ♿ A
- * L8043 Upper facial prosthesis, provided by a non-physician Ⓑ Qp Qh ♿ A
- * L8044 Hemi-facial prosthesis, provided by a non-physician Ⓑ Qp Qh ♿ A
- * L8045 Auricular prosthesis, provided by a non-physician Ⓑ Qp Qh ♿ A
- * L8046 Partial facial prosthesis, provided by a non-physician Ⓑ Qp Qh ♿ A
- * L8047 Nasal septal prosthesis, provided by a non-physician Ⓑ Qp Qh ♿ A
- * L8048 Unspecified maxillofacial prosthesis, by report, provided by a non-physician Ⓑ Qp Qh A
- * L8049 Repair or modification of maxillofacial prosthesis, labor component, 15 minute increments, provided by a non-physician Ⓑ Qp A

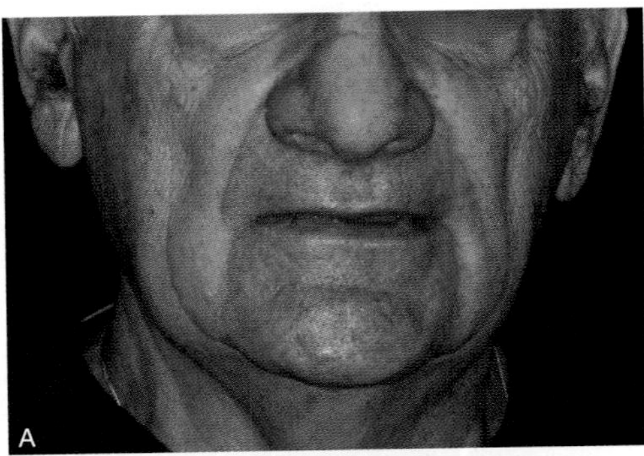
A

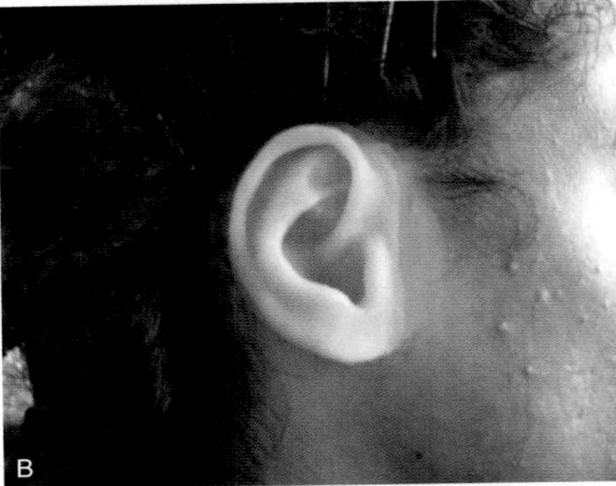
B

Figure 44 (A) Nasal prosthesis, (B) Auricular prosthesis.

Trusses

L8300 Truss, single with standard pad Qp Qh A
IOM: 100-02, 15, 120; 100-03, 4, 280.11; 100-03, 4, 280.12; 100-04, 4, 240

L8310 Truss, double with standard pads Qp Qh A
IOM: 100-02, 15, 120; 100-03, 4, 280.11; 100-03, 4, 280.12; 100-04, 4, 240

L8320 Truss, addition to standard pad, water pad Qp Qh A
IOM: 100-02, 15, 120; 100-03, 4, 280.11; 100-03, 4, 280.12; 100-04, 4, 240

L8330 Truss, addition to standard pad, scrotal pad Qp Qh ♂ A
IOM: 100-02, 15, 120; 100-03, 4, 280.11; 100-03, 4, 280.12; 100-04, 4, 240

Prosthetic Socks

L8400 Prosthetic sheath, below knee, each Qp A
IOM: 100-02, 15, 200

L8410 Prosthetic sheath, above knee, each Qp A
IOM: 100-02, 15, 200

L8415 Prosthetic sheath, upper limb, each Qp A
IOM: 100-02, 15, 200

* **L8417** Prosthetic sheath/sock, including a gel cushion layer, below knee or above knee, each Qp A

L8420 Prosthetic sock, multiple ply, below knee, each Qp A
IOM: 100-02, 15, 200

L8430 Prosthetic sock, multiple ply, above knee, each Qp A
IOM: 100-02, 15, 200

L8435 Prosthetic sock, multiple ply, upper limb, each Qp A
IOM: 100-02, 15, 200

L8440 Prosthetic shrinker, below knee, each Qp A
IOM: 100-02, 15, 200

L8460 Prosthetic shrinker, above knee, each Qp A
IOM: 100-02, 15, 200

L8465 Prosthetic shrinker, upper limb, each Qp A
IOM: 100-02, 15, 200

L8470 Prosthetic sock, single ply, fitting, below knee, each Qp A
IOM: 100-02, 15, 200

L8480 Prosthetic sock, single ply, fitting, above knee, each Qp A
IOM: 100-02, 15, 200

L8485 Prosthetic sock, single ply, fitting, upper limb, each Qp A
IOM: 100-02, 15, 200

Unlisted

* **L8499** Unlisted procedure for miscellaneous prosthetic services A

Prosthetic Implants (L8500-L9900)

Larynx, Tracheoesophageal

L8500 Artificial larynx, any type Qp Qh A
IOM: 100-02, 15, 120; 100-03, 1, 50.2; 100-04, 4, 240

L8501 Tracheostomy speaking valve Qp Qh A
IOM: 100-03, 1, 50.4

* **L8505** Artificial larynx replacement battery/accessory, any type A

* **L8507** Tracheo-esophageal voice prosthesis, patient inserted, any type, each Qp Qh A

* **L8509** Tracheo-esophageal voice prosthesis, inserted by a licensed health care provider, any type Qp Qh A

L8510 Voice amplifier Qp Qh A
IOM: 100-03, 1, 50.2

* **L8511** Insert for indwelling tracheoesophageal prosthesis, with or without valve, replacement only, each Qp Qh A

* **L8512** Gelatin capsules or equivalent, for use with tracheoesophageal voice prosthesis, replacement only, per 10 A

* **L8513** Cleaning device used with tracheoesophageal voice prosthesis, pipet, brush, or equal, replacement only, each A

MIPS | Qp Quantity Physician | Qh Quantity Hospital | ♀ Female only
♂ Male only | A Age | DMEPOS | A2-Z3 ASC Payment Indicator | A-Y ASC Status Indicator | Coding Clinic

✻ **L8514** Tracheoesophageal puncture dilator, replacement only, each Ⓑ Ⓔ Qp Qh ♿ A

✻ **L8515** Gelatin capsule, application device for use with tracheoesophageal voice prosthesis, each Ⓑ Ⓔ Qp Qh ♿ A

Breast

L8600 Implantable breast prosthesis, silicone or equal Ⓑ Qp Qh ♀ ♿ N1 N

IOM: 100-02, 15, 120; 100-3, 2, 140.2

Bulking Agents

L8603 Injectable bulking agent, collagen implant, urinary tract, 2.5 ml syringe, includes shipping and necessary supplies Ⓑ ♿ N1 N

Bill on paper, acquisition cost invoice required

IOM: 100-03, 4, 280.1

✻ **L8604** Injectable bulking agent, dextranomer/ hyaluronic acid copolymer implant, urinary tract, 1 ml, includes shipping and necessary supplies Ⓑ Qp Qh N1 N

✻ **L8605** Injectable bulking agent, dextranomer/ hyaluronic acid copolymer implant, anal canal, 1 ml, includes shipping and necessary supplies Ⓑ Qp Qh ♿ N1 N

L8606 Injectable bulking agent, synthetic implant, urinary tract, 1 ml syringe, includes shipping and necessary supplies Ⓑ Qp Qh ♿ N1 N

Bill on paper, acquisition cost invoice required

IOM: 100-03, 4, 280.1

L8607 Injectable bulking agent for vocal cord medialization, 0.1 ml, includes shipping and necessary supplies Ⓑ Qp Qh ♿ N1 N

IOM: 100-03, 4, 280.1

Eye and Ear

✻ **L8608** Miscellaneous external component, supply or accessory for use with the Argus II retinal prosthesis system N

✻ **L8609** Artificial cornea Ⓑ Qp Qh ♿ N1 N

L8610 Ocular implant Ⓑ Qp Qh ♿ N1 N

IOM: 100-02, 15, 120

L8612 Aqueous shunt Ⓑ Qp Qh ♿ N1 N

IOM: 100-02, 15, 120

Cross Reference Q0074

L8613 Ossicula implant Ⓑ Qp Qh ♿ N1 N

IOM: 100-02, 15, 120

L8614 Cochlear device, includes all internal and external components Ⓑ Qp Qh ♿ N1 N

IOM: 100-02, 15, 120; 100-03, 1, 50.3

L8615 Headset/headpiece for use with cochlear implant device, replacement Ⓑ Qp Qh ♿ A

IOM: 100-03, 1, 50.3

L8616 Microphone for use with cochlear implant device, replacement Ⓑ Qp Qh ♿ A

IOM: 100-03, 1, 50.3

L8617 Transmitting coil for use with cochlear implant device, replacement Ⓑ Qp Qh ♿ A

IOM: 100-03, 1, 50.3

L8618 Transmitter cable for use with cochlear implant device or auditory osseointegrated device, replacement Ⓑ Qp Qh ♿ A

IOM: 100-03, 1, 50.3

L8619 Cochlear implant, external speech processor and controller, integrated system, replacement Ⓑ Qp Qh ♿ A

IOM: 100-03, 1, 50.3

✻ **L8621** Zinc air battery for use with cochlear implant device and auditory osseointegrated sound processors, replacement, each Ⓑ Qp Qh ♿ A

✻ **L8622** Alkaline battery for use with cochlear implant device, any size, replacement, each Ⓑ Qp Qh ♿ A

✻ **L8623** Lithium ion battery for use with cochlear implant device speech processor, other than ear level, replacement, each Ⓑ ♿ A

✻ **L8624** Lithium ion battery for use with cochlear implant or auditory osseointegrated device speech processor, ear level, replacement, each Ⓑ ♿ A

L8625 External recharging system for battery for use with cochlear implant or auditory osseointegrated device, replacement only, each A

IOM: 103-03, PART 1, 50.3

L8627 Cochlear implant, external speech processor, component, replacement Ⓑ Qp Qh ♿ A

IOM: 103-03, PART 1, 50.3

L8628 Cochlear implant, external controller component, replacement Ⓑ Qp Qh ♿ A

IOM: 103-03, PART 1, 50.3

L8629 Transmitting coil and cable, integrated, for use with cochlear implant device, replacement Ⓑ Qp Qh ♿ A

IOM: 103-03, PART 1, 50.3

Hand and Foot

L8630 Metacarpophalangeal joint implant Ⓑ ♿ N1 N

IOM: 100-02, 15, 120

L8631 Metacarpal phalangeal joint replacement, two or more pieces, metal (e.g., stainless steel or cobalt chrome), ceramic-like material (e.g., pyrocarbon), for surgical implantation (all sizes, includes entire system) Ⓑ Qp Qh ♿ N1 N

IOM: 100-02, 15, 120

L8641 Metatarsal joint implant Ⓑ Qp Qh ♿ N1 N

IOM: 100-02, 15, 120

L8642 Hallux implant Ⓑ Qp Qh ♿ N1 N

May be billed by ambulatory surgical center or surgeon

IOM: 100-02, 15, 120

Cross Reference Q0073

L8658 Interphalangeal joint spacer, silicone or equal, each Ⓑ Qp Qh ♿ N1 N

IOM: 100-02, 15, 120

L8659 Interphalangeal finger joint replacement, 2 or more pieces, metal (e.g., stainless steel or cobalt chrome), ceramic-like material (e.g., pyrocarbon) for surgical implantation, any size Ⓑ Qp Qh ♿ N1 N

IOM: 100-02, 15, 120

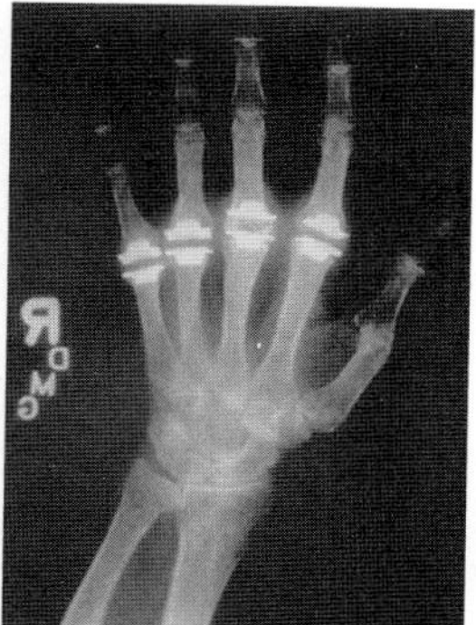

Figure 45 Metacarpophalangeal implant.

Vascular

L8670 Vascular graft material, synthetic, implant Ⓑ Qp Qh ♿ N1 N

IOM: 100-02, 15, 120

Neurostimulator

L8679 Implantable neurostimulator, pulse generator, any type Ⓑ Qp Qh ♿ N1 N

IOM: 100-03, 4, 280.4

⃠ **L8680** Implantable neurostimulator electrode, each Ⓑ Qh E1

Related CPT codes: 43647, 63650, 63655, 64553, 64555, 64560, 64561, 64565, 64573, 64575, 64577, 64580, 64581.

L8681 Patient programmer (external) for use with implantable programmable neurostimulator pulse generator, replacement only Ⓑ Qp Qh ♿ A

IOM: 100-03, 4, 280.4

L8682 Implantable neurostimulator radiofrequency receiver Ⓑ Qp Qh ♿ N1 N

IOM: 100-03, 4, 280.4

L8683 Radiofrequency transmitter (external) for use with implantable neurostimulator radiofrequency receiver Ⓑ Qp Qh ♿ A

IOM: 100-03, 4, 280.4

L8684 Radiofrequency transmitter (external) for use with implantable sacral root neurostimulator receiver for bowel and bladder management, replacement Ⓑ Qp Qh ♿ A

IOM: 100-03, 4, 280.4

⃠ **L8685** Implantable neurostimulator pulse generator, single array, rechargeable, includes extension Ⓑ Qp Qh E1

Related CPT codes: 61885, 64590, 63685.

⃠ **L8686** Implantable neurostimulator pulse generator, single array, non-rechargeable, includes extension Ⓑ Qp Qh E1

Related CPT codes: 61885, 64590, 63685.

⃠ **L8687** Implantable neurostimulator pulse generator, dual array, rechargeable, includes extension Ⓑ Qp Qh E1

Related CPT codes: 64590, 63685, 61886.

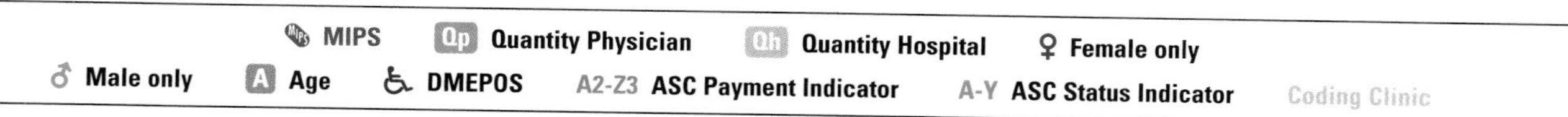
MIPS
Qp Quantity Physician
Qh Quantity Hospital
♀ Female only
♂ Male only
A Age
♿ DMEPOS
A2-Z3 ASC Payment Indicator
A-Y ASC Status Indicator
Coding Clinic

⊘ **L8688** Implantable neurostimulator pulse generator, dual array, non-rechargeable, includes extension Ⓑ Op Qh E1

Related CPT codes: 61885, 64590, 63685.

L8689 External recharging system for battery (internal) for use with implantable neurostimulator, replacement only Ⓑ Op Qh ♿ A

IOM: 100-03, 4, 280.4

Miscellaneous Orthotic and Prosthetic Components, Services, and Supplies

* **L8690** Auditory osseointegrated device, includes all internal and external components Ⓑ Op Qh ♿ N1 N

Related CPT codes: 69714, 69715, 69717, 69718.

* **L8691** Auditory osseointegrated device, external sound processor, excludes transducer/actuator, replacement only, each Ⓑ Op Qh ♿ A

⊘ **L8692** Auditory osseointegrated device, external sound processor, used without osseointegration, body worn, includes headband or other means of external attachment Ⓑ Op Qh E1

Medicare Statute 1862(a)(7)

* **L8693** Auditory osseointegrated device abutment, any length, replacement only Ⓑ Op Qh ♿ A

* **L8694** Auditory osseointegrated device, transducer/actuator, replacement only, each A

L8695 External recharging system for battery (external) for use with implantable neurostimulator, replacement only Ⓑ Op Qh ♿ A

IOM: 100-03, 4, 280.4

L8696 Antenna (external) for use with implantable diaphragmatic/phrenic nerve stimulation device, replacement, each Ⓑ Op Qh ♿ A

L8698 Miscellaneous component, supply or accessory for use with total artificial heart system Ⓑ A

* **L8699** Prosthetic implant, not otherwise specified Ⓑ N1 N

↩ * **L8701** Elbow, wrist, hand device, powered. with single or double upright(s), any type joint(s), includes microprocessor, sensors, all components and accessories Ⓔ A

↩ * **L8702** Elbow, wrist, hand, finger device, powered, with single or double upright(s), any type joint(s), includes microprocessor, sensors, all components and accessories Ⓔ A

* **L9900** Orthotic and prosthetic supply, accessory, and/or service component of another HCPCS "L" code Ⓑ Ⓔ N1 N

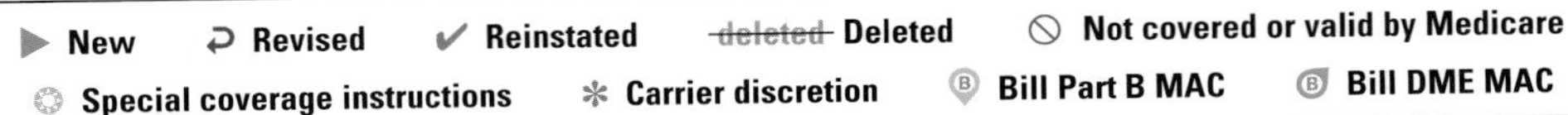
▶ New
↩ Revised
✔ Reinstated
~~deleted~~ Deleted
⊘ Not covered or valid by Medicare
Special coverage instructions
* Carrier discretion
Ⓑ Bill Part B MAC
Ⓔ Bill DME MAC

OTHER MEDICAL SERVICES (M0000-M0301)

⊘ **M0075** Cellular therapy Ⓑ E1

⊘ **M0076** Prolotherapy Ⓑ E1

Prolotherapy stimulates production of new ligament tissue. Not covered by Medicare.

⊘ **M0100** Intragastric hypothermia using gastric freezing Ⓑ E1

▶⊘ **M0239** Intravenous infusion, bamlanivimab-xxxx, includes infusion and post administration monitoring S

▶⊘ **M0243** Intravenous infusion, casirivimab and imdevimab includes infusion and post administration monitoring S

⊘ **M0300** IV chelation therapy (chemical endarterectomy) Ⓑ E1

⊘ **M0301** Fabric wrapping of abdominal aneurysm Ⓑ E1

Treatment for abdominal aneurysms that involves wrapping aneurysms with cellophane or fascia lata. Fabric wrapping of abdominal aneurysms is not a covered Medicare procedure.

⮌ * **M1003** TB screening performed and results interpreted within twelve months prior to initiation of first-time biologic disease modifying anti-rheumatic drug therapy Ⓑ M

* **M1004** Documentation of medical reason for not screening for TB or interpreting results (i.e., patient positive for TB and documentation of past treatment; patient who has recently completed a course of anti-TB therapy) Ⓑ M

* **M1005** TB screening not performed or results not interpreted, reason not given Ⓑ M

* **M1006** Disease activity not assessed, reason not given Ⓑ M

* **M1007** >=50% of total number of a patient's outpatient RA encounters assessed Ⓑ M

* **M1008** <50% of total number of a patient's outpatient RA encounters assessed Ⓑ M

* **M1009** Discharge/discontinuation of the episode of care documented in the medical record Ⓑ M

* **M1010** Discharge/discontinuation of the episode of care documented in the medical record Ⓑ M

* **M1011** Discharge/discontinuation of the episode of care documented in the medical record Ⓑ M

* **M1012** Discharge/discontinuation of the episode of care documented in the medical record Ⓑ M

* **M1013** Discharge/discontinuation of the episode of care documented in the medical record Ⓑ M

* **M1014** Discharge/discontinuation of the episode of care documented in the medical record Ⓑ M

~~M1015 Discharge/discontinuation of the episode of care documented in the medical record~~ ✖

* **M1016** Female patients unable to bear children Ⓑ M

* **M1017** Patient admitted to palliative care services Ⓑ M

* **M1018** Patients with an active diagnosis or history of cancer (except basal cell and squamous cell skin carcinoma), patients who are heavy tobacco smokers, lung cancer screening patients Ⓑ M

* **M1019** Adolescent patients 12 to 17 years of age with major depression or dysthymia who reached remission at twelve months as demonstrated by a twelve month (+/-60 days) PHQ-9 or PHQ-9m score of less than five Ⓑ M

* **M1020** Adolescent patients 12 to 17 years of age with major depression or dysthymia who did not reach remission at twelve months as demonstrated by a twelve month (+/-60 days) PHQ-9 or PHQ-9m score of less than 5. Either PHQ-9 or PHQ-9m score was not assessed or is greater than or equal to 5 Ⓑ M

* **M1021** Patient had only urgent care visits during the performance period Ⓑ M

* **M1022** Patients who were in hospice at any time during the performance period Ⓑ M

~~M1023 Adolescent patients 12 to 17 years of age with major depression or dysthymia who reached remission at six months as demonstrated by a six month (+/-60 days) PHQ-9 or PHQ-9m score of less than five~~ ✖

~~M1024 Adolescent patients 12 to 17 years of age with major depression or dysthymia who did not reach remission at six months as demonstrated by a six month (+/-60 days) PHQ-9 or PHQ-9m score of less than five. Either PHQ-9 or PHQ-9m score was not assessed or is greater than or equal to five~~ ✖

MIPS | Qp Quantity Physician | Qh Quantity Hospital | ♀ Female only | ♂ Male only | A Age | DMEPOS | A2-Z3 ASC Payment Indicator | A-Y ASC Status Indicator | Coding Clinic

* **M1025** Patients who were in hospice at any time during the performance period Ⓑ M

* **M1026** Patients who were in hospice at any time during the performance period Ⓑ M

* **M1027** Imaging of the head (CT or MRI) was obtained Ⓑ M

* **M1028** Documentation of patients with primary headache diagnosis and imaging other than CT or MRI obtained Ⓑ M

* **M1029** Imaging of the head (CT or MRI) was not obtained, reason not given Ⓑ M

* **M1031** Patients with no clinical indications for imaging of the head Ⓑ M

* **M1032** Adults currently taking pharmacotherapy for OUD Ⓑ M

~~M1033 Pharmacotherapy for OUD initiated after June 30th of performance period~~ ✖

* **M1034** Adults who have at least 180 days of continuous pharmacotherapy with a medication prescribed for OUD without a gap of more than seven days Ⓑ M

* **M1035** Adults who are deliberately phased out of medication assisted treatment (MAT) prior to 180 days of continuous treatment Ⓑ M

* **M1036** Adults who have not had at least 180 days of continuous pharmacotherapy with a medication prescribed for oud without a gap of more than seven days Ⓑ M

* **M1037** Patients with a diagnosis of lumbar spine region cancer at the time of the procedure Ⓑ M

* **M1038** Patients with a diagnosis of lumbar spine region fracture at the time of the procedure Ⓑ M

* **M1039** Patients with a diagnosis of lumbar spine region infection at the time of the procedure Ⓑ M

* **M1040** Patients with a diagnosis of lumbar idiopathic or congenital scoliosis Ⓑ M

↩ * **M1041** Patient had cancer, acute fracture or infection related to the lumbar spine or patient had neuromuscular, idiopathic or congenital lumbar scoliosis Ⓑ M

* **M1043** Functional status was not measured by the Oswestry Disability Index (ODI version 2.1a) at one year (9 to 15 months) postoperatively Ⓑ M

↩ * **M1045** Functional status measured by the Oxford Knee Score (OKS) at one year (9 to 15 months) postoperatively was greater than or equal to 37 or knee injury and osteoarthritis outcome score joint replacement (Koos, jr.) was greater than or equal to 71 Ⓑ M

↩ * **M1046** Functional status the Oxford Knee Score (OKS) at one year (9 to 15 months) postoperatively was less than 37 or the knee injury and osteoarthritis outcome score joint replacement (Koos, jr.) was less than 71 postoperatively Ⓑ M

* **M1049** Functional status was not measured by the Oswestry Disability Index (ODI version 2.1a) at three months (6 to 20 weeks) postoperatively Ⓑ M

↩ * **M1051** Patient had cancer, acute fracture or infection related to the lumbar spine or patient had neuromuscular, idiopathic or congenital lumbar scoliosis Ⓑ M

* **M1052** Leg pain was not measured by the Visual Analog Scale (VAS) at one year (9 to 15 months) postoperatively Ⓑ M

* **M1054** Patient had only urgent care visits during the performance period Ⓑ M

* **M1055** Aspirin or another antiplatelet therapy used Ⓑ M

* **M1056** Prescribed anticoagulant medication during the performance period, history of GI bleeding, history of intracranial bleeding, bleeding disorder and specific provider documented reasons: allergy to aspirin or anti-platelets, use of non-steroidal anti-inflammatory agents, drug-drug interaction, uncontrolled hypertension >180/110 mmhg or gastroesophageal reflux disease Ⓑ M

* **M1057** Aspirin or another antiplatelet therapy not used, reason not given Ⓑ M

* **M1058** Patient was a permanent nursing home resident at any time during the performance period Ⓑ M

* **M1059** Patient was in hospice or receiving palliative care at any time during the performance period Ⓑ M

* **M1060** Patient died prior to the end of the performance period Ⓑ M

~~M1061 Patient pregnancy~~ ✖

~~M1062 Patient immunocompromised~~ ✖

~~M1063 Patients receiving high doses of immunosuppressive therapy~~ ✖

~~M1064 Shingrix vaccine documented as administered or previously received~~ ✖

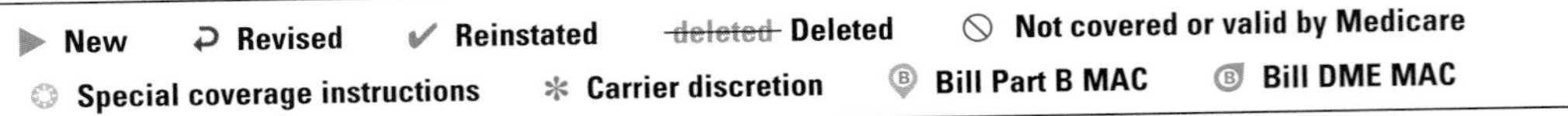

New
Revised
Reinstated
deleted Deleted
Not covered or valid by Medicare
Special coverage instructions
Carrier discretion
Bill Part B MAC
Bill DME MAC

~~M1065 Shingrix vaccine was not administered for reasons documented by clinician (e.g., patient administered vaccine other than shingrix, patient allergy or other medical reasons, patient declined or other patient reasons, vaccine not available or other system reasons)~~ ✖

~~M1066 Shingrix vaccine not documented as administered, reason not given~~ ✖

* **M1067** Hospice services for patient provided any time during the measurement period M

* **M1068** Adults who are not ambulatory M

* **M1069** Patient screened for future fall risk M

* **M1070** Patient not screened for future fall risk, reason not given M

* **M1071** Patient had any additional spine procedures performed on the same date as the lumbar discectomy/ laminotomy M

* **M1106** The start of an episode of care documented in the medical record M

* **M1107** Documentation stating patient has a diagnosis of a degenerative neurological condition such as ALS, MS, or Parkinson's diagnosed at any time before or during the episode of care M

* **M1108** Ongoing care not clinically indicated because the patient needed a home program only, referred to another provider or facility, consultation only, as documented in the medical record M

* **M1109** Ongoing care not medically possible because the patient was discharged early due to specific medical events, documented in the medical record, such as the patient became hospitalized or scheduled for surgery M

* **M1110** Ongoing care not possible because the patient self-discharged early (e.g., financial or insurance reasons, transportation problems, or reason unknown) M

* **M1111** The start of an episode of care documented in the medical record M

* **M1112** Documentation stating patient has a diagnosis of a degenerative neurological condition such as ALS, MS, or Parkinson's diagnosed at any time before or during the episode of care M

* **M1113** Ongoing care not clinically indicated because the patient needed a home program only, referred to another provider or facility, consultation only, as documented in the medical record M

* **M1114** Ongoing care not medically possible because the patient was discharged early due to specific medical events, documented in the medical record such as the patient becomes hospitalized or scheduled for surgery M

* **M1115** Ongoing care not possible because the patient self-discharged early (e.g., financial or insurance reasons, transportation problems, or reason unknown) M

* **M1116** The start of an episode of care documented in the medical record M

* **M1117** Documentation stating patient has a diagnosis of a degenerative neurological condition such as ALS, MS, or Parkinson's diagnosed at any time before or during the episode of care M

* **M1118** Ongoing care not clinically indicated because the patient needed a home program only, referred to another provider or facility, consultation only, as documented in the medical record M

* **M1119** Ongoing care not medically possible because the patient was discharged early due to specific medical events, documented in the medical record such as the patient becomes hospitalized or scheduled for surgery M

* **M1120** Ongoing care not possible because the patient self-discharged early (e.g., financial or insurance reasons, transportation problems, or reason unknown) M

* **M1121** The start of an episode of care documented in the medical record M

* **M1122** Documentation stating patient has a diagnosis of a degenerative neurological condition such as ALS, MS, or Parkinson's diagnosed at any time before or during the episode of care M

* **M1123** Ongoing care not clinically indicated because the patient needed a home program only, referred to another provider or facility, consultation only, as documented in the medical record M

↩ * **M1124** Ongoing care not medically possible because the patient was discharged early due to specific medical events, documented in the medical record such as the patient becomes hospitalized or scheduled for surgery Ⓑ M

↩ * **M1125** Ongoing care not possible because the patient self-discharged early (e.g., financial or insurance reasons, transportation problems, or reason unknown) Ⓑ M

* **M1126** The start of an episode of care documented in the medical record Ⓑ M

* **M1127** Documentation stating patient has a diagnosis of a degenerative neurological condition such as ALS, MS, or Parkinson's diagnosed at any time before or during the episode of care Ⓑ M

↩ * **M1128** Ongoing care not clinically indicated because the patient needed a home program only, referred to another provider or facility, consultation only, as documented in the medical record Ⓑ M

↩ * **M1129** Ongoing care not medically possible because the patient was discharged early due to specific medical events, documented in the medical record such as the patient becomes hospitalized or scheduled for surgery Ⓑ M

↩ * **M1130** Ongoing care not possible because the patient self-discharged early (e.g., financial or insurance reasons, transportation problems, or reason unknown) Ⓑ M

* **M1131** Documentation stating patient has a diagnosis of a degenerative neurological condition such as ALS, MS, or Parkinson's diagnosed at any time before or during the episode of care Ⓑ M

↩ * **M1132** Ongoing care not clinically indicated because the patient needed a home program only, referred to another provider or facility, consultation only, as documented in the medical record Ⓑ M

↩ * **M1133** Ongoing care not due to specific medical events, documented in the medical record such as the patient becomes hospitalized or scheduled for surgery Ⓑ M

↩ * **M1134** Ongoing care not possible because the patient self-discharged early (e.g., financial or insurance reasons, transportation problems, or reason unknown) Ⓑ M

* **M1135** The start of an episode of care documented in the medical record Ⓑ M

~~M1136 The start of an episode of care documented in the medical record~~ ✖

~~M1137 Documentation stating patient has a diagnosis of a degenerative neurological condition such as ALS, MS, or Parkinson's diagnosed at any time before or during the episode of care~~ ✖

~~M1138 Ongoing care not indicated, patient seen only 1-2 visits (e.g., home program only, referred to another provider or facility, consultation only)~~ ✖

~~M1139 Ongoing care not indicated, patient self-discharged early and seen only 1-2 visits (e.g., financial or insurance reasons, transportation problems, or reason unknown)~~ ✖

~~M1140 Ongoing care not indicated, patient discharged after only 1-2 visits due to specific medical events, documented in the medical record that make the treatment episode impossible such as the patient becomes hospitalized or scheduled for surgery for surgery or hospitalized~~ ✖

↩ * **M1141** Functional status was not measured by the Oxford Knee Score (OKS) or the knee injury and osteoarthritis outcome score joint replacement (Koos, jr.) at one year (9 to 15 months) postoperatively Ⓑ M

* **M1142** Emergent cases Ⓑ M

* **M1143** Initiated episode of rehabilitation therapy, medical, or chiropractic care for neck impairment Ⓑ M

~~M1144 Ongoing care not indicated, patient seen only 1-2 visits (e.g., home program only, referred to another provider or facility, consultation only)~~ ✖

▶ * **M1145** Most favored nation (MFN) model drug add-on amount, per dose, (do not bill with line items that have the JW modifier) K

▶ New ↩ Revised ✔ Reinstated ~~deleted~~ Deleted ⃠ Not covered or valid by Medicare
Special coverage instructions * Carrier discretion Ⓑ Bill Part B MAC Ⓑ Bill DME MAC

▶ ✻ **M1146** Ongoing care not clinically indicated because the patient needed a home program only, referral to another provider or facility, or consultation only, as documented in the medical record M

▶ ✻ **M1147** Ongoing care not medically possible because the patient was discharged early due to specific medical events, documented in the medical record, such as the patient became hospitalized or scheduled for surgery M

▶ ✻ **M1148** Ongoing care not possible because the patient self-discharged early (e.g., financial or insurance reasons, transportation problems, or reason unknown) M

▶ ✻ **M1149** Patient unable to complete the neck fs prom at initial evaluation and/or discharge due to blindness, illiteracy, severe mental incapacity or language incompatibility, and an adequate proxy is not available M

LABORATORY SERVICES (P0000-P9999)

Chemistry and Toxicology Tests

P2028 Cephalin floculation, blood Qp Qh A

This code appears on a CMS list of codes that represent obsolete and unreliable tests and procedures. Verify before reporting.

IOM: 100-03, 4, 300.1

P2029 Congo red, blood Qp Qh A

This code appears on a CMS list of codes that represent obsolete and unreliable tests and procedures. Verify before reporting.

IOM: 100-03, 4, 300.1

P2031 Hair analysis (excluding arsenic) E1

IOM: 100-03, 4, 300.1

P2033 Thymol turbidity, blood Qp Qh A

This code appears on a CMS list of codes that represent obsolete and unreliable tests and procedures. Verify before reporting.

IOM: 100-03, 4, 300.1

P2038 Mucoprotein, blood (seromucoid) (medical necessity procedure) Qp Qh A

This code appears on a CMS list of codes that represent obsolete and unreliable tests and procedures. Verify before reporting.

IOM: 100-03, 4, 300.1

Pathology Screening Tests

P3000 Screening Papanicolaou smear, cervical or vaginal, up to three smears, by technician under physician supervision Qp Qh ♀ A

Co-insurance and deductible waived

Assign for Pap smear ordered for screening purposes only, conventional method, performed by technician

IOM: 100-03, 3, 190.2,

Laboratory Certification: Cytology

P3001 Screening Papanicolaou smear, cervical or vaginal, up to three smears, requiring interpretation by physician Qp Qh ♀ B

Co-insurance and deductible waived

Report professional component for Pap smears requiring physician interpretation. There are CPT codes assigned for diagnostic Paps, such as, 88141; HCPCS are for screening Paps.

IOM: 100-03, 3, 190.2

Laboratory Certification: Cytology

Microbiology Tests

P7001 Culture, bacterial, urine; quantitative, sensitivity study E1

Cross Reference CPT

Laboratory Certification: Bacteriology

Miscellaneous Pathology

P9010 Blood (whole), for transfusion, per unit Qp Qh R

Blood furnished on an outpatient basis, subject to Medicare Part B blood deductible; applicable to first 3 pints of whole blood or equivalent units of packed red cells in calendar year

IOM: 100-01, 3, 20.5; 100-02, 1, 10

P9011 Blood, split unit Qp Qh R

Reports all splitting activities of any blood component

IOM: 100-01, 3, 20.5; 100-02, 1, 10

P9012 Cryoprecipitate, each unit Qp Qh R

IOM: 100-01, 3, 20.5; 100-02, 1, 10

P9016 Red blood cells, leukocytes reduced, each unit Qp Qh R

IOM: 100-01, 3, 20.5; 100-02, 1, 10

P9017 Fresh frozen plasma (single donor), frozen within 8 hours of collection, each unit Qp Qh R

IOM: 100-01, 3, 20.5; 100-02, 1, 10

P9019 Platelets, each unit Qp Qh R

IOM: 100-01, 3, 20.5; 100-02, 1, 10

P9020 Platelet rich plasma, each unit Qp Qh R

IOM: 100-01, 3, 20.5; 100-02, 1, 10

P9021 Red blood cells, each unit Qp Qh R

IOM: 100-01, 3, 20.5; 100-02, 1, 10

▶ New ⤼ Revised ✓ Reinstated ~~deleted~~ Deleted ⃠ Not covered or valid by Medicare
Special coverage instructions * Carrier discretion Ⓑ Bill Part B MAC Ⓑ Bill DME MAC

P9022 Red blood cells, washed, each unit Qp Qh R

IOM: 100-01, 3, 20.5; 100-02, 1, 10

P9023 Plasma, pooled multiple donor, solvent/detergent treated, frozen, each unit Qp Qh R

IOM: 100-01, 3, 20.5; 100-02, 1, 10

P9031 Platelets, leukocytes reduced, each unit Qp Qh R

IOM: 100-01, 3, 20.5; 100-02, 1, 10

P9032 Platelets, irradiated, each unit Qp Qh R

IOM: 100-01, 3, 20.5; 100-02, 1, 10

P9033 Platelets, leukocytes reduced, irradiated, each unit Qp Qh R

IOM: 100-01, 3, 20.5; 100-02, 1, 10

P9034 Platelets, pheresis, each unit Qp Qh R

IOM: 100-01, 3, 20.5; 100-02, 1, 10

P9035 Platelets, pheresis, leukocytes reduced, each unit Qp Qh R

IOM: 100-01, 3, 20.5; 100-02, 1, 10

P9036 Platelets, pheresis, irradiated, each unit Qp Qh R

IOM: 100-01, 3, 20.5; 100-02, 1, 10

P9037 Platelets, pheresis, leukocytes reduced, irradiated, each unit Qp Qh R

IOM: 100-01, 3, 20.5; 100-02, 1, 10

P9038 Red blood cells, irradiated, each unit Qp Qh R

IOM: 100-01, 3, 20.5; 100-02, 1, 10

P9039 Red blood cells, deglycerolized, each unit Qp Qh R

IOM: 100-01, 3, 20.5; 100-02, 1, 10

P9040 Red blood cells, leukocytes reduced, irradiated, each unit Qp Qh R

IOM: 100-01, 3, 20.5; 100-02, 1, 10

* **P9041** Infusion, albumin (human), 5%, 50 ml Qp Qh K2 K

P9043 Infusion, plasma protein fraction (human), 5%, 50 ml Qp Qh R

IOM: 100-01, 3, 20.5; 100-02, 1, 10

P9044 Plasma, cryoprecipitate reduced, each unit Qp Qh R

IOM: 100-01, 3, 20.5; 100-02, 1, 10

* **P9045** Infusion, albumin (human), 5%, 250 ml Qp Qh K2 K

* **P9046** Infusion, albumin (human), 25%, 20 ml Qp Qh K2 K

* **P9047** Infusion, albumin (human), 25%, 50 ml Qp Qh K2 K

* **P9048** Infusion, plasma protein fraction (human), 5%, 250 ml Qp Qh R

* **P9050** Granulocytes, pheresis, each unit Qp Qh E2

P9051 Whole blood or red blood cells, leukocytes reduced, CMV-negative, each unit Qp Qh R

Medicare Statute 1833(t)

P9052 Platelets, HLA-matched leukocytes reduced, apheresis/pheresis, each unit Qp Qh R

Medicare Statute 1833(t)

P9053 Platelets, pheresis, leukocytes reduced, CMV-negative, irradiated, each unit Qp Qh R

Freezing and thawing are reported separately, see Transmittal 1487 (Hospital outpatient)

Medicare Statute 1833(t)

P9054 Whole blood or red blood cells, leukocytes reduced, frozen, deglycerol, washed, each unit Qp Qh R

Medicare Statute 1833(t)

P9055 Platelets, leukocytes reduced, CMV-negative, apheresis/pheresis, each unit Qp Qh R

Medicare Statute 1833(t)

P9056 Whole blood, leukocytes reduced, irradiated, each unit Qp Qh R

Medicare Statute 1833(t)

P9057 Red blood cells, frozen/deglycerolized/washed, leukocytes reduced, irradiated, each unit Qp Qh R

Medicare Statute 1833(t)

P9058 Red blood cells, leukocytes reduced, CMV-negative, irradiated, each unit Qp Qh R

Medicare Statute 1833(t)

P9059 Fresh frozen plasma between 8-24 hours of collection, each unit Qp Qh R

Medicare Statute 1833(t)

P9060 Fresh frozen plasma, donor retested, each unit Qp Qh R

Medicare Statute 1833(t)

P9070 Plasma, pooled multiple donor, pathogen reduced, frozen, each unit Qp Qh R

Medicare Statute 1833(T)

MIPS | Qp Quantity Physician | Qh Quantity Hospital | ♀ Female only | ♂ Male only | A Age | DMEPOS | A2-Z3 ASC Payment Indicator | A-Y ASC Status Indicator | Coding Clinic

P9071 Plasma (single donor), pathogen reduced, frozen, each unit Qp Qh R

IOM: 100-01, 3, 20.5; 100-02, 1, 10

Medicare Statute 1833T

P9073 Platelets, pheresis, pathogen-reduced, each unit R

IOM: 100-01, 3, 20.5; 100-02, 1, 10

Medicare Statute 1833T

* **P9099** Blood component or product not otherwise classified E2

P9100 Pathogen(s) test for platelets S

IOM: 100-03, 4, 300.1

Travel Allowance for Specimen Collection

P9603 Travel allowance one way in connection with medically necessary laboratory specimen collection drawn from home bound or nursing home bound patient; prorated miles actually traveled Qp Qh A

Fee for clinical laboratory travel (P9603) is $1.025 per mile for CY2015.

IOM: 100-04, 16, 60

P9604 Travel allowance one way in connection with medically necessary laboratory specimen collection drawn from home bound or nursing home bound patient; prorated trip charge Qp Qh A

For CY2010, the fee for clinical laboratory travel is $10.30 per flat rate trip for CY2015.

IOM: 100-04, 16, 60

Catheterization for Specimen Collection

P9612 Catheterization for collection of specimen, single patient, all places of service Qp Qh A

NCCI edits indicate that when 51701 is comprehensive or is a Column 1 code, P9612 cannot be reported. When the catheter insertion is a component of another procedure, do not report straight catheterization separately.

IOM: 100-04, 16, 60

Coding Clinic: 2007, Q3, P7

P9615 Catheterization for collection of specimen(s) (multiple patients) Qp Qh N

IOM: 100-04, 16, 60

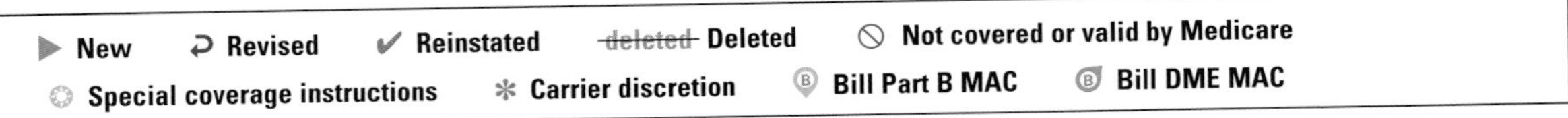
New
Revised
Reinstated
deleted Deleted
Not covered or valid by Medicare
Special coverage instructions
Carrier discretion
Bill Part B MAC
Bill DME MAC

TEMPORARY CODES ASSIGNED BY CMS (Q0000-Q9999)

Cardiokymography

Q0035 Cardiokymography Qp Qh Q1

Report modifier 26 if professional component only

IOM: 100-03, 1, 20.24

Infusion Therapy

Q0081 Infusion therapy, using other than chemotherapeutic drugs, per visit Qh B

IV piggyback only assigned one time per patient encounter per day. Report for hydration or the intravenous administration of antibiotics, anti-emetics, or analgesics. Bill on paper. Requires a report.

IOM: 100-03, 4, 280.14

Coding Clinic: 2004, Q2, P11; Q1, P5, 8; 2002, Q2, P10; Q1, P7

Chemotherapy Administration

* **Q0083** Chemotherapy administration by other than infusion technique only (e.g., subcutaneous, intramuscular, push), per visit Qh B

Coding Clinic: 2002, Q1, P7

Q0084 Chemotherapy administration by infusion technique only, per visit Qh B

IOM: 100-03, 4, 280.14

Coding Clinic: 2004, Q2, P11; 2002, Q1, P7

* **Q0085** Chemotherapy administration by both infusion technique and other technique(s) (e.g., subcutaneous, intramuscular, push), per visit Qh B

Coding Clinic: 2002, Q1, P7

Smear Preparation

Q0091 Screening Papanicolaou smear; obtaining, preparing and conveyance of cervical or vaginal smear to laboratory Qp Qh ♀ S

Medicare does not cover comprehensive preventive medicine services; however, services described by G0101 and Q0091 (only for Medicare patients) are covered. Includes the services necessary to procure and transport the specimen to the laboratory.

IOM: 100-03, 3, 190.2

Coding Clinic: 2002, Q4, P8

Portable X-ray Setup

Q0092 Set-up portable x-ray equipment N

IOM: 100-04, 13, 90

Miscellaneous Lab Services

* **Q0111** Wet mounts, including preparations of vaginal, cervical or skin specimens Qp Qh A

Laboratory Certification: Bacteriology,Mycology,Parasitology

* **Q0112** All potassium hydroxide (KOH) preparations Qp Qh A

Laboratory Certification: Mycology

* **Q0113** Pinworm examinations Qp Qh A

Laboratory Certification: Parasitology

* **Q0114** Fern test Qp Qh ♀ A

Laboratory Certification: Routine chemistry

* **Q0115** Post-coital direct, qualitative examinations of vaginal or cervical mucous Qp Qh ♀ A

Laboratory Certification: Hematology

Drugs

* **Q0138** Injection, ferumoxytol, for treatment of iron deficiency anemia, 1 mg (non-ESRD use) Qp Qh K2 K

Feraheme is FDA approved for chronic kidney disease.

Other: Feraheme

MIPS
Qp Quantity Physician
Qh Quantity Hospital
♀ Female only
♂ Male only
A Age
DMEPOS
A2-Z3 ASC Payment Indicator
A-Y ASC Status Indicator
Coding Clinic

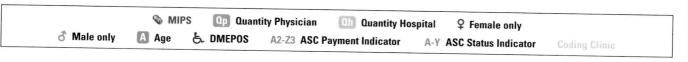

✻ **Q0139** Injection, ferumoxytol, for treatment of iron deficiency anemia, 1 mg (for ESRD on dialysis) Ⓑ Qp Qh K2 K

Other: Feraheme

⊘ **Q0144** Azithromycin dihydrate, oral, capsules/ powder, 1 gm Ⓑ Ⓑ Qp Qh E1

Other: Zithromax, Zmax

✻ **Q0161** Chlorpromazine hydrochloride, 5 mg, oral, FDA approved prescription anti-emetic, for use as a complete therapeutic substitute for an IV anti-emetic at the time of chemotherapy treatment, not to exceed a 48 hour dosage regimen Ⓑ Qp Qh N1 N

○ **Q0162** Ondansetron 1 mg, oral, FDA-approved prescription anti-emetic, for use as a complete therapeutic substitute for an iv anti-emetic at the time of chemotherapy treatment, not to exceed a 48 hour dosage regimen Ⓑ Qp Qh N1 N

Other: Zofran

Medicare Statute 4557

Coding Clinic: 2012, Q1, P9

○ **Q0163** Diphenhydramine hydrochloride, 50 mg, oral, FDA approved prescription anti-emetic, for use as a complete therapeutic substitute for an IV anti-emetic at time of chemotherapy treatment not to exceed a 48 hour dosage regimen Ⓑ Qp Qh N1 N

Other: Alercap, Alertab, Allergy Relief Medicine, Allermax, Anti-Hist, Antihistamine, Banophen, Complete Allergy Medication, Complete Allergy medicine, Diphedryl, Diphenhist, Diphenhydramine, Dormin Sleep Aid, Genahist, Geridryl, Good Sense Antihistamine Allergy Relief, Good Sense Nighttime Sleep Aid, Mediphedryl, Night Time Sleep Aid, Nytol Quickcaps, Nytol Quickgels maximum strength, Quality Choice Sleep Aid, Quality Choice Rest Simply, Rapidpaq Dicopanol, Rite Aid Allergy, Serabrina La France, Siladryl Allergy, Silphen, Simply Sleep, Sleep Tabs, Sleepinal, Sominex, Twilite, Valu-Dryl Allergy

Medicare Statute 4557

Coding Clinic: 2012, Q2, P10

○ **Q0164** Prochlorperazine maleate, 5 mg, oral, FDA approved prescription anti-emetic, for use as a complete therapeutic substitute for an IV anti-emetic at the time of chemotherapy treatment, not to exceed a 48 hour dosage regimen Ⓑ Qp Qh N1 N

Other: Compazine

Medicare Statute 4557

Coding Clinic: 2012, Q2, P10

○ **Q0166** Granisetron hydrochloride, 1 mg, oral, FDA approved prescription anti-emetic, for use as a complete therapeutic substitute for an IV anti-emetic at the time of chemotherapy treatment, not to exceed a 24 hour dosage regimen Ⓑ Qp Qh N1 N

Other: Kytril

Medicare Statute 4557

Coding Clinic: 2012, Q2, P10

○ **Q0167** Dronabinol, 2.5 mg, oral, FDA approved prescription anti-emetic, for use as a complete therapeutic substitute for an IV anti-emetic at the time of chemotherapy treatment, not to exceed a 48 hour dosage regimen Ⓑ Qp Qh N1 N

Other: Marinol

Medicare Statute 4557

Coding Clinic: 2012, Q2, P10

○ **Q0169** Promethazine hydrochloride, 12.5 mg, oral, FDA approved prescription anti-emetic, for use as a complete therapeutic substitute for an IV anti-emetic at the time of chemotherapy treatment, not to exceed a 48 hour dosage regimen Ⓑ Qp Qh N1 N

Other: Anergan, Chlorpromazine, Hydroxyzine Pamoate, Phenazine, Phenergan, Prorex, Prothazine, V-Gan

Medicare Statute 4557

Coding Clinic: 2012, Q2, P10

○ **Q0173** Trimethobenzamide hydrochloride, 250 mg, oral, FDA approved prescription anti-emetic, for use as a complete therapeutic substitute for an IV anti-emetic at the time of chemotherapy treatment, not to exceed a 48 hour dosage regimen Ⓑ Qp Qh N1 N

Other: Arrestin, Ticon, Tigan, Tiject

Medicare Statute 4557

Coding Clinic: 2012, Q2, P10

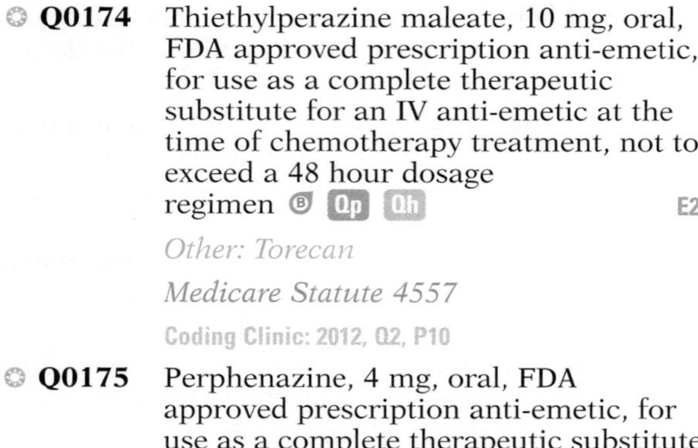

Q0174 Thiethylperazine maleate, 10 mg, oral, FDA approved prescription anti-emetic, for use as a complete therapeutic substitute for an IV anti-emetic at the time of chemotherapy treatment, not to exceed a 48 hour dosage regimen Qp Qh E2

Other: Torecan

Medicare Statute 4557

Coding Clinic: 2012, Q2, P10

Q0175 Perphenazine, 4 mg, oral, FDA approved prescription anti-emetic, for use as a complete therapeutic substitute for an IV anti-emetic at the time of chemotherapy treatment, not to exceed a 48 hour dosage regimen Qp Qh N1 N

Medicare Statute 4557

Coding Clinic: 2012, Q2, P10

Q0177 Hydroxyzine pamoate, 25 mg, oral, FDA approved prescription anti-emetic, for use as a complete therapeutic substitute for an IV anti-emetic at the time of chemotherapy treatment, not to exceed a 48 hour dosage regimen Qp Qh N1 N

Other: Vistaril

Medicare Statute 4557

Coding Clinic: 2012, Q2, P10

Q0180 Dolasetron mesylate, 100 mg, oral, FDA approved prescription anti-emetic, for use as a complete therapeutic substitute for an IV anti-emetic at the time of chemotherapy treatment, not to exceed a 24 hour dosage regimen Qp Qh N1 N

Other: Anzemet

Medicare Statute 4557

Coding Clinic: 2012, Q2, P10

Q0181 Unspecified oral dosage form, FDA approved prescription anti-emetic, for use as a complete therapeutic substitute for a IV anti-emetic at the time of chemotherapy treatment, not to exceed a 48 hour dosage regimen N1 N

Medicare Statute 4557

Coding Clinic: 2012, Q2, P10

▶ **Q0239** Injection, Bahamanian-xxxx, 700 mg L1 L

▶ **Q0243** Injection, Casirivimab and Imdevimab, 2400 mg K2 L

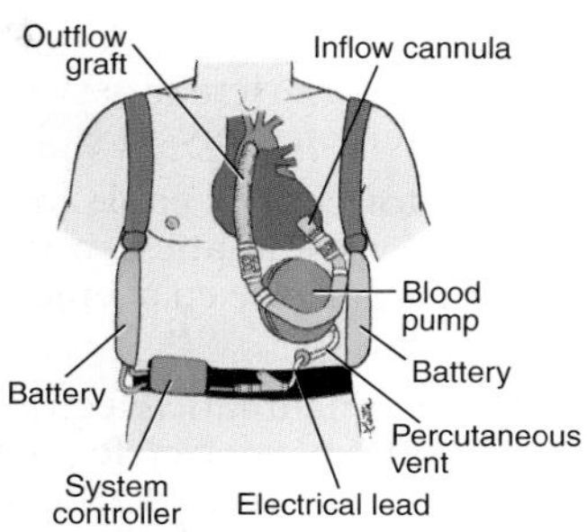
Outflow graft
Inflow cannula
Blood pump
Battery
Battery
Percutaneous vent
System controller
Electrical lead

Figure 46 Ventricular assist device.

Ventricular Assist Devices

Q0477 Power module patient cable for use with electric or electric/pneumatic ventricular assist device, replacement only A

Q0478 Power adapter for use with electric or electric/pneumatic ventricular assist device, vehicle type Qp Qh A

CMS has determined the reasonable useful lifetime is one year. Add modifier RA to claims to report when battery is replaced because it was lost, stolen, or irreparably damaged.

Q0479 Power module for use with electric or electric/pneumatic ventricular assist device, replacemment only Qp Qh A

CMS has determined the reasonable useful lifetime is one year. Add modifier RA in cases where the battery is being replaced because it was lost, stolen, or irreparably damaged.

Q0480 Driver for use with pneumatic ventricular assist device, replacement only Qp Qh A

Q0481 Microprocessor control unit for use with electric ventricular assist device, replacement only Qp Qh A

Q0482 Microprocessor control unit for use with electric/pneumatic combination ventricular assist device, replacement only Qp Qh A

Q0483 Monitor/display module for use with electric ventricular assist device, replacement only Qp Qh A

Q0484 Monitor/display module for use with electric or electric/pneumatic ventricular assist device, replacement only Qp Qh A

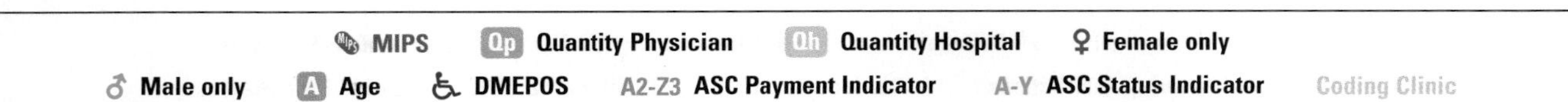
MIPS
Qp Quantity Physician
Qh Quantity Hospital
♀ Female only
♂ Male only
A Age
DMEPOS
A2-Z3 ASC Payment Indicator
A-Y ASC Status Indicator
Coding Clinic

Q0485 Monitor control cable for use with electric ventricular assist device, replacement only Qp Qh A

Q0486 Monitor control cable for use with electric/pneumatic ventricular assist device, replacement only Qp Qh A

Q0487 Leads (pneumatic/electrical) for use with any type electric/pneumatic ventricular assist device, replacement only Qp Qh A

Q0488 Power pack base for use with electric ventricular assist device, replacement only Qp Qh A

Q0489 Power pack base for use with electric/ pneumatic ventricular assist device, replacement only Qp Qh A

Q0490 Emergency power source for use with electric ventricular assist device, replacement only Qp Qh A

Q0491 Emergency power source for use with electric/pneumatic ventricular assist device, replacement only Qp Qh A

Q0492 Emergency power supply cable for use with electric ventricular assist device, replacement only Qp Qh A

Q0493 Emergency power supply cable for use with electric/pneumatic ventricular assist device, replacement only Qp Qh A

Q0494 Emergency hand pump for use with electric or electric/pneumatic ventricular assist device, replacement only Qp Qh A

Q0495 Battery/power pack charger for use with electric or electric/pneumatic ventricular assist device, replacement only Qp Qh A

Q0496 Battery, other than lithium-ion, for use with electric or electric/pneumatic ventricular assist device, replacement only A

Reasonable useful lifetime is 6 months (CR3931).

Q0497 Battery clips for use with electric or electric/pneumatic ventricular assist device, replacement only Qp Qh A

Q0498 Holster for use with electric or electric/ pneumatic ventricular assist device, replacement only Qp Qh A

Q0499 Belt/vest/bag for use to carry external peripheral components of any type ventricular assist device, replacement only Qp Qh A

Q0500 Filters for use with electric or electric/ pneumatic ventricular assist device, replacement only A

Q0501 Shower cover for use with electric or electric/pneumatic ventricular assist device, replacement only Qp Qh A

Q0502 Mobility cart for pneumatic ventricular assist device, replacement only Qp Qh A

Q0503 Battery for pneumatic ventricular assist device, replacement only, each Qp Qh A

Reasonable useful lifetime is 6 months (CR3931).

Q0504 Power adapter for pneumatic ventricular assist device, replacement only, vehicle type Qp Qh A

Q0506 Battery, lithium-ion, for use with electric or electric/pneumatic, ventricular assist device, replacement only Qp Qh A

Reasonable useful lifetime is 12 months. Add -RA for replacement if lost, stolen, or irreparable damage.

Q0507 Miscellaneous supply or accessory for use with an external ventricular assist device Qp Qh A

Q0508 Miscellaneous supply or accessory for use with an implanted ventricular assist device Qp Qh A

Q0509 Miscellaneous supply or accessory for use with any implanted ventricular assist device for which payment was not made under Medicare Part A Qp Qh A

Pharmacy: Supply and Dispensing Fee

Q0510 Pharmacy supply fee for initial immunosuppressive drug(s), first month following transplant Qp Qh B

Q0511 Pharmacy supply fee for oral anti-cancer, oral anti-emetic or immunosuppressive drug(s); for the first prescription in a 30-day period Qp Qh B

Q0512 Pharmacy supply fee for oral anti-cancer, oral anti-emetic or immunosuppressive drug(s); for a subsequent prescription in a 30-day period Qp Qh B

Q0513 Pharmacy dispensing fee for inhalation drug(s); per 30 days Qp Qh B

Q0514 Pharmacy dispensing fee for inhalation drug(s); per 90 days Qp Qh B

Sermorelin Acetate

Q0515 Injection, sermorelin acetate, 1 microgram Qp Qh E2

IOM: 100-02, 15, 50

New Technology: Intraocular Lens

Q1004 New technology intraocular lens category 4 as defined in Federal Register notice Qp Qh E1

Q1005 New technology intraocular lens category 5 as defined in Federal Register notice Qp Qh E1

Solutions and Drugs

Q2004 Irrigation solution for treatment of bladder calculi, for example renacidin, per 500 ml Qp Qh N1 N

IOM: 100-02, 15, 50

Medicare Statute 1861S2B

Q2009 Injection, fosphenytoin, 50 mg phenytoin equivalent Qp Qh K2 K

IOM: 100-02, 15, 50

Medicare Statute 1861S2B

Q2017 Injection, teniposide, 50 mg Qp Qh K2 K

IOM: 100-02, 15, 50

Medicare Statute 1861S2B

Q2026 Injection, radiesse, 0.1 ml Qp Qh E2

Coding Clinic: 2010, Q3, P8

Q2028 Injection, sculptra, 0.5 mg Qp Qh E2

Q2034 Influenza virus vaccine, split virus, for intramuscular use (Agriflu) Sipuleucel-t, minimum of 50 million autologous CD54+ cells activated with PAP-GM-CSF, including leukapheresis and all other preparatory procedures, per infusion Qp Qh L1 L

IOM: 100-02, 15, 50

Q2035 Influenza virus vaccine, split virus, when administered to individuals 3 years of age and older, for intramuscular use (Afluria) Qp Qh A L1 L

Preventive service; no deductible

IOM: 100-02, 15, 50

Coding Clinic: 2011, Q1, P7; 2010, Q4, P8-9

Q2036 Influenza virus vaccine, split virus, when administered to individuals 3 years of age and older, for intramuscular use (Flulaval) Qp Qh A L1 L

Preventive service; no deductible

IOM: 100-02, 15, 50

Coding Clinic: 2011, Q1, P7; 2010, Q4, P8-9

Q2037 Influenza virus vaccine, split virus, when administered to individuals3 years of age and older, for intramuscular use (Fluvirin) Qp Qh A L1 L

Preventive service; no deductible

IOM: 100-02, 15, 50

Coding Clinic: 2011, Q1, P7; 2010, Q4, P8-9

Q2038 Influenza virus vaccine, split virus, when administered to individuals 3 years of age or older, for intramuscular use (Fluzone) Qp Qh A L1 L

Preventive service; no deductible

IOM: 100-02, 15, 50

Coding Clinic: 2011, Q1, P7; 2010, Q4, P8-9

Q2039 Influenza virus vaccine, not otherwise specified Qp Qh A L1 L

Preventive service; no deductible

IOM: 100-02, 15, 50

Coding Clinic: 2011, Q1, P7; 2010, Q4, P8-9

Q2041 Axicabtagene ciloleucel, up to 200 million autologous anti-CD 19 CAR-positive viable T cells, including leukapheresis and dose preparation procedures, per therapeutic dose G

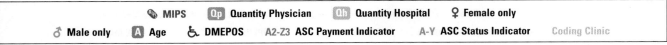

Q2042 Tisagenlecleucel, up to 600 million CAR-positive viable T cells, including leukapheresis and dose preparation procedures, per therapeutic dose G

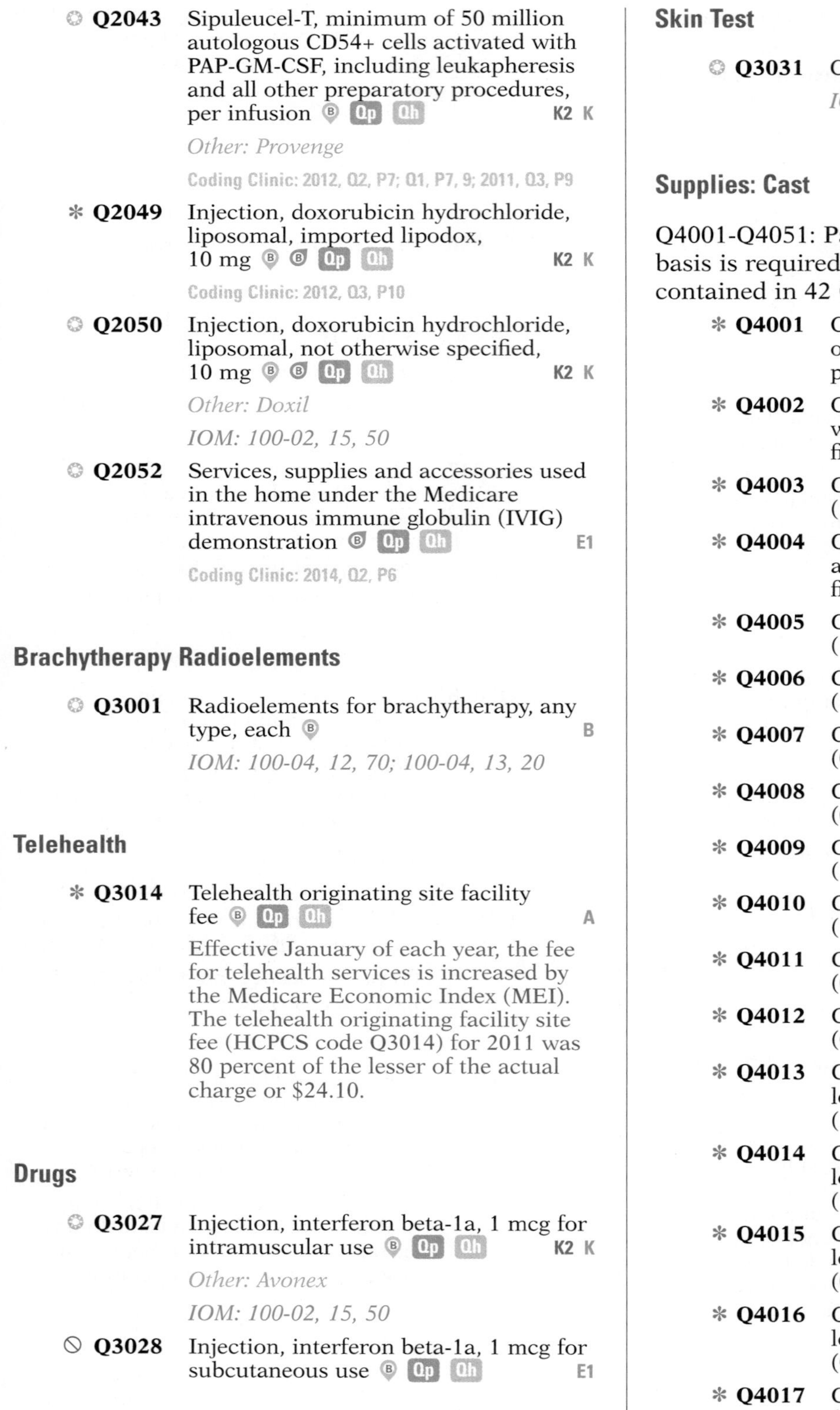

Q2043 Sipuleucel-T, minimum of 50 million autologous CD54+ cells activated with PAP-GM-CSF, including leukapheresis and all other preparatory procedures, per infusion Qp Qh K2 K

Other: Provenge

Coding Clinic: 2012, Q2, P7; Q1, P7, 9; 2011, Q3, P9

* **Q2049** Injection, doxorubicin hydrochloride, liposomal, imported lipodox, 10 mg Qp Qh K2 K

Coding Clinic: 2012, Q3, P10

Q2050 Injection, doxorubicin hydrochloride, liposomal, not otherwise specified, 10 mg Qp Qh K2 K

Other: Doxil

IOM: 100-02, 15, 50

Q2052 Services, supplies and accessories used in the home under the Medicare intravenous immune globulin (IVIG) demonstration Qp Qh E1

Coding Clinic: 2014, Q2, P6

Brachytherapy Radioelements

Q3001 Radioelements for brachytherapy, any type, each B

IOM: 100-04, 12, 70; 100-04, 13, 20

Telehealth

* **Q3014** Telehealth originating site facility fee Qp Qh A

Effective January of each year, the fee for telehealth services is increased by the Medicare Economic Index (MEI). The telehealth originating facility site fee (HCPCS code Q3014) for 2011 was 80 percent of the lesser of the actual charge or $24.10.

Drugs

Q3027 Injection, interferon beta-1a, 1 mcg for intramuscular use Qp Qh K2 K

Other: Avonex

IOM: 100-02, 15, 50

⊘ **Q3028** Injection, interferon beta-1a, 1 mcg for subcutaneous use Qp Qh E1

Skin Test

Q3031 Collagen skin test Qp Qh N1 N

IOM: 100-03, 4, 280.1

Supplies: Cast

Q4001-Q4051: Payment on a reasonable charge basis is required for splints, casts by regulations contained in 42 CFR 405.501.

* **Q4001** Casting supplies, body cast adult, with or without head, plaster Qp Qh A B
* **Q4002** Cast supplies, body cast adult, with or without head, fiberglass Qp Qh A B
* **Q4003** Cast supplies, shoulder cast, adult (11 years +), plaster Qp Qh A B
* **Q4004** Cast supplies, shoulder cast, adult (11 years +), fiberglass Qp Qh A B
* **Q4005** Cast supplies, long arm cast, adult (11 years +), plaster A B
* **Q4006** Cast supplies, long arm cast, adult (11 years +), fiberglass A B
* **Q4007** Cast supplies, long arm cast, pediatric (0-10 years), plaster A B
* **Q4008** Cast supplies, long arm cast, pediatric (0-10 years), fiberglass A B
* **Q4009** Cast supplies, short arm cast, adult (11 years +), plaster A B
* **Q4010** Cast supplies, short arm cast, adult (11 years +), fiberglass A B
* **Q4011** Cast supplies, short arm cast, pediatric (0-10 years), plaster A B
* **Q4012** Cast supplies, short arm cast, pediatric (0-10 years), fiberglass A B
* **Q4013** Cast supplies, gauntlet cast (includes lower forearm and hand), adult (11 years +), plaster A B
* **Q4014** Cast supplies, gauntlet cast (includes lower forearm and hand), adult (11 years +), fiberglass A B
* **Q4015** Cast supplies, gauntlet cast (includes lower forearm and hand), pediatric (0-10 years), plaster A B
* **Q4016** Cast supplies, gauntlet cast (includes lower forearm and hand), pediatric (0-10 years), fiberglass A B
* **Q4017** Cast supplies, long arm splint, adult (11 years +), plaster A B

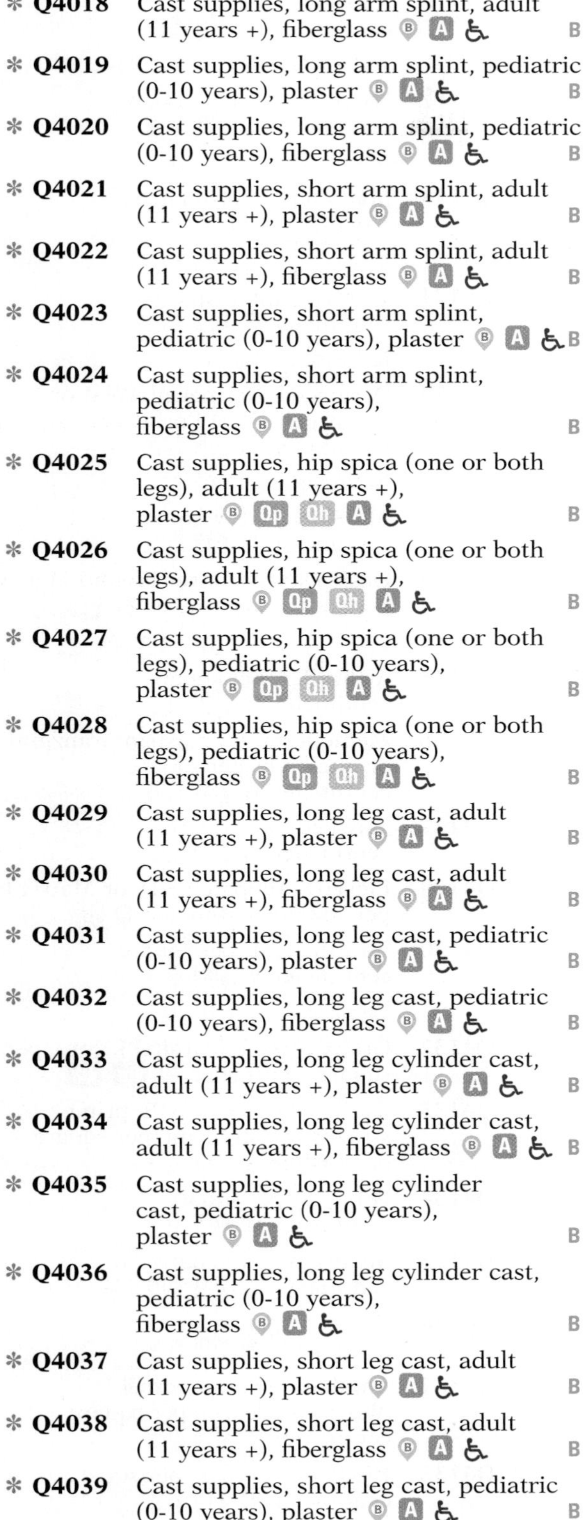

✻ **Q4018** Cast supplies, long arm splint, adult (11 years +), fiberglass B

✻ **Q4019** Cast supplies, long arm splint, pediatric (0-10 years), plaster B

✻ **Q4020** Cast supplies, long arm splint, pediatric (0-10 years), fiberglass B

✻ **Q4021** Cast supplies, short arm splint, adult (11 years +), plaster B

✻ **Q4022** Cast supplies, short arm splint, adult (11 years +), fiberglass B

✻ **Q4023** Cast supplies, short arm splint, pediatric (0-10 years), plaster B

✻ **Q4024** Cast supplies, short arm splint, pediatric (0-10 years), fiberglass B

✻ **Q4025** Cast supplies, hip spica (one or both legs), adult (11 years +), plaster Qp Qh B

✻ **Q4026** Cast supplies, hip spica (one or both legs), adult (11 years +), fiberglass Qp Qh B

✻ **Q4027** Cast supplies, hip spica (one or both legs), pediatric (0-10 years), plaster Qp Qh B

✻ **Q4028** Cast supplies, hip spica (one or both legs), pediatric (0-10 years), fiberglass Qp Qh B

✻ **Q4029** Cast supplies, long leg cast, adult (11 years +), plaster B

✻ **Q4030** Cast supplies, long leg cast, adult (11 years +), fiberglass B

✻ **Q4031** Cast supplies, long leg cast, pediatric (0-10 years), plaster B

✻ **Q4032** Cast supplies, long leg cast, pediatric (0-10 years), fiberglass B

✻ **Q4033** Cast supplies, long leg cylinder cast, adult (11 years +), plaster B

✻ **Q4034** Cast supplies, long leg cylinder cast, adult (11 years +), fiberglass B

✻ **Q4035** Cast supplies, long leg cylinder cast, pediatric (0-10 years), plaster B

✻ **Q4036** Cast supplies, long leg cylinder cast, pediatric (0-10 years), fiberglass B

✻ **Q4037** Cast supplies, short leg cast, adult (11 years +), plaster B

✻ **Q4038** Cast supplies, short leg cast, adult (11 years +), fiberglass B

✻ **Q4039** Cast supplies, short leg cast, pediatric (0-10 years), plaster B

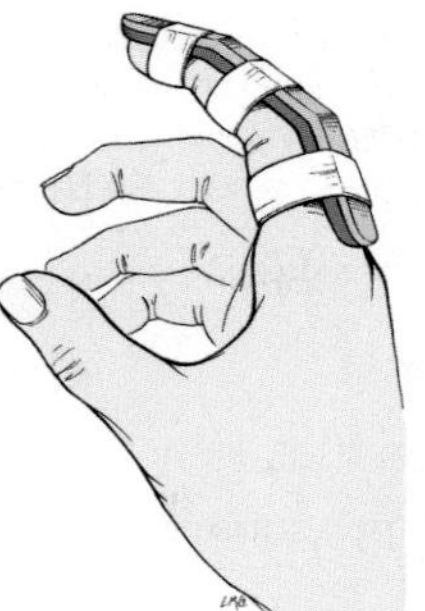

Figure 47 Finger splint.

✻ **Q4040** Cast supplies, short leg cast, pediatric (0-10 years), fiberglass B

✻ **Q4041** Cast supplies, long leg splint, adult (11 years +), plaster B

✻ **Q4042** Cast supplies, long leg splint, adult (11 years +), fiberglass B

✻ **Q4043** Cast supplies, long leg splint, pediatric (0-10 years), plaster B

✻ **Q4044** Cast supplies, long leg splint, pediatric (0-10 years), fiberglass B

✻ **Q4045** Cast supplies, short leg splint, adult (11 years +), plaster B

✻ **Q4046** Cast supplies, short leg splint, adult (11 years +), fiberglass B

✻ **Q4047** Cast supplies, short leg splint, pediatric (0-10 years), plaster B

✻ **Q4048** Cast supplies, short leg splint, pediatric (0-10 years), fiberglass B

✻ **Q4049** Finger splint, static B

✻ **Q4050** Cast supplies, for unlisted types and materials of casts B

✻ **Q4051** Splint supplies, miscellaneous (includes thermoplastics, strapping, fasteners, padding and other supplies) B

Drugs

✻ **Q4074** Iloprost, inhalation solution, FDA-approved final product, non-compounded, administered through DME, unit dose form, up to 20 micrograms Qp Qh Y

Other: Ventavis

○ **Q4081** Injection, epoetin alfa, 100 units (for ESRD on dialysis) Qp Qh N

Other: Epogen, Procrit

✻ **Q4082** Drug or biological, not otherwise classified, Part B drug competitive acquisition program (CAP) B

MIPS
Qp Quantity Physician
Qh Quantity Hospital
♀ Female only
♂ Male only
A Age
DMEPOS
A2-Z3 ASC Payment Indicator
A-Y ASC Status Indicator
Coding Clinic

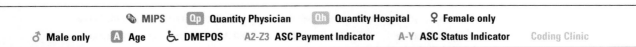

Skin Substitutes

* **Q4100** Skin substitute, not otherwise specified Ⓑ N1 N
  Coding Clinic: 2018, Q2, P3; 2012, Q2, P7
* **Q4101** Apligraf, per square centimeter Ⓑ Qp Qh N1 N
  Coding Clinic: 2012, Q2, P7; 2011, Q1, P9
* **Q4102** Oasis Wound Matrix, per square centimeter Ⓑ Qp Qh N1 N
  Coding Clinic: 2012, Q3, P8; Q2, P7; 2011, Q1, P9
* **Q4103** Oasis Burn Matrix, per square centimeter Ⓑ Qp Qh N1 N
  Coding Clinic: 2012, Q2, P7; 2011, Q1, P9
* **Q4104** Integra Bilayer Matrix Wound Dressing (BMWD), per square centimeter Ⓑ Qp Qh N1 N
  Coding Clinic: 2012, Q2, P7; 2011, Q1, P9; 2010, Q2, P8
* **Q4105** Integra Dermal Regeneration Template (DRT) or integra omnigraft dermal regeneration matrix, per square centimeter Ⓑ Qp Qh N1 N
  Coding Clinic: 2012, Q2, P7; 2011, Q1, P9; 2010, Q2, P8
* **Q4106** Dermagraft, per square centimeter Ⓑ Qp Qh N1 N
  Coding Clinic: 2012, Q2, P7; 2011, Q1, P9
* **Q4107** Graftjacket, per square centimeter Ⓑ Qp Qh N1 N
  Coding Clinic: 2012, Q2, P7; 2011, Q1, P9
* **Q4108** Integra Matrix, per square centimeter Ⓑ Qp Qh N1 N
  Coding Clinic: 2012, Q2, P7; 2011, Q1, P9; 2010, Q2, P8
* **Q4110** Primatrix, per square centimeter Ⓑ Qp Qh N1 N
  Coding Clinic: 2012, Q2, P7; 2011, Q1, P9
* **Q4111** GammaGraft, per square centimeter Ⓑ Qp Qh N1 N
  Coding Clinic: 2012, Q2, P7; 2011, Q1, P9
* **Q4112** Cymetra, injectable, 1 cc Ⓑ Qp Qh N1 N
  Coding Clinic: 2012, Q2, P7; 2011, Q1, P9
* **Q4113** GraftJacket Xpress, injectable, 1 cc Ⓑ Qp Qh N1 N
  Coding Clinic: 2012, Q2, P7; 2011, Q1, P9
* **Q4114** Integra Flowable Wound Matrix, injectable, 1 cc Ⓑ Qp Qh N1 N
  Coding Clinic: 2012, Q2, P7; 2010, Q2, P8
* **Q4115** Alloskin, per square centimeter Ⓑ Qp Qh N1 N
  Coding Clinic: 2012, Q2, P7; 2011, Q1, P9
* **Q4116** Alloderm, per square centimeter Ⓑ Qp Qh N1 N
  Coding Clinic: 2012, Q2, P7; 2011, Q1, P9
* **Q4117** Hyalomatrix, per square centimeter Ⓑ Qp Qh N1 N
  IOM: 100-02, 15, 50
* **Q4118** Matristem micromatrix, 1 mg Ⓑ Qp Qh N1 N
  Coding Clinic: 2013, Q4, P2; 2012, Q2, P7; 2011, Q1, P6
* **Q4121** Theraskin, per square centimeter Ⓑ Qp Qh N1 N
  Coding Clinic: 2012, Q2, P7; 2011, Q1, P6
* **Q4122** Dermacell, Dermacell AWM or Dermacell AWM Porous, per square centimeter Ⓑ Qp Qh N1 N
  Coding Clinic: 2012, Q2, P7; Q1, P8
* **Q4123** AlloSkin RT, per square centimeter Ⓑ Qp Qh N1 N
* **Q4124** Oasis Ultra Tri-layer Wound Matrix, per square centimeter Ⓑ Qp Qh N1 N
  Coding Clinic: 2012, Q2, P7; Q1, P9
* **Q4125** Arthroflex, per square centimeter Ⓑ Qp Qh N1 N
* **Q4126** Memoderm, dermaspan, tranzgraft or integuply, per square centimeter Ⓑ Qp Qh N1 N
* **Q4127** Talymed, per square centimeter Ⓑ Qp Qh N1 N
* **Q4128** FlexHD, Allopatch HD, or Matrix HD, per square centimeter Ⓑ Qp Qh N1 N
* **Q4130** Strattice TM, per square centimeter Ⓑ Qp Qh N1 N
  Coding Clinic: 2012, Q2, P7
* **Q4132** Grafix core and GrafixPL core, per square centimeter Ⓑ Qp Qh N1 N
* **Q4133** Grafix prime, GrafixPL prime, stravix and stravixpl, per square centimeter Ⓑ Qp Qh N1 N
* **Q4134** Hmatrix, per square centimeter Ⓑ Qp Qh N1 N
* **Q4135** Mediskin, per square centimeter Ⓑ Qp Qh N1 N
* **Q4136** Ez-derm, per square centimeter Ⓑ Qp Qh N1 N
* **Q4137** Amnioexcel, amnioexcel plus or biodexcel, per square centimeter Ⓑ Qp Qh N1 N
* **Q4138** Biodfence dryflex, per square centimeter Ⓑ Qp Qh N1 N

* **Q4139** Amniomatrix or biodmatrix, injectable, 1 cc Qp Qh N1 N
* **Q4140** Biodfence, per square centimeter Qp Qh N1 N
* **Q4141** Alloskin ac, per square centimeter Qp Qh N1 N
* **Q4142** XCM biologic tissue matrix, per square centimeter Qp Qh N1 N
* **Q4143** Repriza, per square centimeter Qp Qh N1 N
* **Q4145** Epifix, injectable, 1 mg Qp Qh N1 N
* **Q4146** Tensix, per square centimeter Qp Qh N1 N
* **Q4147** Architect, architect PX, or architect FX, extracellular matrix, per square centimeter Qp Qh N1 N
* **Q4148** Neox cord 1K, Neox cord RT, or Clarix cord 1K, per square centimeter Qp Qh N1 N
* **Q4149** Excellagen, 0.1 cc Qp Qh N1 N
* **Q4150** AlloWrap DS or dry, per square centimeter Qp Qh N1 N
* **Q4151** Amnioband or guardian, per square centimeter Qp Qh N1 N
* **Q4152** DermaPure, per square centimeter Qp Qh N1 N
* **Q4153** Dermavest and Plurivest, per square centimeter Qp Qh N1 N
* **Q4154** Biovance, per square centimeter Qp Qh N1 N
* **Q4155** Neoxflo or clarixflo, 1 mg Qp Qh N1 N
* **Q4156** Neox 100 or Clarix 100, per square centimeter Qp Qh N1 N
* **Q4157** Revitalon, per square centimeter Qp Qh N1 N
* **Q4158** Kerecis Omega3, per square centimeter Qp Qh N1 N
* **Q4159** Affinity, per square centimeter Qp Qh N1 N
* **Q4160** Nushield, per square centimeter Qp Qh N1 N
* **Q4161** Bio-ConneKt Wound Matrix, per square centimeter Qp Qh N1 N
* **Q4162** Woundex flow, BioSkin flow 0.5 cc Qp Qh N1 N
* **Q4163** Woundex, BioSkin per square centimeter Qp Qh N1 N
* **Q4164** Helicoll, per square centimeter Qp Qh N1 N
* **Q4165** Keramatrix or kerasorb, per square centimeter Qp Qh N1 N
* **Q4166** Cytal, per square centimeter Qp Qh N1 N
  Coding Clinic: 2017, Q1, P10
* **Q4167** TruSkin, per square centimeter Qp Qh N1 N
  Coding Clinic: 2017, Q1, P10
* **Q4168** AmnioBand, 1 mg Qp Qh N1 N
  Coding Clinic: 2017, Q1, P10
* **Q4169** Artacent wound, per square centimeter Qp Qh N1 N
  Coding Clinic: 2017, Q1, P10
* **Q4170** Cygnus, per square centimeter Qp Qh N1 N
  Coding Clinic: 2017, Q1, P10
* **Q4171** Interfyl, 1 mg Qp Qh N1 N
  Coding Clinic: 2017, Q1, P10
* **Q4173** PalinGen or PalinGen XPlus, per square centimeter Qp Qh N1 N
  Coding Clinic: 2017, Q1, P10
* **Q4174** PalinGen or ProMatrX, 0.36 mg per 0.25 cc Qp Qh N1 N
  Coding Clinic: 2017, Q1, P10
* **Q4175** Miroderm, per square centimeter Qp Qh N1 N
  Coding Clinic: 2017, Q1, P10
* **Q4176** Neopatch or therion, per square centimeter N1 N
* **Q4177** Floweramnioflo, 0.1 cc N1 N
* **Q4178** Floweramniopatch, per square centimeter N1 N
* **Q4179** Flowerderm, per square centimeter N1 N
* **Q4180** Revita, per square centimeter N1 N
* **Q4181** Amnio wound, per square centimeter N1 N
* **Q4182** Transcyte, per square centimeter N1 N
* **Q4183** Surgigraft, per square centimeter N
* **Q4184** Cellesta or cellesta duo, per square centimeter N
* **Q4185** Cellesta flowable amnion (25 mg per cc); per 0.5 cc N
* **Q4186** Epifix, per square centimeter N
* **Q4187** Epicord, per square centimeter N
* **Q4188** Amnioarmor, per square centimeter N
* **Q4189** Artacent ac, 1 mg N
* **Q4190** Artacent ac, per square centimeter N

MIPS | Qp Quantity Physician | Qh Quantity Hospital | ♀ Female only
♂ Male only | A Age | DMEPOS | A2-Z3 ASC Payment Indicator | A-Y ASC Status Indicator | Coding Clinic

* ✻ **Q4191** Restorigin, per square centimeter Ⓑ N
* ✻ **Q4192** Restorigin, 1 cc Ⓑ N
* ✻ **Q4193** Coll-e-derm, per square centimeter Ⓑ N
* ✻ **Q4194** Novachor, per square centimeter Ⓑ N
* ✻ **Q4195** Puraply, per square centimeter Ⓑ G
* ✻ **Q4196** Puraply am, per square centimeter Ⓑ G
* ✻ **Q4197** Puraply xt, per square centimeter Ⓑ N
* ✻ **Q4198** Genesis amniotic membrane, per square centimeter Ⓑ N
* ✻ **Q4200** Skin te, per square centimeter Ⓑ N
* ✻ **Q4201** Matrion, per square centimeter Ⓑ N
* ✻ **Q4202** Keroxx (2.5g/cc), 1cc Ⓑ N
* ✻ **Q4203** Derma-gide, per square centimeter Ⓑ N
* ✻ **Q4204** Xwrap, per square centimeter Ⓑ N
* ✻ **Q4205** Membrane graft or membrane wrap, per square centimeter Ⓑ
* ✻ **Q4206** Fluid flow or fluid Gf, 1 cc Ⓑ N
* ✻ **Q4208** Novafix, per square cenitmeter Ⓑ N
* ✻ **Q4209** Surgraft, per square centimeter Ⓑ N
* ✻ **Q4210** Axolotl graft or axolotl dualgraft, per square centimeter Ⓑ N
* ✻ **Q4211** Amnion bio or axobiomembrane, per square centimeter Ⓑ N
* ✻ **Q4212** Allogen, per cc Ⓑ N
* ✻ **Q4213** Ascent, 0.5 mg Ⓑ N
* ✻ **Q4214** Cellesta cord, per square centimeter Ⓑ N
* ✻ **Q4215** Axolotl ambient or axolotl cryo, 0.1 mg Ⓑ N
* ✻ **Q4216** Artacent cord, per square centimeter Ⓑ N
* ✻ **Q4217** Woundfix, BioWound, Woundfix Plus, BioWound Plus, Woundfix Xplus or BioWound Xplus, per square centimeter Ⓑ N
* ✻ **Q4218** Surgicord, per square centimeter Ⓑ N
* ✻ **Q4219** Surgigraft-dual, per square centimeter Ⓑ N
* ✻ **Q4220** BellaCell HD or Surederm, per square centimeter Ⓑ N
* ✻ **Q4221** Amniowrap2, per square centimeter Ⓑ N
* ✻ **Q4222** Progenamatrix, per square centimeter Ⓑ N
* ✻ **Q4226** MyOwn skin, includes harvesting and preparation procedures, per square centimeter Ⓑ N
* ▶ ✻ **Q4227** Amniocore, per square centimeter N1 N
* ▶ ✻ **Q4228** Bionextpatch, per square centimeter N1 N
* ▶ ✻ **Q4229** Cogenex amniotic membrane, per square centimeter N1 N
* ▶ ✻ **Q4230** Cogenex flowable amnion, per 0.5 cc N1 N
* ▶ ✻ **Q4231** Corplex P, per cc N1 N
* ▶ ✻ **Q4232** Corplex, per square centimeter N1 N
* ▶ ✻ **Q4233** Surfactor or Nudyn, per 0.5 cc N1 N
* ▶ ✻ **Q4234** Xcellerate, per square centimeter N1 N
* ▶ ✻ **Q4235** Amniorepair or Altiply, per square centimeter N1 N
* ▶ ✻ **Q4236** Carepatch, per square centimeter N1 N
* ▶ ✻ **Q4237** Cryo-cord, per square centimeter N1 N
* ▶ ✻ **Q4238** Derm-maxx, per square centimeter N1 N
* ▶ ✻ **Q4239** Amnio-maxx or amnio-maxx lite, per square centimeter N1 N
* ▶ ✻ **Q4240** Corecyte, for topical use only, per 0.5 cc N1 N
* ▶ ✻ **Q4241** Polycyte, for topical use only, per 0.5 cc N1 N
* ▶ ✻ **Q4242** Amniocyte plus, per 0.5 cc N1 N
* ▶ ✻ **Q4244** Procenta, per 200 mg N1 N
* ▶ ✻ **Q4245** Amniotext, per cc N1 N
* ▶ ✻ **Q4246** Coretext or Protext, per cc N1 N
* ▶ ✻ **Q4248** Dermacyte amniotic membrane allograft, per square centimeter N1 N
* ▶ ✻ **Q4249** Amniply, for topical use only, per square centimeter N
* ▶ ✻ **Q4950** Amnioamp-MP, per square centimeter N
* ▶ ✻ **Q4254** Novafix DL, per square centimeter N
* ▶ ✻ **Q4255** Reguard, for topical use only, per square centimeter N

Hospice Care

* ⊙ **Q5001** Hospice or home health care provided in patient's home/residence Ⓑ B
* ⊙ **Q5002** Hospice or home health care provided in assisted living facility Ⓑ B
* ⊙ **Q5003** Hospice care provided in nursing long term care facility (LTC) or non-skilled nursing facility (NF) Ⓑ B
* ⊙ **Q5004** Hospice care provided in skilled nursing facility (SNF) Ⓑ B
* ⊙ **Q5005** Hospice care provided in inpatient hospital Ⓑ B

▶ New ⤾ Revised ✔ Reinstated ~~deleted~~ Deleted ⊘ Not covered or valid by Medicare
⊙ Special coverage instructions ✻ Carrier discretion Ⓑ Bill Part B MAC Ⓔ Bill DME MAC

Q5006 Hospice care provided in inpatient hospice facility B

Hospice care provided in an inpatient hospice facility. These are residential facilities, which are places for patients to live while receiving routine home care or continuous home care. These hospice residential facilities are not certified by Medicare or Medicaid for provision of General Inpatient (GIP) or respite care, and regulations at 42 CFR 418.202(e) do not allow provision of GIP or respite care at hospice residential facilities.

Q5007 Hospice care provided in long term care facility B

Q5008 Hospice care provided in inpatient psychiatric facility B

Q5009 Hospice or home health care provided in place not otherwise specified (NOS) B

Q5010 Hospice home care provided in a hospice facility B

Biosimilar Drugs

Q5101 Injection, filgrastim-sndz, biosimilar, (zarxio), 1 microgram Qp Qh K2 G

Other: Zarxio

Q5103 Injection, infliximab-dyyb, biosimilar, (inflectra), 10 mg G

Other: Remicade, Inflectra, Renflexis

Q5104 Injection, infliximab-abda, biosimilar, (renflexis), 10 mgn K2 G

Other: Remicade

Q5105 Injection, epoetin alfa-epbx, biosimilar, (retacrit) (for ESRD on dialysis) 100 units K2 G

Other: Retacrit

Q5106 Injection, epoetin alfa-epbx, biosimilar (retacrit) (for non-ESRD use), 1000 units G

Other: Retacrit

Q5107 Injection, bevacizumab-awwb, biosimilar (mvasi), 10 mg E2

Other: Avastin

Q5108 Injection, pegfilgrastim-jmdb, biosimilar (fulphila), 0.5 mg K

Other: Neulasta

Q5109 Injection, infliximab-qbtx, biosimilar (ixifi), 10 mg E2

Other: Remicade, Inflectra, Renflexis

Q5110 Injection, filgrastim-aafi, biosimilar (nivestym), 1 microgram K

Other: Nivestym

* **Q5112** Injection, trastuzumab-dttb, biosimilar (ontruzant), 10 mg E2

* **Q5113** Injection, trastuzumab-pkrb, biosimilar (herzuma), 10 mg E2

* **Q5114** Injection, trastuzumab-dkst, biosimilar (ogivri), 10 mg E2

Q5115 Injection, rituximab-abbs, biosimilar (truxima), 10 mg E2

* **Q5116** Injection, trastuzumab-qyyp, biosimilar (trazimera), 10 mg E2

* **Q5117** Injection, trastuzumab-anns, biosimilar (kanjinti), 10 mg K2 G

* **Q5118** Injection, bevacizumab-bvzr, biosimilar (zirabev), 10 mg E2

▶ **Q5119** **Injection, Rituximab-pvvr, Biosimilar, (Ruxience), 10 mg G**

▶ **Q5120** Injection, Pegfilgrastim-bmez, Biosimilar, (Ziextenzo), 0.5 mg K2 G

▶ **Q5121** Injection, Infliximab-axxq, Biosimilar, (Avsola), 10 mg K2 G

▶ **Q5122** Injection, Pegfilgrastim-apgf, Biosimilar, (Nyvepria), 0.5 mg K5 E1

Veteran Services Chaplain

▶ **Q9001** Assessment by department of veterans affairs chaplain services E1

▶ **Q9002** Counseling, individual, by department of veterans affairs chaplain services E1

▶ **Q9003** Counseling, group, by department of veterans affairs chaplain services E1

Contrast Agents

* **Q9950** Injection, sulfur hexafluoride lipid microspheres, per ml Qp Qh N1 N

Other: Lumason

Q9951 Low osmolar contrast material, 400 or greater mg/ml iodine concentration, per ml Qp Qh N1 N

IOM: 100-04, 12, 70; 100-04, 13, 20; 100-04, 13, 90

Coding Clinic: 2012, Q3, P8

MIPS | Qp Quantity Physician | Qh Quantity Hospital | ♀ Female only
♂ Male only | A Age | DMEPOS | A2-Z3 ASC Payment Indicator | A-Y ASC Status Indicator | Coding Clinic

⊙ **Q9953** Injection, iron-based magnetic resonance contrast agent, per ml Ⓑ Qp Qh N1 N

IOM: 100-04, 12, 70; 100-04, 13, 20; 100-04, 13, 90

Coding Clinic: 2012, Q3, P8

⊙ **Q9954** Oral magnetic resonance contrast agent, per 100 ml Ⓑ Qp Qh N1 N

IOM: 100-04, 12, 70; 100-04, 13, 20; 100-04, 13, 90

Coding Clinic: 2012, Q3, P8

* **Q9955** Injection, perflexane lipid microspheres, per ml Ⓑ Qp Qh N1 N

Coding Clinic: 2012, Q3, P8

* **Q9956** Injection, octafluoropropane microspheres, per ml Ⓑ Qp Qh N1 N

Other: Optison

Coding Clinic: 2012, Q3, P8

* **Q9957** Injection, perflutren lipid microspheres, per ml Ⓑ Qp Qh N1 N

Other: Definity

Coding Clinic: 2012, Q3, P8

⊙ **Q9958** High osmolar contrast material, up to 149 mg/ml iodine concentration, per ml Ⓑ Qp Qh N1 N

Other: Conray 30, Cysto-Conray II, Cystografin

IOM: 100-04, 12, 70; 100-04, 13, 20; 100-04, 13, 90

Coding Clinic: 2012, Q3, P8; 2007, Q1, P6

⊙ **Q9959** High osmolar contrast material, 150-199 mg/ml iodine concentration, per ml Ⓑ Qp Qh N1 N

IOM: 100-04, 12, 70; 100-04, 13, 20; 100-04, 13, 90

Coding Clinic: 2012, Q3, P8; 2007, Q1, P6

⊙ **Q9960** High osmolar contrast material, 200-249 mg/mliodine concentration, per ml Ⓑ Qp Qh N1 N

Other: Conray 43

IOM: 100-04, 12, 70; 100-04, 13, 20; 100-04, 13, 90

Coding Clinic: 2012, Q3, P8; 2007, Q1, P6

⊙ **Q9961** High osmolar contrast material, 250-299 mg/mliodine concentration, per ml Ⓑ Qp Qh N1 N

Other: Conray, Cholografin Meglumine

IOM: 100-04, 12, 70; 100-04, 13, 20; 100-04, 13, 90

Coding Clinic: 2012, Q3, P8; 2007, Q1, P6

⊙ **Q9962** High osmolar contrast material, 300-349 mg/ml iodine concentration, per ml Ⓑ Qp Qh N1 N

IOM: 100-04, 12, 70; 100-04, 13, 20; 100-04, 13, 90

Coding Clinic: 2012, Q3, P8; 2007, Q1, P6

⊙ **Q9963** High osmolar contrast material, 350-399 mg/ml iodine concentration, per ml Ⓑ Qp Qh N1 N

Other: Gastrografin, MD-76R, MD Gastroview, Sinografin

IOM: 100-04, 12, 70; 100-04, 13, 20; 100-04, 13, 90

Coding Clinic: 2012, Q3, P8; 2007, Q1, P6

⊙ **Q9964** High osmolar contrast material, 400 or greater mg/ml iodine concentration, per ml Ⓑ Qp Qh N1 N

IOM: 100-04, 12, 70; 100-04, 13, 20; 100-04, 13, 90

Coding Clinic: 2012, Q3, P8; 2007, Q1, P6

⊙ **Q9965** Low osmolar contrast material, 100-199 mg/ml iodine concentration, per ml Ⓑ N1 N

Other: Omnipaque

IOM: 100-04, 12, 70; 100-04, 13, 20; 100-04, 13, 90

Coding Clinic: 2012, Q3, P8

⊙ **Q9966** Low osmolar contrast material, 200-299 mg/ml iodine concentration, per ml Ⓑ Qp Qh N1 N

Other: Isovue, Omnipaque, Optiray, Ultravist 240, Visipaque

IOM: 100-04, 12, 70; 100-04, 13, 20; 100-04, 13, 90

Coding Clinic: 2012, Q3, P8

⊙ **Q9967** Low osmolar contrast material, 300-399 mg/ml iodine concentration, per ml Ⓑ Qp Qh N1 N

Other: Hexabrix 320, Isovue, Omnipaque, Optiray, Oxilan, Ultravist, Vispaque

IOM: 100-04, 12, 70; 100-04, 13, 20; 100-04, 13, 90

Coding Clinic: 2012, Q3, P8

* **Q9968** Injection, non-radioactive, non-contrast, visualization adjunct (e.g., Methylene Blue, Isosulfan Blue), 1 mg Ⓑ K2 K

⊙ **Q9969** Tc-99m from non-highly enriched uranium source, full cost recovery add-on, per study dose Ⓑ Qp Qh K

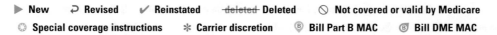

▶ New ⮐ Revised ✔ Reinstated ~~deleted~~ Deleted ⃠ Not covered or valid by Medicare
⊙ Special coverage instructions * Carrier discretion Ⓑ Bill Part B MAC Ⓓ Bill DME MAC

Radiopharmaceuticals

Q9982 Flutemetamol F18, diagnostic, per study dose, up to 5 millicuries Qp Qh K2 G

Other: Vizamyl

Q9983 Florbetaben F18, diagnostic, per study dose, up to 8.1 millicuries Qp Qh K2 G

Other: Neuraceq

* **Q9991** Injection, buprenorphine extended-release (sublocade), less than or equal to 100 mg G

Other: Subutex, Buprenex, Belbuca, Probuphine, Butrans

* **Q9992** Injection, buprenorphine extended-release (sublocade), greater than 100 mg G

Other: Subutex, Buprenex, Belbuca, Probuphine, Butrans

MIPS 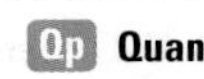 Quantity Physician 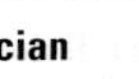 Quantity Hospital 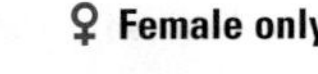 Female only
Male only A Age DMEPOS A2-Z3 ASC Payment Indicator A-Y ASC Status Indicator Coding Clinic

DIAGNOSTIC RADIOLOGY SERVICES (R0000-R9999)

Transportation/Setup of Portable Equipment

R0070 Transportation of portable x-ray equipment and personnel to home or nursing home, per trip to facility or location, one patient seen Qp Qh B

CMS Transmittal B03-049; specific instructions to contractors on pricing

IOM: 100-04, 13, 90; 100-04, 13, 90.3

R0075 Transportation of portable x-ray equipment and personnel to home or nursing home, per trip to facility or location, more than one patient seen Qp Qh B

This code would not apply to the x-ray equipment if stored at the location where the x-ray was performed (e.g., a nursing home).

IOM: 100-04, 13, 90; 100-04, 13, 90.3

R0076 Transportation of portable ECG to facility or location, per patient Qp Qh B

EKG procedure code 93000 or 93005 must be submitted on same claim as transportation code. Bundled status on physician fee schedule

IOM: 100-01, 5, 90.2; 100-02, 15, 80; 100-03, 1, 20.15; 100-04, 13, 90; 100-04, 16, 10; 100-04, 16, 110.4

New | Revised | Reinstated | ~~deleted~~ Deleted | Not covered or valid by Medicare
Special coverage instructions | Carrier discretion | Bill Part B MAC | Bill DME MAC

TEMPORARY NATIONAL CODES ESTABLISHED BY PRIVATE PAYERS (S0000-S9999)

Note: Medicare and other federal payers do not recognize "S" codes; however, S codes may be useful for claims to some private insurers.

Non-Medicare Drugs

⊘ **S0012** Butorphanol tartrate, nasal spray, 25 mg

▶⊘ **S0013** Esketamine, nasal spray, 1 mg

⊘ **S0014** Tacrine hydrochloride, 10 mg

⊘ **S0017** Injection, aminocaproic acid, 5 grams

⊘ **S0020** Injection, bupivacaine hydrochloride, 30 ml

⊘ **S0021** Injection, cefoperazone sodium, 1 gram

⊘ **S0023** Injection, cimetidine hydrochloride, 300 mg

⊘ **S0028** Injection, famotidine, 20 mg

⊘ **S0030** Injection, metronidazole, 500 mg

⊘ **S0032** Injection, nafcillin sodium, 2 grams

⊘ **S0034** Injection, ofloxacin, 400 mg

⊘ **S0039** Injection, sulfamethoxazole and trimethoprim, 10 ml

⊘ **S0040** Injection, ticarcillin disodium and clavulanate potassium, 3.1 grams

⊘ **S0073** Injection, aztreonam, 500 mg

⊘ **S0074** Injection, cefotetan disodium, 500 mg

⊘ **S0077** Injection, clindamycin phosphate, 300 mg

⊘ **S0078** Injection, fosphenytoin sodium, 750 mg

⊘ **S0080** Injection, pentamidine isethionate, 300 mg

⊘ **S0081** Injection, piperacillin sodium, 500 mg

⊘ **S0088** Imatinib, 100 mg

⊘ **S0090** Sildenafil citrate, 25 mg A

⊘ **S0091** Granisetron hydrochloride, 1 mg (for circumstances falling under the Medicare Statute, use Q0166)

⊘ **S0092** Injection, hydromorphone hydrochloride, 250 mg (loading dose for infusion pump)

⊘ **S0093** Injection, morphine sulfate, 500 mg (loading dose for infusion pump)

⊘ **S0104** Zidovudine, oral, 100 mg

⊘ **S0106** Bupropion HCl sustained release tablet, 150 mg, per bottle of 60 tablets

⊘ **S0108** Mercaptopurine, oral, 50 mg

⊘ **S0109** Methadone, oral, 5 mg

⊘ **S0117** Tretinoin, topical, 5 grams

⊘ **S0119** Ondansetron, oral, 4 mg (for circumstances falling under the Medicare statute, use HCPCS Q code)

⊘ **S0122** Injection, menotropins, 75 IU

⊘ **S0126** Injection, follitropin alfa, 75 IU

⊘ **S0128** Injection, follitropin beta, 75 IU

⊘ **S0132** Injection, ganirelix acetate, 250 mcg

⊘ **S0136** Clozapine, 25 mg

⊘ **S0137** Didanosine (DDI), 25 mg

⊘ **S0138** Finasteride, 5 mg

⊘ **S0139** Minoxidil, 10 mg

⊘ **S0140** Saquinavir, 200 mg

⊘ **S0142** Colistimethate sodium, inhalation solution administered through DME, concentrated form, per mg

⊘ **S0145** Injection, pegylated interferon alfa-2a, 180 mcg per ml

⊘ **S0148** Injection, pegylated interferon ALFA-2b, 10 mcg

⊘ **S0155** Sterile dilutant for epoprostenol, 50 ml

⊘ **S0156** Exemestane, 25 mg

⊘ **S0157** Becaplermin gel 0.01%, 0.5 gm

⊘ **S0160** Dextroamphetamine sulfate, 5 mg

⊘ **S0164** Injection, pantoprazole sodium, 40 mg

⊘ **S0166** Injection, olanzapine, 2.5 mg

⊘ **S0169** Calcitrol, 0.25 microgram

⊘ **S0170** Anastrozole, oral, 1 mg

⊘ **S0171** Injection, bumetanide, 0.5 mg

⊘ **S0172** Chlorambucil, oral, 2 mg

⊘ **S0174** Dolasetron mesylate, oral 50 mg (for circumstances falling under the Medicare Statute, use Q0180)

⊘ **S0175** Flutamide, oral, 125 mg

⊘ **S0176** Hydroxyurea, oral, 500 mg

⊘ **S0177** Levamisole hydrochloride, oral, 50 mg

⊘ **S0178** Lomustine, oral, 10 mg

⊘ **S0179** Megestrol acetate, oral, 20 mg

⊘ **S0182** Procarbazine hydrochloride, oral, 50 mg

⊘ **S0183** Prochlorperazine maleate, oral, 5 mg (for circumstances falling under the Medicare Statute, use Q0164)

⊘ **S0187** Tamoxifen citrate, oral, 10 mg

⊘ **S0189** Testosterone pellet, 75 mg

⊘ **S0190** Mifepristone, oral, 200 mg

⊘ **S0191** Misoprostol, oral 200 mcg

⊘ **S0194** Dialysis/stress vitamin supplement, oral, 100 capsules

⊘ **S0197** Prenatal vitamins, 30-day supply ♀

Provider Services

⊘ **S0199** Medically induced abortion by oral ingestion of medication including all associated services and supplies (e.g., patient counseling, office visits, confirmation of pregnancy by HCG, ultrasound to confirm duration of pregnancy, ultrasound to confirm completion of abortion) except drugs ♀

⊘ **S0201** Partial hospitalization services, less than 24 hours, per diem

⊘ **S0207** Paramedic intercept, non-hospital-based ALS service (non-voluntary), non-transport

⊘ **S0208** Paramedic intercept, hospital-based ALS service (non-voluntary), non-transport

⊘ **S0209** Wheelchair van, mileage, per mile

⊘ **S0215** Non-emergency transportation; mileage per mile

⊘ **S0220** Medical conference by a physician with interdisciplinary team of health professionals or representatives of community agencies to coordinate activities of patient care (patient is present); approximately 30 minutes

⊘ **S0221** Medical conference by a physician with interdisciplinary team of health professionals or representatives of community agencies to coordinate activities of patient care (patient is present); approximately 60 minutes

⊘ **S0250** Comprehensive geriatric assessment and treatment planning performed by assessment team A

⊘ **S0255** Hospice referral visit (advising patient and family of care options) performed by nurse, social worker, or other designated staff

⊘ **S0257** Counseling and discussion regarding advance directives or end of life care planning and decisions, with patient and/or surrogate (list separately in addition to code for appropriate evaluation and management service)

⊘ **S0260** History and physical (outpatient or office) related to surgical procedure (list separately in addition to code for appropriate evaluation and management service)

⊘ **S0265** Genetic counseling, under physician supervision, each 15 minutes

⊘ **S0270** Physician management of patient home care, standard monthly case rate (per 30 days)

⊘ **S0271** Physician management of patient home care, hospice monthly case rate (per 30 days)

⊘ **S0272** Physician management of patient home care, episodic care monthly case rate (per 30 days)

⊘ **S0273** Physician visit at member's home, outside of a capitation arrangement

⊘ **S0274** Nurse practitioner visit at member's home, outside of a capitation arrangement

⊘ **S0280** Medical home program, comprehensive care coordination and planning, initial plan

⊘ **S0281** Medical home program, comprehensive care coordination and planning, maintenance of plan

⊘ **S0285** Colonoscopy consultation performed prior to a screening colonoscopy procedure

⊘ **S0302** Completed Early Periodic Screening Diagnosis and Treatment (EPSDT) service (list in addition to code for appropriate evaluation and management service) A

⊘ **S0310** Hospitalist services (list separately in addition to code for appropriate evaluation and management service)

⊘ **S0311** Comprehensive management and care coordination for advanced illness, per calendar month

⊘ **S0315** Disease management program; initial assessment and initiation of the program

⊘ **S0316** Disease management program; follow-up/reassessment

⊘ **S0317** Disease management program; per diem

⊘ **S0320** Telephone calls by a registered nurse to a disease management program member for monitoring purposes; per month

⊘ **S0340** Lifestyle modification program for management of coronary artery disease, including all supportive services; first quarter/stage

⊘ **S0341** Lifestyle modification program for management of coronary artery disease, including all supportive services; second or third quarter/stage

⊘ **S0342** Lifestyle modification program for management of coronary artery disease, including all supportive services; fourth quarter/stage

⊘ **S0353** Treatment planning and care coordination management for cancer, initial treatment

⊘ **S0354** Treatment planning and care coordination management for cancer, established patient with a change of regimen

⊘ **S0390** Routine foot care; removal and/or trimming of corns, calluses and/or nails and preventive maintenance in specific medical conditions (e.g., diabetes), per visit

⊘ **S0395** Impression casting of a foot performed by a practitioner other than the manufacturer of the orthotic

⊘ **S0400** Global fee for extracorporeal shock wave lithotripsy treatment of kidney stone(s)

Vision Supplies

⊘ **S0500** Disposable contact lens, per lens

⊘ **S0504** Single vision prescription lens (safety, athletic, or sunglass), per lens

⊘ **S0506** Bifocal vision prescription lens (safety, athletic, or sunglass), per lens

⊘ **S0508** Trifocal vision prescription lens (safety, athletic, or sunglass), per lens

⊘ **S0510** Non-prescription lens (safety, athletic, or sunglass), per lens

⊘ **S0512** Daily wear specialty contact lens, per lens

⊘ **S0514** Color contact lens, per lens

⊘ **S0515** Scleral lens, liquid bandage device, per lens

⊘ **S0516** Safety eyeglass frames

⊘ **S0518** Sunglasses frames

⊘ **S0580** Polycarbonate lens (list this code in addition to the basic code for the lens)

⊘ **S0581** Nonstandard lens (list this code in addition to the basic code for the lens)

⊘ **S0590** Integral lens service, miscellaneous services reported separately

⊘ **S0592** Comprehensive contact lens evaluation

⊘ **S0595** Dispensing new spectacle lenses for patient supplied frame

⊘ **S0596** Phakic intraocular lens for correction of refractive error

Screening and Examinations

⊘ **S0601** Screening proctoscopy

⊘ **S0610** Annual gynecological examination, new patient ♀

⊘ **S0612** Annual gynecological examination, established patient ♀

⊘ **S0613** Annual gynecological examination; clinical breast examination without pelvic evaluation ♀

⊘ **S0618** Audiometry for hearing aid evaluation to determine the level and degree of hearing loss

⊘ **S0620** Routine ophthalmological examination including refraction; new patient

Many non-Medicare vision plans may require code for routine encounter, no complaints

⊘ **S0621** Routine ophthalmological examination including refraction; established patient

Many non-Medicare vision plans may require code for routine encounter, no complaints

⊘ **S0622** Physical exam for college, new or established patient (list separately) in addition to appropriate evaluation and management code A

Provider Services and Supplies

⊘ **S0630** Removal of sutures; by a physician other than the physician who originally closed the wound

⊘ **S0800** Laser in situ keratomileusis (LASIK)

MIPS
Qp Quantity Physician
Qh Quantity Hospital
♀ Female only
♂ Male only
A Age
DMEPOS
A2-Z3 ASC Payment Indicator
A-Y ASC Status Indicator
Coding Clinic

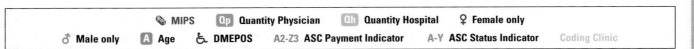

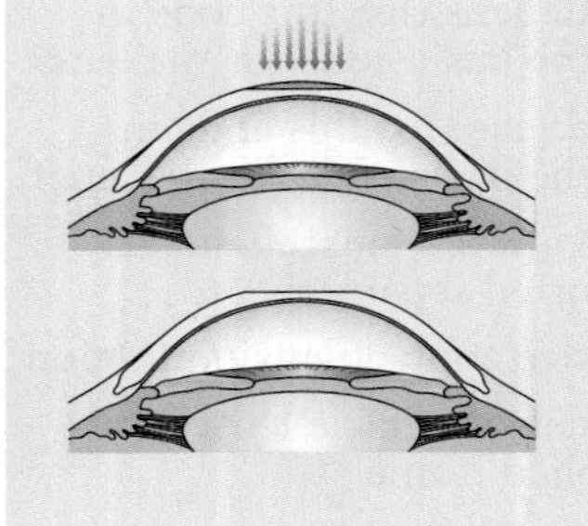

Figure 48 Phototherapeutic keratectomy (PRK).

⊘ **S0810** Photorefractive keratectomy (PRK)

⊘ **S0812** Phototherapeutic keratectomy (PTK)

⊘ **S1001** Deluxe item, patient aware (list in addition to code for basic item)

⊘ **S1002** Customized item (list in addition to code for basic item)

⊘ **S1015** IV tubing extension set

⊘ **S1016** Non-PVC (polyvinyl chloride) intravenous administration set, for use with drugs that are not stable in PVC (e.g., paclitaxel)

⊘ **S1030** Continuous noninvasive glucose monitoring device, purchase (for physician interpretation of data, use CPT code)

⊘ **S1031** Continuous noninvasive glucose monitoring device, rental, including sensor, sensor replacement, and download to monitor (for physician interpretation of data, use CPT code)

⊘ **S1034** Artificial pancreas device system (e.g., low glucose suspend (LGS) feature) including continuous glucose monitor, blood glucose device, insulin pump and computer algorithm that communicates with all of the devices

⊘ **S1035** Sensor; invasive (e.g., subcutaneous), disposable, for use with artificial pancreas device system

⊘ **S1036** Transmitter; external, for use with artificial pancreas device system

⊘ **S1037** Receiver (monitor); external, for use with artificial pancreas device system

⊘ **S1040** Cranial remolding orthosis, pediatric, rigid, with soft interface material, custom fabricated, includes fitting and adjustment(s) A

⊘ **S2053** Transplantation of small intestine and liver allografts

⊘ **S2054** Transplantation of multivisceral organs

⊘ **S2055** Harvesting of donor multivisceral organs, with preparation and maintenance of allografts; from cadaver donor

⊘ **S2060** Lobar lung transplantation

⊘ **S2061** Donor lobectomy (lung) for transplantation, living donor

⊘ **S2065** Simultaneous pancreas kidney transplantation

⊘ **S2066** Breast reconstruction with gluteal artery perforator (GAP) flap, including harvesting of the flap, microvascular transfer, closure of donor site and shaping the flap into a breast, unilateral ♀

⊘ **S2067** Breast reconstruction of a single breast with "stacked" deep inferior epigastric perforator (DIEP) flap(s) and/or gluteal artery perforator (GAP) flap(s), including harvesting of the flap(s), microvascular transfer, closure of donor site(s) and shaping the flap into a breast, unilateral ♀

⊘ **S2068** Breast reconstruction with deep inferior epigastric perforator (DIEP) flap, or superficial inferior epigastric artery (SIEA) flap, including harvesting of the flap, microvascular transfer, closure of donor site and shaping the flap into a breast, unilateral ♀

⊘ **S2070** Cystourethroscopy, with ureteroscopy and/or pyeloscopy; with endoscopic laser treatment of ureteral calculi (includes ureteral catheterization)

⊘ **S2079** Laparoscopic esophagomyotomy (Heller type)

⊘ **S2080** Laser-assisted uvulopalatoplasty (LAUP)

⊘ **S2083** Adjustment of gastric band diameter via subcutaneous port by injection or aspiration of saline

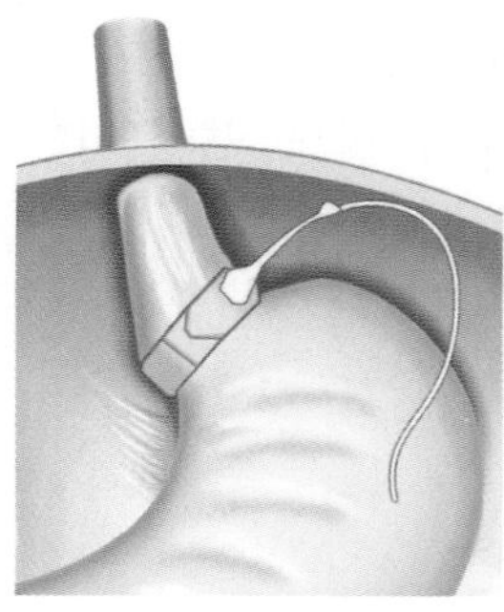

Figure 49 Gastric band.

⊘ **S2095** Transcatheter occlusion or embolization for tumor destruction, percutaneous, any method, using yttrium-90 microspheres

⊘ **S2102** Islet cell tissue transplant from pancreas; allogeneic

⊘ **S2103** Adrenal tissue transplant to brain

⊘ **S2107** Adoptive immunotherapy i.e. development of specific anti-tumor reactivity (e.g., tumor-infiltrating lymphocyte therapy) per course of treatment

⊘ **S2112** Arthroscopy, knee, surgical for harvesting of cartilage (chondrocyte cells)

⊘ **S2115** Osteotomy, periacetabular, with internal fixation

⊘ **S2117** Arthroereisis, subtalar

⊘ **S2118** Metal-on-metal total hip resurfacing, including acetabular and femoral components

⊘ **S2120** Low density lipoprotein (LDL) apheresis using heparin-induced extracorporeal LDL precipitation

⊘ **S2140** Cord blood harvesting for transplantation, allogeneic

⊘ **S2142** Cord blood-derived stem cell transplantation, allogeneic

⊘ **S2150** Bone marrow or blood-derived stem cells (peripheral or umbilical), allogeneic or autologous, harvesting, transplantation, and related complications; including: pheresis and cell preparation/storage; marrow ablative therapy; drugs, supplies, hospitalization with outpatient follow-up; medical/surgical, diagnostic, emergency, and rehabilitative services; and the number of days of pre- and post-transplant care in the global definition

⊘ **S2152** Solid organ(s), complete or segmental, single organ or combination of organs; deceased or living donor(s), procurement, transplantation, and related complications; including: drugs; supplies; hospitalization with outpatient follow-up; medical/surgical, diagnostic, emergency, and rehabilitative services, and the number of days of pre- and post-transplant care in the global definition

⊘ **S2202** Echosclerotherapy

MIPS ⊘ **S2205** Minimally invasive direct coronary artery bypass surgery involving mini-thoracotomy or mini-sternotomy surgery, performed under direct vision; using arterial graft(s), single coronary arterial graft

MIPS ⊘ **S2206** Minimally invasive direct coronary artery bypass surgery involving mini-thoracotomy or mini-sternotomy surgery, performed under direct vision; using arterial graft(s), two coronary arterial grafts

MIPS ⊘ **S2207** Minimally invasive direct coronary artery bypass surgery involving mini-thoracotomy or mini-sternotomy surgery, performed under direct vision; using venous graft only, single coronary venous graft

MIPS ⊘ **S2208** Minimally invasive direct coronary artery bypass surgery involving mini-thoracotomy or mini-sternotomy surgery, performed under direct vision; using single arterial and venous graft(s), single venous graft

MIPS ⊘ **S2209** Minimally invasive direct coronary artery bypass surgery involving mini-thoracotomy or mini-sternotomy surgery, performed under direct vision; using two arterial grafts and single venous graft

⊘ **S2225** Myringotomy, laser-assisted

⊘ **S2230** Implantation of magnetic component of semi-implantable hearing device on ossicles in middle ear

⊘ **S2235** Implantation of auditory brain stem implant

⊘ **S2260** Induced abortion, 17 to 24 weeks ♀

⊘ **S2265** Induced abortion, 25 to 28 weeks ♀

⊘ **S2266** Induced abortion, 29 to 31 weeks ♀

⊘ **S2267** Induced abortion, 32 weeks or greater ♀

⊘ **S2300** Arthroscopy, shoulder, surgical; with thermally-induced capsulorrhaphy

⊘ **S2325** Hip core decompression

Coding Clinic: 2017, Q3, P1

⊘ **S2340** Chemodenervation of abductor muscle(s) of vocal cord

⊘ **S2341** Chemodenervation of adductor muscle(s) of vocal cord

⊘ **S2342** Nasal endoscopy for post-operative debridement following functional endoscopic sinus surgery, nasal and/or sinus cavity(s), unilateral or bilateral

MIPS
Qp Quantity Physician
Qh Quantity Hospital
♀ Female only
♂ Male only
A Age
DMEPOS
A2-Z3 ASC Payment Indicator
A-Y ASC Status Indicator
Coding Clinic

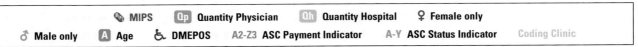

⃠ **S2348** Decompression procedure, percutaneous, of nucleus pulpous of intervertebral disc, using radiofrequency energy, single or multiple levels, lumbar

⃠ **S2350** Diskectomy, anterior, with decompression of spinal cord and/or nerve root(s), including osteophytectomy; lumbar, single interspace

⃠ **S2351** Diskectomy, anterior, with decompression of spinal cord and/or nerve root(s) including osteophytectomy; lumbar, each additional interspace (list separately in addition to code for primary procedure)

⃠ **S2400** Repair, congenital diaphragmatic hernia in the fetus using temporary tracheal occlusion, procedure performed in utero ♀ A

⃠ **S2401** Repair, urinary tract obstruction in the fetus, procedure performed in utero ♀ A

⃠ **S2402** Repair, congenital cystic adenomatoid malformation in the fetus, procedure performed in utero ♀ A

⃠ **S2403** Repair, extralobar pulmonary sequestration in the fetus, procedure performed in utero ♀ A

⃠ **S2404** Repair, myelomeningocele in the fetus, procedure performed in utero ♀ A

⃠ **S2405** Repair of sacrococcygeal teratoma in the fetus, procedure performed in utero ♀ A

⃠ **S2409** Repair, congenital malformation of fetus, procedure performed in utero, not otherwise classified ♀ A

⃠ **S2411** Fetoscopic laser therapy for treatment of twin-to-twin transfusion syndrome A

⃠ **S2900** Surgical techniques requiring use of robotic surgical system (list separately in addition to code for primary procedure)

Coding Clinic: 2010, Q2, P6

⃠ **S3000** Diabetic indicator; retinal eye exam, dilated, bilateral

⃠ **S3005** Performance measurement, evaluation of patient self assessment, depression

⃠ **S3600** STAT laboratory request (situations other than S3601)

⃠ **S3601** Emergency STAT laboratory charge for patient who is homebound or residing in a nursing facility

S3620 Newborn metabolic screening panel, includes test kit, postage and the laboratory tests specified by the state for inclusion in this panel (e.g., galactose; hemoglobin, electrophoresis; hydroxyprogesterone, 17-D; phenylalanine (PKU); and thyroxine, total) A

⃠ **S3630** Eosinophil count, blood, direct

⃠ **S3645** HIV-1 antibody testing of oral mucosal transudate

⃠ **S3650** Saliva test, hormone level; during menopause ♀

⃠ **S3652** Saliva test, hormone level; to assess preterm labor risk ♀

⃠ **S3655** Antisperm antibodies test (immunobead) ♀

⃠ **S3708** Gastrointestinal fat absorption study

⃠ **S3722** Dose optimization by area under the curve (AUC) analysis, for infusional 5-fluorouracil

Genetic Testing

⃠ **S3800** Genetic testing for amyotrophic lateral sclerosis (ALS)

⃠ **S3840** DNA analysis for germline mutations of the RET proto-oncogene for susceptibility to multiple endocrine neoplasia type 2

⃠ **S3841** Genetic testing for retinoblastoma

⃠ **S3842** Genetic testing for von Hippel-Lindau disease

⃠ **S3844** DNA analysis of the connexin 26 gene (GJB2) for susceptibility to congenital, profound deafness

⃠ **S3845** Genetic testing for alpha-thalassemia

⃠ **S3846** Genetic testing for hemoglobin E beta-thalassemia

⃠ **S3849** Genetic testing for Niemann-Pick disease

⃠ **S3850** Genetic testing for sickle cell anemia

⃠ **S3852** DNA analysis for APOE epilson 4 allele for susceptibility to Alzheimer's disease

⃠ **S3853** Genetic testing for myotonic muscular dystrophy

⃠ **S3854** Gene expression profiling panel for use in the management of breast cancer treatment ♀

⃠ **S3861** Genetic testing, sodium channel, voltage-gated, type V, alpha subunit (SCN5A) and variants for suspected Brugada syndrome

⊘ **S3865** Comprehensive gene sequence analysis for hypertrophic cardiomyopathy

⊘ **S3866** Genetic analysis for a specific gene mutation for hypertrophic cardiomyopathy (HCM) in an individual with a known HCM mutation in the family

⊘ **S3870** Comparative genomic hybridization (CGH) microarray testing for developmental delay, autism spectrum disorder and/or intellectual disability

Other Tests

⊘ **S3900** Surface electromyography (EMG)

⊘ **S3902** Ballistrocardiogram

⊘ **S3904** Masters two step

Bill on paper. Requires a report.

Obstetric and Fertility Services

⊘ **S4005** Interim labor facility global (labor occurring but not resulting in delivery) ♀

⊘ **S4011** In vitro fertilization; including but not limited to identification and incubation of mature oocytes, fertilization with sperm, incubation of embryo(s), and subsequent visualization for determination of development ♀

⊘ **S4013** Complete cycle, gamete intrafallopian transfer (GIFT), case rate ♀

⊘ **S4014** Complete cycle, zygote intrafallopian transfer (ZIFT), case rate ♀

⊘ **S4015** Complete in vitro fertilization cycle, not otherwise specified, case rate ♀

⊘ **S4016** Frozen in vitro fertilization cycle, case rate ♀

⊘ **S4017** Incomplete cycle, treatment cancelled prior to stimulation, case rate ♀

⊘ **S4018** Frozen embryo transfer procedure cancelled before transfer, case rate ♀

⊘ **S4020** In vitro fertilization procedure cancelled before aspiration, case rate ♀

⊘ **S4021** In vitro fertilization procedure cancelled after aspiration, case rate ♀

⊘ **S4022** Assisted oocyte fertilization, case rate ♀

⊘ **S4023** Donor egg cycle, incomplete, case rate ♀

⊘ **S4025** Donor services for in vitro fertilization (sperm or embryo), case rate

⊘ **S4026** Procurement of donor sperm from sperm bank ♂

⊘ **S4027** Storage of previously frozen embryos ♀

⊘ **S4028** Microsurgical epididymal sperm aspiration (MESA) ♂

⊘ **S4030** Sperm procurement and cryopreservation services; initial visit ♂

⊘ **S4031** Sperm procurement and cryopreservation services; subsequent visit ♂

⊘ **S4035** Stimulated intrauterine insemination (IUI), case rate ♀

⊘ **S4037** Cryopreserved embryo transfer, case rate ♀

⊘ **S4040** Monitoring and storage of cryopreserved embryos, per 30 days ♀

⊘ **S4042** Management of ovulation induction (interpretation of diagnostic tests and studies, non-face-to-face medical management of the patient), per cycle ♀

⊘ **S4981** Insertion of levonorgestrel-releasing intrauterine system ♀

⊘ **S4989** Contraceptive intrauterine device (e.g., Progestasert IUD), including implants and supplies ♀

Therapeutic Substances and Medications

⊘ **S4990** Nicotine patches, legend

⊘ **S4991** Nicotine patches, non-legend

⊘ **S4993** Contraceptive pills for birth control ♀

Only billed by Family Planning Clinics

⊘ **S4995** Smoking cessation gum

⊘ **S5000** Prescription drug, generic

⊘ **S5001** Prescription drug, brand name

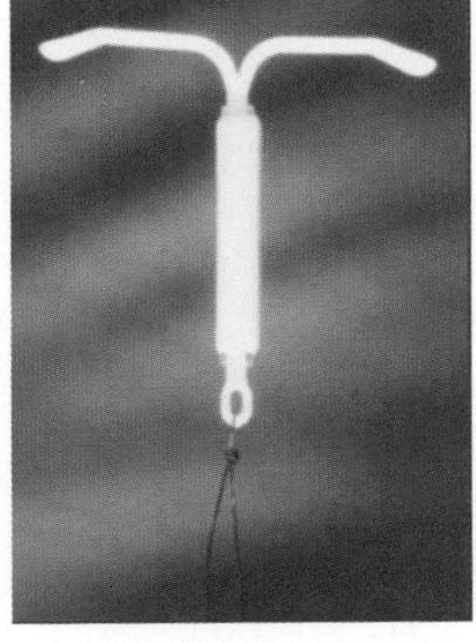

Figure 50 IUD.

⊘ **S5010** 5% dextrose and 0.45% normal saline, 1000 ml

⊘ **S5012** 5% dextrose with potassium chloride, 1000 ml

⊘ **S5013** 5% dextrose/0.45% normal saline with potassium chloride and magnesium sulfate, 1000 ml

⊘ **S5014** 5% dextrose/0.45% normal saline with potassium chloride and magnesium sulfate, 1500 ml

Home Care Services

⊘ **S5035** Home infusion therapy, routine service of infusion device (e.g., pump maintenance)

⊘ **S5036** Home infusion therapy, repair of infusion device (e.g., pump repair)

⊘ **S5100** Day care services, adult; per 15 minutes A

⊘ **S5101** Day care services, adult; per half day A

⊘ **S5102** Day care services, adult; per diem A

⊘ **S5105** Day care services, center-based; services not included in program fee, per diem

⊘ **S5108** Home care training to home care client, per 15 minutes

⊘ **S5109** Home care training to home care client, per session

⊘ **S5110** Home care training, family; per 15 minutes

⊘ **S5111** Home care training, family; per session

⊘ **S5115** Home care training, non-family; per 15 minutes

⊘ **S5116** Home care training, non-family; per session

⊘ **S5120** Chore services; per 15 minutes

⊘ **S5121** Chore services; per diem

⊘ **S5125** Attendant care services; per 15 minutes

⊘ **S5126** Attendant care services; per diem

⊘ **S5130** Homemaker service, NOS; per 15 minutes

⊘ **S5131** Homemaker service, NOS; per diem

⊘ **S5135** Companion care, adult (e.g., IADL/ ADL); per 15 minutes A

⊘ **S5136** Companion care, adult (e.g., IADL/ ADL); per diem A

⊘ **S5140** Foster care, adult; per diem A

⊘ **S5141** Foster care, adult; per month A

⊘ **S5145** Foster care, therapeutic, child; per diem A

⊘ **S5146** Foster care, therapeutic, child; per month A

⊘ **S5150** Unskilled respite care, not hospice; per 15 minutes

⊘ **S5151** Unskilled respite care, not hospice; per diem

⊘ **S5160** Emergency response system; installation and testing

⊘ **S5161** Emergency response system; service fee, per month (excludes installation and testing)

⊘ **S5162** Emergency response system; purchase only

⊘ **S5165** Home modifications; per service

⊘ **S5170** Home delivered meals, including preparation; per meal

⊘ **S5175** Laundry service, external, professional; per order

⊘ **S5180** Home health respiratory therapy, initial evaluation

⊘ **S5181** Home health respiratory therapy, NOS, per diem

⊘ **S5185** Medication reminder service, non-face-to-face; per month

⊘ **S5190** Wellness assessment, performed by non-physician

⊘ **S5199** Personal care item, NOS, each

Home Infusion Therapy

⊘ **S5497** Home infusion therapy, catheter care/ maintenance, not otherwise classified; includes administrative services, professional pharmacy services, care coordination, and all necessary supplies and equipment (drugs and nursing visits coded separately), per diem

⊘ **S5498** Home infusion therapy, catheter care/ maintenance, simple (single lumen), includes administrative services, professional pharmacy services, care coordination and all necessary supplies and equipment, (drugs and nursing visits coded separately), per diem

⊘ **S5501** Home infusion therapy, catheter care/ maintenance, complex (more than one lumen), includes administrative services, professional pharmacy services, care coordination, and all necessary supplies and equipment (drugs and nursing visits coded separately), per diem

⊘ **S5502** Home infusion therapy, catheter care/ maintenance, implanted access device, includes administrative services, professional pharmacy services, care coordination, and all necessary supplies and equipment, (drugs and nursing visits coded separately), per diem (use this code for interim maintenance of vascular access not currently in use)

⊘ **S5517** Home infusion therapy, all supplies necessary for restoration of catheter patency or declotting

⊘ **S5518** Home infusion therapy, all supplies necessary for catheter repair

⊘ **S5520** Home infusion therapy, all supplies (including catheter) necessary for a peripherally inserted central venous catheter (PICC) line insertion

Bill on paper. Requires a report.

⊘ **S5521** Home infusion therapy, all supplies (including catheter) necessary for a midline catheter insertion

⊘ **S5522** Home infusion therapy, insertion of peripherally inserted central venous catheter (PICC), nursing services only (no supplies or catheter included)

⊘ **S5523** Home infusion therapy, insertion of midline central venous catheter, nursing services only (no supplies or catheter included)

Insulin Services

⊘ **S5550** Insulin, rapid onset, 5 units

⊘ **S5551** Insulin, most rapid onset (Lispro or Aspart); 5 units

⊘ **S5552** Insulin, intermediate acting (NPH or Lente); 5 units

⊘ **S5553** Insulin, long acting; 5 units

⊘ **S5560** Insulin delivery device, reusable pen; 1.5 ml size

⊘ **S5561** Insulin delivery device, reusable pen; 3 ml size

⊘ **S5565** Insulin cartridge for use in insulin delivery device other than pump; 150 units

⊘ **S5566** Insulin cartridge for use in insulin delivery device other than pump; 300 units

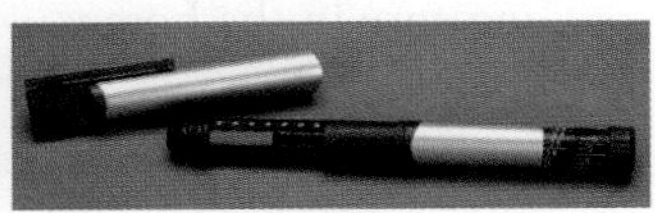

Figure 51 Nova pen.

⊘ **S5570** Insulin delivery device, disposable pen (including insulin); 1.5 ml size

⊘ **S5571** Insulin delivery device, disposable pen (including insulin); 3 ml size

Imaging

⊘ **S8030** Scleral application of tantalum ring(s) for localization of lesions for proton beam therapy

⊘ **S8035** Magnetic source imaging

⊘ **S8037** Magnetic resonance cholangiopancreatography (MRCP)

⊘ **S8040** Topographic brain mapping

⊘ **S8042** Magnetic resonance imaging (MRI), low-field

⊘ **S8055** Ultrasound guidance for multifetal pregnancy reduction(s), technical component (only to be used when the physician doing the reduction procedure does not perform the ultrasound, guidance is included in the CPT code for multifetal pregnancy reduction - 59866) ♀

⊘ **S8080** Scintimammography (radioimmunoscintigraphy of the breast), unilateral, including supply of radiopharmaceutical ♀

⊘ **S8085** Fluorine-18 fluorodeoxyglucose (F-18 FDG) imaging using dual-head coincidence detection system (non-dedicated PET scan)

⊘ **S8092** Electron beam computed tomography (also known as ultrafast CT, cine CT)

Assistive Breathing Supplies

⊘ **S8096** Portable peak flow meter

⊘ **S8097** Asthma kit (including but not limited to portable peak expiratory flow meter, instructional video, brochure, and/or spacer)

⊘ **S8100** Holding chamber or spacer for use with an inhaler or nebulizer; without mask

⊘ **S8101** Holding chamber or spacer for use with an inhaler or nebulizer; with mask

⊘ **S8110** Peak expiratory flow rate (physician services)

⊘ **S8120** Oxygen contents, gaseous, 1 unit equals 1 cubic foot

⊘ **S8121** Oxygen contents, liquid, 1 unit equals 1 pound

MIPS
Qp Quantity Physician
Qh Quantity Hospital
♀ Female only
♂ Male only
A Age
DMEPOS
A2-Z3 ASC Payment Indicator
A-Y ASC Status Indicator
Coding Clinic

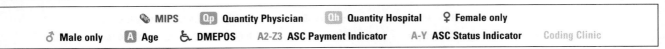

⊘ **S8130** Interferential current stimulator, 2 channel

⊘ **S8131** Interferential current stimulator, 4 channel

⊘ **S8185** Flutter device

⊘ **S8186** Swivel adapter

⊘ **S8189** Tracheostomy supply, not otherwise classified

⊘ **S8210** Mucus trap

Miscellaneous Supplies and Services

⊘ **S8265** Haberman feeder for cleft lip/palate

⊘ **S8270** Enuresis alarm, using auditory buzzer and/or vibration device

⊘ **S8301** Infection control supplies, not otherwise specified

⊘ **S8415** Supplies for home delivery of infant A

⊘ **S8420** Gradient pressure aid (sleeve and glove combination), custom made

⊘ **S8421** Gradient pressure aid (sleeve and glove combination), ready made

⊘ **S8422** Gradient pressure aid (sleeve), custom made, medium weight

⊘ **S8423** Gradient pressure aid (sleeve), custom made, heavy weight

⊘ **S8424** Gradient pressure aid (sleeve), ready made

⊘ **S8425** Gradient pressure aid (glove), custom made, medium weight

⊘ **S8426** Gradient pressure aid (glove), custom made, heavy weight

⊘ **S8427** Gradient pressure aid (glove), ready made

⊘ **S8428** Gradient pressure aid (gauntlet), ready made

⊘ **S8429** Gradient pressure exterior wrap

⊘ **S8430** Padding for compression bandage, roll

⊘ **S8431** Compression bandage, roll

⊘ **S8450** Splint, prefabricated, digit (specify digit by use of modifier)

⊘ **S8451** Splint, prefabricated, wrist or ankle

⊘ **S8452** Splint, prefabricated, elbow

⊘ **S8460** Camisole, post-mastectomy

⊘ **S8490** Insulin syringes (100 syringes, any size)

⊘ **S8930** Electrical stimulation of auricular acupuncture points; each 15 minutes of personal one-on-one contact with the patient

⊘ **S8940** Equestrian/Hippotherapy, per session

⊘ **S8948** Application of a modality (requiring constant provider attendance) to one or more areas; low-level laser; each 15 minutes

⊘ **S8950** Complex lymphedema therapy, each 15 minutes

⊘ **S8990** Physical or manipulative therapy performed for maintenance rather than restoration

⊘ **S8999** Resuscitation bag (for use by patient on artificial respiration during power failure or other catastrophic event)

⊘ **S9001** Home uterine monitor with or without associated nursing services ♀

⊘ **S9007** Ultrafiltration monitor

⊘ **S9024** Paranasal sinus ultrasound

⊘ **S9025** Omnicardiogram/cardiointegram

⊘ **S9034** Extracorporeal shockwave lithotripsy for gall stones (if performed with ERCP, use 43265)

⊘ **S9055** Procuren or other growth factor preparation to promote wound healing

⊘ **S9056** Coma stimulation per diem

⊘ **S9061** Home administration of aerosolized drug therapy (e.g., pentamidine); administrative services, professional pharmacy services, care coordination, all necessary supplies and equipment (drugs and nursing visits coded separately), per diem

⊘ **S9083** Global fee urgent care centers

⊘ **S9088** Services provided in an urgent care center (list in addition to code for service)

⊘ **S9090** Vertebral axial decompression, per session

⊘ **S9097** Home visit for wound care

⊘ **S9098** Home visit, phototherapy services (e.g., Bili-Lite), including equipment rental, nursing services, blood draw, supplies, and other services, per diem

⊘ **S9110** Telemonitoring of patient in their home, including all necessary equipment; computer system, connections, and software; maintenance; patient education and support; per month

⊘ **S9117** Back school, per visit

⊘ **S9122** Home health aide or certified nurse assistant, providing care in the home; per hour

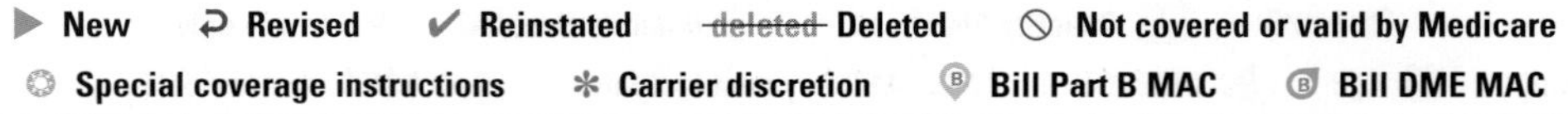

▶ New
Revised
✔ Reinstated
~~deleted~~ Deleted
⊘ Not covered or valid by Medicare
Special coverage instructions
✻ Carrier discretion
Bill Part B MAC
Bill DME MAC

⊘ **S9123** Nursing care, in the home; by registered nurse, per hour (use for general nursing care only, not to be used when CPT codes 99500-99602 can be used)

⊘ **S9124** Nursing care, in the home; by licensed practical nurse, per hour

⊘ **S9125** Respite care, in the home, per diem

⊘ **S9126** Hospice care, in the home, per diem

⊘ **S9127** Social work visit, in the home, per diem

⊘ **S9128** Speech therapy, in the home, per diem

⊘ **S9129** Occupational therapy, in the home, per diem

⊘ **S9131** Physical therapy; in the home, per diem

⊘ **S9140** Diabetic management program, follow-up visit to non-MD provider

⊘ **S9141** Diabetic management program, follow-up visit to MD provider

⊘ **S9145** Insulin pump initiation, instruction in initial use of pump (pump not included)

⊘ **S9150** Evaluation by ocularist

⊘ **S9152** Speech therapy, re-evaluation

Home Management of Pregnancy

⊘ **S9208** Home management of preterm labor, including administrative services, professional pharmacy services, care coordination, and all necessary supplies or equipment (drugs and nursing visits coded separately), per diem (do not use this code with any home infusion per diem code) ♀

⊘ **S9209** Home management of preterm premature rupture of membranes (PPROM), including administrative services, professional pharmacy services, care coordination, and all necessary supplies or equipment (drugs and nursing visits coded separately), per diem (do not use this code with any home infusion per diem code) ♀

⊘ **S9211** Home management of gestational hypertension, includes administrative services, professional pharmacy services, care coordination, and all necessary supplies and equipment (drugs and nursing visits coded separately); per diem (do not use this code with any home infusion per diem code) ♀

⊘ **S9212** Home management of postpartum hypertension, includes administrative services, professional pharmacy services, care coordination, and all necessary supplies and equipment (drugs and nursing visits coded separately), per diem (do not use this code with any home infusion per diem code) ♀

⊘ **S9213** Home management of preeclampsia, includes administrative services, professional pharmacy services, care coordination, and all necessary supplies and equipment (drugs and nursing services coded separately); per diem (do not use this code with any home infusion per diem code) ♀

⊘ **S9214** Home management of gestational diabetes, includes administrative services, professional pharmacy services, care coordination, and all necessary supplies and equipment (drugs and nursing visits coded separately); per diem (do not use this code with any home infusion per diem code) ♀

Home Infusion Therapy

⊘ **S9325** Home infusion therapy, pain management infusion; administrative services, professional pharmacy services, care coordination, and all necessary supplies and equipment, (drugs and nursing visits coded separately), per diem (do not use this code with S9326, S9327 or S9328)

⊘ **S9326** Home infusion therapy, continuous (twenty-four hours or more) pain management infusion; administrative services, professional pharmacy services, care coordination, and all necessary supplies and equipment (drugs and nursing visits coded separately), per diem

⊘ **S9327** Home infusion therapy, intermittent (less than twenty-four hours) pain management infusion; administrative services, professional pharmacy services, care coordination, and all necessary supplies and equipment (drugs and nursing visits coded separately), per diem

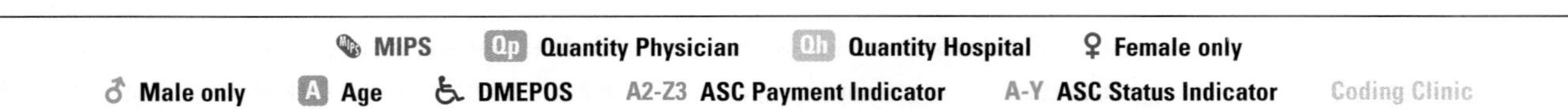
MIPS
Qp Quantity Physician
Qh Quantity Hospital
♀ Female only
♂ Male only
A Age
DMEPOS
A2-Z3 ASC Payment Indicator
A-Y ASC Status Indicator
Coding Clinic

⊘ **S9328** Home infusion therapy, implanted pump pain management infusion; administrative services, professional pharmacy services, care coordination, and all necessary supplies and equipment (drugs and nursing visits coded separately), per diem

⊘ **S9329** Home infusion therapy, chemotherapy infusion; administrative services, professional pharmacy services, care coordination, and all necessary supplies and equipment (drugs and nursing visits coded separately), per diem (do not use this code with S9330 or S9331)

⊘ **S9330** Home infusion therapy, continuous (twenty-four hours or more) chemotherapy infusion; administrative services, professional pharmacy services, care coordination, and all necessary supplies and equipment (drugs and nursing visits coded separately), per diem

⊘ **S9331** Home infusion therapy, intermittent (less than twenty-four hours) chemotherapy infusion; administrative services, professional pharmacy services, care coordination, and all necessary supplies and equipment (drugs and nursing visits coded separately), per diem

⊘ **S9335** Home therapy, hemodialysis; administrative services, professional pharmacy services, care coordination, and all necessary supplies and equipment (drugs and nursing services coded separately), per diem

⊘ **S9336** Home infusion therapy, continuous anticoagulant infusion therapy (e.g., heparin), administrative services, professional pharmacy services, care coordination, and all necessary supplies and equipment (drugs and nursing visits coded separately), per diem

⊘ **S9338** Home infusion therapy, immunotherapy, administrative services, professional pharmacy services, care coordination, and all necessary supplies and equipment (drug and nursing visits coded separately), per diem

⊘ **S9339** Home therapy; peritoneal dialysis, administrative services, professional pharmacy services, care coordination and all necessary supplies and equipment (drugs and nursing visits coded separately), per diem

⊘ **S9340** Home therapy; enteral nutrition; administrative services, professional pharmacy services, care coordination, and all necessary supplies and equipment (enteral formula and nursing visits coded separately), per diem

⊘ **S9341** Home therapy; enteral nutrition via gravity; administrative services, professional pharmacy services, care coordination, and all necessary supplies and equipment (enteral formula and nursing visits coded separately), per diem

⊘ **S9342** Home therapy; enteral nutrition via pump; administrative services, professional pharmacy services, care coordination, and all necessary supplies and equipment (enteral formula and nursing visits coded separately), per diem

⊘ **S9343** Home therapy; enteral nutrition via bolus; administrative services, professional pharmacy services, care coordination, and all necessary supplies and equipment (enteral formula and nursing visits coded separately), per diem

⊘ **S9345** Home infusion therapy, anti-hemophilic agent infusion therapy (e.g., Factor VIII); administrative services, professional pharmacy services, care coordination, and all necessary supplies and equipment (drugs and nursing visits coded separately), per diem

⊘ **S9346** Home infusion therapy, alpha-1-proteinase inhibitor (e.g., Prolastin); administrative services, professional pharmacy services, care coordination, and all necessary supplies and equipment (drugs and nursing visits coded separately), per diem

⊘ **S9347** Home infusion therapy, uninterrupted, long-term, controlled rate intravenous or subcutaneous infusion therapy (e.g., Epoprostenol); administrative services, professional pharmacy services, care coordination, and all necessary supplies and equipment (drugs and nursing visits coded separately), per diem

⊘ **S9348** Home infusion therapy, sympathomimetic/inotropic agent infusion therapy (e.g., Dobutamine); administrative services, professional pharmacy services, care coordination, all necessary supplies and equipment (drugs and nursing visits coded separately), per diem

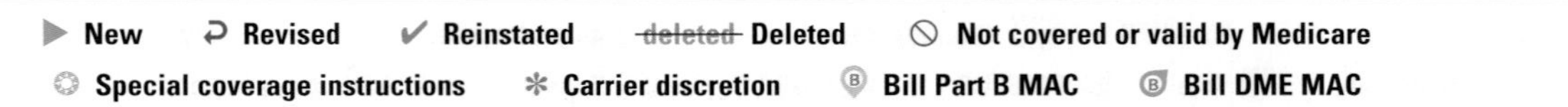

▶ New
↩ Revised
✔ Reinstated
~~deleted~~ Deleted
⊘ Not covered or valid by Medicare
Special coverage instructions
✻ Carrier discretion
Bill Part B MAC
Bill DME MAC

⊘ **S9349** Home infusion therapy, tocolytic infusion therapy; administrative services, professional pharmacy services, care coordination, and all necessary supplies and equipment (drugs and nursing visits coded separately), per diem

⊘ **S9351** Home infusion therapy, continuous or intermittent anti-emetic infusion therapy; administrative services, professional pharmacy services, care coordination, and all necessary supplies and equipment (drugs and visits coded separately), per diem

⊘ **S9353** Home infusion therapy, continuous insulin infusion therapy; administrative services, professional pharmacy services, care coordination, and all necessary supplies and equipment (drugs and nursing visits coded separately), per diem

⊘ **S9355** Home infusion therapy, chelation therapy; administrative services, professional pharmacy services, care coordination, and all necessary supplies and equipment (drugs and nursing visits coded separately), per diem

⊘ **S9357** Home infusion therapy, enzyme replacement intravenous therapy (e.g., Imiglucerase); administrative services, professional pharmacy services, care coordination, and all necessary supplies and equipment (drugs and nursing visits coded separately), per diem

⊘ **S9359** Home infusion therapy, anti-tumor necrosis factor intravenous therapy (e.g., Infliximab); administrative services, professional pharmacy services, care coordination, and all necessary supplies and equipment (drugs and nursing visits coded separately), per diem

⊘ **S9361** Home infusion therapy, diuretic intravenous therapy; administrative services, professional pharmacy services, care coordination, and all necessary supplies and equipment (drugs and nursing visits coded separately), per diem

⊘ **S9363** Home infusion therapy, anti-spasmotic therapy; administrative services, professional pharmacy services, care coordination, and all necessary supplies and equipment (drugs and nursing visits coded separately), per diem

⊘ **S9364** Home infusion therapy, total parenteral nutrition (TPN); administrative services, professional pharmacy services, care coordination, and all necessary supplies and equipment including standard TPN formula (lipids, specialty amino acid formulas, drugs other than in standard formula, and nursing visits coded separately) per diem (do not use with home infusion codes S9365-S9368 using daily volume scales)

⊘ **S9365** Home infusion therapy, total parenteral nutrition (TPN); one liter per day, administrative services, professional pharmacy services, care coordination, and all necessary supplies and equipment including standard TPN formula (lipids, specialty amino acid formulas, drugs other than in standard formula and nursing visits coded separately), per diem

⊘ **S9366** Home infusion therapy, total parenteral nutrition (TPN); more than one liter but no more than two liters per day, administrative services, professional pharmacy services, care coordination, and all necessary supplies and equipment including standard TPN formula (lipids, specialty amino acid formulas, drugs other than in standard formula and nursing visits coded separately), per diem

⊘ **S9367** Home infusion therapy, total parenteral nutrition (TPN); more than two liters but no more than three liters per day, administrative services, professional pharmacy services, care coordination, and all necessary supplies and equipment including standard TPN formula (lipids, specialty amino acid formulas, drugs other than in standard formula and nursing visits coded separately), per diem

⊘ **S9368** Home infusion therapy, total parenteral nutrition (TPN); more than three liters per day, administrative services, professional pharmacy services, care coordination, and all necessary supplies and equipment (including standard TPN formula; lipids, specialty amino acid formulas, drugs other than in standard formula and nursing visits coded separately), per diem

⃠ **S9370** Home therapy, intermittent anti-emetic injection therapy; administrative services, professional pharmacy services, care coordination, and all necessary supplies and equipment (drugs and nursing visits coded separately), per diem

⃠ **S9372** Home therapy; intermittent anticoagulant injection therapy (e.g., heparin); administrative services, professional pharmacy services, care coordination, and all necessary supplies and equipment (drugs and nursing visits coded separately), per diem (do not use this code for flushing of infusion devices with heparin to maintain patency)

⃠ **S9373** Home infusion therapy, hydration therapy; administrative services, professional pharmacy services, care coordination, and all necessary supplies and equipment (drugs and nursing visits coded separately), per diem (do not use with hydration therapy codes S9374-S9377 using daily volume scales)

⃠ **S9374** Home infusion therapy, hydration therapy; one liter per day, administrative services, professional pharmacy services, care coordination, and all necessary supplies and equipment (drugs and nursing visits coded separately), per diem

⃠ **S9375** Home infusion therapy, hydration therapy; more than one liter but no more than two liters per day, administrative services, professional pharmacy services, care coordination, and all necessary supplies and equipment (drugs and nursing visits coded separately), per diem

⃠ **S9376** Home infusion therapy, hydration therapy; more than two liters but no more than three liters per day, administrative services, professional pharmacy services, care coordination, and all necessary supplies and equipment (drugs and nursing visits coded separately), per diem

⃠ **S9377** Home infusion therapy, hydration therapy; more than three liters per day, administrative services, professional pharmacy services, care coordination, and all necessary supplies (drugs and nursing visits coded separately), per diem

⃠ **S9379** Home infusion therapy, infusion therapy, not otherwise classified; administrative services, professional pharmacy services, care coordination, and all necessary supplies and equipment (drugs and nursing visits coded separately), per diem

Miscellaneous Supplies and Services

⃠ **S9381** Delivery or service to high risk areas requiring escort or extra protection, per visit

⃠ **S9401** Anticoagulation clinic, inclusive of all services except laboratory tests, per session

⃠ **S9430** Pharmacy compounding and dispensing services

⃠ **S9433** Medical food nutritionally complete, administered orally, providing 100% of nutritional intake

⃠ **S9434** Modified solid food supplements for inborn errors of metabolism

⃠ **S9435** Medical foods for inborn errors of metabolism

⃠ **S9436** Childbirth preparation/Lamaze classes, non-physician provider, per session ♀

⃠ **S9437** Childbirth refresher classes, non-physician provider, per session ♀

⃠ **S9438** Cesarean birth classes, non-physician provider, per session ♀

⃠ **S9439** VBAC (vaginal birth after cesarean) classes, non-physician provider, per session ♀

⃠ **S9441** Asthma education, non-physician provider, per session

⃠ **S9442** Birthing classes, non-physician provider, per session ♀

⃠ **S9443** Lactation classes, non-physician provider, per session ♀

⃠ **S9444** Parenting classes, non-physician provider, per session

⃠ **S9445** Patient education, not otherwise classified, non-physician provider, individual, per session

⃠ **S9446** Patient education, not otherwise classified, non-physician provider, group, per session

⃠ **S9447** Infant safety (including CPR) classes, non-physician provider, per session

⃠ **S9449** Weight management classes, non-physician provider, per session

⊘ **S9451** Exercise classes, non-physician provider, per session

⊘ **S9452** Nutrition classes, non-physician provider, per session

⊘ **S9453** Smoking cessation classes, non-physician provider, per session

⊘ **S9454** Stress management classes, non-physician provider, per session

⊘ **S9455** Diabetic management program, group session

⊘ **S9460** Diabetic management program, nurse visit

⊘ **S9465** Diabetic management program, dietitian visit

⊘ **S9470** Nutritional counseling, dietitian visit

⊘ **S9472** Cardiac rehabilitation program, non-physician provider, per diem

⊘ **S9473** Pulmonary rehabilitation program, non-physician provider, per diem

⊘ **S9474** Enterostomal therapy by a registered nurse certified in enterostomal therapy, per diem

⊘ **S9475** Ambulatory setting substance abuse treatment or detoxification services, per diem

⊘ **S9476** Vestibular rehabilitation program, non-physician provider, per diem

MIPS ⊘ **S9480** Intensive outpatient psychiatric services, per diem

⊘ **S9482** Family stabilization services, per 15 minutes

MIPS ⊘ **S9484** Crisis intervention mental health services, per hour

MIPS ⊘ **S9485** Crisis intervention mental health services, per diem

Home Therapy Services

⊘ **S9490** Home infusion therapy, corticosteroid infusion; administrative services, professional pharmacy services, care coordination, and all necessary supplies and equipment (drugs and nursing visits coded separately), per diem

⊘ **S9494** Home infusion therapy, antibiotic, antiviral, or antifungal therapy; administrative services, professional pharmacy services, care coordination, and all necessary supplies and equipment (drugs and nursing visits coded separately) per diem (do not use this code with home infusion codes for hourly dosing schedules S9497-S9504)

⊘ **S9497** Home infusion therapy, antibiotic, antiviral, or antifungal therapy; once every 3 hours; administrative services, professional pharmacy services, care coordination, and all necessary supplies and equipment (drugs and nursing visits coded separately), per diem

⊘ **S9500** Home infusion therapy, antibiotic, antiviral, or antifungal therapy; once every 24 hours; administrative services, professional pharmacy services, care coordination, and all necessary supplies and equipment (drugs and nursing visits coded separately), per diem

⊘ **S9501** Home infusion therapy, antibiotic, antiviral, or antifungal therapy; once every 12 hours; administrative services, professional pharmacy services, care coordination, and all necessary supplies and equipment (drugs and nursing visits coded separately), per diem

⊘ **S9502** Home infusion therapy, antibiotic, antiviral, or antifungal therapy; once every 8 hours, administrative services, professional pharmacy services, care coordination, and all necessary supplies and equipment (drugs and nursing visits coded separately), per diem

⊘ **S9503** Home infusion therapy, antibiotic, antiviral, or antifungal; once every 6 hours; administrative services, professional pharmacy services, care coordination, and all necessary supplies and equipment (drugs and nursing visits coded separately), per diem

⊘ **S9504** Home infusion therapy, antibiotic, antiviral, or antifungal; once every 4 hours; administrative services, professional pharmacy services, care coordination, and all necessary supplies and equipment (drugs and nursing visits coded separately), per diem

⊘ **S9529** Routine venipuncture for collection of specimen(s), single home bound, nursing home, or skilled nursing facility patient

⊘ **S9537** Home therapy; hematopoietic hormone injection therapy (e.g., erythropoietin, G-CSF, GM-CSF); administrative services, professional pharmacy services, care coordination, and all necessary supplies and equipment (drugs and nursing visits coded separately), per diem

⦸ **S9538** Home transfusion of blood product(s); administrative services, professional pharmacy services, care coordination, and all necessary supplies and equipment (blood products, drugs, and nursing visits coded separately), per diem

⦸ **S9542** Home injectable therapy; not otherwise classified, including administrative services, professional pharmacy services, care coordination, and all necessary supplies and equipment (drugs and nursing visits coded separately), per diem

⦸ **S9558** Home injectable therapy; growth hormone, including administrative services, professional pharmacy services, care coordination, and all necessary supplies and equipment (drugs and nursing visits coded separately), per diem

⦸ **S9559** Home injectable therapy; interferon, including administrative services, professional pharmacy services, care coordination, and all necessary supplies and equipment (drugs and nursing visits coded separately), per diem

⦸ **S9560** Home injectable therapy; hormonal therapy (e.g., Leuprolide, Goserelin), including administrative services, professional pharmacy services, care coordination, and all necessary supplies and equipment (drugs and nursing visits coded separately), per diem

⦸ **S9562** Home injectable therapy, palivizumab, including administrative services, professional pharmacy services, care coordination, and all necessary supplies and equipment (drugs and nursing visits coded separately), per diem

⦸ **S9590** Home therapy, irrigation therapy (e.g., sterile irrigation of an organ or anatomical cavity); including administrative services, professional pharmacy services, care coordination, and all necessary supplies and equipment (drugs and nursing visits coded separately), per diem

⦸ **S9810** Home therapy; professional pharmacy services for provision of infusion, specialty drug administration, and/or disease state management, not otherwise classified, per hour (do not use this code with any per diem code)

Other Services and Fees

⦸ **S9900** Services by journal-listed Christian Science Practitioner for the purpose of healing, per diem

⦸ **S9901** Services by a journal-listed Christian Science nurse, per hour

⦸ **S9960** Ambulance service, conventional air service, nonemergency transport, one way (fixed wing)

⦸ **S9961** Ambulance service, conventional air service, nonemergency transport, one way (rotary wing)

⦸ **S9970** Health club membership, annual

⦸ **S9975** Transplant related lodging, meals and transportation, per diem

⦸ **S9976** Lodging, per diem, not otherwise classified

⦸ **S9977** Meals, per diem, not otherwise specified

⦸ **S9981** Medical records copying fee, administrative

⦸ **S9982** Medical records copying fee, per page

⦸ **S9986** Not medically necessary service (patient is aware that service not medically necessary)

⦸ **S9988** Services provided as part of a Phase I clinical trial

⦸ **S9989** Services provided outside of the United States of America (list in addition to code(s) for services(s))

⦸ **S9990** Services provided as part of a Phase II clinical trial

⦸ **S9991** Services provided as part of a Phase III clinical trial

⦸ **S9992** Transportation costs to and from trial location and local transportation costs (e.g., fares for taxicab or bus) for clinical trial participant and one caregiver/companion

⦸ **S9994** Lodging costs (e.g., hotel charges) for clinical trial participant and one caregiver/companion

⦸ **S9996** Meals for clinical trial participant and one caregiver/companion

⦸ **S9999** Sales tax

TEMPORARY NATIONAL CODES ESTABLISHED BY MEDICAID (T1000-T9999)

Not Valid For Medicare

⊘ **T1000** Private duty/independent nursing service(s) - licensed, up to 15 minutes

⊘ **T1001** Nursing assessment/evaluation

⊘ **T1002** RN services, up to 15 minutes

⊘ **T1003** LPN/LVN services, up to 15 minutes

⊘ **T1004** Services of a qualified nursing aide, up to 15 minutes

⊘ **T1005** Respite care services, up to 15 minutes

⊘ **T1006** Alcohol and/or substance abuse services, family/couple counseling

⊘ **T1007** Alcohol and/or substance abuse services, treatment plan development and/or modification

⊘ **T1009** Child sitting services for children of the individual receiving alcohol and/or substance abuse services A

⊘ **T1010** Meals for individuals receiving alcohol and/or substance abuse services (when meals not included in the program)

⊘ **T1012** Alcohol and/or substance abuse services, skills development

⊘ **T1013** Sign language or oral interpretive services, per 15 minutes

⊘ **T1014** Telehealth transmission, per minute, professional services bill separately

⊘ **T1015** Clinic visit/encounter, all-inclusive

⊘ **T1016** Case Management, each 15 minutes

⊘ **T1017** Targeted Case Management, each 15 minutes

⊘ **T1018** School-based individualized education program (IEP) services, bundled

⊘ **T1019** Personal care services, per 15 minutes, not for an inpatient or resident of a hospital, nursing facility, ICF/MR or IMD, part of the individualized plan of treatment (code may not be used to identify services provided by home health aide or certified nurse assistant)

⊘ **T1020** Personal care services, per diem, not for an inpatient or resident of a hospital, nursing facility, ICF/MR or IMD, part of the individualized plan of treatment (code may not be used to identify services provided by home health aide or certified nurse assistant)

⊘ **T1021** Home health aide or certified nurse assistant, per visit

⊘ **T1022** Contracted home health agency services, all services provided under contract, per day

⊘ **T1023** Screening to determine the appropriateness of consideration of an individual for participation in a specified program, project or treatment protocol, per encounter

⊘ **T1024** Evaluation and treatment by an integrated, specialty team contracted to provide coordinated care to multiple or severely handicapped children, per encounter A

⊘ **T1025** Intensive, extended multidisciplinary services provided in a clinic setting to children with complex medical, physical, mental and psychosocial impairments, per diem A

⊘ **T1026** Intensive, extended multidisciplinary services provided in a clinic setting to children with complex medical, physical, medical and psychosocial impairments, per hour A

⊘ **T1027** Family training and counseling for child development, per 15 minutes A

⊘ **T1028** Assessment of home, physical and family environment, to determine suitability to meet patient's medical needs

⊘ **T1029** Comprehensive environmental lead investigation, not including laboratory analysis, per dwelling

⊘ **T1030** Nursing care, in the home, by registered nurse, per diem

⊘ **T1031** Nursing care, in the home, by licensed practical nurse, per diem

⊘ **T1040** Medicaid certified community behavioral health clinic services, per diem

⊘ **T1041** Medicaid certified community behavioral health clinic services, per month

⊘ **T1502** Administration of oral, intramuscular and/or subcutaneous medication by health care agency/professional, per visit

⊘ **T1503** Administration of medication, other than oral and/or injectable, by a health care agency/professional, per visit

⊘ **T1505** Electronic medication compliance management device, includes all components and accessories, not otherwise classified

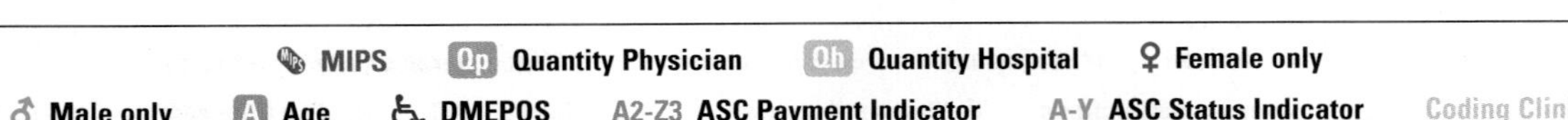
MIPS
Qp Quantity Physician
Qh Quantity Hospital
♀ Female only
♂ Male only
A Age
DMEPOS
A2-Z3 ASC Payment Indicator
A-Y ASC Status Indicator
Coding Clinic

⃠ **T1999** Miscellaneous therapeutic items and supplies, retail purchases, not otherwise classified; identify product in "remarks"

⃠ **T2001** Non-emergency transportation; patient attendant/escort

⃠ **T2002** Non-emergency transportation; per diem

⃠ **T2003** Non-emergency transportation; encounter/trip

⃠ **T2004** Non-emergency transport; commercial carrier, multi-pass

⃠ **T2005** Non-emergency transportation: stretcher van

⃠ **T2007** Transportation waiting time, air ambulance and non-emergency vehicle, one-half (1/2) hour increments

⃠ **T2010** Preadmission screening and resident review (PASRR) level I identification screening, per screen

⃠ **T2011** Preadmission screening and resident review (PASRR) level II evaluation, per evaluation

⃠ **T2012** Habilitation, educational, waiver; per diem

⃠ **T2013** Habilitation, educational, waiver; per hour

⃠ **T2014** Habilitation, prevocational, waiver; per diem

⃠ **T2015** Habilitation, prevocational, waiver; per hour

⃠ **T2016** Habilitation, residential, waiver; per diem

⃠ **T2017** Habilitation, residential, waiver; 15 minutes

⃠ **T2018** Habilitation, supported employment, waiver; per diem

⃠ **T2019** Habilitation, supported employment, waiver; per 15 minutes

⃠ **T2020** Day habilitation, waiver; per diem

⃠ **T2021** Day habilitation, waiver; per 15 minutes

⃠ **T2022** Case management, per month

⃠ **T2023** Targeted case management; per month

⃠ **T2024** Service assessment/plan of care development, waiver

⃠ **T2025** Waiver services; not otherwise specified (NOS)

⃠ **T2026** Specialized childcare, waiver; per diem

⃠ **T2027** Specialized childcare, waiver; per 15 minutes

⃠ **T2028** Specialized supply, not otherwise specified, waiver

⃠ **T2029** Specialized medical equipment, not otherwise specified, waiver

⃠ **T2030** Assisted living, waiver; per month

⃠ **T2031** Assisted living; waiver, per diem

⃠ **T2032** Residential care, not otherwise specified (NOS), waiver; per month

⃠ **T2033** Residential care, not otherwise specified (NOS), waiver; per diem

⃠ **T2034** Crisis intervention, waiver; per diem

⃠ **T2035** Utility services to support medical equipment and assistive technology/ devices, waiver

⃠ **T2036** Therapeutic camping, overnight, waiver; each session

⃠ **T2037** Therapeutic camping, day, waiver; each session

⃠ **T2038** Community transition, waiver; per service

⃠ **T2039** Vehicle modifications, waiver; per service

⃠ **T2040** Financial management, self-directed, waiver; per 15 minutes

⃠ **T2041** Supports brokerage, self-directed, waiver; per 15 minutes

⃠ **T2042** Hospice routine home care; per diem

⃠ **T2043** Hospice continuous home care; per hour

⃠ **T2044** Hospice inpatient respite care; per diem

⃠ **T2045** Hospice general inpatient care; per diem

⃠ **T2046** Hospice long term care, room and board only; per diem

▶ ⃠ **T2047** Habilitation, prevocational, waiver; per 15 minutes

⃠ **T2048** Behavioral health; long-term care residential (non-acute care in a residential treatment program where stay is typically longer than 30 days), with room and board, per diem

⃠ **T2049** Non-emergency transportation; stretcher van, mileage; per mile

⃠ **T2101** Human breast milk processing, storage and distribution only ♀

⃠ **T4521** Adult sized disposable incontinence product, brief/diaper, small, each A

IOM: 100-03, 4, 280.1

▶ New ⮌ Revised ✔ Reinstated ~~deleted~~ Deleted ⃠ Not covered or valid by Medicare
Special coverage instructions ✻ Carrier discretion Ⓑ Bill Part B MAC Ⓔ Bill DME MAC

⊘ **T4522** Adult sized disposable incontinence product, brief/diaper, medium, each A
IOM: 100-03, 4, 280.1

⊘ **T4523** Adult sized disposable incontinence product, brief/diaper, large, each A
IOM: 100-03, 4, 280.1

⊘ **T4524** Adult sized disposable incontinence product, brief/diaper, extra large, each A
IOM: 100-03, 4, 280.1

⊘ **T4525** Adult sized disposable incontinence product, protective underwear/pull-on, small size, each A
IOM: 100-03, 4, 280.1

⊘ **T4526** Adult sized disposable incontinence product, protective underwear/pull-on, medium size, each A
IOM: 100-03, 4, 280.1

⊘ **T4527** Adult sized disposable incontinence product, protective underwear/pull-on, large size, each A
IOM: 100-03, 4, 280.1

⊘ **T4528** Adult sized disposable incontinence product, protective underwear/pull-on, extra large size, each A
IOM: 100-03, 4, 280.1

⊘ **T4529** Pediatric sized disposable incontinence product, brief/diaper, small/medium size, each A
IOM: 100-03, 4, 280.1

⊘ **T4530** Pediatric sized disposable incontinence product, brief/diaper, large size, each A
IOM: 100-03, 4, 280.1

⊘ **T4531** Pediatric sized disposable incontinence product, protective underwear/pull-on, small/medium size, each A
IOM: 100-03, 4, 280.1

⊘ **T4532** Pediatric sized disposable incontinence product, protective underwear/pull-on, large size, each A
IOM: 100-03, 4, 280.1

⊘ **T4533** Youth sized disposable incontinence product, brief/diaper, each A
IOM: 100-03, 4, 280.1

⊘ **T4534** Youth sized disposable incontinence product, protective underwear/pull-on, each A
IOM: 100-03, 4, 280.1

⊘ **T4535** Disposable liner/shield/guard/pad/undergarment, for incontinence, each
IOM: 100-03, 4, 280.1

⊘ **T4536** Incontinence product, protective underwear/pull-on, reusable, any size, each
IOM: 100-03, 4, 280.1

⊘ **T4537** Incontinence product, protective underpad, reusable, bed size, each
IOM: 100-03, 4, 280.1

⊘ **T4538** Diaper service, reusable diaper, each diaper
IOM: 100-03, 4, 280.1

⊘ **T4539** Incontinence product, diaper/brief, reusable, any size, each
IOM: 100-03, 4, 280.1

⊘ **T4540** Incontinence product, protective underpad, reusable, chair size, each
IOM: 100-03, 4, 280.1

⊘ **T4541** Incontinence product, disposable underpad, large, each

⊘ **T4542** Incontinence product, disposable underpad, small size, each

⊘ **T4543** Adult sized disposable incontinence product, protective brief/diaper, above extra large, each A
IOM: 100-03, 4, 280.1

⊘ **T4544** Adult sized disposable incontinence product, protective underwear/pull-on, above extra large, each A
IOM: 100-03, 4, 280.1

⊘ **T4545** Incontinence product, disposable, penile wrap, each ♂

⊘ **T5001** Positioning seat for persons with special orthopedic needs, supply, not otherwise specified

⊘ **T5999** Supply, not otherwise specified

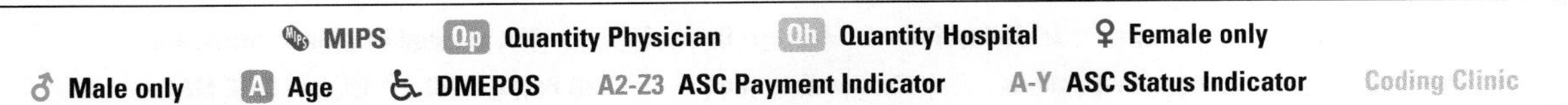
MIPS
Qp Quantity Physician
Qh Quantity Hospital
♀ Female only
♂ Male only
A Age
DMEPOS
A2-Z3 ASC Payment Indicator
A-Y ASC Status Indicator
Coding Clinic

CORONAVIRUS DIAGNOSTIC PANEL (U0001-U0004

▶ **U0001** CDC 2019 novel coronavirus (2019-nCoV) real-time RT-PCR diagnostic panel A

▶ **U0002** 2019-nCoV coronavirus, SARS-CoV-2/2019-nCoV (COVID-19), any technique, multiple types or subtypes (includes all targets), non-CDC A

▶ **U0003** Infectious agent detection by nucleic acid (DNA or RNA); severe acute respiratory syndrome coronavirus 2 (SARS-CoV-2) (Coronavirus disease [COVID-19]), amplified probe technique, making use of high throughput technologies as described by CMS-2020-01-R A

▶ **U0004** 2019-nCoV Coronavirus, SARS-CoV-2/2019-nCoV (COVID-19), any technique, multiple types or subtypes (includes all targets), non-CDC, making use of high throughput technologies as described by CMS-2020-01-R A

▶ **U0005** Infectious agent detection by nucleic acid (DNA or RNA); severe acute respiratory syndrome coronavirus 2 (SARS-CoV-2) (Coronavirus disease [COVID-19]), amplified probe technique, CDC or non-CDC, making use of high throughput technologies, completed within 2 calendar days from date of specimen collection (list separately in addition to either HCPCS code U0003 or U0004) as described by CMS-2020-01-R2 A

VISION SERVICES (V0000-V2999)

Frames

V2020 Frames, purchases Qp Qh A
Includes cost of frame/replacement and dispensing fee. One unit of service represents one pair of eyeglass frames.
IOM: 100-02, 15, 120

V2025 Deluxe frame Qp Qh E1
Not a benefit. Billing deluxe frames-submit V2020 on one line; V2025 on second line.
IOM: 100-04, 1, 30.3.5

If a CPT procedure code for supply of spectacles or a permanent prosthesis is reported, recode with the specific lens type listed below.

Single Vision Lenses

* **V2100** Sphere, single vision, plano to plus or minus 4.00, per lens Qp Qh A
* **V2101** Sphere, single vision, plus or minus 4.12 to plus or minus 7.00d, per lens Qp Qh A
* **V2102** Sphere, single vision, plus or minus 7.12 to plus or minus 20.00d, per lens Qp Qh A
* **V2103** Spherocylinder, single vision, plano to plus or minus 4.00d sphere, .12 to 2.00d cylinder, per lens Qp Qh A
* **V2104** Spherocylinder, single vision, plano to plus or minus 4.00d sphere, 2.12 to 4.00d cylinder, per lens Qp Qh A
* **V2105** Spherocylinder, single vision, plano to plus or minus 4.00d sphere, 4.25 to 6.00d cylinder, per lens Qp Qh A
* **V2106** Spherocylinder, single vision, plano to plus or minus 4.00d sphere, over 6.00d cylinder, per lens Qp Qh A
* **V2107** Spherocylinder, single vision, plus or minus 4.25 to plus or minus 7.00 sphere, .12 to 2.00d cylinder, per lens Qp Qh A
* **V2108** Spherocylinder, single vision, plus or minus 4.25d to plus or minus 7.00d sphere, 2.12 to 4.00d cylinder, per lens Qp Qh A
* **V2109** Spherocylinder, single vision, plus or minus 4.25 to plus or minus 7.00d sphere, 4.25 to 6.00d cylinder, per lens Qp Qh A
* **V2110** Sperocylinder, single vision, plus or minus 4.25 to 7.00d sphere, over 6.00d cylinder, per lens Qp Qh A
* **V2111** Spherocylinder, single vision, plus or minus 7.25 to plus or minus 12.00d sphere, .25 to 2.25d cylinder, per lens Qp Qh A
* **V2112** Spherocylinder, single vision, plus or minus 7.25 to plus or minus 12.00d sphere, 2.25d to 4.00d cylinder, per lens Qp Qh A
* **V2113** Spherocylinder, single vision, plus or minus 7.25 to plus or minus 12.00d sphere, 4.25 to 6.00d cylinder, per lens Qp Qh A
* **V2114** Spherocylinder, single vision, sphere over plus or minus 12.00d, per lens Qp Qh A
* **V2115** Lenticular, (myodisc), per lens, single vision Qp Qh A
* **V2118** Aniseikonic lens, single vision Qp Qh A

V2121 Lenticular lens, per lens, single Qp Qh A
IOM: 100-02, 15, 120; 100-04, 3, 10.4

* **V2199** Not otherwise classified, single vision lens Qp Qh A
Bill on paper. Requires report of type of single vision lens and optical lab invoice.

Bifocal Lenses

* **V2200** Sphere, bifocal, plano to plus or minus 4.00d, per lens Qp Qh A
* **V2201** Sphere, bifocal, plus or minus 4.12 to plus or minus 7.00d, per lens Qp Qh A
* **V2202** Sphere, bifocal, plus or minus 7.12 to plus or minus 20.00d, per lens Qp Qh A
* **V2203** Spherocylinder, bifocal, plano to plus or minus 4.00d sphere, .12 to 2.00d cylinder, per lens Qp Qh A
* **V2204** Spherocylinder, bifocal, plano to plus or minus 4.00d sphere, 2.12 to 4.00d cylinder, per lens Qp Qh A
* **V2205** Spherocylinder, bifocal, plano to plus or minus 4.00d sphere, 4.25 to 6.00d cylinder, per lens Qp Qh A
* **V2206** Spherocylinder, bifocal, plano to plus or minus 4.00d sphere, over 6.00d cylinder, per lens Qp Qh A

* **V2207** Spherocylinder, bifocal, plus or minus 4.25 to plus or minus 7.00d sphere, .12 to 2.00d cylinder, per lens Ⓑ Qp Qh ♿ A
* **V2208** Spherocylinder, bifocal, plus or minus 4.25 to plus or minus 7.00d sphere, 2.12 to 4.00d cylinder, per lens Ⓑ Qp Qh ♿ A
* **V2209** Spherocylinder, bifocal, plus or minus 4.25 to plus or minus 7.00d sphere, 4.25 to 6.00d cylinder, per lens Ⓑ Qp Qh ♿ A
* **V2210** Spherocylinder, bifocal, plus or minus 4.25 to plus or minus 7.00d sphere, over 6.00d cylinder, per lens Ⓑ Qp Qh ♿ A
* **V2211** Spherocylinder, bifocal, plus or minus 7.25 to plus or minus 12.00d sphere, .25 to 2.25d cylinder, per lens Ⓑ Qp Qh ♿ A
* **V2212** Spherocylinder, bifocal, plus or minus 7.25 to plus or minus 12.00d sphere, 2.25 to 4.00d cylinder, per lens Ⓑ Qp Qh ♿ A
* **V2213** Spherocylinder, bifocal, plus or minus 7.25 to plus or minus 12.00d sphere, 4.25 to 6.00d cylinder, per lens Ⓑ Qp Qh ♿ A
* **V2214** Spherocylinder, bifocal, sphere over plus or minus 12.00d, per lens Ⓑ Qp Qh ♿ A
* **V2215** Lenticular (myodisc), per lens, bifocal Ⓑ Qp Qh ♿ A
* **V2218** Aniseikonic, per lens, bifocal Ⓑ Qp Qh ♿ A
* **V2219** Bifocal seg width over 28 mm Ⓑ Qp Qh ♿ A
* **V2220** Bifocal add over 3.25d Ⓑ Qp Qh ♿ A

○ **V2221** Lenticular lens, per lens, bifocal Ⓑ Qp Qh ♿ A

IOM: 100-02, 15, 120; 100-04, 3, 10.4

* **V2299** Specialty bifocal (by report) Ⓑ Qp Qh A

Bill on paper. Requires report of type of specialty bifocal lens and optical lab invoice.

Trifocal Lenses

* **V2300** Sphere, trifocal, plano to plus or minus 4.00d, per lens Ⓑ Qp Qh ♿ A
* **V2301** Sphere, trifocal, plus or minus 4.12 to plus or minus 7.00d per lens Ⓑ Qp Qh ♿ A
* **V2302** Sphere, trifocal, plus or minus 7.12 to plus or minus 20.00, per lens Ⓑ Qp Qh ♿ A
* **V2303** Spherocylinder, trifocal, plano to plus or minus 4.00d sphere, .12 to 2.00d cylinder, per lens Ⓑ Qp Qh ♿ A
* **V2304** Spherocylinder, trifocal, plano to plus or minus 4.00d sphere, 2.25-4.00d cylinder, per lens Ⓑ Qp Qh ♿ A
* **V2305** Spherocylinder, trifocal, plano to plus or minus 4.00d sphere, 4.25 to 6.00 cylinder, per lens Ⓑ Qp Qh ♿ A
* **V2306** Spherocylinder, trifocal, plano to plus or minus 4.00d sphere, over 6.00d cylinder, per lens Ⓑ Qp Qh ♿ A
* **V2307** Spherocylinder, trifocal, plus or minus 4.25 to plus or minus 7.00d sphere, .12 to 2.00d cylinder, per lens Ⓑ Qp Qh ♿ A
* **V2308** Spherocylinder, trifocal, plus or minus 4.25 to plus or minus 7.00d sphere, 2.12 to 4.00d cylinder, per lens Ⓑ Qp Qh ♿ A
* **V2309** Spherocylinder, trifocal, plus or minus 4.25 to plus or minus 7.00d sphere, 4.25 to 6.00d cylinder, per lens Ⓑ Qp Qh ♿ A
* **V2310** Spherocylinder, trifocal, plus or minus 4.25 to plus or minus 7.00d sphere, over 6.00d cylinder, per lens Ⓑ Qp Qh ♿ A
* **V2311** Spherocylinder, trifocal, plus or minus 7.25 to plus or minus 12.00d sphere, .25 to 2.25d cylinder, per lens Ⓑ Qp Qh ♿ A
* **V2312** Spherocylinder, trifocal, plus or minus 7.25 to plus or minus 12.00d sphere, 2.25 to 4.00d cylinder, per lens Ⓑ Qp Qh ♿ A
* **V2313** Spherocylinder, trifocal, plus or minus 7.25 to plus or minus 12.00d sphere, 4.25 to 6.00d cylinder, per lens Ⓑ Qp Qh ♿ A
* **V2314** Spherocylinder, trifocal, sphere over plus or minus 12.00d, per lens Ⓑ Qp Qh ♿ A
* **V2315** Lenticular, (myodisc), per lens, trifocal Ⓑ Qp Qh ♿ A
* **V2318** Aniseikonic lens, trifocal Ⓑ Qp Qh ♿ A
* **V2319** Trifocal seg width over 28 mm Ⓑ Qp Qh ♿ A
* **V2320** Trifocal add over 3.25d Ⓑ Qp Qh ♿ A

▶ New ↩ Revised ✔ Reinstated ~~deleted~~ Deleted ⊘ Not covered or valid by Medicare
○ Special coverage instructions * Carrier discretion Ⓑ Bill Part B MAC Ⓑ Bill DME MAC

V2321 Lenticular lens, per lens, trifocal A

IOM: 100-02, 15, 120; 100-04, 3, 10.4

* V2399 Specialty trifocal (by report) A

Bill on paper. Requires report of type of trifocal lens and optical lab invoice.

Variable Asphericity/Sphericity Lenses

* V2410 Variable asphericity lens, single vision, full field, glass or plastic, per lens A
* V2430 Variable asphericity lens, bifocal, full field, glass or plastic, per lens A
* V2499 Variable sphericity lens, other type A

Bill on paper. Requires report of other ptical lab invoice.

Contact Lenses

If a CPT procedure code for supply of contact lens is reported, recode with specific lens type listed below (per lens).

* V2500 Contact lens, PMMA, spherical, per lens A

Requires prior authorization for patients under age 21.

* V2501 Contact lens, PMMA, toric or prism ballast, per lens A

Requires prior authorization for clients under age 21.

* V2502 Contact lens, PMMA, bifocal, per lens A

Requires prior authorization for clients under age 21. Bill on paper. Requires optical lab invoice.

* V2503 Contact lens PMMA, color vision deficiency, per lens A

Requires prior authorization for clients under age 21. Bill on paper. Requires optical lab invoice.

* V2510 Contact lens, gas permeable, spherical, per lens A

Requires prior authorization for clients under age 21.

* V2511 Contact lens, gas permeable, toric, prism ballast, per lens A

Requires prior authorization for clients under age 21.

* V2512 Contact lens, gas permeable, bifocal, per lens A

Requires prior authorization for clients under age 21.

* V2513 Contact lens, gas permeable, extended wear, per lens A

Requires prior authorization for clients under age 21.

V2520 Contact lens, hydrophilic, spherical, per lens A

Requires prior authorization for clients under age 21.

IOM: 100-03, 1, 80.1; 100-03, 1, 80.4

V2521 Contact lens, hydrophilic, toric, or prism ballast, per lens A

Requires prior authorization for clients under age 21.

IOM: 100-03, 1, 80.1; 100-03, 1, 80.4

V2522 Contact lens, hydrophilic, bifocal, per lens A

Requires prior authorization for clients under age 21.

IOM: 100-03, 1, 80.1; 100-03, 1, 80.4

V2523 Contact lens, hydrophilic, extended wear, per lens A

Requires prior authorization for clients under age 21.

IOM: 100-03, 1, 80.1; 100-03, 1, 80.4

▶ V2524 Contact lens, hydrophilic, spherical, photochromic additive, per lens A

* V2530 Contact lens, scleral, gas impermeable, per lens (for contact lens modification, *see* 92325) A

Requires prior authorization for clients under age 21.

V2531 Contact lens, scleral, gas permeable, per lens (for contact lens modification, see 92325) A

Requires prior authorization for clients under age 21. Bill on paper. Requires optical lab invoice.

IOM: 100-03, 1, 80.5

* V2599 Contact lens, other type A

Requires prior authorization for clients under age 21. Bill on paper. Requires report of other type of contact lens and optical invoice.

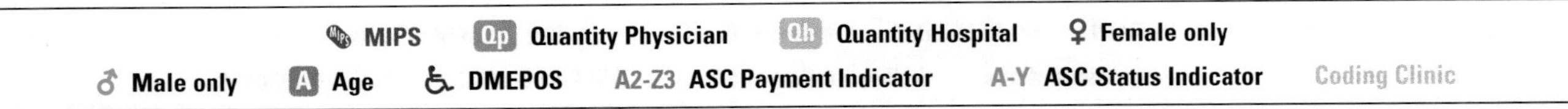
MIPS
Qp Quantity Physician
Qh Quantity Hospital
♀ Female only
♂ Male only
A Age
DMEPOS
A2-Z3 ASC Payment Indicator
A-Y ASC Status Indicator
Coding Clinic

Low Vision Aids

If a CPT procedure code for supply of low vision aid is reported, recode with specific systems listed below.

* **V2600** Hand held low vision aids and other nonspectacle mounted aids Ⓑ Qp Qh — A
  Requires prior authorization.
* **V2610** Single lens spectacle mounted low vision aids Ⓑ Qp Qh — A
  Requires prior authorization.
* **V2615** Telescopic and other compound lens system, including distance vision telescopic, near vision telescopes and compound microscopic lens system Ⓑ Qp Qh — A
  Requires prior authorization. Bill on paper. Requires optical lab invoice.

Prosthetic Eye

○ **V2623** Prosthetic eye, plastic, custom Ⓑ Qp Qh ♿ — A
  DME regional carrier. Requires prior authorization. Bill on paper. Requires optical lab invoice.

* **V2624** Polishing/resurfacing of ocular prosthesis Ⓑ Qp Qh ♿ — A
  Requires prior authorization. Bill on paper. Requires optical lab invoice.
* **V2625** Enlargement of ocular prosthesis Ⓑ Qp Qh ♿ — A
  Requires prior authorization. Bill on paper. Requires optical lab invoice.
* **V2626** Reduction of ocular prosthesis Ⓑ Qp Qh ♿ — A
  Requires prior authorization. Bill on paper. Requires optical lab invoice.

○ **V2627** Scleral cover shell Ⓑ Qp Qh ♿ — A
  DME regional carrier
  Requires prior authorization. Bill on paper. Requires optical lab invoice.
  IOM: 100-03, 4, 280.2

* **V2628** Fabrication and fitting of ocular conformer Ⓑ Qp Qh ♿ — A
  Requires prior authorization. Bill on paper. Requires optical lab invoice.
* **V2629** Prosthetic eye, other type Ⓑ Qp Qh — A
  Requires prior authorization. Bill on paper. Requires optical lab invoice.

Intraocular Lenses

○ **V2630** Anterior chamber intraocular lens Ⓑ Qp Qh ♿ — N1 N
  IOM: 100-02, 15, 120

○ **V2631** Iris supported intraocular lens Ⓑ Qp Qh ♿ — N1 N
  IOM: 100-02, 15, 120

○ **V2632** Posterior chamber intraocular lens Ⓑ Qp Qh ♿ — N1 N
  IOM: 100-02, 15, 120

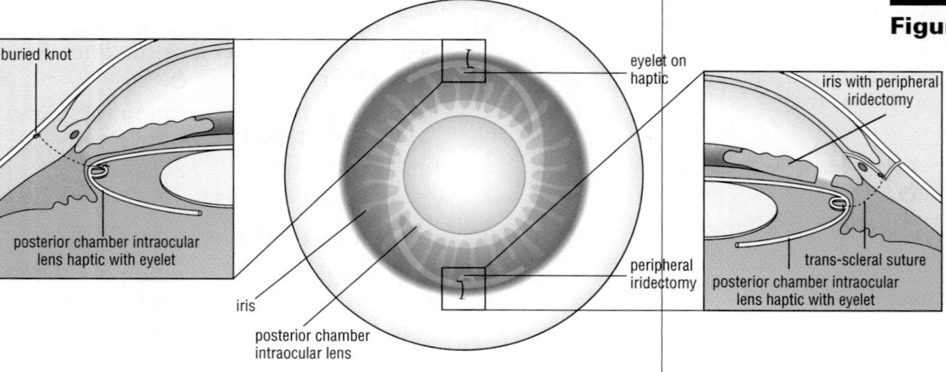

buried knot
posterior chamber intraocular lens haptic with eyelet
iris
posterior chamber intraocular lens
eyelet on haptic
peripheral iridectomy
iris with peripheral iridectomy
trans-scleral suture
posterior chamber intraocular lens haptic with eyelet

Figure 52 Posterior intraocular lens.

▶ New ⮌ Revised ✔ Reinstated ~~deleted~~ Deleted ⊘ Not covered or valid by Medicare
○ Special coverage instructions * Carrier discretion Ⓑ Bill Part B MAC Ⓑ Bill DME MAC

Miscellaneous Vision Services

V2700 Balance lens, per lens Qp Qh A

V2702 Deluxe lens feature Qp Qh E1

IOM: 100-02, 15, 120; 100-04, 3, 10.4

V2710 Slab off prism, glass or plastic, per lens Qp Qh A

V2715 Prism, per lens Qp Qh A

V2718 Press-on lens, Fresnel prism, per lens Qp Qh A

V2730 Special base curve, glass or plastic, per lens Qp Qh A

V2744 Tint, photochromatic, per lens Qp Qh A

Requires prior authorization.

IOM: 100-02, 15, 120; 100-04, 3, 10.4

V2745 Addition to lens, tint, any color, solid, gradient or equal, excludes photochroatic, any lens material, per lens Qp Qh A

Includes photochromatic lenses (V2744) used as sunglasses, which are prescribed in addition to regular prosthetic lenses for aphakic patient will be denied as not medically necessary.

IOM: 100-02, 15, 120; 100-04, 3, 10.4

V2750 Anti-reflective coating, per lens Qp Qh A

Requires prior authorization.

IOM: 100-02, 15, 120; 100-04, 3, 10.4

V2755 U-V lens, per lens Qp Qh A

IOM: 100-02, 15, 120; 100-04, 3, 10.4

V2756 Eye glass case Qp Qh E1

V2760 Scratch resistant coating, per lens Qp Qh E1

V2761 Mirror coating, any type, solid, gradient or equal, any lens material, per lens Qp Qh B

IOM: 100-02, 15, 120; 100-04, 3, 10.4

V2762 Polarization, any lens material, per lens Qp Qh E1

IOM: 100-02, 15, 120; 100-04, 3, 10.4

V2770 Occluder lens, per lens Qp Qh A

Requires prior authorization.

V2780 Oversize lens, per lens Qp Qh A

Requires prior authorization.

V2781 Progressive lens, per lens Qp Qh B

Requires prior authorization.

V2782 Lens, index 1.54 to 1.65 plastic or 1.60 to 1.79 glass, excludes polycarbonate, per lens Qp Qh A

Do not bill in addition to V2784

IOM: 100-02, 15, 120; 100-04, 3, 10.4

V2783 Lens, index greater than or equal to 1.66 plastic or greater than or equal to 1.80 glass, excludes polycarbonate, per lens Qp Qh A

Do not bill in addition to V2784

IOM: 100-02, 15, 120; 100-04, 3, 10.4

V2784 Lens, polycarbonate or equal, any index, per lens Qp Qh A

Covered only for patients with functional vision in one eye-in this situation, an impact-resistant material is covered for both lenses if eyeglasses are covered. Claims with V2784 that do not meet this coverage criterion will be denied as not medically necessary.

IOM: 100-02, 15, 120; 100-04, 3, 10.4

V2785 Processing, preserving and transporting corneal tissue Qp Qh F4 F

For ASC, bill on paper. Must attach eye bank invoice to claim.

For Hospitals, bill charges for corneal tissue to receive cost based reimbursement.

IOM: 100- 4, 4, 200.1

V2786 Specialty occupational multifocal lens, per lens Qp Qh E1

IOM: 100-02, 15, 120; 100-04, 3, 10.4

V2787 Astigmatism correcting function of intraocular lens E1

Medicare Statute 1862(a)(7)

V2788 Presbyopia correcting function of intraocular lens E1

Medicare Statute 1862a7

V2790 Amniotic membrane for surgical reconstruction, per procedure Qp Qh N1 N

V2797 Vision supply, accessory and/or service component of another HCPCS vision code Qp Qh E1

V2799 Vision item or service, miscellaneous A

Bill on paper. Requires report of miscellaneous service and optical lab invoice.

MIPS | Qp Quantity Physician | Qh Quantity Hospital | Female only
Male only | A Age | DMEPOS | A2-Z3 ASC Payment Indicator | A-Y ASC Status Indicator | Coding Clinic

HEARING SERVICES (V5000-V5999)

These codes are for non-physician services.

Assessments and Evaluations

⃠ **V5008** Hearing screening Ⓑ Qp Qh E1
IOM: 100-02, 16, 90

⃠ **V5010** Assessment for hearing aid Ⓑ Qp Qh E1
Medicare Statute 1862a7

⃠ **V5011** Fitting/orientation/checking of hearing aid Ⓑ Qp Qh E1
Medicare Statute 1862a7

⃠ **V5014** Repair/modification of a hearing aid Ⓑ E1
Medicare Statute 1862a7

⃠ **V5020** Conformity evaluation Ⓑ E1
Medicare Statute 1862a7

Monaural Hearing Aid

⃠ **V5030** Hearing aid, monaural, body worn, air conduction Ⓑ E1
Medicare Statute 1862a7

⃠ **V5040** Hearing aid, monaural, body worn, bone conduction Ⓑ E1
Medicare Statute 1862a7

⃠ **V5050** Hearing aid, monaural, in the ear Ⓑ E1
Medicare Statute 1862a7

⃠ **V5060** Hearing aid, monaural, behind the ear Ⓑ E1
Medicare Statute 1862a7

Miscellaneous Services and Supplies

⃠ **V5070** Glasses, air conduction Ⓑ E1
Medicare Statute 1862a7

⃠ **V5080** Glasses, bone conduction Ⓑ E1
Medicare Statute 1862a7

⃠ **V5090** Dispensing fee, unspecified hearing aid Ⓑ E1
Medicare Statute 1862a7

⃠ **V5095** Semi-implantable middle ear hearing prosthesis Ⓑ E1
Medicare Statute 1862a7

⃠ **V5100** Hearing aid, bilateral, body worn Ⓑ E1
Medicare Statute 1862a7

⃠ **V5110** Dispensing fee, bilateral Ⓑ E1
Medicare Statute 1862a7

Hearing Aids

⃠ **V5120** Binaural, body Ⓑ E1
Medicare Statute 1862a7

⃠ **V5130** Binaural, in the ear Ⓑ E1
Medicare Statute 1862a7

⃠ **V5140** Binaural, behind the ear Ⓑ E1
Medicare Statute 1862a7

⃠ **V5150** Binaural, glasses Ⓑ E1
Medicare Statute 1862a7

⃠ **V5160** Dispensing fee, binaural Ⓑ E1
Medicare Statute 1862a7

⃠ **V5171** Hearing aid, contralateral routing device, monaural, in the ear (ITE) E1
Medicare Statute 1862a7

⃠ **V5172** Hearing aid, contralateral routing device, monaural, in the canal (ITC) E1
Medicare Statute 1862a7

⃠ **V5181** Hearing aid, contralateral routing device, monaural, behind the ear (BTE) E1
Medicare Statute 1862a7

⃠ **V5190** Hearing aid, contralateral routing, monaural, glasses Ⓑ E1
Medicare Statute 1862a7

⃠ **V5200** Dispensing fee, contralateral, monaural Ⓑ E1
Medicare Statute 1862a7

⃠ **V5211** Hearing aid, contralateral routing system, binaural, ITE/ITE E1
Medicare Statute 1862a7

⃠ **V5212** Hearing aid, contralateral routing system, binaural, ITE/ITC E1
Medicare Statute 1862a7

⃠ **V5213** Hearing aid, contralateral routing system, binaural, ITE/BTE E1
Medicare Statute 1862a7

▶ New ⮌ Revised ✔ Reinstated ~~deleted~~ Deleted ⃠ Not covered or valid by Medicare
Special coverage instructions ✻ Carrier discretion Ⓑ Bill Part B MAC Ⓑ Bill DME MAC

V5214 Hearing aid, contralateral routing system, binaural, ITC/ITC E1
Medicare Statute 1862a7

V5215 Hearing aid, contralateral routing system, binaural, ITC/BTE E1
Medicare Statute 1862a7

V5221 Hearing aid, contralateral routing system, binaural, BTE/BTE E1
Medicare Statute 1862a7

V5230 Hearing aid, contralateral routing system, binaural, glasses E1
Medicare Statute 1862a7

V5240 Dispensing fee, contralateral routing system, binaural E1
Medicare Statute 1862a7

V5241 Dispensing fee, monaural hearing aid, any type E1
Medicare Statute 1862a7

V5242 Hearing aid, analog, monaural, CIC (completely in the ear canal) E1
Medicare Statute 1862a7

V5243 Hearing aid, analog, monaural, ITC (in the canal) E1
Medicare Statute 1862a9

V5244 Hearing aid, digitally programmable analog, monaural, CIC E1
Medicare Statute 1862a7

V5245 Hearing aid, digitally programmable, analog, monaural, ITC E1
Medicare Statute 1862a7

V5246 Hearing aid, digitally programmable analog, monaural, ITE (in the ear) E1
Medicare Statute 1862a7

V5247 Hearing aid, digitally programmable analog, monaural, BTE (behind the ear) E1
Medicare Statute 1862a7

V5248 Hearing aid, analog, binaural, CIC E1
Medicare Statute 1862a7

V5249 Hearing aid, analog, binaural, ITC E1
Medicare Statute 1862a7

V5250 Hearing aid, digitally programmable analog, binaural, CIC E1
Medicare Statute 1862a7

V5251 Hearing aid, digitally programmable analog, binaural, ITC E1
Medicare Statute 1862a7

V5252 Hearing aid, digitally programmable, binaural, ITE E1
Medicare Statute 1862a7

V5253 Hearing aid, digitally programmable, binaural, BTE E1
Medicare Statute 1862a7

V5254 Hearing aid, digital, monaural, CIC E1
Medicare Statute 1862a7

V5255 Hearing aid, digital, monaural, ITC E1
Medicare Statute 1862a7

V5256 Hearing aid, digital, monaural, ITE E1
Medicare Statute 1862a7

V5257 Hearing aid, digital, monaural, BTE E1
Medicare Statute 1862a7

V5258 Hearing aid, digital, binaural, CIC E1
Medicare Statute 1862a7

V5259 Hearing aid, digital, binaural, ITC E1
Medicare Statute 1862a7

V5260 Hearing aid, digital, binaural, ITE E1
Medicare Statute 1862a7

V5261 Hearing aid, digital, binaural, BTE E1
Medicare Statute 1862a7

V5262 Hearing aid, disposable, any type, monaural E1
Medicare Statute 1862a7

V5263 Hearing aid, disposable, any type, binaural E1
Medicare Statute 1862a7

V5264 Ear mold/insert, not disposable, any type E1
Medicare Statute 1862a7

V5265 Ear mold/insert, disposable, any type E1
Medicare Statute 1862a7

V5266 Battery for use in hearing device E1
Medicare Statute 1862a7

V5267 Hearing aid or assistive listening device/supplies/accessories, not otherwise specified E1
Medicare Statute 1862a7

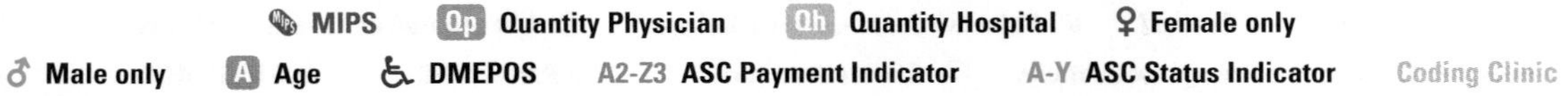
MIPS
Qp Quantity Physician
Qh Quantity Hospital
Female only
Male only
A Age
DMEPOS
A2-Z3 ASC Payment Indicator
A-Y ASC Status Indicator
Coding Clinic

Assistive Listening Devices

⃠ **V5268** Assistive listening device, telephone amplifier, any type Ⓑ E1
Medicare Statute 1862a7

⃠ **V5269** Assistive listening device, alerting, any type Ⓑ E1
Medicare Statute 1862a7

⃠ **V5270** Assistive listening device, television amplifier, any type Ⓑ E1
Medicare Statute 1862a7

⃠ **V5271** Assistive listening device, television caption decoder Ⓑ E1
Medicare Statute 1862a7

⃠ **V5272** Assistive listening device, TDD Ⓑ E1
Medicare Statute 1862a7

⃠ **V5273** Assistive listening device, for use with cochlear implant Ⓑ E1
Medicare Statute 1862a7

⃠ **V5274** Assistive listening device, not otherwise specified Ⓑ Qp Qh E1
Medicare Statute 1862a7

⃠ **V5275** Ear impression, each Ⓑ E1
Medicare Statute 1862a7

⃠ **V5281** Assistive listening device, personal FM/DM system, monaural (1 receiver, transmitter, microphone), any type Ⓑ Qp Qh E1
Medicare Statute 1862a7

⃠ **V5282** Assistive listening device, personal FM/DM system, binaural (2 receivers, transmitter, microphone), any type Ⓑ Qp Qh E1
Medicare Statute 1862a7

⃠ **V5283** Assistive listening device, personal FM/DM neck, loop induction receiver Ⓑ Qp Qh E1
Medicare Statute 1862a7

⃠ **V5284** Assistive listening device, personal FM/DM, ear level receiver Ⓑ Qp Qh E1
Medicare Statute 1862a7

⃠ **V5285** Assistive listening device, personal FM/DM, direct audio input receiver Ⓑ Qp Qh E1
Medicare Statute 1862a7

⃠ **V5286** Assistive listening device, personal Bluetooth FM/DM receiver Ⓑ Qp Qh E1
Medicare Statute 1862a7

⃠ **V5287** Assistive listening device, personal FM/DM receiver, not otherwise specified Ⓑ Qp Qh E1
Medicare Statute 1862a7

⃠ **V5288** Assistive listening device, personal FM/DM transmitter assistive listening device Ⓑ Qp Qh E1
Medicare Statute 1862a7

⃠ **V5289** Assistive listening device, personal FM/DM adapter/boot coupling device for receiver, any type Ⓑ Qp Qh E1
Medicare Statute 1862a7

⃠ **V5290** Assistive listening device, transmitter microphone, any type Ⓑ Qp Qh E1
Medicare Statute 1862a7

Other Supllies and Miscellaneous Services

⃠ **V5298** Hearing aid, not otherwise classified Ⓑ E1
Medicare Statute 1862a7

✪ **V5299** Hearing service, miscellaneous Ⓑ B
IOM: 100-02, 16, 90

Repair/Modification

⃠ **V5336** Repair/modification of augmentative communicative system or device (excludes adaptive hearing aid) Ⓓ E1
Medicare Statute 1862a7

Speech, Language, and Pathology Screening

These codes are for non-physician services.

⃠ **V5362** Speech screening Ⓑ E1
Medicare Statute 1862a7

⃠ **V5363** Language screening Ⓑ E1
Medicare Statute 1862a7

⃠ **V5364** Dysphagia screening Ⓑ E1
Medicare Statute 1862a7

▶ New ⟲ Revised ✔ Reinstated ~~deleted~~ Deleted ⃠ Not covered or valid by Medicare
✪ Special coverage instructions ✻ Carrier discretion Ⓑ Bill Part B MAC Ⓓ Bill DME MAC

APPENDIX A

Jurisdiction List for DMEPOS HCPCS Codes

Deleted codes are valid for dates of service on or before the date of deletion. The jurisdiction list includes codes that are not payable by Medicare. Please consult the Medicare contractor in whose jurisdiction a claim would be filed in order to determine coverage under Medicare.

NOTE: All Local Carrier language has been changed to Part B MAC

HCPCS	DESCRIPTION	JURISDICTION
A0021 - A0999	Ambulance Services	Part B MAC
A4206 - A4209	Medical, Surgical, and Self-Administered Injection Supplies	Part B MAC if incident to a physician's service (not separately payable). If other, DME MAC.
A4210	Needle Free Injection Device	DME MAC
A4211	Medical, Surgical, and Self-Administered Injection Supplies	Part B MAC if incident to a physician's service (not separately payable). If other, DME MAC.
A4212	Non Coring Needle or Stylet with or without Catheter	Part B MAC
A4213 - A4215	Medical, Surgical, and Self-Administered Injection Supplies	Part B MAC if incident to a physician's service (not separately payable). If other, DME MAC.
A4216 - A4218	Saline	Part B MAC if incident to a physician's service (not separately payable). If other, DME MAC.
A4220	Refill Kit for Implantable Pump	Part B MAC
A4221 - A4236	Self-Administered Injection and Diabetic Supplies	DME MAC
A4244 - A4250	Medical, Surgical, and Self-Administered Injection Supplies	Part B MAC if incident to a physician's service (not separately payable). If other, DME MAC.
A4252 - A4259	Diabetic Supplies	DME MAC
A4261	Cervical Cap for Contraceptive Use	Part B MAC
A4262 - A4263	Lacrimal Duct Implants	Part B MAC
A4264	Contraceptive Implant	Part B MAC
A4265	Paraffin	Part B MAC if incident to a physician's service (not separately payable). If other, DME MAC.
A4266 - A4269	Contraceptives	Part B MAC
A4270	Endoscope Sheath	Part B MAC
A4280	Accessory for Breast Prosthesis	DME MAC
A4281 - A4286	Accessory for Breast Pump	DME MAC
A4290	Sacral Nerve Stimulation Test Lead	Part B MAC
A4300 - A4301	Implantable Catheter	Part B MAC
A4305 - A4306	Disposable Drug Delivery System	Part B MAC if incident to a physician's service (not separately payable). If other, DME MAC.

HCPCS	DESCRIPTION	JURISDICTION
A4310 - A4358	Incontinence Supplies/ Urinary Supplies	If provided in the physician's office for a temporary condition, the item is incident to the physician's service & billed to the Part B MAC. If provided in the physician's office or other place of service for a permanent condition, the item is a prosthetic device & billed to the DME MAC.
A4360 - A4435	Urinary Supplies	If provided in the physician's office for a temporary condition, the item is incident to the physician's service & billed to the Part B MAC. If provided in the physician's office or other place of service for a permanent condition, the item is a prosthetic device & billed to the DME MAC.
A4450 - A4456	Tape; Adhesive Remover	Part B MAC if incident to a physician's service (not separately payable), or if supply for implanted prosthetic device. If other, DME MAC.
A4458-A4459	Enema Bag/System	DME MAC
A4461-A4463	Surgical Dressing Holders	Part B MAC if incident to a physician's service (not separately payable). If other, DME MAC.
A4465 - A4467	Non-elastic Binder and Garment, Strap, Covering	DME MAC
A4470	Gravlee Jet Washer	Part B MAC
A4480	Vabra Aspirator	Part B MAC
A4481	Tracheostomy Supply	Part B MAC if incident to a physician's service (not separately payable). If other, DME MAC.
A4483	Moisture Exchanger	DME MAC
A4490 - A4510	Surgical Stockings	DME MAC
A4520	Diapers	DME MAC
A4550	Surgical Trays	Part B MAC
A4553 - A4554	Underpads	DME MAC
A4555 - A4558	Electrodes; Lead Wires; Conductive Paste	Part B MAC if incident to a physician's service (not separately payable). If other, DME MAC.
A4559	Coupling Gel	Part B MAC if incident to a physician's service (not separately payable). If other, DME MAC.
A4561 - A4563	Pessary; Vaginal Insert	Part B MAC

HCPCS	DESCRIPTION	JURISDICTION
A4565-A4566	Sling	Part B MAC
A4570	Splint	Part B MAC
A4575	Topical Hyperbaric Oxygen Chamber, Disposable	DME MAC
A4580 - A4590	Casting Supplies & Material	Part B MAC
A4595	TENS Supplies	Part B MAC if incident to a physician's service (not separately payable). If other, DME MAC.
A4600	Sleeve for Intermittent Limb Compression Device	DME MAC
A4601-A4602	Lithium Replacement Batteries	DME MAC
A4604	Tubing for Positive Airway Pressure Device	DME MAC
A4605	Tracheal Suction Catheter	DME MAC
A4606	Oxygen Probe for Oximeter	DME MAC
A4608	Transtracheal Oxygen Catheter	DME MAC
A4611 - A4613	Oxygen Equipment Batteries and Supplies	DME MAC
A4614	Peak Flow Rate Meter	Part B MAC if incident to a physician's service (not separately payable). If other, DME MAC.
A4615 - A4629	Oxygen & Tracheostomy Supplies	Part B MAC if incident to a physician's service (not separately payable). If other, DME MAC.
A4630 - A4640	DME Supplies	DME MAC
A4641 - A4642	Imaging Agent; Contrast Material	Part B MAC
A4648	Tissue Marker, Implanted	Part B MAC
A4649	Miscellaneous Surgical Supplies	Part B MAC if incident to a physician's service (not separately payable), or if supply for implanted prosthetic device or implanted DME. If other, DME MAC.
A4650	Implantable Radiation Dosimeter	Part B MAC
A4651 - A4932	Supplies for ESRD	DME MAC (not separately payable)
A5051 - A5093	Additional Ostomy Supplies	If provided in the physician's office for a temporary condition, the item is incident to the physician's service & billed to the Part B MAC. If provided in the physician's office or other place of service for a permanent condition, the item is a prosthetic device & billed to the DME MAC.

HCPCS	DESCRIPTION	JURISDICTION
A5102 - A5200	Additional Incontinence and Ostomy Supplies	If provided in the physician's office for a temporary condition, the item is incident to the physician's service & billed to the Part B MAC. If provided in the physician's office or other place of service for a permanent condition, the item is a prosthetic device & billed to the DME MAC.
A5500 - A5514	Therapeutic Shoes	DME MAC
A6000	Non-Contact Wound Warming Cover	DME MAC
A6010-A6024	Surgical Dressing	Part B MAC if incident to a physician's service (not separately payable) or if supply for implanted prosthetic device or implanted DME. If other, DME MAC.
A6025	Silicone Gel Sheet	Part B MAC if incident to a physician's service (not separately payable) or if supply for implanted prosthetic device or implanted DME. If other, DME MAC.
A6154 - A6411	Surgical Dressing	Part B MAC if incident to a physician's service (not separately payable) or if supply for implanted prosthetic device or implanted DME. If other, DME MAC.
A6412	Eye Patch	Part B MAC if incident to a physician's service (not separately payable) or if supply for implanted prosthetic device or implanted DME. If other, DME MAC.
A6413	Adhesive Bandage	Part B MAC if incident to a physician's service (not separately payable) or if supply for implanted prosthetic device or implanted DME. If other, DME MAC.
A6441 - A6457	Surgical Dressing	Part B MAC if incident to a physician's service (not separately payable) or if supply for implanted prosthetic device or implanted DME. If other, DME MAC.
A6460 - A6461	Surgical Dressing	Part B MAC
A6501 - A6512	Surgical Dressing	Part B MAC if incident to a physician's service (not separately payable) or if supply for implanted prosthetic device or implanted DME. If other, DME MAC.
A6513	Compression Burn Mask	DME MAC
A6530 - A6549	Compression Gradient Stockings	DME MAC
A6550	Supplies for Negative Pressure Wound Therapy Electrical Pump	DME MAC
A7000 - A7002	Accessories for Suction Pumps	DME MAC
A7003 - A7039	Accessories for Nebulizers, Aspirators and Ventilators	DME MAC

HCPCS	DESCRIPTION	JURISDICTION
A7040 - A7041	Chest Drainage Supplies	Part B MAC
A7044 - A7047	Respiratory Accessories	DME MAC
A7048	Vacuum Drainage Supply	Part B MAC
A7501-A7527	Tracheostomy Supplies	DME MAC
A8000-A8004	Protective Helmets	DME MAC
A9150	Non-Prescription Drugs	Part B MAC
A9152 - A9153	Vitamins	Part B MAC
A9155	Artificial Saliva	Part B MAC
A9180	Lice Infestation Treatment	Part B MAC
A9270	Noncovered Items or Services	DME MAC
A9272	Disposable Wound Suction Pump	DME MAC
A9273	Hot Water Bottles, Ice Caps or Collars, and Heat and/or Cold Wraps	DME MAC
A9274 - A9278	Glucose Monitoring	DME MAC
A9279	Monitoring Feature/ Device	DME MAC
A9280	Alarm Device	DME MAC
A9281	Reaching/Grabbing Device	DME MAC
A9282	Wig	DME MAC
A9283	Foot Off Loading Device	DME MAC
A9284- A9286	Non-electric Spirometer, Inversion Devices and Hygienic Items	DME MAC
A9300	Exercise Equipment	DME MAC
A9500 - A9700	Supplies for Radiology Procedures	Part B MAC
A9900	Miscellaneous DME Supply or Accessory	Part B MAC if used with implanted DME. If other, DME MAC.
A9901	Delivery	DME MAC
A9999	Miscellaneous DME Supply or Accessory	Part B MAC if used with implanted DME. If other, DME MAC.
B4034 - B9999	Enteral and Parenteral Therapy	DME MAC
D0120 - D9999	Dental Procedures	Part B MAC
E0100 - E0105	Canes	DME MAC
E0110 - E0118	Crutches	DME MAC
E0130 - E0159	Walkers	DME MAC
E0160 - E0175	Commodes	DME MAC
E0181 - E0199	Decubitus Care Equipment	DME MAC
E0200 - E0239	Heat/Cold Applications	DME MAC
E0240 - E0248	Bath and Toilet Aids	DME MAC
E0249	Pad for Heating Unit	DME MAC

HCPCS	DESCRIPTION	JURISDICTION
E0250 - E0304	Hospital Beds	DME MAC
E0305 - E0326	Hospital Bed Accessories	DME MAC
E0328 - E0329	Pediatric Hospital Beds	DME MAC
E0350 - E0352	Electronic Bowel Irrigation System	DME MAC
E0370	Heel Pad	DME MAC
E0371 - E0373	Decubitus Care Equipment	DME MAC
E0424 - E0484	Oxygen and Related Respiratory Equipment	DME MAC
E0485 - E0486	Oral Device to Reduce Airway Collapsibility	DME MAC
E0487	Electric Spirometer	DME MAC
E0500	IPPB Machine	DME MAC
E0550 - E0585	Compressors/Nebulizers	DME MAC
E0600	Suction Pump	DME MAC
E0601	CPAP Device	DME MAC
E0602 - E0604	Breast Pump	DME MAC
E0605	Vaporizer	DME MAC
E0606	Drainage Board	DME MAC
E0607	Home Blood Glucose Monitor	DME MAC
E0610 - E0615	Pacemaker Monitor	DME MAC
E0616	Implantable Cardiac Event Recorder	Part B MAC
E0617	External Defibrillator	DME MAC
E0618 - E0619	Apnea Monitor	DME MAC
E0620	Skin Piercing Device	DME MAC
E0621 - E0636	Patient Lifts	DME MAC
E0637 - E0642	Standing Devices/Lifts	DME MAC
E0650 - E0676	Pneumatic Compressor and Appliances	DME MAC
E0691 - E0694	Ultraviolet Light Therapy Systems	DME MAC
E0700	Safety Equipment	DME MAC
E0705	Transfer Board	DME MAC
E0710	Restraints	DME MAC
E0720 - E0745	Electrical Nerve Stimulators	DME MAC
E0746	EMG Device	Part B MAC
E0747 - E0748	Osteogenic Stimulators	DME MAC
E0749	Implantable Osteogenic Stimulators	Part B MAC
E0755- E0770	Stimulation Devices	DME MAC
E0776	IV Pole	DME MAC
E0779 - E0780	External Infusion Pumps	DME MAC
E0781	Ambulatory Infusion Pump	DME MAC

HCPCS	DESCRIPTION	JURISDICTION
E0782 - E0783	Infusion Pumps, Implantable	Part B MAC
E0784	Infusion Pumps, insulin	DME MAC
E0785 - E0786	Implantable Infusion Pump Catheter	Part B MAC
E0787	Infusion Pump, Insulin	DME MAC
E0791	Parenteral Infusion Pump	DME MAC
E0830	Ambulatory Traction Device	DME MAC
E0840 - E0900	Traction Equipment	DME MAC
E0910 - E0930	Trapeze/Fracture Frame	DME MAC
E0935 - E0936	Passive Motion Exercise Device	DME MAC
E0940	Trapeze Equipment	DME MAC
E0941	Traction Equipment	DME MAC
E0942 - E0945	Orthopedic Devices	DME MAC
E0946 - E0948	Fracture Frame	DME MAC
E0950 - E1298	Wheelchairs	DME MAC
E1300 - E1310	Whirlpool Equipment	DME MAC
E1352 - E1392	Additional Oxygen Related Equipment	DME MAC
E1399	Miscellaneous DME	Part B MAC if implanted DME. If other, DME MAC.
E1405 - E1406	Additional Oxygen Equipment	DME MAC
E1500 - E1699	Artificial Kidney Machines and Accessories	DME MAC (not separately payable)
E1700 - E1702	TMJ Device and Supplies	DME MAC
E1800 - E1841	Dynamic Flexion Devices	DME MAC
E1902	Communication Board	DME MAC
E2000	Gastric Suction Pump	DME MAC
E2100 - E2101	Blood Glucose Monitors with Special Features	DME MAC
E2120	Pulse Generator for Tympanic Treatment of Inner Ear	DME MAC
E2201 - E2397	Wheelchair Accessories	DME MAC
E2402	Negative Pressure Wound Therapy Pump	DME MAC
E2500 - E2599	Speech Generating Device	DME MAC
E2601 - E2633	Wheelchair Cushions and Accessories	DME MAC
E8000 - E8002	Gait Trainers	DME MAC
G0008 - G0067	Misc. Professional Services	Part B MAC
G0068 - G0070	Infusion Drug Professional Services	DME MAC

HCPCS	DESCRIPTION	JURISDICTION
G0071 - G0329	Misc. Professional Services	Part B MAC
G0333	Dispensing Fee	DME MAC
G0337 - G0364	Misc. Professional Services	Part B MAC
G0372	Misc. Professional Services	Part B MAC
G0378 - G0490 G0491-G9987	Misc. Professional Services	Part B MAC
J0120 - J1094	Injection	Part B MAC if incident to a physician's service or used in an implanted infusion pump. If other, DME MAC.
J1095 - J1097	Ophthalmic Drug	Part B MAC
J1100 - J2786	Injection	Part B MAC if incident to a physician's service or used in an implanted infusion pump. If other, DME MAC.
J2787	Ophthalmic Drug	Part B MAC
J2788 - J3570	Injection	Part B MAC if incident to a physician's service or used in an implanted infusion pump. If other, DME MAC.
J3590 - J9591	Unclassified Biologicals	Part B MAC
J7030 - J7131	Miscellaneous Drugs and Solutions	Part B MAC if incident to a physician's service or used in an implanted infusion pump. If other, DME MAC.
J7170 - J7179	Clotting Factors	Part B MAC
J7180 - J7195	Antihemophilic Factor	Part B MAC
J7196 - J7197	Antithrombin III	Part B MAC
J7198	Anti-inhibitor; per I.U.	Part B MAC
J7199 - J7211	Other Hemophilia Clotting Factors	Part B MAC
J7296 - J7307	Contraceptives	Part B MAC
J7308 - J7309	Aminolevulinic Acid HCL	Part B MAC
J7310	Ganciclovir, Long-Acting Implant	Part B MAC
J7311 - J7316	Ophthalmic Drugs	Part B MAC
J7318 - J7329	Hyaluronan	Part B MAC
J7330	Autologous Cultured Chondrocytes, Implant	Part B MAC
J7331-J7332	Hyaluronan	Part B MAC
J7336	Capsaicin	Part B MAC
J7340	Carbidopa/Levodopa	Part B MAC if incident to a physician's service or used in an implanted infusion pump. If other, DME MAC.
J7342 - J7345	Ciprofloxacin otic & Topical Aminolevulinic Acid	Part B MAC
J7401	Sinus Implant	Part B MAC

HCPCS	DESCRIPTION	JURISDICTION
J7500 - J7599	Immunosuppressive Drugs	Part B MAC if incident to a physician's service or used in an implanted infusion pump. If other, DME MAC.
J7604 - J7699	Inhalation Solutions	Part B MAC if incident to a physician's service. If other, DME MAC.
J7799 -J7999	NOC Drugs, Other than Inhalation Drugs	Part B MAC if incident to a physician's service or used in an implanted infusion pump. If other, DME MAC.
J8498	Anti-emetic Drug	DME MAC
J8499	Prescription Drug, Oral, Non Chemotherapeutic	Part B MAC if incident to a physician's service. If other, DME MAC.
J8501 - J8999	Oral Anti-Cancer Drugs	DME MAC
J9000 - J9999	Chemotherapy Drugs	Part B MAC if incident to a physician's service or used in an implanted infusion pump. If other, DME MAC.
K0001 - K0108	Wheelchairs	DME MAC
K0195	Elevating Leg Rests	DME MAC
K0455	Infusion Pump used for Uninterrupted Administration of Epoprostenal	DME MAC
K0462	Loaner Equipment	DME MAC
K0552 - K0605	External Infusion Pump Supplies & Continuous Glucose Monitor	DME MAC
K0606 - K0609	Defibrillator Accessories	DME MAC
K0669	Wheelchair Cushion	DME MAC
K0672	Soft Interface for Orthosis	DME MAC
K0730	Inhalation Drug Delivery System	DME MAC
K0733	Power Wheelchair Accessory	DME MAC
K0738	Oxygen Equipment	DME MAC
K0739	Repair or Nonroutine Service for DME	Part B MAC if implanted DME. If other, DME MAC.
K0740	Repair or Nonroutine Service for Oxygen Equipment	DME MAC
K0743 - K0746	Suction Pump and Dressings	DME MAC
K0800 - K0899	Power Mobility Devices	DME MAC
K0900	Custom DME, other than Wheelchair	DME MAC
K1001-K1003	Devices	DME MAC
K1004	Device	Part B MAC
K1005	Device Accessory	DME MAC
L0112 - L4631	Orthotics & Devices	DME MAC
L5000 - L5999	Lower Limb Prosthetics	DME MAC
L6000 - L7499	Upper Limb Prosthetics	DME MAC

HCPCS	DESCRIPTION	JURISDICTION
L7510 - L7520	Repair of Prosthetic Device	Part B MAC if repair of implanted prosthetic device. If other, DME MAC.
L7600 - L8485	Prosthetics	DME MAC
L8499	Unlisted Procedure for Miscellaneous Prosthetic Services	Part B MAC if implanted prosthetic device. If other, DME MAC.
L8500 - L8501	Artificial Larynx; Tracheostomy Speaking Valve	DME MAC
L8505	Artificial Larynx Accessory	DME MAC
L8507	Voice Prosthesis, Patient Inserted	DME MAC
L8509	Voice Prosthesis, Inserted by a Licensed Health Care Provider	Part B MAC for dates of service on or after 10/01/2010. DME MAC for dates of service prior to 10/01/2010
L8510	Voice Prosthesis	DME MAC
L8511 - L8515	Voice Prosthesis	Part B MAC if used with tracheoesophageal voice prostheses inserted by a licensed health care provider. If other, DME MAC
L8701 - L8702	Assist Device	DME MAC
L8600 - L8699	Prosthetic Implants	Part B MAC
L9900	Miscellaneous Orthotic or Prosthetic Component or Accessory	Part B MAC if used with implanted prosthetic device. If other, DME MAC.
M0075 - M1143	Medical Services	Part B MAC
P2028 - P9615	Laboratory Tests	Part B MAC
Q0035	Cardio-kymography	Part B MAC
Q0081	Infusion Therapy	Part B MAC
Q0083 - Q0085	Chemotherapy Administration	Part B MAC
Q0091	Smear Preparation	Part B MAC
Q0092	Portable X-ray Setup	Part B MAC
Q0111 - Q0115	Miscellaneous Lab Services	Part B MAC
Q0138-Q0139	Ferumoxytol Injection	Part B MAC
Q0144	Azithromycin Dihydrate	Part B MAC if incident to a physician's service. If other, DME MAC.
Q0161 - Q0181	Anti-emetic	DME MAC
Q0477 - Q0509	Ventricular Assist Devices	Part B MAC
Q0510 - Q0514	Drug Dispensing Fees	DME MAC
Q0515	Sermorelin Acetate	Part B MAC
Q1004 - Q1005	New Technology IOL	Part B MAC
Q2004	Irrigation Solution	Part B MAC
Q2009	Fosphenytoin	Part B MAC
Q2017	Teniposide	Part B MAC
Q2026-Q2028	Injectable Dermal Fillers	Part B MAC

HCPCS	DESCRIPTION	JURISDICTION
Q2034 - Q2039	Influenza Vaccine	Part B MAC
Q2041 - Q2043	Cellular Immunotherapy	Part B MAC
Q2049-Q2050	Doxorubicin	Part B MAC if incident to a physician's service or used in an implanted infusion pump. If other, DME MAC.
Q2052	IVIG Demonstration	DME MAC
Q3001	Supplies for Radiology Procedures	Part B MAC
Q3014	Telehealth Originating Site Facility Fee	Part B MAC
Q3027 - Q3028	Vaccines	Part B MAC
Q3031	Collagen Skin Test	Part B MAC
Q4001 - Q4051	Splints and Casts	Part B MAC
Q4074	Inhalation Drug	Part B MAC if incident to a physician's service. If other, DME MAC.
Q4081	Epoetin	Part B MAC
Q4082	Drug Subject to Competitive Acquisition Program	Part B MAC
Q4100 - Q4226	Skin Substitutes	Part B MAC
Q5001 - Q5010	Hospice Services	Part B MAC
Q5101-Q5118	Injection	Part B MAC if incident to a physician's service or used in an implanted infusion pump. If other, DME MAC.
Q9950 - Q9954	Imaging Agents	Part B MAC
Q9955 - Q9957	Microspheres	Part B MAC
Q9958 - Q9983	Imaging Agents & Radiology Supplies	Part B MAC
Q9991 - Q9992	Injection	Part B MAC if incident to a physician's service or used in an implanted infusion pump. If other, DME MAC.

HCPCS	DESCRIPTION	JURISDICTION
R0070 - R0076	Diagnostic Radiology Services	Part B MAC
V2020 - V2025	Frames	DME MAC
V2100 - V2513	Lenses	DME MAC
V2520 - V2523	Hydrophilic Contact Lenses	Part B MAC if incident to a physician's service. If other, DME MAC.
V2530 - V2531	Contact Lenses, Scleral	DME MAC
V2599	Contact Lens, Other Type	Part B MAC if incident to a physician's service. If other, DME MAC.
V2600 - V2615	Low Vision Aids	DME MAC
V2623 - V2629	Prosthetic Eyes	DME MAC
V2630 - V2632	Intraocular Lenses	Part B MAC
V2700 - V2780	Miscellaneous Vision Service	DME MAC
V2781	Progressive Lens	DME MAC
V2782 - V2784	Lenses	DME MAC
V2785	Processing—Corneal Tissue	Part B MAC
V2786	Lens	DME MAC
V2787 - V2788	Intraocular Lenses	Part B MAC
V2790	Amniotic Membrane	Part B MAC
V2797	Vision Supply	DME MAC
V2799	Miscellaneous Vision Service	Part B MAC if supply for an implanted prosthetic device. If other, DME MAC
V5008 - V5299	Hearing Services	Part B MAC
V5336	Repair/Modification of Augmentative Communicative System or Device	DME MAC
V5362 - V5364	Speech Screening	Part B MAC

APPENDIX B

GENERAL CORRECT CODING POLICIES FOR NATIONAL CORRECT CODING INITIATIVE POLICY MANUAL FOR MEDICARE SERVICES

Chapter I

Revision Date 1/1/2020

GENERAL CORRECT CODING POLICIES

A. Introduction

Healthcare providers *use* HCPCS/CPT codes to report medical services performed on patients to MACs. HCPCS (Healthcare Common Procedure Coding System) consists of Level I CPT (Current Procedural Terminology) codes and Level II codes. CPT codes are defined in the American Medical Association's (AMA*'s*) *CPT Manual,* which is updated and published annually. HCPCS Level II codes are defined by the Centers for Medicare & Medicaid Services (CMS) and are updated throughout the year as necessary. Changes in CPT codes are approved by the AMA CPT Editorial Panel which meets three times per year.

CPT and HCPCS Level II codes define medical and surgical procedures performed on patients. Some procedure codes are very specific *in* defining a single service [e.g., CPT code 93000 (electrocardiogram)], while other codes define procedures consisting of many services [e.g., CPT code 58263 (vaginal hysterectomy with removal of tube(s) and ovary(s) and repair of enterocele)]. Because many procedures can be performed by different approaches, different methods, or in combination with other procedures, there are often multiple HCPCS/CPT codes defining similar or related procedures.

CPT and HCPCS Level II code descriptors usually do not define all services included in a procedure. There are often services inherent in a procedure or group of procedures. For example, anesthesia services include certain preparation and monitoring services.

The CMS developed the NCCI *program* to prevent inappropriate payment of services that should not be reported together. Prior to April 1, 2012, NCCI PTP edits were placed into either the "Column One/Column Two Correct Coding Edit Table" or the "Mutually Exclusive Edit Table." However, on April 1, 2012, the edits in the "Mutually Exclusive Edit Table" were moved to the "Column One/Column Two Correct Coding Edit Table" so that all the NCCI PTP edits are currently contained in this single table. Combining the two tables simplifies researching NCCI edits and online use of NCCI tables.

Each edit table contains edits which are pairs of HCPCS/CPT codes that in general should not be reported together. Each edit has a Column One and Column Two HCPCS/CPT code. If a provider reports the two codes of an edit pair, the Column Two code is denied, and the Column One code is eligible for payment. However, if it is clinically appropriate to *use* an NCCI *PTP*-associated modifier, both the Column One and Column Two codes are eligible for payment. (NCCI *PTP*-associated modifiers and their appropriate use are discussed elsewhere in this chapter.)

When the NCCI was first established and during its early years, the "Column One/Column Two Correct Coding Edit Table" was termed the "Comprehensive/Component Edit Table." This latter terminology was a misnomer. Although the Column Two code is often a component of a more comprehensive Column One code, this relationship is not true for many edits. In the latter type of edit the code pair edit simply represents two codes that should not be reported together. For example, a provider shall not report a vaginal hysterectomy code and total abdominal hysterectomy code together.

In this chapter, Sections B–Q address various issues relating to NCCI PTP edits.

Medically Unlikely Edits (MUEs) prevent payment for a *potentially* inappropriate number/quantity of the same service on a single day. An MUE for a HCPCS/CPT code is the maximum number of units of service (UOS) *reportable* under most circumstances by the same provider for the same beneficiary on the same date of service. The ideal MUE value for a HCPCS/CPT code is one that allows the vast majority of appropriately coded claims to pass the MUE. *For more* information concerning MUEs, *see* Section V of this chapter.

In this Manual many policies are described *using* the term "physician." Unless *otherwise* indicated the use of this term does not restrict the *application of* policies to physicians only. *Rather, the policies apply* to all practitioners, hospitals, providers, or suppliers eligible to bill the relevant HCPCS/CPT codes pursuant to applicable portions of the Social Security Act (SSA) of 1965, the Code of Federal Regulations (CFR), and Medicare rules. In some sections of this Manual, the term "physician" would not include some of these entities because specific rules do not apply to them. For example, Anesthesia Rules [e.g., CMS Internet-only Manual Publication 100-04 (Medicare Claims Processing Manual), Chapter 12 (Physician/Nonphysician Practitioners), Section 50 (Payment for Anesthesiology Services)] and Global Surgery Rules [e.g., CMS Internet-only Manual, Publication 100-04 (Medicare Claims Processing Manual), Chapter 12 (Physician/Nonphysician Practitioners), Section 40 (Surgeons and Global Surgery)] do not apply to hospitals.

Providers reporting services under Medicare's hospital Outpatient Prospective Payment System (OPPS) shall report all services in accordance with appropriate Medicare Internet-only Manual (IOM) instructions.

Physicians must report services correctly. This manual discusses general coding principles in Chapter I and principles more relevant to other specific groups of HCPCS/CPT codes in the other chapters. There are certain types of improper coding that physicians must avoid.

Procedures shall be reported with the most comprehensive CPT code that describes the services performed. Physicians must not unbundle the services described by a HCPCS/CPT code. Some examples follow:

- A physician shall not report multiple HCPCS/CPT codes when a single comprehensive HCPCS/CPT code describes these services. For example if a physician performs a vaginal hysterectomy on a uterus weighing less than 250 grams with bilateral salpingo-oophorectomy, the physician shall report CPT code 58262 (Vaginal hysterectomy, for uterus 250 g or less; with removal of tube(s), and/or ovary(s)). The physician shall not report CPT code 58260 (Vaginal hysterectomy, for uterus 250 g or less;) plus CPT code 58720 (Salpingo-oophorectomy, complete or partial, unilateral or bilateral (separate procedure)).
- A physician shall not fragment a procedure into component parts. For example, if a physician performs an anal endoscopy with biopsy, the physician shall report CPT code 46606 (Anoscopy; with biopsy, single or multiple). It is improper to unbundle this procedure and report CPT code 46600 (Anoscopy; diagnostic,...) plus CPT code 45100 (Biopsy of anorectal wall, anal approach...). The latter code is not intended to be utilized with an endoscopic procedure code.
- A physician shall not unbundle a bilateral procedure code into two unilateral procedure codes. For example if a physician performs bilateral mammography, the physician shall report CPT code 77066 (Diagnostic mammography . . . bilateral). The physician shall not report CPT code 77065 (Diagnostic mammography . . . unilateral) with two *UOS* or 77065LT plus 77065RT.
- A physician shall not unbundle services that are integral to a more comprehensive procedure. For example, surgical access is integral to a surgical procedure. A physician shall not report CPT code 49000 (Exploratory laparotomy,...) when performing an open abdominal procedure such as a total abdominal colectomy (e.g., CPT code 44150).

Physicians must avoid downcoding. If a HCPCS/CPT code exists that describes the services performed, the physician must report this code rather than report a less comprehensive code with other codes describing the services not included in the less comprehensive code. For example if a physician performs a unilateral partial mastectomy with axillary lymphadenectomy, the provider shall report CPT code 19302 (Mastectomy, partial...; with axillary lymphadenectomy). A physician shall not report CPT code 19301 (Mastectomy, partial...) plus CPT code 38745 (Axillary lymphadenectomy; complete).

Physicians must avoid upcoding. A HCPCS/CPT code may be reported only if all services described by that code have been performed. For example, if a physician performs a superficial axillary lymphadenectomy (CPT code 38740), the physician shall not report CPT code 38745 (Axillary lymphadenectomy; complete).

Physicians must report *UOS* correctly. Each HCPCS/CPT code has a defined unit of service for reporting purposes. A physician shall not report *UOS* for a HCPCS/CPT code using a criterion that differs from the code's defined unit of service. For example, some therapy codes are reported in fifteen minute increments (e.g., CPT codes 97110-97124). Others are reported per session (e.g., CPT codes 92507, 92508). A physician shall not report a "per session" code using fifteen minute increments. CPT code 92507 or 92508 should be reported with one unit of service on a single date of service.

MUE and NCCI PTP edits are based on services provided by the same physician to the same beneficiary on the same date of service. Physicians shall not inconvenience beneficiaries nor increase risks to beneficiaries by performing services on different dates of service to avoid MUE or NCCI PTP edits.

In 2010 the *CPT Manual* modified the numbering of codes so that the sequence of codes as they appear in the *CPT Manual* does not necessarily correspond to a sequential numbering of codes. In the *National Correct Coding Initiative Policy Manual for Medicare Services,* use of a numerical range of codes reflects all codes that numerically fall within the range regardless of their sequential order in the *CPT Manual*.

This chapter addresses general coding principles, issues, and policies. Many of these principles, issues, and policies are addressed further in subsequent chapters dealing with specific groups of HCPCS/CPT codes. In this chapter examples are often *used* to clarify principles, issues, or policies. The examples do not represent the only codes to which the principles, issues, or policies apply.

B. Coding Based on Standards of Medical/ Surgical Practice

Most HCPCS/CPT code defined procedures include services that are integral to them. Some of these integral services have specific CPT codes for reporting the service when not performed as an integral part of another procedure. For example, CPT code 36000 (Introduction of needle or intracatheter into a vein) is integral to all nuclear medicine procedures requiring injection of a radiopharmaceutical into a vein. CPT code 36000 is not separately reportable with these types of nuclear medicine procedures. However, CPT code 36000 may be reported alone if the only service provided is the introduction of a needle into a vein. Other integral services do not have specific CPT codes. (For example, wound irrigation is integral to the treatment of all wounds and does not have a HCPCS/CPT code.) Services integral to HCPCS/CPT code defined procedures are included in those procedures based *upon* the standards of medical/surgical practice. It is inappropriate to separately report services that are integral to another procedure with that procedure.

Many NCCI PTP edits are based *upon* the standards of medical/ surgical practice. Services that are integral to another service are component parts of the more comprehensive service. When integral component services have their own HCPCS/CPT codes, NCCI PTP edits place the comprehensive service in column one and the component service in column two. Since a component service integral to a comprehensive service is not separately reportable, the column two code is not separately reportable with the column one code.

Some services are integral to large numbers of procedures. Other services are integral to a more limited number of procedures. Examples of services integral to a large number of procedures include:

- Cleansing, shaving and prepping of skin
- Draping and positioning of patient
- Insertion of intravenous access for medication administration

- Insertion of urinary catheter
- Sedative administration by the physician performing a procedure (see Chapter II, Anesthesia Services)
- Local, topical or regional anesthesia administered by the physician performing the procedure
- Surgical approach including identification of anatomical landmarks, incision, evaluation of the surgical field, debridement of traumatized tissue, lysis of adhesions, and isolation of structures limiting access to the surgical field such as bone, blood vessels, nerve, and muscles including stimulation for identification or monitoring
- Surgical cultures
- Wound irrigation
- Insertion and removal of drains, suction devices, and pumps into same site
- Surgical closure and dressings
- Application, management, and removal of postoperative dressings and analgesic devices (peri-incisional)
- Application of TENS unit
- Institution of Patient Controlled Anesthesia
- Preoperative, intraoperative and postoperative documentation, including photographs, drawings, dictation, or transcription as necessary to document the services provided
- *Imaging and/or ultrasound guidance*
- Surgical supplies, except for specific situations where CMS policy permits separate payment

Although other chapters in this Manual further address issues related to the standards of medical/surgical practice for the procedures covered by that chapter, it is not possible to discuss all NCCI PTP edits based *upon* the principle of the standards of medical/surgical practice *due to space limitations*. However, there are several general principles that can be applied to the edits as follows:

1. The component service is an accepted standard of care when performing the comprehensive service.
2. The component service is usually necessary to complete the comprehensive service.
3. The component service is not a separately distinguishable procedure when performed with the comprehensive service.

Specific examples of services that are not separately reportable because they are components of more comprehensive services follow:

Medical:

1. Since interpretation of cardiac rhythm is an integral component of the interpretation of an electrocardiogram, a rhythm strip is not separately reportable.
2. Since determination of ankle/brachial indices requires both upper and lower extremity Doppler studies, an upper extremity Doppler study is not separately reportable.
3. Since a cardiac stress test includes multiple electrocardiograms, an electrocardiogram is not separately reportable.

Surgical:

1. Since a myringotomy requires access to the tympanic membrane through the external auditory canal, removal of impacted cerumen from the external auditory canal is not separately reportable.
2. A "scout" bronchoscopy to assess the surgical field, anatomic landmarks, extent of disease, etc., is not separately reportable with an open pulmonary procedure such as a pulmonary lobectomy. By contrast, an initial diagnostic bronchoscopy is separately reportable. If the diagnostic bronchoscopy is performed at the same patient encounter as the open pulmonary procedure and does not duplicate an earlier diagnostic bronchoscopy by the same or another physician, the diagnostic bronchoscopy may be reported with modifier –58 appended to the open pulmonary procedure code to indicate a staged procedure. A cursory examination of the upper airway during a bronchoscopy with the bronchoscope shall not be reported separately as a laryngoscopy. However, separate endoscopies of anatomically distinct areas with different endoscopes may be reported separately (e.g., thoracoscopy and mediastinoscopy).
3. If an endoscopic procedure is performed at the same patient encounter as a non-endoscopic procedure to ensure no intraoperative injury occurred or verify the procedure was performed correctly, the endoscopic procedure is not separately reportable with the non-endoscopic procedure.
4. Since a colectomy requires exposure of the colon, the laparotomy and adhesiolysis to expose the colon are not separately reportable.

C. Medical/Surgical Package

Most medical and surgical procedures include pre-procedure, intra-procedure, and post-procedure work. When multiple procedures are performed at the same patient encounter, there is often overlap of the pre-procedure and post-procedure work. Payment methodologies for surgical procedures account for the overlap of the pre-procedure and post-procedure work.

The component elements of the pre-procedure and post-procedure work for each procedure are included component services of that procedure as a standard of medical/surgical practice. Some general guidelines follow:

1. Many invasive procedures require vascular and/or airway access. The work associated with obtaining the required access is included in the pre-procedure or intra-procedure work. The work associated with returning a patient to the appropriate post-procedure state is included in the post-procedure work.

Airway access is necessary for general anesthesia and is not separately reportable. There is no CPT code for elective endotracheal intubation. CPT code 31500 describes an emergency endotracheal intubation and shall not be reported for elective endotracheal intubation. Visualization of the airway is a component part of an endotracheal intubation, and CPT codes describing procedures that visualize the airway (e.g., nasal endoscopy, laryngoscopy, bronchoscopy) shall not be reported with an endotracheal intubation. These CPT codes describe diagnostic and therapeutic endoscopies, and it is a misuse of these codes to report visualization of the airway for endotracheal intubation.

Intravenous access (e.g., CPT codes 36000, 36400, 36410) is not separately reportable when performed with many types of procedures (e.g., surgical procedures, anesthesia procedures, radiological procedures requiring intravenous contrast, nuclear medicine procedures requiring intravenous radiopharmaceutical).

After vascular access is achieved, the access must be maintained by a slow infusion (e.g., saline) or injection of heparin or saline into a "lock." Since these services are necessary for maintenance of the vascular access, they are not separately reportable with the vascular access CPT codes or procedures requiring vascular access as a standard of medical/surgical practice. CPT codes 37211-37214 (Transcatheter therapy with infusion for thrombolysis) shall not be reported for use of an anticoagulant to maintain vascular access.

The global surgical package includes the administration of fluids and drugs during the operative procedure. CPT codes 96360-96377 shall not be reported separately for that operative procedure. Under OPPS, the administration of fluids and drugs during or for an operative procedure are included services and are not separately reportable (e.g., CPT codes 96360-96377).

When a procedure requires more invasive vascular access services (e.g., central venous access, pulmonary artery access), the more invasive vascular service is separately reportable if it is not typical of the procedure and the work of the more invasive vascular service has not been included in the valuation of the procedure.

Insertion of a central venous access device (e.g., central venous catheter, pulmonary artery catheter) requires passage of a catheter through central venous vessels and, in the case of a pulmonary artery catheter, through the right atrium and ventricle. These services often require the use of fluoroscopic guidance. Separate reporting of CPT codes for right heart catheterization, selective venous catheterization, or pulmonary artery catheterization is not appropriate when reporting a CPT code for insertion of a central venous access device. Since CPT code 77001 describes fluoroscopic guidance for central venous access device procedures, CPT codes for more general fluoroscopy (e.g., 76000, 76001, 77002) shall not be reported separately. (CPT code 76001 was deleted January 1, 2019.)

2. Medicare Anesthesia Rules prevent separate payment for anesthesia services by the same physician performing a surgical or medical procedure. The physician performing a surgical or medical procedure shall not report CPT codes 96360-96377 for the administration of anesthetic agents during the procedure. If it is medically reasonable and necessary that a separate provider (anesthesia practitioner) perform anesthesia services (e.g., monitored anesthesia care) for a surgical or medical procedure, a separate anesthesia service may be reported by the second provider.

Under *the* OPPS, anesthesia for a surgical procedure is an included service and is not separately reportable. For example, a provider shall not report CPT codes 96360-96377 for anesthesia services.

When anesthesia services are not separately reportable, physicians and facilities shall not unbundle components of anesthesia and report them in lieu of an anesthesia code.

3. If an endoscopic procedure is performed at the same patient encounter as a non-endoscopic procedure to ensure *that* no intraoperative injury occurred or *to* verify *that* the procedure was performed correctly, the endoscopic procedure is not separately reportable with the non-endoscopic procedure.
4. Many procedures require cardiopulmonary monitoring either by the physician performing the procedure or an anesthesia practitioner. Since these services are integral to the procedure, they are not separately reportable. Examples of these services include cardiac monitoring, pulse oximetry, and ventilation management (e.g., 93000-93010, 93040-93042, 94760, 94761, 94770).
5. A biopsy performed at the time of another more extensive procedure (e.g., excision, destruction, removal) is separately reportable under specific circumstances.

If the biopsy is performed on a separate lesion, it is separately reportable. This situation may be reported with anatomic modifiers or modifier -59 *or XS*.

The biopsy is not separately reportable if *used* for the purpose of assessing margins of resection or verifying resectability.

If a biopsy is performed and submitted for pathologic evaluation that will be completed after the more extensive procedure is performed, the biopsy is not separately reportable with the more extensive procedure.

6. Exposure and exploration of the surgical field is integral to an operative procedure and is not separately reportable. For example, an exploratory laparotomy (CPT code 49000) is not separately reportable with an intra-abdominal procedure. If exploration of the surgical field results in additional procedures other than the primary procedure, the additional procedures may generally be reported separately. However, a procedure designated by the CPT code descriptor as a "separate procedure" is not separately reportable if performed in a region anatomically related to the other procedure(s) through the same skin incision, orifice, or surgical approach.
7. If a definitive surgical procedure requires access through diseased tissue (e.g., necrotic skin, abscess, hematoma, seroma), a separate service for this access (e.g., debridement, incision and drainage) is not separately reportable. Types of procedures to which this principle applies include, but are not limited to, -ectomy, -otomy, excision, resection, -plasty, insertion, revision, replacement, relocation, removal or closure. For example, debridement of skin and subcutaneous tissue at the site of an abdominal incision made to perform an intra-abdominal procedure is not separately reportable. (See Chapter IV, Section H (General Policy Statements), Subsection #11 for guidance on reporting debridement with open fractures and dislocations.)
8. If removal, destruction, or other form of elimination of a lesion requires coincidental elimination of other pathology, only the primary procedure may be reported. For example, if an area of pilonidal disease contains an abscess, incision and drainage of the abscess during the procedure to excise the area of pilonidal disease is not separately reportable.
9. An excision and removal (–ectomy) includes the incision and opening (–otomy) of the organ. A HCPCS/CPT code for an –otomy procedure shall not be reported with an –ectomy code for the same organ.
10. Multiple approaches to the same procedure are mutually exclusive of one another and shall not be reported separately.

For example, both a vaginal hysterectomy and abdominal hysterectomy should not be reported separately.

11. If a procedure *using* one approach fails and is converted to a procedure *using* a different approach, only the completed procedure may be reported. For example, if a laparoscopic hysterectomy is converted to an open hysterectomy, only the open hysterectomy procedure code may be reported.
12. If a laparoscopic procedure fails and is converted to an open procedure, the physician shall not report a diagnostic laparoscopy in lieu of the failed laparoscopic procedure. For example, if a laparoscopic cholecystectomy is converted to an open cholecystectomy, the physician shall not report the failed laparoscopic cholecystectomy nor a diagnostic laparoscopy.

13. If a diagnostic endoscopy is the basis for and precedes an open procedure, the diagnostic endoscopy may be reported with modifier -58 appended to the open procedure code. However, the medical record must document the medical reasonableness and necessity for the diagnostic endoscopy. A scout endoscopy to assess anatomic landmarks and extent of disease is not separately reportable with an open procedure. When an endoscopic procedure fails and is converted to another surgical procedure, only the completed surgical procedure may be reported. The endoscopic procedure is not separately reportable with the completed surgical procedure.
14. Treatment of complications of primary surgical procedures is separately reportable with some limitations. The global surgical package for an operative procedure includes all intra-operative services that are normally a usual and necessary part of the procedure. Additionally the global surgical package includes all medical and surgical services required of the surgeon during the postoperative period of the surgery to treat complications that do not require return to the operating room. Thus, treatment of a complication of a primary surgical procedure is not separately reportable (1) if it represents usual and necessary care in the operating room during the procedure or (2) if it occurs postoperatively and does not require return to the operating room. For example, control of hemorrhage is a usual and necessary component of a surgical procedure in the operating room and is not separately reportable. Control of postoperative hemorrhage is also not separately reportable unless the patient must be returned to the operating room for treatment. In the latter case, the control of hemorrhage may be separately reportable with modifier -78.

D. Evaluation and Management (E&M) Services

Medicare Global Surgery Rules define the rules for reporting evaluation and management (E&M) services with procedures covered by these rules. This section summarizes some of the rules.

All procedures on the Medicare Physician Fee Schedule are assigned a global period of 000, 010, 090, XXX, YYY, ZZZ, or MMM. The global concept does not apply to XXX procedures. The global period for YYY procedures is defined by the *MAC*. All procedures with a global period of ZZZ are related to another procedure, and the applicable global period for the ZZZ code is determined by the related procedure. Procedures with a global period of MMM are maternity procedures.

Since NCCI PTP edits are applied to same day services by the same provider to the same beneficiary, certain Global Surgery Rules are applicable to NCCI. An E&M service is separately reportable on the same date of service as a procedure with a global period of 000, 010, or 090 under limited circumstances.

If a procedure has a global period of 090 days, it is defined as a major surgical procedure. If an E&M *service* is performed on the same date of service as a major surgical procedure for the purpose of deciding whether to perform this surgical procedure, the E&M service is separately reportable with modifier -57. Other preoperative E&M services on the same date of service as a major surgical procedure are included in the global payment for the procedure and are not separately reportable. NCCI does not contain edits based on this rule because *MACs* have separate edits.

If a procedure has a global period of 000 or 010 days, it is defined as a minor surgical procedure. In general, E&M services *performed* on *a* same date of service as the minor surgical procedure are included in the payment for the procedure. The decision to perform a minor surgical procedure is included in the payment for the minor surgical procedure and shall not be reported separately as an E&M service. However, a significant and separately identifiable E&M service unrelated to the decision to perform the minor surgical procedure is separately reportable with modifier -25. The E&M service and minor surgical procedure do not require different diagnoses. If a minor surgical procedure is performed on a new patient, the same rules for reporting E&M services apply. The fact that the patient is "new" to the provider is not sufficient alone to justify reporting an E&M service on the same date of service as a minor surgical procedure. NCCI contains many, but not all, possible edits based on these principles.

Example: If a physician determines that a new patient with head trauma requires sutures, confirms the allergy and immunization status, obtains informed consent, and performs the repair, an E&M service is not separately reportable. However, if the physician also performs a medically reasonable and necessary full neurological examination, an E&M service may be separately reportable.

For major and minor surgical procedures, postoperative E&M services related to recovery from the surgical procedure during the postoperative period are included in the global surgical package as are E&M services related to complications of the surgery. Postoperative visits unrelated to the diagnosis for which the surgical procedure was performed unless related to a complication of surgery may be reported separately on the same day as a surgical procedure with modifier -24 ("Unrelated Evaluation and Management Service by the Same Physician or Other Qualified Health Care Professional During a Postoperative Period").

Procedures with a global surgery indicator of "XXX" are not covered by these rules. Many of these "XXX" procedures are performed by physicians and have inherent pre-procedure, intra-procedure, and post-procedure work usually performed each time the procedure is completed. This work shall not be reported as a separate E&M code. Other "XXX" procedures are not usually performed by a physician and have no physician work relative value units associated with them. A physician shall not report a separate E&M code with these procedures for the supervision of others performing the procedure or for the interpretation of the procedure. With most "XXX" procedures, the physician may, however, perform a significant and separately identifiable E&M service on the same date of service which may be reported by appending modifier -25 to the E&M code. This E&M service may be related to the same diagnosis necessitating performance of the "XXX" procedure but cannot include any work inherent in the "XXX" procedure, supervision of others performing the "XXX" procedure, or time for interpreting the result of the "XXX" procedure. Appending modifier -25 to a significant, separately identifiable E&M service when performed on the same date of service as an "XXX" procedure is correct coding.

E. Modifiers and Modifier Indicators

1. The AMA *CPT Manual* and CMS define modifiers that may be appended to HCPCS/CPT codes to provide additional information about the services rendered. Modifiers consist of two alphanumeric characters.

Modifiers may be appended to HCPCS/CPT codes only if the clinical circumstances justify the use of the modifier. A modifier shall not be appended to a HCPCS/CPT code solely to bypass an NCCI PTP edit if the clinical circumstances do not justify its use. If the Medicare program imposes restrictions on the use of a modifier, the modifier may only be used to bypass an NCCI PTP edit if the Medicare restrictions are fulfilled.

Modifiers that may be used under appropriate clinical circumstances to bypass an NCCI edit include:

Anatomic modifiers: E1-E4, FA, F1-F9, TA, T1-T9, LT, RT, LC, LD, RC, LM, RI

Global surgery modifiers: -24, -25, -57, -58, -78, -79

Other modifiers: -27,-59, -91, XE, XS, XP, XU

Modifiers -76 ("Repeat Procedure or Service by Same Physician") and 77 ("Repeat Procedure by Another Physician") are not NCCI *PTP*-associated modifiers. Use of either of these modifiers does not bypass an NCCI PTP edit.

Each NCCI PTP edit has an assigned modifier indicator. A modifier indicator of "0" indicates that NCCI *PTP*-associated modifiers cannot be used to bypass the edit. A modifier indicator of "1" indicates that NCCI *PTP*-associated modifiers may be used to bypass an edit under appropriate circumstances. A modifier indicator of "9" indicates that the edit has been deleted, and the modifier indicator is not relevant.

It is very important that NCCI *PTP*-associated modifiers only be used when appropriate. In general these circumstances relate to separate patient encounters, separate anatomic sites or separate specimens. (See subsequent discussion of modifiers in this section.) Most edits involving paired organs or structures (e.g., eyes, ears, extremities, lungs, kidneys) have NCCI PTP modifier indicators of "1" because the two codes of the code pair edit may be reported if performed on the contralateral organs or structures. Most of these code pairs should not be reported with NCCI *PTP*-associated modifiers when performed on the ipsilateral organ or structure unless there is a specific coding rationale to bypass the edit. The existence of the NCCI PTP edit indicates that the two codes generally cannot be reported together unless the two corresponding procedures are performed at two separate patient encounters or two separate anatomic locations. However, if the two corresponding procedures are performed at the same patient encounter and in contiguous structures *in the same organ or anatomic region*, NCCI *PTP*-associated modifiers generally should not be *used*.

The appropriate use of most of these modifiers is straightforward. However, further explanation is provided about modifiers -25, -58, and -59. Although modifier -22 is not a modifier that bypasses an NCCI PTP edit, its use is occasionally relevant to an NCCI PTP edit and is discussed below.

a) **Modifier -22:** Modifier -22 is defined by the *CPT Manual* as "Increased Procedural Services." This modifier shall not be reported unless the service(s) performed is(are) substantially more extensive than the usual service(s) included in the procedure described by the HCPCS/CPT code reported.

Occasionally, a provider may perform two procedures that should not be reported together based on an NCCI PTP edit. If the edit allows use of NCCI *PTP*-associated modifiers to bypass it and the clinical circumstances justify use of one of these modifiers, both services may be reported with the NCCI-associated modifier. However, if the NCCI PTP edit does not allow use of NCCI *PTP*-associated modifiers to bypass it and the procedure qualifies as an unusual procedural service, the physician may report the Column One HCPCS/CPT code of the NCCI PTP edit with modifier -22. The MAC may then evaluate the unusual procedural service to determine whether additional payment is justified.

For example, CMS limits payment for CPT code 69990 (Microsurgical techniques, requiring use of operating microscope . . .) to procedures listed in the Internet-only Manual (IOM) (*Claims Processing Manual*, Publication 100-04, 12-§20.4.5). If a physician reports CPT code 69990 with two other CPT codes and one of the codes is not on this list, an NCCI PTP edit with the code not on the list will prevent payment for CPT code 69990. Claims processing systems do not determine which procedure is linked with CPT code 69990. In situations such as this, the physician may submit his claim to the local MAC for readjudication appending modifier -22 to the CPT code. Although the MAC cannot override an NCCI PTP edit that does not allow use of NCCI *PTP*-associated modifiers, the MAC has discretion to adjust payment to include use of the operating microscope based on modifier -22.

b) **Modifier -25:** The *CPT Manual* defines modifier -25 as a "Significant, Separately Identifiable Evaluation and Management Service by the Same Physician or Other Qualified Health Care Professional on the Same Day of the Procedure or Other Service." Modifier -25 may be appended to an evaluation and management (E&M) CPT code to indicate that the E&M service is significant and separately identifiable from other services reported on the same date of service. The E&M service may be related to the same or different diagnosis as the other procedure(s).

Modifier -25 may be appended to E&M services reported with minor surgical procedures (*with* global period*s* of 000 or 010 days) or procedures not covered by *Global Surgery rules (with a* global indicator of XXX). Since minor surgical procedures and XXX procedures include pre-procedure, intra-procedure, and post-procedure work inherent in the procedure, the provider shall not report an E&M service for this work. Furthermore, Medicare Global Surgery Rules prevent the reporting of a separate E&M service for the work associated with the decision to perform a minor surgical procedure *regardless of* whether the patient is a new or established patient.

c) **Modifier -58:** Modifier -58 is defined by the *CPT Manual* as a "Staged or Related Procedure or Service by the Same Physician or Other Qualified Health Care Professional During the Postoperative Period." It may be used to indicate that a procedure was followed by a second procedure during the post-operative period of the first procedure. This situation may occur because the second procedure was planned prospectively, was more extensive than the first procedure, or was therapy after a diagnostic surgical service. Use of modifier -58 will bypass NCCI PTP edits that allow use of NCCI *PTP*-associated modifiers.

If a diagnostic endoscopic procedure results in the decision to perform an open procedure, both procedures may be reported with modifier -58 appended to the HCPCS/CPT code for the open procedure. However, if the endoscopic procedure preceding an open procedure is a "scout" procedure to assess anatomic landmarks and/or extent of disease, it is not separately reportable.

Diagnostic endoscopy is never separately reportable with another endoscopic procedure of the same organ(s) *or anatomic region* when performed at the same patient encounter. Similarly, diagnostic laparoscopy is never separately reportable with a surgical laparoscopic procedure of the same body cavity when performed at the same patient encounter.

If a planned laparoscopic procedure fails and is converted to an open procedure, only the open procedure may be reported. The failed laparoscopic procedure is not separately reportable. The NCCI contains many, but not all, edits bundling laparoscopic procedures into open procedures. Since the number of possible code combinations bundling a laparoscopic procedure into an open procedure is much greater than the number of such edits in NCCI, the principle stated in this paragraph is applicable regardless of whether the selected code pair combination is included in the NCCI tables. A provider shall not select laparoscopic and open HCPCS/CPT codes to report because the combination is not included in the NCCI tables.

d) Modifier -59: Modifier -59 is an important NCCI *PTP*-associated modifier that is often used incorrectly. For the NCCI its primary purpose is to indicate that two or more procedures are performed at different anatomic sites or different patient encounters. One function of NCCI PTP edits is to prevent payment for codes that report overlapping services except in those instances where the services are "separate and distinct." Modifier -59 shall only be used if no other modifier more appropriately describes the relationships of the two or more procedure codes. The *CPT Manual* defines modifier -59 as follows:

Modifier -59: Distinct Procedural Service: Under certain circumstances, it may be necessary to indicate that a procedure or service was distinct or independent from other non E/M services performed on the same day. Modifier -59 is used to identify procedures/services other than E/M services that are not normally reported together, but are appropriate under the circumstances. Documentation must support a different session, different procedure or surgery, different site or organ system, separate incision/excision, separate lesion, or separate injury (or area of injury in extensive injuries) not ordinarily encountered or performed on the same day by the same individual. However, when another already established modifier is appropriate, it should be used rather than modifier -59. Only if no more descriptive modifier is available, and the use of modifier -59 best explains the circumstances, should modifier -59 be used. Note: Modifier -59 should not be appended to an E/M service. To report a separate and distinct E/M service with a non-E/M service performed on the same date, see modifier -25.

Modifier -59 and other NCCI-associated modifiers should ***NOT*** *be used to bypass a PTP edit unless the proper criteria for use of the modifier are met. Documentation in the medical record must satisfy the criteria required by any NCCI-associated modifier that is used.*

Modifier -59 or XS is used appropriately for different anatomic sites during the same encounter only when procedures which are not ordinarily performed or encountered on the same day are performed on different organs, or different anatomic regions, or in limited situations on different, non-contiguous lesions in different anatomic regions of the same organ.

NCCI PTP edits define when two procedure HCPCS/CPT codes may not be reported together except under special circumstances. If an edit allows use of NCCI *PTP*-associated modifiers, the two procedure codes may be reported together when the two procedures are performed at different anatomic sites or different patient encounters. MAC processing systems *use* NCCI *PTP*-associated modifiers to allow payment of both codes of an edit. Modifier -59 and other NCCI *PTP*-associated modifiers shall NOT be used to bypass an NCCI PTP edit unless the proper criteria for use of the modifier are met. Documentation in the medical record must satisfy the criteria required by any NCCI *PTP*-associated modifier used.

Some examples of the appropriate use of modifier -59 are contained in the individual chapter policies.

One of the common misuses of modifier -59 is related to the portion of the definition of modifier -59 allowing its use to describe "different procedure or surgery." The code descriptors of the two codes of a code pair edit usually represent different procedures or surgeries. The edit indicates that the two procedures/surgeries cannot be reported together if performed at the same anatomic site and same patient encounter. The provider cannot use modifier -59 for such an edit based on the two codes being different procedures/surgeries. However, if the two procedures/surgeries are performed at separate anatomic sites or at separate patient encounters on the same date of service, modifier -59 may be appended to indicate that they are different procedures/surgeries on that date of service.

There are several exceptions to this general principle about misuse of modifier -59 that apply to some code pair edits for procedures performed at the same patient encounter.

(1) When a diagnostic procedure precedes a surgical or non-surgical therapeutic procedure and is the basis on which the decision to perform the surgical or non-surgical therapeutic procedure is made, that diagnostic procedure may be considered to be a separate and distinct procedure as long as (a) it occurs before the therapeutic procedure and is not interspersed with services that are required for the therapeutic intervention; (b) it clearly provides the information needed to decide whether to proceed with the therapeutic procedure; and (c) it does not constitute a service that would have otherwise been required during the therapeutic intervention. If the diagnostic procedure is an inherent component of the surgical or non-surgical therapeutic procedure, it shall not be reported separately.
(2) When a diagnostic procedure follows a surgical procedure or non-surgical therapeutic procedure, that diagnostic procedure may be considered to be a separate and distinct procedure as long as (a) it occurs after the completion of the therapeutic procedure and is not interspersed with or otherwise commingled with services that are only required for the therapeutic intervention, and (b) it does not constitute a service that would have otherwise been required during the therapeutic intervention. If the post-procedure diagnostic procedure is an inherent component or otherwise included (or not separately payable) post-procedure service of the surgical procedure or non-surgical therapeutic procedure, it shall not be reported separately.
(3) There is an appropriate use for modifier -59 that is applicable only to codes for which the unit of service is a measure of time (e.g., per 15 minutes, per hour). If two separate and distinct timed services are provided in separate and distinct time blocks, modifier -59 may be used to

identify the services. The separate and distinct time blocks for the two services may be sequential to one another or split. When the two services are split, the time block for one service may be followed by a time block for the second service followed by another time block for the first service. All Medicare rules for reporting timed services are applicable. For example, the total time is calculated for all related timed services performed. The number of reportable *UOS* is based on the total time, and these *UOS* are allocated between the HCPCS/CPT codes for the individual services performed. The physician is not permitted to perform multiple services, each for the minimal reportable time, and report each of these as separate *UOS* (e.g., a physician or therapist performs eight minutes of neuromuscular reeducation (CPT code 97112) and eight minutes of therapeutic exercises (CPT code 97110). Since the physician or therapist performed 16 minutes of related timed services, only one unit of service may be reported for one, not each, of these codes.)

Use of modifier -59 to indicate different procedures/surgeries does not require a different diagnosis for each HCPCS/CPT coded procedure/surgery. Additionally, different diagnoses are not adequate criteria for use of modifier -59. The HCPCS/CPT codes remain bundled unless the procedures/surgeries are performed at different anatomic sites or separate patient encounters.

From an NCCI perspective, the definition of different anatomic sites includes different organs, different anatomic regions, or different lesions in the same organ. It does not include treatment of contiguous structures *in* the same organ *or anatomic region*. For example, treatment of the nail, nail bed, and adjacent soft tissue constitutes treatment of a single anatomic site. Treatment of posterior segment structures in the ipsilateral eye constitutes treatment of a single anatomic site.

If the same procedure is performed at different anatomic sites, it does not necessarily imply that a HCPCS/CPT code may be reported with more than one unit of service for the procedure. Determining whether additional UOS may be reported depends in part upon the HCPCS/CPT code descriptor including the definition of the code's unit of service, when present.

Example #1: The Column One/Column Two code edit with column one CPT code 38221 (Diagnostic bone marrow biopsy) and Column Two CPT code 38220 (Diagnostic bone marrow, aspiration) includes two distinct procedures when performed at separate anatomic sites (e.g., contralateral iliac bones) or separate patient encounters. In these circumstances, it would be acceptable to use modifier -59. However, if both 38221 and 38220 are performed on the same iliac bone at the same patient encounter which is the usual practice, modifier -59 shall NOT be used. Although CMS does not allow separate payment for CPT code 38220 with CPT code 38221 when bone marrow aspiration and biopsy are performed on the same iliac bone at a single patient encounter, a physician may report CPT code 38222 Diagnostic bone marrow; biopsy(ies) and aspiration(s).

Example #2: The *PTP* edit with Column One CPT code 11055 (paring or cutting of benign hyperkeratotic lesion ...) and Column Two CPT code 11720 (Debridement of nail(s) by any method; 1 to 5) may be bypassed with modifier -59 only if the paring/cutting of a benign hyperkeratotic lesion is performed on a different digit (e.g., toe) than one that has nail debridement. Modifier -59 shall not be used to bypass the edit if the two procedures are performed on the same digit.

e) Modifiers XE, XS, XP, XU: These modifiers were effective January 1, 2015. These modifiers were developed to provide greater reporting specificity in situations where modifier -59 was previously reported and may be utilized in lieu of modifier -59 whenever possible. (Modifier -59 should only be *used* if no other more specific modifier is appropriate.) Although NCCI will eventually require use of these modifiers rather than modifier -59 with certain edits, physicians may begin using them for claims with dates of service on or after January 1, 2015. The modifiers are defined as follows:

XE – "Separate Encounter, A service that is distinct because it occurred during a separate encounter" This modifier shall only be used to describe separate encounters on the same date of service.

XS – "Separate Structure, A service that is distinct because it was performed on a separate organ/structure"

XP – "Separate Practitioner, A service that is distinct because it was performed by a different practitioner"

XU – "Unusual Non-Overlapping Service, The use of a service that is distinct because it does not overlap usual components of the main service"

F. Standard Preparation/Monitoring Services for Anesthesia

With few exceptions anesthesia HCPCS/CPT codes do not specify the mode of anesthesia for a particular procedure. Regardless of the mode of anesthesia, preparation and monitoring services are not separately reportable with anesthesia service HCPCS/CPT codes when performed in association with the anesthesia service. However, if the provider of the anesthesia service performs one or more of these services prior to and unrelated to the anticipated anesthesia service or after the patient is released from the anesthesia practitioner's postoperative care, the service may be separately reportable with modifier*s* -59 *or X {EU}*.

G. Anesthesia Service Included in the Surgical Procedure

Under the CMS Anesthesia Rules, with limited exceptions, Medicare does not allow separate payment for anesthesia services performed by the physician who also furnishes the medical or surgical service. In this case, payment for the anesthesia service is included in the payment for the medical or surgical procedure. For example, separate payment is not allowed for the physician's performance of local, regional, or most other anesthesia including nerve blocks if the physician also performs the medical or surgical procedure. However, Medicare allows separate reporting for moderate conscious sedation services (CPT codes 99151-99153) when provided by same physician performing a medical or surgical procedure except for those procedures listed in Appendix G of the *CPT Manual*.

CPT codes describing anesthesia services (00100-01999) or services that are bundled into anesthesia shall not be reported in addition to the surgical or medical procedure requiring the anesthesia services if performed by the same physician. Examples of improperly reported services that are bundled into the anesthesia service when anesthesia is provided by the physician performing the medical or surgical procedure include introduction of needle or intracatheter into a vein (CPT code 36000), venipuncture (CPT code 36410), intravenous infusion/injection (CPT codes 96360-96368, 96374-96377) or cardiac assessment (e.g., CPT codes 93000-93010, 93040-93042). However, if these services are not related to the delivery of an anesthetic agent, or are not an inherent component of the procedure or global service, they may be reported separately.

The physician performing a surgical or medical procedure shall not report an epidural/subarachnoid injection (CPT codes 62320-62327) or nerve block (CPT codes 64400-64530) for anesthesia for that procedure.

H. HCPCS/CPT Procedure Code Definition

The HCPCS/CPT code descriptors of two codes are often the basis of an NCCI PTP edit. If two HCPCS/CPT codes describe redundant services, they shall not be reported separately. Several general principles follow:

1. A family of CPT codes may include a CPT code followed by one or more indented CPT codes. The first CPT code descriptor includes a semicolon. The portion of the descriptor of the first code in the family preceding the semicolon is a common part of the descriptor for each subsequent code of the family. For example,

   CPT code 70120   Radiologic examination, mastoids; less than 3 views per side
   CPT code 70130   Complete, minimum of 3 views per side

   The portion of the descriptor preceding the semicolon ("Radiologic examination, mastoids") is common to both CPT codes 70120 and 70130. The difference between the two codes is the portion of the descriptors following the semicolon. Often as in this case, two codes from a family may not be reported separately. A physician cannot report CPT codes 70120 and 70130 for a procedure performed on ipsilateral mastoids at the same patient encounter. It is important to recognize, however, that there are numerous circumstances when it may be appropriate to report more than one code from a family of codes. For example, CPT codes 70120 and 70130 may be reported separately if the two procedures are performed on contralateral mastoids or at two separate patient encounters on the same date of service.

2. If a HCPCS/CPT code is reported, it includes all components of the procedure defined by the descriptor. For example, CPT code 58291 includes a vaginal hysterectomy with "removal of tube(s) and/or ovary(s)." A physician cannot report a salpingo-oophorectomy (CPT code 58720) separately with CPT code 58291.
3. CPT code descriptors often define correct coding relationships where two codes may not be reported separately with one another at the same anatomic site and/or same patient encounter. A few examples follow:
   a) A "partial" procedure is not separately reportable with a "complete" procedure.
   b) A "partial" procedure is not separately reportable with a "total" procedure.
   c) A "unilateral" procedure is not separately reportable with a "bilateral" procedure.
   d) A "single" procedure is not separately reportable with a "multiple" procedure.
   e) A "with" procedure is not separately reportable with a "without" procedure.
   f) An "initial" procedure is not separately reportable with a "subsequent" procedure.

I. *CPT Manual* and CMS Coding Manual Instructions

CMS often publishes coding instructions in its rules, manuals, and notices. Physicians must utilize these instructions when reporting services rendered to Medicare patients.

The *CPT Manual* also includes coding instructions which may be found in the "Introduction," individual chapters, and appendices. In individual chapters the instructions may appear at the beginning of a chapter, at the beginning of a subsection of the chapter, or after specific CPT codes. Physicians should follow *CPT Manual* instructions unless CMS has provided different coding or reporting instructions.

The American Medical Association publishes *CPT Assistant* which contains coding guidelines. CMS does not review nor approve the information in this publication. In the development of NCCI PTP edits, CMS occasionally disagrees with the information in this publication. If a physician *uses* information from *CPT Assistant* to report services rendered to Medicare patients, it is possible that MACs may *use* different criteria to process claims.

J. CPT "Separate Procedure" Definition

If a CPT code descriptor includes the term "separate procedure," the CPT code may not be reported separately with a related procedure. CMS interprets this designation to prohibit the separate reporting of a "separate procedure" when performed with another procedure in an anatomically related region often through the same skin incision, orifice, or surgical approach.

A CPT code with the "separate procedure" designation may be reported with another procedure if it is performed at a separate patient encounter on the same date of service or at the same patient encounter in an anatomically unrelated area often through a separate skin incision, orifice, or surgical approach. Modifiers -59 or *-X {ES} (or* a more specific modifier e.g., anatomic modifier) may be appended to the "separate procedure" CPT code to indicate that it qualifies as a separately reportable service.

K. Family of Codes

The *CPT Manual* often contains a group of codes that describe related procedures that may be performed in various combinations. Some codes describe limited component services, and other codes describe various combinations of component services. Physicians must *use* several principles in selecting the correct code to report:

1. A HCPCS/CPT code may be reported if and only if all services described by the code are performed.

2. The HCPCS/CPT code describing the services performed shall be reported. A physician shall not report multiple codes corresponding to component services if a single comprehensive code describes the services performed. There are limited exceptions to this rule which are specifically identified in this Manual.
3. HCPCS/CPT code(s) corresponding to component service(s) of other more comprehensive HCPCS/CPT code(s) shall not be reported separately with the more comprehensive HCPCS/CPT code(s) that include the component service(s).
4. If the HCPCS/CPT codes do not correctly describe the procedure(s) performed, the physician shall report a "not otherwise specified" CPT code rather than a HCPCS/CPT code that most closely describes the procedure(s) performed.

L. More Extensive Procedure

The *CPT Manual* often describes groups of similar codes differing in the complexity of the service. Unless services are performed at separate patient encounters or at separate anatomic sites, the less complex service is included in the more complex service and is not separately reportable. Several examples of this principle follow:

1. If two procedures only differ in that one is described as a "simple" procedure and the other as a "complex" procedure, the "simple" procedure is included in the "complex" procedure and is not separately reportable unless the two procedures are performed at separate patient encounters or at separate anatomic sites.
2. If two procedures only differ in that one is described as a "simple" procedure and the other as a "complicated" procedure, the "simple" procedure is included in the "complicated" procedure and is not separately reportable unless the two procedures are performed at separate patient encounters or at separate anatomic sites.
3. If two procedures only differ in that one is described as a "limited" procedure and the other as a "complete" procedure, the "limited" procedure is included in the "complete" procedure and is not separately reportable unless the two procedures are performed at separate patient encounters or at separate anatomic sites.
4. If two procedures only differ in that one is described as an "intermediate" procedure and the other as a "comprehensive" procedure, the "intermediate" procedure is included in the "comprehensive" procedure and is not separately reportable unless the two procedures are performed at separate patient encounters or at separate anatomic sites.
5. If two procedures only differ in that one is described as a "superficial" procedure and the other as a "deep" procedure, the "superficial" procedure is included in the "deep" procedure and is not separately reportable unless the two procedures are performed at separate patient encounters or at separate anatomic sites.
6. If two procedures only differ in that one is described as an "incomplete" procedure and the other as a "complete" procedure, the "incomplete" procedure is included in the "complete" procedure and is not separately reportable unless the two procedures are performed at separate patient encounters or at separate anatomic sites.
7. If two procedures only differ in that one is described as an "external" procedure and the other as an "internal" procedure, the "external" procedure is included in the "internal" procedure and is not separately reportable unless the two procedures are performed at separate patient encounters or at separate anatomic sites.

M. Sequential Procedure

Some surgical procedures may be performed by different surgical approaches. If an initial surgical approach to a procedure fails and a second surgical approach is *used* at the same patient encounter, only the HCPCS/CPT code corresponding to the second surgical approach may be reported. If there are different HCPCS/CPT codes for the two different surgical approaches, the two procedures are considered "sequential," and only the HCPCS/CPT code corresponding to the second surgical approach may be reported. For example, a physician may begin a cholecystectomy procedure utilizing a laparoscopic approach and have to convert the procedure to an open abdominal approach. Only the CPT code for the open cholecystectomy may be reported. The CPT code for the failed laparoscopic cholecystectomy is not separately reportable.

N. Laboratory Panel

The *CPT Manual* defines organ and disease specific panels of laboratory tests. If a laboratory performs all tests included in one of these panels, the laboratory shall report the CPT code for the panel. If the laboratory repeats one of these component tests as a medically reasonable and necessary service on the same date of service, the CPT code corresponding to the repeat laboratory test may be reported with modifier -91 appended (See Chapter X, Section C [Organ or Disease Oriented Panels]).

O. Misuse of Column Two Code with Column One Code (Misuse of Code Edit Rationale)

CMS manuals and instructions often describe groups of HCPCS/CPT codes that should not be reported together for the Medicare program. Edits based on these instructions are often included as misuse of Column Two code with Column One code.

A HCPCS/CPT code descriptor does not include exhaustive information about the code. Physicians who are not familiar with a HCPCS/CPT code may incorrectly report the code in a context different than intended. The NCCI has identified HCPCS/CPT codes that are incorrectly reported with other HCPCS/CPT codes as a result of the misuse of the Column Two code with the Column One code. If these edits allow use of NCCI *PTP*-associated modifiers (modifier indicator of "1"), there are limited circumstances when the Column Two code may be reported on the same date of service as the Column One code. Two examples follow:

1. Three or more HCPCS/CPT codes may be reported on the same date of service. Although the Column Two code is misused if reported as a service associated with the Column One code, the Column Two code may be appropriately reported with a third HCPCS/CPT code reported on the same date of service. For example, CMS limits separate payment for use of the operating microscope for microsurgical techniques (CPT code 69990) to a group of procedures listed in the online *Claims Processing Manual* (Chapter 12, Section 20.4.5

(Allowable Adjustments)). The NCCI has edits with Column One codes of surgical procedures not listed in this section of the manual and Column Two CPT code of 69990. Some of these edits allow use of NCCI *PTP*-associated modifiers because the two services listed in the edit may be performed at the same patient encounter as a third procedure for which CPT code 69990 is separately reportable.

2. There may be limited circumstances when the Column Two code is separately reportable with the Column One code. For example, the NCCI has an edit with Column One CPT code of 80061 (lipid profile) and Column Two CPT code of 83721 (LDL cholesterol by direct measurement). If the triglyceride level is less than 400 mg/dl, the LDL is a calculated value *using* the results from the lipid profile for the calculation, and CPT code 83721 is not separately reportable. However, if the triglyceride level is greater than 400 mg/dl, the LDL may be measured directly and may be separately reportable with CPT code 83721 utilizing an NCCI *PTP*-associated modifier to bypass the edit.

Misuse of code as an edit rationale may be applied to procedure to procedure edits where the Column Two code is not separately reportable with the Column One code based on the nature of the Column One coded procedure. This edit rationale may also be applied to code pairs where use of the Column Two code with the Column One code is deemed to be a coding error.

P. Mutually Exclusive Procedures

Many procedure codes cannot be reported together because they are mutually exclusive of each other. Mutually exclusive procedures cannot reasonably be performed at the same anatomic site or same patient encounter. An example of a mutually exclusive situation is the repair of an organ that can be performed by two different methods. Only one method can be chosen to repair the organ. A second example is a service that can be reported as an "initial" service or a "subsequent" service. With the exception of drug administration services, the initial service and subsequent service cannot be reported at the same patient encounter.

Q. Gender-Specific Procedures (formerly Designation of Sex)

The descriptor of some HCPCS/CPT codes includes a gender-specific restriction on the use of the code. HCPCS/CPT codes specific for one gender should not be reported with HCPCS/CPT codes for the opposite gender. For example, CPT code 53210 describes a total urethrectomy including cystostomy in a female, and CPT code 53215 describes the same procedure in a male. Since the patient cannot have both the male and female procedures performed, the two CPT codes cannot be reported together.

R. Add-on Codes

Some codes in the *CPT Manual* are identified as "add-on" codes *(AOCs)*, which describe a service that can only be reported in addition to a primary procedure. *CPT Manual* instructions specify the primary procedure code(s) for most *AOCs*. For other *AOCs*, the primary procedure code(s) is(are) not specified. When the *CPT Manual* identifies specific primary codes, the *AOC* shall not be reported as a supplemental service for other HCPCS/CPT codes not listed as a primary code.

AOCs permit the reporting of significant supplemental services commonly performed in addition to the primary procedure. By contrast, incidental services that are necessary to accomplish the primary procedure (e.g., lysis of adhesions in the course of an open cholecystectomy) are not separately reportable with an *AOC*. Similarly, complications inherent in an invasive procedure occurring during the procedure are not separately reportable. For example, control of bleeding during an invasive procedure is considered part of the procedure and is not separately reportable.

In general, NCCI procedure to procedure edits do not include edits with most *AOCs* because edits related to the primary procedure(s) are adequate to prevent inappropriate payment for an *AOC* procedure. (i.e., if an edit prevents payment of the primary procedure code, the *AOC* shall not be paid). However, NCCI does include edits for some *AOCs* when coding edits related to the primary procedures must be supplemented. Examples include edits with add-on HCPCS/CPT codes 69990 (Microsurgical techniques requiring use of operating microscope) and 95940/95941/G0453 (Intraoperative neurophysiology testing).

HCPCS/CPT codes that are not designated as *AOCs* shall not be misused as an *AOC* to report a supplemental service. A HCPCS/CPT code may be reported if and only if all services described by the CPT code are performed. A HCPCS/CPT code shall not be reported with another service because a portion of the service described by the HCPCS/CPT code was performed with the other procedure. For example: If an ejection fraction is estimated from an echocardiogram study, it would be inappropriate to additionally report CPT code 78472 (Cardiac blood pool imaging with ejection fraction) with the echocardiography (CPT code 93307). Although the procedure described by CPT code 78472 includes an ejection fraction, it is measured by gated equilibrium with a radionuclide which is not *used* in echocardiography.

S. Excluded Service

The NCCI does not address issues related to HCPCS/CPT codes describing services that are excluded from Medicare coverage or are not otherwise recognized for payment under the Medicare program.

T. Unlisted Procedure Codes

The *CPT Manual* includes codes to identify services or procedures not described by other HCPCS/CPT codes. These unlisted procedure codes are generally identified as XXX99 or XXXX9 codes and are located at the end of each section or subsection of the Manual. If a physician provides a service that is not accurately described by other HCPCS/CPT codes, the service shall be reported *using* an unlisted procedure code. A physician shall not report a CPT code for a specific procedure if it does not accurately describe the service performed. It is inappropriate to report the best fit HCPCS/CPT code unless it accurately describes the service performed, and all components of the HCPCS/CPT code were performed. Since unlisted procedure codes may be reported for a very diverse group of services, the NCCI generally does not include edits with these codes.

U. Modified, Deleted, and Added Code Pairs/Edits

Information moved to Introduction chapter, Section (Purpose), Page Intro-5 of this Manual.

V. Medically Unlikely Edits (MUEs)

To lower the Medicare Fee-For-Service Paid Claims Error Rate, CMS has established units of service edits referred to as Medically Unlikely Edit(s) (MUEs).

An MUE for a HCPCS/CPT code is the maximum number of units of service (UOS) under most circumstances allowable by the same provider for the same beneficiary on the same date of service. The ideal MUE value for a HCPCS/CPT code is the unit of service that allows the vast majority of appropriately coded claims to pass the MUE.

All practitioner claims submitted to MACs, outpatient facility services claims (Type of Bill 13X, 14X, 85X), and supplier claims submitted to Durable Medical Equipment (DME) MACs are tested against MUEs.

Prior to April 1, 2013, each line of a claim was adjudicated separately against the MUE value for the HCPCS/CPT code reported on that claim line. If the *UOS* on that claim line exceeded the MUE value, the entire claim line was denied.

In the April 1, 2013 version of MUEs, CMS began introducing date of service (DOS) MUEs. Over time CMS will convert many, but not all, MUEs to DOS MUEs. Since April 1, 2013, MUEs are adjudicated either as claim line edits or DOS edits. If the MUE is adjudicated as a claim line edit, the UOS on each claim line are compared to the MUE value for the HCPCS/CPT code on that claim line. If the UOS exceed the MUE value, all UOS on that claim line are denied. If the MUE is adjudicated as a DOS MUE, all UOS on each claim line for the same date of service for the same HCPCS/CPT code are summed, and the sum is compared to the MUE value. If the summed UOS exceed the MUE value, all UOS for the HCPCS/CPT code for that date of service are denied. Denials due to claim line MUEs or DOS MUEs may be appealed to the local claims processing contractor. DOS MUEs are *used* for HCPCS/CPT codes where it would be extremely unlikely that more UOS than the MUE value would ever be performed on the same date of service for the same patient.

The MUE files on the CMS NCCI website display an "MUE Adjudication Indicator" (MAI) for each HCPCS/CPT code. An MAI of "1" indicates that the edit is a claim line MUE. An MAI of "2" or "3" indicates that the edit is a DOS MUE.

If a HCPCS/CPT code has an MUE that is adjudicated as a claim line edit, appropriate use of CPT modifiers (e.g., -59, -76, -77, -91, anatomic) may be used to the same HCPCS/CPT code on separate lines of a claim. Each line of the claim with that HCPCS/CPT code will be separately adjudicated against the MUE value for that HCPCS/CPT code. Claims processing contractors have rules limiting use of these modifiers with some HCPCS/CPT codes.

MUEs for HCPCS codes with an MAI of "2" are absolute date of service edits. These are "per day edits based on policy." HCPCS codes with an MAI of "2" have been rigorously reviewed and vetted within CMS and obtain this MAI designation because UOS on the same date of service (DOS) in excess of the MUE value would be considered impossible because it was contrary to statute, regulation or subregulatory guidance. This subregulatory guidance includes clear correct coding policy that is binding on both providers and CMS claims processing contractors. Limitations created by anatomical or coding limitations are incorporated in correct coding policy, both in the HIPAA mandated coding descriptors and CMS approved coding guidance as well as specific guidance in CMS and NCCI manuals. For example, it would be contrary to correct coding policy to report more than one unit of service for CPT 94002 *(Ventilation* assist and management . . . initial *day)* because such *use* could not accurately describe two initial days of management occurring on the same date of service as would be required by the code descriptor. As a result, claims processing contractors are instructed that an MAI of "2" denotes a claims processing restriction for which override during processing, reopening, or redetermination would be contrary to CMS policy.

MUEs for HCPCS codes with an MAI of "3" are "per day edits based on clinical benchmarks." MUEs assigned an MAI of "3" are based on criteria (e.g., nature of service, prescribing information) combined with data such that it would be possible but medically highly unlikely that higher values would represent correctly reported medically necessary services. If contractors have evidence (e.g., medical review) that UOS in excess of the MUE value were actually provided, were correctly coded and were medically necessary, the contractor may bypass the MUE for a HCPCS code with an MAI of "3" during claim processing, reopening or redetermination, or in response to effectuation instructions from a reconsideration or higher level appeal.

Both the MAI and MUE value for each HCPCS/CPT code are based on one or more of the following criteria:

(1) Anatomic considerations may limit *UOS* based on anatomic structures. For example:
   a) The MUE value for an appendectomy is "1" since there is only one appendix.
   b) The MUE for a knee brace is "2" because there are two knees and Medicare policy does not cover back-up equipment.
   c) The MUE value for a lumbar spine procedure reported per lumbar vertebra or per lumbar interspace cannot exceed "5" since there are only five lumbar vertebrae or interspaces.
   d) The MUE value for a procedure reported per lung lobe cannot exceed "5" since there are only five lung lobes (three in right lung and two in left lung).

(2) CPT code descriptors/CPT coding instructions in the *CPT Manual* may limit *UOS*. For example,
   a) A procedure described as the "initial 30 minutes" would have an MUE value of 1 because of the use of the term "initial." A different code may be reported for additional time.
   b) If a code descriptor uses the plural form of the procedure, it must not be reported with multiple *UOS*. For example, if the code descriptor states "biopsies," the code is reported with "1" unit of service regardless of the number of biopsies performed.
   c) The MUE value for a procedure with "per day," "per week," or "per month" in its code descriptor is "1" because MUEs are based on number of services per day of service.

d) The MUE value of a code for a procedure described as "unilateral" is "1" if there is a different code for the procedure described as "bilateral."

e) The code descriptors of a family of codes may define different levels of service, each having an MUE of "1."
For example, CPT codes 78102-78104 describe bone marrow imaging. CPT code 78102 is reported for imaging a "limited area." CPT code 78103 is reported for imaging "multiple areas." CPT code 78104 is reported for imaging the "whole body."

f) The MUE value for CPT code 86021 (Antibody identification; leukocyte antibodies) is "1" because the code descriptor is plural including testing for any and all leukocyte antibodies. On a single date of service only one specimen from a patient would be tested for leukocyte antibodies.

(3) Edits based on established CMS policies may limit UOS. For example:

a) The MUE value for a surgical or diagnostic procedure may be based on the bilateral surgery indicator on the Medicare Physician Fee Schedule Database(MPFSDB)

i. If the bilateral surgery indicator is "0," a bilateral procedure must be reported with "1" *unit of service*. There is no additional payment for the code if reported as a unilateral or bilateral procedure because of anatomy or physiology. Alternatively, the code descriptor may specifically state that the procedure is a unilateral procedure, and there is a separate code for a bilateral procedure.

ii. If the bilateral surgery indicator is "1," a bilateral surgical procedure must be reported with "1" *unit of service* and modifier -50 (bilateral modifier). A bilateral diagnostic procedure may be reported with "2" *unit of service* on one claim line, "1" *unit of service* and modifier -50 on one claim line, or "1" *unit of service* with modifier RT on one claim line plus "1" *unit of service* and modifier LT on a second claim line.

iii. If the bilateral surgery indicator is "2," a bilateral procedure must be reported with "1" *unit of service*. The procedure is priced as a bilateral procedure because (1) the code descriptor defines the procedure as bilateral; (2) the code descriptor states that the procedure is performed unilaterally or bilaterally; or (3) the procedure is usually performed as a bilateral procedure.

iv. If the bilateral surgery indicator is "3," a bilateral surgical procedure must be reported with "1" *unit of service* and modifier -50 (bilateral modifier). A bilateral diagnostic procedure may be reported with "2" *unit of service* on one claim line, "1" *unit of service* and modifier -50 on one claim line, or 1 *unit of service* with modifier RT on one claim line plus "1" *unit of service* and modifier LT on a second claim line.

b) The MUE value for a code may be "1" where the code descriptor does not specify a UOS and CMS considers the default UOS to be "per day."

c) The MUE value for a code may be "0" because the code is listed as invalid, not covered, bundled, not separately payable, statutorily excluded, not reasonable and necessary, etc. based on

i. The Medicare Physician Fee Schedule Database
ii. Outpatient Prospective Payment System Addendum B
iii. Alpha-Numeric HCPCS Code File
iv. DMEPOS Jurisdiction List
v. Medicare Internet-Only Manual

(4) The nature of an analyte may limit *UOS* and is in general determined by: The nature of the specimen may limit the *UOS*. For example, CPT code 82575 describes a creatinine clearance test and has an MUE of "1" because the test requires a *twenty-four* hour urine collection
a); or b) The physiology, pathophysiology, or clinical application of the analyte is such that a maximum unit of service for a single date of service can be determined. For example, the MUE for CPT code 82747 (RBC folic acid) is "1" because the test result would not be expected to change during a single day, and thus it is not necessary to perform the test more than once on a single date of service.

(5) The nature of a procedure/service may limit *UOS* and is in general determined by the amount of time required to perform a procedure/service (e.g., overnight sleep studies) or clinical application of a procedure/service (e.g., motion analysis tests).

a) The MUE for many surgical or medical procedures is "1" because the procedure is rarely, if ever, performed more than one time per day (e.g., colonoscopy, motion analysis tests).

b) The MUE value for a procedure is "1" because of the amount of time required to perform the procedure (e.g., overnight sleep study).

(6) The nature of equipment may limit *UOS* and is in general determined by the number of items of equipment that would be *used* (e.g., cochlear implant or wheelchair). For example, the MUE value for a wheelchair code is "1" because only one wheelchair is used at one time and Medicare policy does not cover back-up equipment.

(7) Although clinical judgment considerations and determinations are based on input from numerous physicians and certified coders are sometimes initially *used* to establish some MUE values, these values are subsequently validated or changed based on submitted and/or paid claims data.

(8) Prescribing information is based on FDA labeling as well as off-label information published in CMS approved drug compendia. See below for additional information about how prescribing information is *used* in determining MUE values.

(9) Submitted and paid claims data (100%) from a six month period is *used* to ascertain the distribution pattern of UOS typically reported for a given HCPCS/CPT code.

(10) Published policies of the Durable Medical Equipment (DME) Medicare Administrative Contractors (MACs) may limit *UOS* for some durable medical equipment, prosthetics, orthotics, and supplies (DMEPOS). For example,

a) The MUE values for many ostomy and urological supply codes, nebulizer codes, and CPAP accessory codes are typically based on a three month supply of items.

b) The MUE values for surgical dressings, parenteral and enteral nutrition, immunosuppressive drugs, and oral anti-cancer drugs are typically based on a one month supply.

c) The MUE values take into account the requirement for reporting certain codes with date spans.

d) The MUE value of a code may be 0 if the item is non-covered, not medically necessary, or not separately payable.

e) The MUE value of a code may be 0 if the code is invalid for claim submission to the DME MAC.

UOS denied based on an MUE may be appealed. Because a denial of services due to an MUE is a coding denial, not a medical necessity denial, the presence of an Advanced Beneficiary Notice of Noncoverage (ABN) shall not shift liability to the beneficiary for UOS denied based on an MUE. If during reopening or redetermination medical records are provided with respect to an MUE denial for an edit with an MAI of "3," contractors will review the records to determine if the provider actually furnished units in excess of the MUE, if the codes were used correctly, and whether the services were medically reasonable and necessary. If the units were actually provided but one of the other conditions is not met, a change in denial reason may be warranted (for example, a change from the MUE denial based on incorrect coding to a determination that the item/service is not reasonable and necessary under section 1862(a)(1)). This may also be true for certain edits with an MAI of "1." CMS interprets the notice delivery requirements under §1879 of the Social Security Act (the Act) as applying to situations in which a provider expects the initial claim determination to be a reasonable and necessary denial. Consistent with NCCI guidance, denials resulting from MUEs are not based on any of the statutory provisions that give liability protection to beneficiaries under Section 1879 of the Act. Thus, ABN issuance based on an MUE is NOT appropriate. A provider/ supplier may not issue an ABN in connection with services denied due to an MUE and cannot bill the beneficiary for *UOS* denied based on an MUE.

HCPCS J code and drug related C and Q code MUEs are based on prescribing information and 100% claims data for a six month period of time. *Using* the prescribing information the highest total daily dose for each drug was determined. This dose and its corresponding units of service were evaluated against paid and submitted claims data. Some of the guiding principles *used* in developing these edits are as follows:

(1) If the prescribing information defined a maximum daily dose, this value was used to determine the MUE value. For some drugs there is an absolute maximum daily dose. For others there is a maximum "recommended" or "usual" dose. In the latter of the two cases, the daily dose calculation was evaluated against claims data.
(2) If the maximum daily dose calculation is based on actual body weight, a dose based on a weight range of 110-150 kg was evaluated against the claims data. If the maximum daily dose calculation is based on ideal body weight, a dose based on a weight range of 90-110 kg was evaluated against claims data. If the maximum daily dose calculation is based on body surface area (BSA), a dose based on a BSA range of 2.4-3.0 square meters was evaluated against claims data.
(3) For "as needed" (PRN) drugs and drugs where maximum daily dose is based on patient response, prescribing information and claims data were *used* to establish MUE values.
(4) Published off label *use* of a drug was considered for the maximum daily dose calculation.
(5) The MUE values for some drug codes are set to 0. The rationale for such values include but are not limited to: discontinued manufacture of drug, non-FDA approved compounded drug, practitioner MUE values for oral antineoplastic, oral anti-emetic, and oral immune suppressive drugs which should be billed to the DME MACs, and outpatient hospital MUE values for inhalation drugs which should be billed to the DME MACs, and Practitioner/ASC MUE values for HCPCS C codes describing medications that would not be related to a procedure performed in an ASC.

Non-drug related HCPCS/CPT codes may be assigned an MUE of 0 for a variety of reasons including, but not limited to: outpatient hospital MUE value for surgical procedure only performed as an inpatient procedure, noncovered service, bundled service, or packaged service.

The MUE files on the CMS NCCI website display an "Edit Rationale" for each HCPCS/CPT code. Although an MUE may be based on several rationales, only one is displayed on the website. One of the listed rationales is "Data." This rationale indicates that 100% claims data from a six month period of time was the major factor in determining the MUE value. If a physician appeals an MUE denial for a HCPCS/CPT code where the MUE is based on "Data," the reviewer will usually confirm that (1) the correct code is reported; (2) the correct UOS is *used*; (3) the number of reported UOS were performed; and (4) all UOS were medically reasonable and necessary.

The first MUEs were implemented January 1, 2007. Additional MUEs are added on a quarterly basis on the same schedule as NCCI updates. Prior to implementation proposed MUEs are sent to numerous national healthcare organizations for a sixty day review and comment period.

Many surgical procedures may be performed bilaterally. Instructions in the CMS *Internet-only Manual* (Publication 100-04 *Medicare Claims Processing Manual,* Chapter 12 (Physicians/Nonphysician Practitioners), Section 40.7.B. and Chapter 4 (Part B Hospital (Including Inpatient Hospital Part B and OPPS)), Section 20.6.2 require that bilateral surgical procedures be reported using modifier -50 with one unit of service unless the code descriptor defines the procedure as "bilateral." If the code descriptor defines the procedure as a "bilateral" procedure, it shall be reported with one unit of service without modifier -50. If a bilateral surgical procedure is performed at different sites bilaterally, one unit of service may be reported for each site. That is, the HCPCS/CPT code may be reported with modifier -50 and one unit of service for each site at which it was performed bilaterally.

Some A/B MACs allow providers to report repetitive services performed over a range of dates on a single line of a claim with multiple *UOS*. If a provider reports services in this fashion, the provider should report the "from date" and "to date" on the claim line. Contractors are instructed to divide the *UOS* reported on the claim line by the number of days in the date span and round to the nearest whole number. This number is compared to the MUE value for the code on the claim line.

Suppliers billing services to the DME MACs typically report some HCPCS codes for supply items for a period exceeding a single day. The DME MACs have billing rules for these codes. For some codes the DME MACs require that the "from date" and "to date" be reported. The MUEs for these codes are based on the maximum number of *UOS* that may be reported for a single date of service. For other codes the DME MACs permit multiple days' supply items to be reported on a single claim line where the "from date" and "to date" are the same. The DME MACs have rules allowing supply items for a maximum number of days to be reported at one time for each of these types of codes. The MUE values for these codes are based on the maximum number of days that may be reported at one time. As with all MUEs, the MUE value does not represent a utilization guideline. Suppliers shall not assume that they may report *UOS* up to the MUE value on each date of service. Suppliers may only report supply items that are medically reasonable and necessary.

Most MUE values are set so that a provider or supplier would only very occasionally have a claim line denied. If a provider encounters a code with frequent denials due to the MUE, or frequent use of a CPT modifier to bypass the MUE, the provider or supplier should consider the following: (1) Is the HCPCS/CPT code being used correctly? (2) Is the unit of service being counted correctly? (3) Are all reported services medically reasonable and necessary? and (4) Why does the provider's or supplier's practice differ from national patterns? A provider or supplier may choose to discuss these questions with the local Medicare contractor or a national healthcare organization whose members frequently perform the procedure.

Most MUE values are published on the CMS MUE webpage (https://www.cms.gov/Medicare/Coding/NationalCorrectCodInitEd/MUE.html). However, some MUE values are not published and are confidential. These values shall not be published in oral or written form by any party that acquires one or more of them.

MUEs are not utilization edits. Although the MUE value for some codes may represent the commonly reported *UOS* (e.g., MUE of "1" for appendectomy), the usual *UOS* for many HCPCS/CPT codes is less than the MUE value. Claims reporting *UOS* less than the MUE value may be subject to review by claims processing contractors, *Unified Program Integrity Contractor (UPICS),* Recovery Audit Contractors (RACs), and Department of Justice (DOJ).

Since MUEs are coding edits rather than medical necessity edits, claims processing contractors may have *UOS* edits that are more restrictive than MUEs. In such cases, the more restrictive claims processing contractor edit would be applied to the claim. Similarly, if the MUE is more restrictive than a claims processing contractor edit, the more restrictive MUE would apply.

A *national*, healthcare organization, *provider/supplier,* or other interested *third* party may request *a* reconsideration of an MUE value for a HCPCS/CPT code *by submitting a written request to: NCCIPTPMUE@cms.hhs. The written request should include a rationale for consideration, as well a a suggested remedy.*

W. Add-on Code Edit Tables

Add-on codes *(AOCs)* are discussed in Chapter I, Section R (Add-on Codes). CMS publishes a list of *AOCs* and their primary codes annually prior to January 1. The list is updated quarterly based on the AMA's "CPT Errata" documents or implementation of new HCPCS/CPT add-on codes. CMS identifies *AOCs* and their primary codes based on CPT Manual instructions, CMS interpretation of HCPCS/CPT codes, and CMS coding instructions.

The NCCI program includes three *AOC* Edit Tables, one table for each of three "Types" of *AOCs*. Each table lists the add-on code with its primary codes. An *AOC*, with one exception, is eligible for payment if and only if one of its primary codes is also eligible for payment.

The "Type I *AOC* Edit Table" lists *AOCs* for which the CPT Manual or HCPCS tables define all acceptable primary codes. Claims processing contractors should not allow other primary codes with Type I *AOCs*. CPT code 99292 (Critical care, evaluation and management of the critically ill or critically injured patient; each additional 30 minutes (List separately in addition to code for primary service)) is included as a Type I *AOC* since its only primary code is CPT code 99291 (Critical care, evaluation and management of the critically ill or critically injured patient; first 30-74 minutes). For Medicare purposes, CPT code 99292 may be eligible for payment to a physician without CPT code 99291 if another physician of the same specialty and physician group reports and is paid for CPT code 99291.

The "Type II *AOC* Edit Table" lists *AOCs* for which the CPT Manual and HCPCS tables do not define any primary codes. Claims processing contractors should develop their own lists of acceptable primary codes.

The "Type III *AOC* Edit Table" lists *AOCs* for which the CPT Manual or HCPCS tables define some, but not all, acceptable primary codes. Claims processing contractors should allow the listed primary codes for these *AOCs* but may develop their own lists of additional acceptable primary codes.

Although the *AOC* and primary code are normally reported for the same date of service, there are unusual circumstances where the two services may be reported for different dates of service (e.g., CPT codes 99291 and 99292).

The first *AOC* edit tables were implemented April 1, 2013. For subsequent years, new *AOC* edit tables will be published to be effective for January 1 of the new year based on changes in the new year's CPT Manual. CMS also issues quarterly updates to the Add-On Code edit tables if required due to publication of new HCPCS/CPT codes or changes in add-on codes or their primary codes. The changes in the quarterly update files (April 1, July 1, or October 1) are retroactive to the implementation date of that year's annual *AOC* edit files unless the files specify a different effective date for a change. Since the first Add-On Code edit files were implemented on April 1, 2013, changes in the July 1 and October 1 quarterly updates for 2013 were retroactive to April 1, 2013 unless the files specified a different effective date for a change.

FIGURE CREDITS

1. From Little J, et al: *Dental Management of the Medically Compromised Patient,* ed 9, St. Louis, 2017, Mosby. *(Courtesy Medtronic, Minneapolis)*
2. From Franklin I, Dawson P, Rodway A: *Essentials of Clinical Surgery*, ed 2, St. Louis, 2012, Saunders.
3. Modified from Grosfeld J, et al: *Pediatric Surgery,* ed 7, Philadelphia, 2012, Mosby.
4. Modified from Hsu J, Michael J, Fisk J: *AAOS Atlas of Orthoses and Assistive Devices,* ed 4, Philadelphia, 2008, Mosby.
5. From Wold G: *Basic Geriatric Nursing*, ed 5, St. Louis, 2011, Mosby.
6. Modified from Roberts J, Hedges J: *Clinical Procedures in Emergency Medicine,* ed 6, St. Louis, 2013, Saunders.
7. From Auerbach P: *Wilderness Medicine,* ed 7, Philadelphia, 2016, Mosby. (Courtesy Black Diamond Equipment, Ltd.)
8. *(Original to book).*
9. Modified from Abeloff M, et al: *Clinical Oncology,* ed 5, Philadelphia, 2013, Churchill Livingstone.
10. *(Original to book).*
11. Modified from Duthie E, Katz P, Malone M: *Practice of Geriatrics,* ed 4, Philadelphia, 2007, Saunders.
12. Modified from Roberts J, Hedges J: *Clinical Procedures in Emergency Medicine,* ed 6, St. Louis, 2013, Saunders.
13. From Young A, Proctor D: *Kinn's The Medical Assistant,* ed 13, St. Louis, 2016, Saunders.
14. From Bonewit-West K: *Clinical Procedures for Medical Assistants,* ed 9, Philadelphia, 2015, WB Saunders.
15. From Roberts J, Hedges J: *Clinical Procedures in Emergency Medicine,* ed 6, St. Louis, 2013, Saunders.
16. From Yeo: *Shackelford's Surgery of the Alimentary Tract,* ed 7, Philadelphia, 2012, Saunders.
17. Redrawn from Bragg D, Rubin P, Hricak H: *Oncologic Imaging,* ed 2, 2002, Saunders.
18. From Roberts J, Hedges J: *Clinical Procedures in Emergency Medicine,* ed 6, St. Louis, 2013, Saunders. *(Courtesy Atrium Medical Corp., Hudson, NH 03051)*
19. **A** From Auerbach P: *Wilderness Medicine,* ed 7, Philadelphia, 2016, Mosby. **B** Modified from Hsu J, Michael J, Fisk J: *AAOS Atlas of Orthoses and Assistive Devices,* ed 4, Philadelphia, 2008, Mosby.
20. Modified from Lusardi M, Nielsen C: *Orthotics and Prosthetics in Rehabilitation,* ed 3, St. Louis, 2013, Butterworth-Heinemann.
21. Modified from Lusardi M, Nielsen C: *Orthotics and Prosthetics in Rehabilitation,* ed 3, St. Louis, 2013, Butterworth-Heinemann.
22. Modified from Lusardi M, Nielsen C: *Orthotics and Prosthetics in Rehabilitation,* ed 3, St. Louis, 2013, Butterworth-Heinemann.
23. From Buck C: *The Next Step, Advanced Medical Coding 2021-2022 edition,* St. Louis, 2021, Saunders.
24. From Jardins T: *Clinical Manifestations and Assessment of Respiratory Disease,* ed 7, St. Louis, 2015, Elsevier.
25. From Hsu J, Michael J, Fisk J: *AAOS Atlas of Orthoses and Assistive Devices,* ed 4, Philadelphia, 2008, Mosby.
26. Modified from Hsu J, Michael J, Fisk J: *AAOS Atlas of Orthoses and Assistive Devices,* ed 4, Philadelphia, 2008, Mosby.
27. Modified from Hsu J, Michael J, Fisk J: *AAOS Atlas of Orthoses and Assistive Devices,* ed 4, Philadelphia, 2008, Mosby.
28. From Didomenico L, Gatlyak N: "End-Stage Ankle Arthritis." *Clinics in Podiatric Medicine and Surgery* 29.3 (2012): 391-412.
29. Cameron M, Monroe L: *Physical Rehabilitation for the Physical Therapist Assistant,* ed 1, St. Louis, 2011, Saunders.
30. From Rowe D, Jadhav A: "Care of the Adolescent with Spina Bifida." *Pediatric Clinics of North America* 55.6 (2008): 1359-374.
31. Modified from Lusardi M, Nielsen C: *Orthotics and Prosthetics in Rehabilitation,* ed 3, St. Louis, 2013, Butterworth-Heinemann.
32. From Hsu J, Michael J, Fisk J: *AAOS Atlas of Orthoses and Assistive Devices,* ed 4, Philadelphia, 2008, Mosby.
33. *(Original to book.)*
34. From Hochberg M: *Rheumatology,* ed 5, Philadelphia, 2011, Mosby.
35. Modified from Hsu J, Michael J, Fisk J: *AAOS Atlas of Orthoses and Assistive Devices,* ed 4, Philadelphia, 2008, Mosby.
36. From Coughlin M, Mann R, Saltzman C: *Surgery of the Foot and Ankle,* ed 9, Philadelphia, 2013, Mosby.
37. From Canale S: *Campbell's Operative Orthopaedics,* ed 12, St. Louis, 2012, Mosby.
38. From Sorrentino S, Gorek B: *Mosby's Textbook for Long-term Care Nursing Assistants,* ed 7, St. Louis, 2014, Mosby.
39. From Pedretti L, Pendleton H, Schultz-Krohn W: *Pedretti's Occupational Therapy: Practice Skills for Physical Dysfunction,* ed 7, St. Louis, 2013, Elsevier.
40. From Skirven T: *Rehabilitation of the Hand and Upper Extremity,* ed 6, Philadelphia, 2010, Mosby.
41. From Lusardi M, Nielsen C: *Orthotics and Prosthetics in Rehabilitation,* ed 3, St. Louis, 2013, Butterworth-Heinemann. *(Courtesy Michael Curtain)*
42. Schickendantz M: "Diagnosis and Treatment of Elbow Disorders in the Overhead Athlete." *Hand Clinics* 18.1 (2002): 65-75.
43. Modified from Bland K, Copeland E: *The Breast: Comprehensive Management of Benign and Malignant Disorders,* ed 4, St. Louis, 2009, Saunders.
44. From Shah J, Patel S, Singh B, Shah J: *Jatin Shah's Head and Neck Surgery and Oncology,* ed 4, Philadelphia, 2012, Mosby, 2012. From Subburaj K, Nair C, Rajesh S, Ravi B: "Rapid Development of Auricular Prosthesis Using CAD and Rapid Prototyping Technologies." *International Journal of Oral and Maxillofacial Surgery* 36.10 (2007): 938-43.
45. From Weinzweig J: *Plastic Surgery Secrets,* ed 2, Philadelphia, 2010, Hanley & Belfus, p 543.
46. Modified from Mann D: *Heart Failure: A Companion to Braunwald's Heart Disease,* ed 3, Philadelphia, 2015, Saunders.
47. Modified from Roberts J, Hedges J: *Clinical Procedures in Emergency Medicine,* ed 6, Philadelphia, 2013, Saunders.
48. From Yanoff M, Duker J: *Ophthalmology,* ed 4, St. Louis, 2014, Mosby.
49. From Feldman M, Friedman L, Brandt L: *Sleisenger and Fordtran's Gastrointestinal and Liver Disease,* ed 10, Philadelphia, 2015, Saunders.
50. From Katz V, et al: *Comprehensive Gynecology,* ed 7, Philadelphia, 2016, Mosby.
51. From Young A, Proctor D: *Kinn's The Medical Assistant,* ed 13, St. Louis, 2016, Saunders.
52. From Yanoff M, Duker J: *Ophthalmology,* ed 4, St. Louis, 2014, Mosby.